OXFORD MEDICAL PUBLICATIONS

SOCIETY, STRESS, AND DISEASE

VOLUME 4

WORKING LIFE

SOCIETY, STRESS,

The symposium on which this volume is based was sponsored jointly

by

THE UNIVERSITY OF UPPSALA

and

THE WORLD HEALTH ORGANIZATION

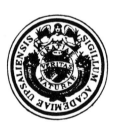 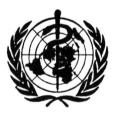

Oxford   OXFORD UNIVERSITY

AND DISEASE

VOLUME 4

WORKING LIFE

Edited by LENNART LEVI, M.D.

Director, Laboratory for Clinical Stress Research,
Karolinska Institute, Stockholm

PRESS   *New York, Toronto 1981*

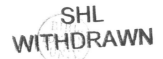

Oxford University Press, Walton Street, Oxford OX2 6DP

London Glasgow New York Toronto
Delhi Bombay Calcutta Madras Karachi
Kuala Lumpur Singapore Hong Kong Tokyo
Nairobi Dar es Salaam Cape Town
Melbourne Wellington

and associate companies in
Beirut Berlin Ibadan Mexico City

© *Oxford University Press 1981*

British Library Cataloguing in Publication Data

Society, stress and disease.
   Vol. 4: Working life. − (Oxford medical
publications).
   1. Medicine, Psychosomatic − Congresses
   2. Stress (Physiology) − Congresses
   I. Levi, Lennart II. Series
   616.08   RC49   81-40338

   ISBN 0-19-264421-1

The symposium on which this volume is based
was made possible through the generosity of
The Trygg–Hansa Insurance Group,
Stockholm

Typeset by Oxprint Ltd., Oxford
Printed and bound in Great Britian by
William Clowes (Beccles) Limited, Beccles and London

CONTENTS

SESSION 1

DEFINITIONS OF PROBLEMS AND OBJECTIVES

SESSION 2

POTENTIALLY PATHOGENIC PSYCHOSOCIAL STRESSORS IN MODERN WORKING LIFE

SESSION 3

MENTAL, PHYSICAL, AND SOCIAL DISABILITY POSSIBLY ASSOCIATED WITH PSYCHOSOCIAL STRESSORS AT WORK

SESSION 4

HEALTH PROTECTION AND PROMOTION THROUGH PSYCHOSOCIAL FACTORS

SESSION 5

OBJECTIVES AND METHODOLOGY FOR FUTURE RESEARCH

LIST OF CONTRIBUTORS

TORBJÖRN ÅKERSTEDT, Ph.D., Associate Professor, Laboratory for Clinical Stress Research, Box 60205, S-104 01 Stockholm, Sweden.

MAUREEN A. BAILEY, Ph.D., Consultant, Behavioral Sciences, Office of Mental Health, World Health Organization, CH-1211 Geneva 27, Switzerland. Present address: c/o Ross, 309 Calle Mira Mar, Sarasota, Florida, USA.

M. A. EL BATAWI, M.D., M.P.H., D.Sc., Chief Medical Officer, Office for Occupational Health, World Health Organization, CH-1211 Geneva 27, Switzerland.

VICTOR P. BELOV, Professor, Director, Central Research Insitute for Evaluation of Working Capacity and Vocational Assistance to Disabled Persons of the Ministry of Social Security, CIETIN, Ostryakova, 3, 125057 Mosocow, USSR.

ERIK BOLINDER, M.D., Medical Adviser to the Swedish Trade Union Confederation (LO), Barnhusgatan 18, S-105 53 Stockholm, Sweden.

M. HARVEY BRENNER, Ph.D., Professor, Operations Research and Behavioral Sciences, Department of Health Services Administration, The John Hopkins University, 615 North Wolfe Street, Baltimore, Maryland 21205, USA.

SAMUEL A. CORSON, Ph.D., B.S., M.S., Professor, Early and Middle Childhood Education, Ohio State University, 1945 North High Street, Columbus, Ohio 43210, USA.

BÖRJE CRONHOLM, M.D., Professor Emeritus, Department of Psychiatry, Karolinska sjukhuset, S-104 01 Stockholm 60, Sweden.

LARS DAHLGREN, Ph.D., formerly Managing Director, Trygg-Hansa Insurance Group, S-106 26 Stockholm, Sweden. Present address: Värtavägen 14, S-115 24 Stockholm, Sweden.

GUNNAR DANIELSON, LL.B., Director-General, Swedish National Board of Occupational Safety and Health, S-171 84 Solna, Sweden.

RENÉ DUBOS, Ph.D., Professor, The Rockefeller University, New York, N.Y. 100 21, USA.

BENGT EDGREN, M.A., M.Sc., Senior Researcher, Laboratory for Clinical Stress Research, Box 60205, S-104 01 Stockholm 60, Sweden.

RICARDO EDSTRÖM, M.D., Medical Director, Stiftelsen Samhällsföretag, Box 123, S-14501 Norsborg, Sweden.

ARNE ENGSTRÖM, M.D., Professor, Secretary, Swedish Science Advisory Council, Ministry of Education, S-103 33 Stockholm, Sweden. Present position and address: Director-General, the National Swedish Food Administration, Box 622, S-751 Uppsala, Sweden.

AMITAI ETZIONI, Ph.D., Professor, Director, Center for Policy Research, 475 Riverside Drive, New York, N.Y. 100 27, USA.

JAN FORSLIN, Ph.D., Research Fellow, Swedish Council for Personnel Administration, Box 5157, S-102 44 Stockholm 5, Sweden. Present address: Blåklintstigen 4 S-13700 Västerhaninge, Sweden.

S. FORSSMAN, M.D., Professor, formerly Chief Technical Adviser, Regional Office for Europe, World Health Organization, 8 Scherfigsvej, DK-2100 Copenhagen Ö, Denmark. Present address: Brunnsbacken 7, S-190 30 Sigtuna, Sweden.

MARIANNE FRANKENHAEUSER, Ph.D., Professor, Department of Psychology, Karolinska institutet, Box 6706, S-113 85 Stockholm, Sweden.

BJÖRN FRANZÉN, M.D., Medical Director, Gränges Metallverken, S-721 88 Västerås, Sweden.

JOHN R.P. FRENCH, JR., M.A. Ph.D., Program Director, Institute for Social Research, University of Michigan, Ann Arbor, Michigan 48106, USA.

JAN E. FRÖBERG, Ph.D., Associate Professor, National Defence Research Institute, FOA 541, Fack, S-104 50 Stockholm, Sweden.

BERTIL GARDELL, Ph.D., Professor of Occupational Psychology, Psychological Laboratories, University of Stockholm, Box 6706, S-113 85 Stockholm, Sweden.

N. GAVRILESCU, M.D., D.P.H., D.O.H., D.I.H., Chief, Department of Occupational Medicine, Occupational Safety and Health Branch, International Labour Office, CH-1211 Geneva, Switzerland.

J. J. Groen, M.D., F.R.C.P., Professor, Academisch Zieknhuis Leiden, Afdeling K.N.O., Rijnsburgerweg 10, 2333 AA Leiden, The Netherlands.

Beatrix A. Hamburg, A.B., M.D., Medical Officer and Senior Research Psychiatrist, Laboratory of Developmental Psychology, National Institute of Mental Health, 9000 Rockville Pike, Bethesda, Maryland 20205, USA.

David A. Hamburg, M.D., B.A., Professor, Director, Division of Health Policy Research and Education, John F. Kennedy School of Government, Harvard University, 79 Boylston Street, Cambridge, Massachusetts 02138, USA.

James P. Henry, M.D., Ph.D., Professor, Department of Physiology, University of Southern California, 815 W., 37th Street, Los Angeles, California 90007, USA.

Milan Horváth, Dr. rer.nat., Ph.D., Associate Professor, Head, Laboratory for Physiology of Higher Nervous Functions at the Centre for Industrial Hygiene and Occupational Diseases, Institute of Hygiene and Epidemiology, Srobárova 48, 10042 Prague, Czechoslovakia.

Gunn Johansson, Ph.D., Psychological Laboratories, University of Stockholm, Box 6706, S-113 85 Stockholm, Sweden.

Aubrey R. Kagan, M.B., B.S., M.R.C.P., D.P.H. (Lon.), Visiting Professor, WHO Collaborating Research and Training Centre on Psychosocial Factors and Health, Box 60205, S-104 01 Stockholm, Sweden.

Claes-Göran Karlsson, M.Sc., Pl 9146, S-71100 Lindesberg, Sweden.

W. Kroes, Ph.D., Ma, B.S, formerly Chief, Stress Research Section, National Institute for Occupational Safety and Health, 1014 Broadway, Cincinnati, Ohio 45202, USA.

Thomas A. Lambo, M.B., Ch.B. (Birmingham), M.D. (Birm.), F.R.C.P., D.P.M. (Eng.), Hon. D.Sc. (A.B.U.), Hon. LL.D. (K.S.U.), Hon. LL.D. (Birm.), Deputy Director-General, World Health Organization, CH-1211 Geneva 27, Switzerland.

R. S. Lazarus, Ph.D., Professor, Department of Psychology, Tolman Hall, University of California, Berkeley, California 94720, USA.

Anna-Greta Leijon, MP, formerly Cabinet Minister, Riksdagen, Fack, S-100 12 Stockholm, Sweden.

Lennart Levi, M.D., Professor and Chairman, Laboratory for Clinical Stress Research (WHO Collaborating Research and Training Centre on Psychosocial Factors and Health), Box 60205, S-104 01 Stockholm, Sweden.

H. Levinson, B.S., M.S., Ph.D., Professor, College of Business Administration, Boston University, Box 95, Cambridge, Massachusetts 02138, USA.

Evy Lind, B.Sc., Researcher, WHO Collaborating Research and Training Centre on Psychosocial Factors and Health, Box 60205, S-104 01 Stockholm, Sweden.

Nils Lundgren, M.D., Professor, Head, Department of Occupational Health, National Board of Occupational Safety and Health, S-171 84 Solna, Sweden.

Ulf Lundberg, Ph.D., Research psychologist, Psychological Laboratories, University of Stockholm, Box 6706, S-113 85 Stockholm, Sweden.

Alan A. McLean, M.D., Associate Professor, Eastern Area Medical Director for the IBM Corporation, One Citicorp Center, 153 East 53rd Street, New York, N.Y. 10022, USA.

Nils Masreliez, M.D., Medical Adviser to the Swedish Employers' Confederation, P.O. Box 16 120, 103 23 Stockholm, Sweden.

Ernest Mastromatteo, M.D., D.P.H., D.I.H., formerly Chief, Occupational Safety and Health Branch, International Labour Office, CH-1211 Geneva, Switzerland.

Evelyn E. Meyer, Ph.D., Technical Adviser, Office of Mental Health, World Health Organization, CH-1211 Geneva 27, Switzerland.

Erland Mindus, M.D., Medical Director, Swedish National Road Board, Fack, S-102 20 Stockholm 12, Sweden.

Gunnar Nerell, M.D., Medical Adviser to the Swedish Central Organization of Salaried Employees, Box 5252, S-102 45 Stockholm, Sweden.

Carina Nilsson, Ph.D., Psychological Adviser to the Swedish Trade Union Confederation (LO), Barnhusgatan 18, S-105 53 Stockholm, Sweden.

GÖRAN OLHAGEN, Ph.D., Chief, Division of Sociology, Laboratory for Clinical Stress Research, Box 60205, S-104 01 Stockholm, Sweden.

BO OSCARSSON, M.D., Managing Director, Swedish Work Environment Fund, Box 1122, S-111 81 Stockholm, Sweden.

INGEMAR PETERSÉN, M.D., Ph.D., Professor, Head, Department of Clinical Neurophysiology, Sahlgrenska sjukhuset, S-413 45 Gothenburg, Sweden.

WILLIAM PETERSON, Ph.D. Adviser to the Swedish Confederation of Professional Associations. Researcher, Swedish Council for Personnel Administration, Box 5157, S-102 44 Stockholm 5, Sweden.

TORGNY SEGERSTEDET, Ph.D., Professor Emeritus, Formerly Rector Magnificus of Uppsala University, Box 256, S-751 05 Uppsala, Sweden.

HANS SELYE, M.D., Ph.D., D.Sc., D.Sc.(hon.), M.D.(hon.), F.N.A.(hon.), F.R.S.C., F.I.C.S.(hon.), Professor, President, International Institute of Stress, Université de Montréal, 2900 Boul. Edouard-Montpetit, Montréal, Canada H3C 3J7.

F. E. SPANER, B.S., M.S., Ph.D., Psychologist, Division of Mental Health Service Programs, National Institute of Mental Health, 5600 Fishers Lane, Rockville, Maryland 20852, USA.

OOLE SVANE, M.D., Physician-in-Chief, The Labour Inspectorate, (Arbejdstilsynet), Rosenvaengets Allé 16–18, 2100 Copenhagen, Denmark.

TÖRES THEORELL, M.D., Associate Professor, National Swedish Institute for Psychosocial Factors and Health (IPM), Box 60210, S-104 01 Stockholm, Sweden.

INGRID WAHLUND, Ph.D., Psychological Adviser to the Swedish Central Organization of Salaried Employees, Box 5252, S-102 45 Stockholm, Sweden.

PREFACE

Man's psychophysiological reaction patterns, his genetically determined 'psychobiological program', have remained essentially unchanged over the last 100 000 years. Over the same period, environmental demands on this 'program' have changed dramatically. The resulting discrepancy between environmental demands and opportunities at work on the one hand and man's genetically determined abilities and needs on the other, and his psychological, behavioural, and physiological *reactions* to these discrepancies, constitute the subject matter of this, fourth, volume in a series of five, on *Society, stress, and disease* throughout the entire life span. The volumes are based on international, interdisciplinary symposia, jointly sponsored by the World Health Organization and the University of Uppsala, organized by the Laboratory of Clinical Stress Research (WHO Psychosocial Center) of the Karaolinska Institute in Stockholm, and made possible through the generosity of the Trygg–Hansa Insurance Group.

The first symposium in this series aimed at a bird's-eye view of the entire area of man's psychosocial environment and his morbidity and mortality in psychosomatic diseases (Levi 1971). The second symposium focused on problems specific to the most formative years, namely childhood and adolescence (Levi 1975). The third symposium concerned itself with problems due to change in male/female roles and relationships (Levi 1978). The fourth one dealt with the problems specific to working life. The proceedings of this fourth symposium are now presented in an expanded and updated form.

The organizers have aimed to bring together researchers, practitioners, and decision-makers from many disciplines and parts of the world to discuss many aspects of *occupational* environments, roles and relationships as psychosocial human stressors, and their possible influences on health and well-being. The participants were chosen to represent many different fields of knowledge and many different methods of scientific and practical approach. No attempts were made to reach any consensus of opinion. It is hoped, however, that this volume does present not only a selection, but also a meaningful *pattern*, of facts, theories, hypotheses, speculations, and value judgements concerning the various components of the 'psycho-social–factors–stress–disease' system and their interrelationship, with particular references to problems specific to working life.

During the last century, work has changed from being the completion of a well-defined job activity with a clearly recognized end-product, to a breakdown of activities into narrow and highly specified sub-units, bearing little apparent relation to the end-product. The growing size of factory units now tends to result in a long chain of command between management and the individual worker, giving rise to a situation of remoteness between the two groups. The worker becomes remote also from the consumer, since rapid elaborations for marketing, distribution, and selling interpose many steps between producer and consumer (WHO 1973).

Mass production normally involves not only a pronounced fragmentation of the work process but also a decrease in worker control of the work process, partly because work organization, worker content, and pace are determined by the machine system, partly because of the detailed preplanning that is necessary in such systems. All this usually results in monotony, social isolation, lack of freedom, and time pressure, with possible long-term effects on health and well-being.

Mass production also favours the introduction of piece wages. In addition, heavy investment in machinery, alone or combined with shorter hours of work, has increased the proportion of people working in shifts. These and related problems are analysed in the present volume.

Another focus of discussion concerns the important question whether occupational health and well-being will improve and the strain on the workers diminish by a transition to *automated production systems*, where the repetitive, manual elements are taken over by machines, and the workers are left with mainly supervisory controlling functions. This kind of work is generally rather skilled, it is not regulated in detail, and the worker is free to move about (cf. Levi, Frankenaeuser, and Gardell 1981).

Accordingly, the introduction of automation is generally considered to be a positive step, partly because it eliminates many of the disadvantages of the mass production technique. However, this holds true mainly for those stages of automation where the operator is, indeed, assisted by the computer and maintains some control over its services. If, however, operator skills and knowledge are gradually taken over by the computer—a likely development if decision-making is left to economists and technologists—a new impoverishment of the work may result, with reintroduction of monotony, social isolation, and lack of control. With the striving toward maximum automation, man may again become the tool—of his own tools!

Until very recently, such problems of adaptation have been dealt with by financial compensation for the resulting suffering and health hazards. A complementary approach has been the traditional medical one, according to which the worker is offered surgical, pharmacological, and/or psychological intervention to eliminate some of the ill effects that constitute the cost for this adaptation.

However, the entire ideology of this series of symposia in general and of the contributions to this volume in particular point to the emerging complementary approach of adapting occupational structures and processes to the workers' abilities and needs to facilitate a good person–environment fit. This must be the major emphasis in our joint future endeavours.

This has also been the goal of recent Scandinavian legislation, e.g. of the *Norwegian* Work Environment Act, which expresses the following provisions:

1. *General requirements*: Technology, work organization, work time (e.g., shift plans) and payment systems are to be designed so that negative physiological or psychological effects for employees are avoided as well as negative influence on the alertness necessary to the observance of safety considerations. Employees are to be given possibilities for personal development and for the maintenance and development of skills.

2. *Design of jobs*: In the planning of work and design of jobs, possibilities for employee self-determination and maintenance of skills are to be considered. Monotonous, repetitive work and work that is bound by machine or assembly line, in such a way that no room is left for variation in work rhythm should be avoided.

Jobs should be designed so as to give possibilities for variation, for contact with others, for understanding of the interdependence between elements that constitute a job, and for information and feedback to employees concerning production requirements and results.

3. *Systems for planning and control* (e.g. automatic data processing systems): Employees or their elected representatives are to be kept informed about systems used for planning and control, and for changes in such systems. They are to be given the training necessary to understand the systems and the right to influence their design.

4. *Mode of remuneration and risk to safety*: Piece rate payment and related forms of payment are not to be used if salaried systems can increase the safety level (cf. WHO 1980).

The *Swedish* legislative approach is twofold. A new Work Environment Act came into force on 1 July, 1978. It is an open-frame law with general statements such as 'working conditions shall be adapted to man's mental and physical capacities', and 'jobs shall be designed so that the employees themselves may influence their work situation'.

This frame is complemented by specifications from two sources, the National Board of Occupational Safety and Health (1980), and, perhaps even more important for mental health purposes, the Co-determination Act (1976). The latter act requires that information be given to employee union representatives on all matters, and at all levels, about working conditions. It entitles local unions to negotiate on any matter that may influence their job situation. The parties themselves, the managers and the employees at the local plants, shall agree on the job specifications they consider suitable. In order to guide local action, the Swedish Confederation of Trade Unions has endorsed a special action programme on psychosocial aspects of the work environment (LO 1980).

As can be seen the contents of this volume, many ideas exist for a better adaptation of man's total environment to his abilities and needs, and about ways to accomplish this. Needless to say, many of these ideas need to be tested out on model scale and the outcome evaluated using an interdisciplinary and systems approach.

For example, it seems reasonable to investigate whether steps taken to:

increase an individual worker's control of his/her own work arrangements;

take part in decision making on the organization of work;

avoid monotonous, machine-paced, short but frequently repeated work actions;

optimize (not maximize) automation;

see his/her work in relation to the total product;

avoid quantitative over- and underload;

feel that it is easy to communicate with, and give or receive support from workmates and others;

will in most cases improve health and well-being of workers and families, without reducing (and perhaps with improvement of) productivity (Levi, Frankenhauser, and Gardell 1981).

Some people might regard the goals underlying many of the proposals presented in this book as clearly Utopian, and no doubt they are in many parts of the world. Still, these goals, although certainly not reached overnight, indicate the *direction* for our endeavours (cf. Levi 1979, 1980).

According to a Persian proverb 'one pound of learning requires ten pounds of common sense to apply it'. Although problems of application were extensively discussed and a number of proposals put forward, it will be up to the reader to provide the 'ten pounds' and to consider, in each specific case, the possibilities for application.

This book is intended to furnish a *smörgåsbord* of ideas and information. It is hoped that a wide variety of readers will be able to chose from it in accordance with their specific background and needs.

I would like to express my deep gratitude to the two sponsors of the symposia series and particularly to its President, Professor Torgny Segerstedt. I am further indebted to the publishers of the proceedings of the entire series, the Oxford University Press, for their helpfulness and co-operation.

The English in some of the chapters has been revised by Mr Patrick Hort, M.A., whose help is gratefully acknowledged. Last but not least, I would like to express deep indebtedness to Dr Aubrey R. Kagan and Mrs Gun Nerje for their personal involvement and invaluable work in the organization of this symposium and in the compilation of the proceedings.

Laboratory for Clinical Stress Research LENNART LEVI
Box 60205
S-104 01 Stockholm, Sweden
January 1981

REFERENCES

Co-determination Act, Swedish. The Swedish Code of Statutes, 1976, No. 580.

LEVI, L. (ed.) (1971). *Society, stress, and disease*, Vol. I: *The Psychosocial environment and psychosomatic diseases*. Oxford University Press.

—— (ed.) (1975). *Society, stress, and disease*, Vol. II: *Childhood and adolescence*. Oxford University Press.

—— (ed.) (1978). *Society, stress, and disease*, Vol. III: *The productive and reproductive age—male/female roles and relationships*. Oxford University Press.

——, (1979). Psychosocial factors in preventive medicine. In *Healthy people*. The Surgeon General's Report on Health Promotion and Disease Prevention. Background papers. (ed. D. A. Hamburg, E. O. Nightingale, and V. Kalmar). Superintendent of Documents, US Government Printing Office, Washington DC.

——, (1980). *Preventing work stress*. Addison-Wesley, Reading, Massachusetts.

——, FRANKENHAEUSER, M., and GARDELL, B. *Work stress related to social structures and processes*. Paper for the Insitute of Medicine, National Academy of Sciences, Committee on research on stress in health and disease, Washington DC (in press).

LO (Swedish Trade Union Confederation) (1980). *Mental and social hazards to health in the working environment. Programme of Action*. LO, Stockholm.

NATIONAL BOARD OF OCCUPATIONAL SAFETY AND HEALTH (1980). *Psykiska och sociala aspekter på arbetsmiljön*. (Mental and social aspects of the work environment.) Arbetarskddsstyrelsens för-fattningssamling, Stockholm AFS 1980:14.

Work Environment Act, Swedish. The Swedish Code of Statutes. 1977, No. 1160.

WORLD HEALTH ORGANIZATION (1973). *Occupational mental health*. Maule, H. G., Levi, L., McLean, A., Pardon, N., and Savicevic, M. Geneve: WHO/OH/73.13.

——, (1980). *Health aspects of wellbeing in working places*. Report on a WHO working group. EURO Reports and Studies 31. World Health Organization, Regional Office for Europe, Copenhagen.

ACKNOWLEDGEMENTS

Chapter 12 is part of the scientific evidence delivered to the Swedish Government in preparation of the Work Environment Act, made effective 1 July 1978. The chapter has been shortened, revised, and up-dated for this volume.

The research on which Chapter 13 is based was supported by grants from the Swedish Work Environment Fund, the Swedish Medical Research Council (contract No. B78-26P-4316-06), the Swedish Delegation for Applied Medical Defence Research, and the Folksam Insurance Group, Stockholm.

The authors of Chapter 14 gratefully acknowledge the financial support from the Swedish Work Environment Fund (Project No. 55/73) and the Swedish Medical Research Council (Project No. 997).

The authors of Chapter 20 are indebted to the Commonwealth Fund for making their work possible.

The research on which Chapter 21 is based was supported by Götaverken Ltd., Göteborg, the Swedish Medical Research Council, Grant No. B74-19X-825-09A, and the Swedish Work Environment Fund.

Chapter 22 was originally published† in the *International Journal of Psychiatry in Medicine* and is reproduced by kind permission of the Baywood Publishing Company, Inc.

The authors of Chapter 23 gratefully acknowledge the support they have received from the National Institutes of Health, Bethesda, Maryland under Grant HL 17706-01 from the National Heart, Lung, and Blood Institute.

The research on which Chapter 29 is based was supported in part by the Ohio State University Graduate School Biomedical Research Support Grant, United States Public Health Service Grant HL 20861, and the Grant Foundation. The authors wish to express their appreciation and gratitude to Roland Dartau for his meticulous checking of the bibliography and to Linda Weiss for her careful typing and proof-reading.

Chapter 30 is a revised version of 'Influence of the social environment on psychopathology: the historical perspective; a paper presented at the Annual Meeting of the American Psychopathological Association, Boston, March 1978, and to be published in *Stress and mental disorder* (ed. J. E. Barrett, R. M. Rose, and G. L. Klerman). Raven Press, New York (1979). Dr. Brenner gratefully acknowledges support for this research under National Institute of Mental Health No. MH 26154, entitled Economic Change and Social Pathologies in Urban Areas, under the Centre for the Studies of Metropolitan Problems.

Part of Chapter 32 is adapted from McLean, A. A. (1966). Occupational mental health: review of an emerging art. *Amer. J. Psychiat.*, **1222** (9), 961–76.

The views and opinions expressed in Chapter 36 are those of the author, Fred E. Spaner, and do not necessarily reflect those of the National Institute of Mental Health or the government of the United States of America.

The research on which Chapter 38 is based was supported by grants from the Swedish Work Environment Fund, the Swedish Medical Research Council (contract No. B78-26P-4316-06), the Swedish Delegation for Applied Medical Defence Research, and the Folksam Insurance Group, Stockholm. Chapter 39 is based, in part, on a report presented by the author at the ILO Symposium on 'New trends in the optimization of the working environment', Istanbul (ILO, Geneva, 1980).

---

† Lazarus, R. (1974). Psychological stress and coping in psychosomatic illness. *Int. J. Psychiat. Med.*, **5**, 321–3.

INTRODUCTION: INAUGURAL SPEECHES

THOMAS A. LAMBO

Mr Chairman, the Honourable Minister, distinguished ladies and gentlemen. It gives me great pleasure on behalf of the Director General of the World Health Organization to welcome the distinguished participants to this Symposium on Society, Stress, and Disease in Working Life. Four years ago the first international symposium on stress was held in this country, and this occasion will mark the fourth meeting jointly sponsored by the University of Uppsala and the World Health Organization. Therefore, we take special pride in the fact that this is the first such symposium to be organized by the newly designated WHO Research and Training Centre on Psychosocial Factors and Health. This is very important to all of us, especially to our organization which is undergoing, at the moment, a creative evolution in order to set itself new perspectives, new philosophies, and critical challenges. Our commitment is to engage in a broad combined strategy of social and health action and economic advances which will improve the conditions of people at the bottom of social and economic pyramid in many of our contemporary societies. In other words, the human context has become a major challenge to the World Health Organization.

In May 1974, the World Health Assembly in Geneva adopted a resolution calling for the establishment of a psychosocial programme and emphasizing the need to study man and social environmental factors as they affected the health of individuals and groups. The adoption of the resolution was preceded by two days of fascinating and productive discussion in which member states detailed their special needs in this long neglected field. I am sure it will be a great reward to the World Health Organization to have your views not only on such perennial topics as organization in medical sociology, social class and illness, but also on such stimulating topics as the existential view of man, his universal inner needs, his subjective consciousness, his alienation. A lot of criticisms were implied in the statements from many member states about the effect of modern industry on man and about the blind and confused character of this society which is dominated essentially by purely economic relationships.

Mr Chairman, I am sure that Marx and Freud and a host of lesser men have destroyed the belief in the competence of reason to arrive at ultimate truth, but in spite of this many people have tried to find what in society was destructive of the human person. Among these giants are Thomas Carlyle, in his essays and later John Ruskin in *Until the Last*. Perhaps more than anybody, Carlyle tried to give us the clue. We must remember that this was the time when economists were laying down the principles upon which the new industrial society of our times was being built. Ricardo, John Stuart Mill, and Michael Lodge, all gave us a system of automatically operating economic law based on self-interest. It was earlier believed that business naturally was the way to maximize prosperity for all of us. But its laws worked automatically and mechanically and were no more to be tampered with than the laws which regulated the operation of a steam engine. But then it was realized that these laws worked in a very odd way. Sometime they put us all to work. Sometimes they threw all of us out of work. Sometimes they allowed wages to rise. Sometimes they required them to fall. Sometimes they produced too much to sell profitably, but never too much to satisfy human need. There were economic crises, trade wars, and finally poverty amid plenty, until desperate men everywhere began to ask themselves; would the maggots starve because the apple was too big?

Time has not changed a bit and human nature remains essentially the same. Professor Haiyak, a pillar of economic orthodoxy wrote that individuals in participating in the social processes must be ready and willing to adjust themselves to changes and to submit to conventions which are not the result of intelligent design whose justification may not be rcognizable and which to him will often appear unintelligible and irrational.

Thus the designation of the WHO Research and Training Centre on Psychosocial Factors and Health should be seen as part of the World Health Organization's very firm and growing commitment to the new philosophy of man. It should be made clear that this commitment is not made principally to broaden our horizons, although broadened they will be. We simply recognize that our basic role cannot be fulfilled unless social and psychological factors are taken fully into account.

Aside from the new and promising collaborative work which this meeting will discuss the symposium will deal, I hope, with an area where the WHO's programme are particularly vigorous and intelligently aggressive and where psychosocial factors have already been given some prominence: the area of occupational health. In the last few years the World Health Assembly has resolved to promote its occupational health programme to meet the increasing demand as developing countries become industrialized. The WHO has, therefore, expanded its work in occupational health by providing assistance to countries in all regions. There is also a vital trend, which the organization wishes to communicate to occupational health institutions all over the world, towards dealing with workers' total health and towards the study and control not only of physical, chemical, and biological factors at work, but also of the psychosocial working environment. There is strong evidence everywhere that unless special attention is given to psychosocial factors at work we may miss the opportunity of providing and improving the total well-being of working populations everywhere, through the humanization of work and we would instead be likely to witness increasing mental and psychosomatic disorder at all levels of our populations.

This symposium will explore all facets of the epidemiological evidence that relates to physical, mental, and social pathology, arising from stress in the working environment. However, better understanding and control of factors which contribute to such condition as, creeping neurosis, alcoholism, crime, hypertensive disease, ulcers, and so on, may not lead as directly as we would hope to the development of a work environment that promotes or strengthens feelings of well-being. We must therefore keep in mind that satisfaction and contentment are certainly not merely the absence of anomy. And so I hope that the potential capacity of the working environment to contribute to positive health will receive special attention in your deliberations. If working environments ever prove capable of strengthening man's sense of competence and feelings of well-being many significant health problems will, we hope, be substantially resolved.

Today, groups and groups' ideals, philosophers, works of art and literature, and scientists everywhere can express without compromise the fears and hopes of humanity against prevailing social and economic conditions. They are no longer in subjection to economic conditions. The ideology of necessary poverty and social injustice can be dislodged from its institutional as well as its rational ground. We can today unhesitatingly subscribe to Marx's doctrine in his introduction to the *Critique of Hegel's 'philosophy of right'* that there is a categorical imperative to overthrow all conditions in which man is humilated, enslaved, or exploited. Central to our own present philosophy, therefore, is that man individually and collectively, is a process. Prevention and control of all adverse material, social, spiritual, and cultural conditions is therefore for us the *modus operandi* to a fuller quality of life.

ANNA-GRETA LEIJON

Mr Chairman, ladies and gentlemen. On behalf of the Swedish government I have the pleasure to wish you all welcome to Sweden. Conditions in working life are attracting great international interest. Unfortunately, this interest has, in many cases, been formulated in terms of negative behaviour among employees. Large turn-over of staff, high percentages of absenteeism, and strikes have been said to be typical of such behaviour. We in Sweden have become acquainted with these problems. However, I should like to point out some other information which has to a great extent made the question of working life the centre of general political interest. At the end of the 1960s, two commission reports were published in Sweden. The first dealt with conditions of life and described how one part of the population, the salaried employees, successfully built up their knowledge and value through their work, whilst another group the manual workers, are being worn out and broken down in their work. This gap between different groups of citizens is inconsistent with democratic ideals. Another investigation carried out by the Swedish Confederation of Trade Unions showed that more than 80 per cent of the members were of the opinion that their health was threatened by a dangerous working environment. The Swedish government has allocated funds to a large programme of reforms in the field of working life, and we have then chosen industrial democracy as a general conception. By industrial democracy, we mean that employees should have influence over their own work and place of work and the enterprise where they work. By giving the employees directly and through their organizations, a greater influence over their working conditions these conditions will be better adapted to their wishes. We hope to achieve job satisfaction for the employees in two ways: on the one hand through changes in working conditions, on the other through the fact that participation in decision-making is, in itself, a source of work satisfaction. This programme of reforms has already been decided by parliament to a great extent. A new law on the working environment has been introduced. It gives the 80 000 safety officers elected by the employees more influence over the purchase of new machines, as well as a right to stop production if workers' security is threatened, among other things. A law on security of employment will diminish the risk of arbitrary sacking and also improve the position of the elderly and handicapped who would otherwise be threatened by being set apart from regular working life. Claims of employees for the right to participate in management have been duly considered through a law on workers' representatives on company boards and through provisions for greater insight into company accounts. These new laws put increasing demands on the union representatives. Through a special law they have been given a better security against deterioration of their working conditions resulting from their union work, and also the right of carrying out their union work during paid working hours. Our programme is intended to give the employees and their organizations a better position. It should, however, for the sake of completeness be mentioned that measures to improve environment have been primarily directed toward the physical environment, while factors contributing to mental stress have been relatively neglected. These days we talk a lot about the quality of life and how to improve it. One of the most important elements in man's life is work and the conditions thereof. Work is a means of earning a substantial livelihood, but work has also a specific quality of paving the way towards social communication. Work is the answer to the basic human need to develop and enrich one's existence. I think it is essential that we have those facts in mind when discussing the issues of stress and disease in working life. Once again, I wish you all welcome to Sweden, and I hope our work will be successful.

LARS DAHLGREN

Mrs Cabinet Minister, representatives from the World Health Organization, ladies and gentlemen. As a general manager of the Trygg–Hansa Insurance Group, I have pleasure in greeting you at this fourth symposium in the series, *Society, stress, and disease*, which was first conceived not so long ago. I well remember the talks and conferences we had on this subject in the winter of 1969 to 1970. Dr Levi, an energetic man and a talented organizer, has succeeded in developing a line of co-operation with our group in the field of activities related to environmental questions, a field no doubt of even higher importance now than in the 1960s. Dr Levi succeeded in the double diplomatic task of making us willing to pay—for something that we really believed in, of course—and the WHO willing to accept our doing so, while still remaining the good-humoured patron saint of this series. I think Dr Kissinger has got something of the same talents of dealing with great powers. For us, this engagement is thoroughly natural, however, being responsible for one fourth of the total insurance market of Sweden. Thus it is our tradition to support activities which can help prevent the damages to our millions of clients, to their persons, or their material belongings. The stress problem, a symptom of deep underlying technical, economical, or social factors is strongly related to the insurance field.

Have the previous three symposia been successful? Have we reached the goals of 1969 so far? Of course, the world on the whole is not yet affected by what has happened within these four walls during those weeks. We are still confused, but on a higher level, I think the old saying goes. But the understanding, both between different disciplines and scientists and between these, the mass media, and the politicians is no doubt better today than five years ago. To this, these symposia no doubt have contributed, as well as to the founding of the World Health Organization Collaborating Research and Training Centre on Psychosocial Factors and Health here in Stockholm. I wish you a successful continuity of this important and useful work.

SESSION 1

Definitions of problems and objectives

1. MAN ADAPTING TO WORKING CONDITIONS

RENÉ DUBOS

INTRODUCTION

I see no evidence that modern man is less resistant to environmental stresses than his Stone Age ancestors. In our century, millions of normal human beings have survived the frightful ordeals of combat in the trenches of the First World War or among the devilish electronic weapons of more recent conflicts. Many have survived for years under the bestial conditions of concentration camps. All over the world men and women now spend much of their adult years working in the noisy and traumatic environments, either of industrial plants contaminated with chemical fumes or of offices clouded with tobacco smoke. Spectacular increases of populations are occurring in areas where living and working conditions are detestable from all points of view. And even though most human beings suffer in the modern urban environment, the most polluted and congested agglomerations have great appeal for people of all races and ages.

Mankind is thus displaying now, as it has always displayed in the past, a startling ability to survive and function in environments which are highly unnatural and hostile to its biological and psychological nature—including the environments created by scientific technology and urban complexity. The long-range cost of this adaptability however is the emergence of new disease patterns and an impoverishment of emotional life. The theme of this chapter is that modern man is not on his way to extinction, but that the quality of his life will undergo progressive degradation if he does not design environments better suited than the present ones to his unchangeable biological and psychological nature. I shall emphasize the effects of working conditions on physical and mental health.

ADAPTATION TO AN OBJECTIONABLE ENVIRONMENT

Concern for a better environment is widespread in all technological countries, but surprisingly little attention is given to the fact that factories and offices commonly expose workers to working conditions which are not only unpleasant but also potentially dangerous. There is, of course, much information concerning workers who are killed on the job or made obviously sick by their professional activities but this represents only a very small part of the influence of working life on health and disease. Toxic materials, noise and other stimuli, stresses, or monotony, may not cause obvious disturbances at the time they are experienced. In many cases, however, conditions which appear tolerable exert deleterious effects that do not become manifest until long after the initial exposure. A large percentage of the chronic diseases that now plague our society—the so-called diseases of civilization—can probably be traced to the fact that modern man has made some form of *adaptation* to environments which are fundamentally objectionable, although they are tolerable. I have emphasized the word *adaptation* because its misuse is at the origin of many medical and behavioural problems. I shall first illustrate this statement with examples not necessarily related to working conditions.

A few years ago, an American medical journal carried an article entitled 'Villagers adapting to their arsenic-filled water'. According to this article, the underground water of a certain Mexican village is so heavily contaminated with arsenic that two-thirds of the inhabitants exhibit skin lesions, blood protein abnormalities, neurological disorders, and other signs and symptoms of chronic arsenic poisoning. Yet, most of the villagers so affected are able to work and go about the usual activities of Mexican life. The author of the article used the word *adapting* in the title to convey the notion that, in his words, the villagers 'appeared well accustomed to their disorder'. What he really meant of course was that they had come to accept chronic arsenic poisoning as an inescapable fact of life.

Long-range deleterious effects

Tolerance of environments that are deleterious is a common occurrence. Since the beginning of the Industrial Revolution, for example, the air in many parts of Northern Europe has been contaminated with a variety of pollutants from coal smoke and chemical fumes. These pollutants are made even more unpleasant and dangerous by the inclemency of the Atlantic climate. On the whole, however, the inhabitants of industrial Northern Europe have 'adapted' to their dismal atmosphere; they have multiplied, produced great economic wealth, and contributed to knowledge. The price has been that, as a consequence of exposure to air pollution, a large percentage of Northern Europeans suffer from chronic pulmonary disease—which they tend to accept as a matter of course much as the above-mentioned Mexican villagers accept chronic arsenic poisoning. The various forms of chronic pulmonary disease are increasing also in North America and in all other parts of the world which are heavily industrialized.

Similarly, most people become 'adapted' to loud

noises. In this case, 'adaptation' is achieved through a decrease in the ability to perceive certain sounds by impairment of the hearing apparatus and therefore at the cost of the enjoyment of music and of the finer qualities of the human voice. People also become 'adapted' to working and living in crowded and confused environments; this kind of adaptation means in reality developing protective attitudes and behavioural patterns of which the ultimate outcome is to restrict pleasurable social contacts and to impoverish human relationships.

Countless other examples could be provided to illustrate that the word adaptation, as commonly used, denotes processes that have some initial protective value against environmental insults but that commonly result in long-range deleterious effects. In most cases, the exposed person is not even aware of these long-range dangers because the physiological or psychological insult is of a low level, and the protective response is sufficiently effective to mask the effects of the initial exposure.

Difficulties in recognizing environmental dangers

The recognition of environmental insults is especially difficult when these cannot be perceived by the senses, as is increasingly common in the world of modern technology. We still function anatomically and physiologically with the equipment of our Stone Age ancestors and our evolutionary past has not provided us with any biological mechanisms to warn us of the dangers lurking in an invisible beam of radiation or in an odourless kind of vapour. Neither instinct nor biological experience can make us detect the environmental threats that cannot be perceived by our senses and that do not produce immediate deleterious effects readily linked to their cause.

The following substances are among those generally regarded as constituting major health hazards in the modern environment: carbon monoxide, sulphur oxides, nitrogen oxides, nitrates and nitrites, DDT and related pesticides, polychlorinated biphenyls (PCB), mercury, manganese, lead, asbestos, mycotoxins—and of course ionizing radiations. All the items in this list are associated with industrial or agricultural operations and since most of them escape detection by the senses, they present difficult problems for the protection of the workers.

Increased vulnerability as a result of stress

A further difficulty in the identification of environmental stresses is that substances and situations that exert no apparent ill effect under normal conditions may become dangerous under stress. For example, lead stored in the bones can be suddenly released into the general circulation during episodes of pneumonia. Many toxic or carcinogenic compounds are stored in a harmless state in the liver by conjunction with glucuronic acid; however, the process of detoxification can be impaired by liver disease, it can be swamped by overload with other ligands, and it can be reversed by glucu-

ronidase. DDT, dieldrin, and other halogenated pesticides which do not cause obvious damage when stored away in body fats can generate gross and even fatal pathologies when they are suddenly released into the general circulation. Release can occur in various forms of physiological stress such as pregnancy, lactation, food deprivation, intoxication, or acute infection, or even as a result of emotional disturbances. Synergistic effects have been described in several other situations—for example, in experimental systems involving a polychorinated biphenyl hydrocarbon (PDB) and the duck hepatitis virus. Thus, many different kinds of physiological or infectious stresses can act as triggers to activate potential toxicities that would otherwise remain unmanifested under usual conditions.

PSYCHOLOGICAL STRESSES IN WORKING LIFE

Environmental insults of a physicochemical nature have been the ones most extensively studied, in part because they have probably been the most important aetiological agents of disease in industrial work until a few decades ago and also because methods for their control can be formulated at least within economic limitations. Under modern conditions of industrial and office work, however, environmental insults of psychological character are becoming increasingly important.

Sudden changes

It has long been known that most sudden changes are stressful. When Hippocrates wrote, 'It is changes that are chiefly responsible for diseases, especially . . . the violent alterations'; he was referring to seasonal changes. However, this statement applied also to other kinds of changes as suggested by the passage in the same text that 'gradual changes of any regimen' are safer than abrupt changes.

Experience has in fact repeatedly confirmed that sudden changes in working conditions or life situations are likely to be stressful; they do not allow for the orderly emergence of the progressive adaptive mechanisms required for a satisfactory adjustment to new conditions. An example of physiological disturbances caused by abrupt changes in the routine of life has been recently provided by Levi (1964, 1972) in his studies of the effect of piece work on the urine flow and hormonal balance of healthy Swedish women. When extraneous stimuli of physical or psychosocial nature were introduced into their lives, these women experienced subjective disturbances such as fatigue and discomfort and also objective measurable changes in their urine flow and in their excretion of epinephrine, norepinephrine, and creatinine.

Deprivation of stimuli

While sudden changes and overstimulation commonly have a variety of traumatic effects, deprivation of stimuli seems paradoxically to be becoming a more common

4

cause of pathology under modern conditions of work. The reason is that a certain amount of diversity is essential for mental well-being and probably also for physical health.

In the course of evolution, human beings have been exposed to a wide variety of stimuli, in part because their physical environment was complex and changeable and more importantly because their own activities constantly modified their relationships to the external world. It will suffice to mention here that while the human species emerged in a semitropical savannah kind of country, it has now colonized all types of climatic and topographic zones on earth. Since environmental stimuli have affected all aspects of human evolutionary development, it can be expected that some forms of stimulation are essential for the normal performance of physiological and psychological processes. This evolutionary conditioning is reflected in the fact that in animals and man a constant bombardment by a variety of stimuli is essential for successful development and function.

There is much empirical experience concerning the effects of restricted stimulation on adults. For example, mental aberrations are common among prisoners in solitary confinement, or among people who are isolated during long periods of time, either for accidental or for professional reasons. People who are completely isolated are likely to experience abnormalities in feeling states, deterioration of ability to think, perceptual distortions, even hallucinations and delusions. Empirical findings of this nature have been confirmed and extended by studies of sensory deprivation in experimental animals. Such experiments have revealed, for example, that both the development and the maintenance of nerve tissue are dependent on metabolic phenomena conditioned by a proper intensity of stimulation. The atrophic changes caused by removal of stimuli can be reversed if the stimulation is resumed soon enough but they can become permanent if deprivation is prolonged. In human beings objective evidence of the damage done by sensory deprivation has been provided by electroencephalographic studies—showing a decrease in the alpha range of brain waves—and also by physiological studies—revealing disturbances of epinephrine and norepinephrine excretion.

Needless to say, the physiological and psychological effects of sensory deprivation have their counterpart in the disturbances associated with the monotony of automated work and dial-watching tasks. It is possible and indeed probable that workers can become 'adapted' to such monotonous working conditions, in the sense that they tolerate them to earn better wages. As in the case of exposure to low levels of environmental pollutants, however, such tolerance has long-range deleterious effects. The various forms of assembly line work are objectionable not only because monotonous activity is boring but perhaps even more because monotony can generate physiological and behavioural disorders. Diversity is not only the salt of life; it is an essential element of physical and mental health.

IMPOSSIBILITY OF TRUE ADAPTATION TO MANY TECHNOLOGICAL PROBLEMS

I have focused my remarks on certain types of working environments that appear almost innocuous and the pathological effects of which are delayed and indirect. Under such conditions, it is extremely difficult if not impossible to demonstrate convincingly a link between cause and effect. Asbestos, lead, pesticides, and countless other potentially toxic and mutagenic substances are absorbed by the tissues without the exposed person being aware of their presence in his environment. Dial-watching or repetitive tasks appear only boring to the operator, who is usually unaware of the fact that continued monotony may generate physiological and behavioural disturbances.

The classical mechanisms of protective organismic response to injury do not operate in such situations. A truly adaptive response is one which brings into action metabolic, hormonal, and mental processes which correct the disturbing effects of outside forces on the body and the mind, thus reestablishing the equilibrium state. This is the process W. B. Cannon (1932) called homeostasis in his book *The wisdom of the body*. Such responses were developed in the course of evolution to deal with the environmental insults that primitive man encountered in his daily life. The human body, however, has no 'wisdom' for the new kinds of insults created by modern technology, because there was no counterpart for most of them in the evolutionary experience of the human species. Even when the response to an insult of the technological environment has some protective value at the time it occurs, commonly it has delayed consequences that are deleterious. With regard to the technological world, the wisdom of the body is at best shortsighted. Air pollution elicits from the lungs an overproduction of mucus which at first protects its tissues against the pollutants, but this eventually results in emphysema and chronic bronchitis; and similar misdirected compensatory processes are elicited by the new physical and psychical insults of the modern environment. These insults rarely destroy life outright, but they spoil its later years.

No genetic adaptation possible

Furthermore, there is no chance for a genetic adaptation to the threats of the modern technological environment. Since they usually do not have marked effects on health until a long period after exposure, they do not interfere with reproductive ability and therefore provide no chance for genetic selection against them. For example, if a certain environmental factor is a cause of cancer, the chances are very great that the person so affected will produce children long before being incapacitated by the disease. In consequence, these children will not be better adapted than their parents to the undesirable environmental conditions which produced the cancer. In any case, adaptive changes resulting from alteration of the genetic apparatus are extremely slow, and would require many generations before making a significant difference. Even if it were true that we can become adapted to industrial fumes, to the noises of jackhammers, or to the traumatic experiences of the 'rat race' and competitive life, it would take more than ten generations before the genes making for adaptation to these insults become established in society as a whole.

No 'wisdom of the body'

The widespread acceptance of the phrase 'The wisdom of the body' among pathologists, and of 'Nature knows best' among ecologists, is the expression of the Pollyanna attitude in which we have been raised and which makes us expect that good is the normal state of affairs, whereas in reality any kind of change implies danger. It is not pessimism to believe that there cannot be any lasting security; it is simple realism. Modern industrial and office work requires eternal vigilance, but the individual worker cannot possibly take the responsibility for his own health in a complex world which he cannot apprehend and which the experts themselves do not fully understand.

The time has therefore come to devote as much thought and research to the health hazards of working conditions as is devoted to engineering design, purchase specifications, or sales policies. It must be emphasized, however, that the usual methods of medical research and practice are not well suited to this type of pathological problem. In many cases, the victim does not perceive the threat to which he is exposed, the epidemiologist has no simple way of detecting exposure, and the physician can recognize the signs and symptoms only when the pathological process is far advanced.

THE ROLE OF MEDICINE

A medical alarm system

It is unrealistic furthermore to hope that safety measures and other improvements in working conditions could completely prevent industrial and office pathology even if they were based on much greater knowledge than we now have. New substances and new working techniques are constantly being introduced so rapidly that there is no chance to evaluate their potential health dangers before they have affected large numbers of people. The only way to deal with this unfortunate but inevitable state of affairs is to carry out systematically a great variety of tests on samples of the working population, in the hope of detecting evidences of pathological changes as early as possible. This approach, which could be regarded as a form of prospective epidemiology or as a medical alarm system, would of course be cumbersome and costly, but the inconvenience would be small compared with the medical load now being created by the chronic disabilities resulting from undesirable working conditions. In a truly civilized society, protection of the health of the worker should be regarded—both for humanitarian and economic reasons—as the most essential and irreducible aspect of production cost.

Further prophylactic possibilites for industrial medicine

I shall briefly mention a few recent technological developments which illustrate the urgency, and also the possibility, of greatly strengthening the prophylactic aspects of industrial medicine.

Near Louisville, Kentucky, at least six workers in a single plant have recently died of angiosarcoma of the liver, an unusual type of cancer. They had been exposed to vinyl chloride monomer, the building block of the ubiquitous polyvinyl plastics. Earlier research had indicated that vinyl chloride can cause a wide variety of tumours in experimental animals; furthermore, a human case of angiosarcoma had been known to occur at a plant of Imperial Chemical Industries in the United Kingdom. It is not known whether the hazard posed by the vinyl chloride monomer extends to the polyvinyl chloride (PVC) products, but the question is of enormous practical importance because PVC is used in the manufacture of a wide range of consumer products such as pipes, bottles, dentures, flooring materials, food packaging, pharmaceutical compounds, etc. In a responsible technological civilization, the knowledge that was available concerning the potential dangers of vinyl chloride should have served as a warning to develop more information and techniques for the protection of the workers and consumers likely to come into contact with the monomer raw materials and their derivatives.

As a result of the forthcoming shortages and higher prices of petroleum products, it can be taken for granted that there will be much increase in the use of coal and of derivatives prepared from it, and probably also in the use of other fossil fuels such as those derived from shale oil deposits. It is known that every year for several decades more than 200 miners have died of mine accidents in the United States, but little attention is paid to the fact that a large percentage of miners suffer from the coal dust in their lungs. Even though good statistical evidence is not available, the likelihood is great that the life expectancy of miners is rather short even when they are not killed or maimed in mining accidents. There are also definite signs that various pathologies can result from exposure to the aerosols that are released when shale is processed to release the fuels it contains. Extensive epidemiological, experimental, and clinical studies are therefore urgently needed to determine the dangers associated with coal mining, with the extraction of oil from shale, and with all other related technologies, before large-scale operations are undertaken as is likely to occur in the near future.

EXAMPLES OF FAULTY ADAPTATION

There is more to the problems of health and disease than the physical and psychological quality of working conditions. Emotional, aesthetic, and other values should also be considered when judging the working environment. In the final analysis, the human environment means everything that is experienced by man and it is the total nature of this experience that determines the quality of life. Since I do not have the necessary background to discuss these problems from the point of view of environmental quality in factories and offices, I shall briefly illustrate with other aspects of life that faulty adaptation can occur with regard to perceptual quality, as it does with problems of health.

I spent my school years in Paris at a time when the historical buildings of the city were covered with a layer of soot and dirt deposited by domestic and industrial smoke. It used to be thought that the prevailing greyness gave a distinguished and refined quality to the Parisian atmosphere. Indeed, there was an outcry of anger when André Malraux ordered that the buildings be washed. Then a miracle happened. When the grey layer was removed from the monuments, their surfaces revealed the golden hue of the stone work, as subtle as that of young human flesh. For more than a century Parisians and the rest of the world had become accustomed—'adapted'—to the somber tonality created by the soot and the dirt of the Industrial Revolution. Perceptual life had thus been impoverished by a century of unconscious conditioning—of so called adaptation—to an environmental defect. Instructed by this experience, I now feel sorrow and indignation at seeing people in American cities being everywhere exposed to noise, ugliness, and garbage in the street. By 'adapting' to this kind of environment, the American public progressively accepts messiness and squalor as the normal state of affairs—in factories and offices as well as in the street.

REFUSAL TO 'ADAPT'—A HEALTHY SIGN

Fortunately, there are reasons not to end on such a gloomy note. Many people in all age and social groups are refusing to 'adapt' to undesirable conditions. The campaign for a better environment is gaining momentum and it is not limited to the health aspects of the environmental problem; it has begun to encompass emotional and aesthetic qualities. Sooner or later, the environmental crusade will spread to working conditions in factories and offices. In fact, labour unions are beginning to take an active part in this campaign both inside and outside working places. For example, labour unions in Australia have recently put a 'green ban' on the construction of some industrial plants until the proper steps

have been taken to provide adequate pollution controls. They even refused to build a certain parking lot near the new Sydney Opera House because this would have required the cutting down of three magnificent fig trees that had an emotional value for the local citizens.

Many people, I know, believe that concern for the quality of the environment is just a fad that will vanish when the economic cost and inconveniences of effective control measures become apparent. But there is a new factor in the situation. A large part of the public has come to regard a good environment as a *natural right* of man—just as civil rights, the right to education, and the right to medical care are natural rights. And it is obvious that a good environment will have to include healthy and pleasant working conditions. The environmental movement cannot be merely a fad, because history shows that there has never been a lasting retreat from the recognition of a natural right of man.

SUMMARY

In advanced technological countries, most working environments are now sufficiently well controlled to prevent or at least minimize the occurrence of obviously toxic or disabling situations. As a result, workers are usually willing to tolerate conditions that are fundamentally undesirable but appear acceptable because they do not grossly interfere with social and economic life.

Such tolerance, however, commonly has indirect consequences which are deleterious in the long run even though they are not recognized at the time of initial exposure. The ultimate effects are various types of chronic disorders—of either physiological of psychological nature.

From a long-range point of view, there cannot be any true adaptation to the environments, especially those created by modern technology, that do not conform to the biological and psychological nature of the human species; what is called adaptation is usually achieved at the cost of impairment of function.

Since man cannot successfully 'adapt' to injurious artificial conditions, he should protect himself from contact with them, or preferably design environments that are really adapted to his nature.

REFERENCES

Cannon, W. B. (1932). *The widsom of the body*, New York.
Levi, L. (1964). The stress of everyday life as reflected in productiveness, subjective feelings, and urinary excretion of adrenaline and noradrenaline under salaried and piece-work conditions. *J. Psychosom. Res.* **8**, 199.

——— (1972). Stress and distress in response to psychosocial stimuli. Laboratory and real life studies on sympathoadrenomedullary and related reactions. *Acta med. scand.*, Suppl. **528**, 106–18.

2. A PRACTICAL MODEL OF THE PSYCHOSOCIAL–STRESS–HEALTH SYSTEM

AUBREY R. KAGAN

THE THEME OF THE SERIES

The underlying premises of the series of volumes on *Society, stress, and disease* are that:

Stimuli arising from changing psychosocial situations may promote health or cause disease;

If such situations are adapted to the organism's needs or the organism can adapt to the situation, health ensues; if not, disease results;

When changes are slow, e.g., over periods of 100 000 years or so, natural selection and survival of the fittest is nature's method of adaptation;

Our innate characteristics must still carry the lessons of our formative aeons up to a few thousand years ago;

When changes are faster, but still over periods of two or three generations, the process of adaptation depends much on man-made efforts. The time honoured method is to see trouble coming or, more usually, after it has come, and to make corrections. This has sometimes been described as 'planning from crisis to crisis'.

The fear today is that changes are so fast and so extensive that ill effects might occur on too large a scale with too little warning to be able to make a rational correction in time;

This is the prospect of people in developing and developed countries today. Environmental change—physical, social, and psychical—is frequent, extensive, often incomplete, and, when planned, its significance is, at best, only partly known;

The rate of social change is probably still increasing;

Since these changes are man-made, we can, in theory, reduce risk by trying to slow the tempo or by obtaining a better understanding of the effects of environmental change and introducing rational control.

PURPOSE

The purpose of *this series* of volumes is to consider whether psychosocial stimuli arising through social situations cause or prevent disease. If so, what health actions can be recommended on the basis of present knowledge, and what are the priorities in increasing our knowledge?

The purpose of *this volume* is to consider all this from the point of view of psychosocial stimuli arising from social relations specific to working life. Working life includes much more than work, e.g. there are marital and child-rearing problems and often problems of looking after the dependent aged as well. In addition there are problems related to change of location, migration, urbanization. Stress due to marital relations and child rearing has already been considered in Vols. 2 and 3 of this series and will therefore be given less emphasis here.

DEFINITIONS

The notion of a psychosocial–stress–health system has arisen through our work and through previous symposia. This has proved to be of value in deciding what kind of studies need to be carried out, how they might be carried out, and the kind of observations that need to be made.

In the hope that it may be of use to others I define below the elements in the system depicted in the model (Fig. 2.1, p. 11) and indicate briefly how these relate to working life.

Social situations

These are the environmental structures and rules imposed by society. Structure may be considered the anatomical form of the social situation while the social rules are the physiology or mode of function. We are concerned with social situations which, because they demand adaptation on the part of members, or 'would-be' members, of the society, are likely to give rise to psychological stimuli. Examples relevant to working life are structures and rules by which:

Work is obtained;
Employment is retained;
Promotion in responsibility, or payment, is made;
Participation with others is possible;
The family is supported;
Food, housing, health, transport is provided;
Education is obtained;
Recreation is enjoyed;
Decisions are made.

Similar structures do not necessarily imply similar rules. Several societies may share a similar type of employment bureau. But in one priority may be given to the handicapped and in another the rules may prevent such people from being employed at all. A similar structure for promotion may exist in many societies, but in one the rules may ensure promotion on the basis of duration of employment, in another on ability and in a third on being a 'friend of the minister'.

Structures and rules may differ independently and change independently between societies and within societies over a period of time. It is particularly when one or other or both change, or are not understood, or become unfamiliar, that psychosocial stimuli (see below) are likely to arise.

Psychosocial stimuli

These are stimuli, suspected of being able to cause disease, which originate in social situations (i.e., in the environment) and affect the organism through the medium of higher nervous processes. [Kagan and Levi 1974]

Psychological stimuli that may arise from social situations include deprivation, excess, or threat to:

Physiological needs or safety of the individual, family, or community;
Sense of belonging;
Self-esteem and status;
Sense of purpose and self-realization.

In relation to work these may be considered as:

Means of obtaining minimum needs for the worker and his family;
A sense of mutual interest and support with and from the working group or institution;
Matching the work and responsibility with the worker's aspirations;
The work itself providing a main interest and source of satisfaction and enabling him to utilize his capabilities in a satisfactory manner.

Threat must be perceived, but need not be real. The degree of psychological stimulus would be expected to depend to a large extent on the difference between expectation and the situation as perceived. Such a stimulus is likely to be common to many social situations, but its intensity would depend on the psychobiological programme (see below). A person who cannot obtain the bare necessities of life for himself and his family is not likely to be stimulated by thoughts of self-esteem and status. However once subsistence level is reached he may be much concerned by threat to opportunities of better relations with co-workers, more satisfaction from doing a job, higher pay, participation in management, etc. Nevertheless whether this will be the case or not for a particular individual once minimum essential needs are obtained, depends on his present status or psychobiological programme to which a large variety of factors contribute.

The stimulus is likely to be enhanced or prolonged when the psychobiological programme provides no guidelines or rules to decision or correct action. This is particularly likely to occur when the situation is new, when the rules are changing, when they appear irrational, or when there is no accepted leadership. Such must be the case in developed countries where notions of the relationship between employer and employee are in flux and even more so in developing countries when industrialization is first introduced.

Psychobiological programme

By this we mean a propensity to react in accordance with a certain pattern, e.g., when solving a problem, or adapting to an environment. Determinants of this programme in an organism are genetic factors, and earlier environmental influences. [Kagan and Levi 1974]

Thus, although there is a fixed genetic element, the psychobiological programme is continuously altered by 'feedback' in the form of education and experience. The 'programme' will determine what is expected from a given situation at particular time and also how the situation is perceived. It determines whether a given social situation produces a psychological stimulus and the intensity of the stimulus.

The programme may also have a modifying effect on the output side (see 'Mechanism' below). Thus different subjects exposed to the same stimulus respond biologically to a different extent. This has been well demonstrated for adrenal secretions in humans and is probably an inherited characteristic. There is a growing body of evidence to show that such functions might be influenced in a controlled manner by learned behaviour.

Mechanisms

These are reactions in the organism, induced by psychosocial stimuli, which, under some conditions of intensity, frequency or duration, and in the presence or absence of certain, interacting variables, will lead to disease.

A number of processes are suspected of being mechanisms whereby psychosocial stimuli cause disease, e.g., mental, endocrine, immunological, social. Relatively little is known about them. Most is known about hypothalamo-adrenomedullary and hypophyseal-adrenocortical reactions. These are characterized by increased catecholamine and 17-OH Corticosteroid secretion respectively, and are often assessed by measurement of these substances excreted in the urine. These reactions, which involve other endocrine secretions and other systems, are often referred to as 'Selye stress' but would be more correctly described as 'Selye strain'.

They occur with most, perhaps all forms of stimulation, whether the latter are physical or mental pleasant or unpleasant. Their relation to a wide variety of precursors of disease, e.g., anxiety, raised blood pressure, increased rate of platelet aggregation, attenuated immune response, has been demonstrated in man and animals.

The process parallels 'arousal', a useful preparation for adaptation to the needs of fight or flight, and is phylogenetically an ancient reaction. Whether it is the mechanism by which psychosocial stimuli cause disease is not known. It is strongly suspected that this is so, however, because of its known relationship to precursors of disease and because the normal response for which it prepares him is rarely indulged in by modern man. The man or woman threatened by the dissatisfaction of the supervisor can neither fight or run away from the situation. Similarly those inspired to work with zeal and vigour are often frustrated in doing so by management or workmates.

Possibilities are:

1. That 'Selye stress' is the common pathway by which stimuli cause disease;
2. That disease occurs only if 'Selye stress' is prolonged or frequent;
3. That disease occurs only if the normal response to Selye stress—fight or flight—is not allowed to follow;
4. That Selye stress is not a disease mechanism at all, but is an index of response to stimulus.

Precursors of disease

These are malfunctions in mental or physical systems which have not resulted in disability but, if continued, are likely to do so. [Kagan and Levi 1974]

Malfunctions identical with precursors of disease, but of short duration, are known to be caused by Selye stress (or strain), e.g. anxiety, rapid heart rate, hypertension, increased blood glucose, decreased blood clotting time. Evidence for association of 'Selye stress' with other malfunctions is accruing but a causal relationship has not yet been proven, e.g. diminished immunological response, raised blood cholesterol.

Prospective studies have shown that subjects with these malfunctions but without any apparent disability (see below) are at high risk to subsequent disease. But whilst all subjects with disease have some malfunction there are many who have malfunction but no disease (e.g. recent surveys in the United States, England and Wales, Australia, and Yugoslavia show that 10–15 per cent of men and women in the productive age have severe disability whilst 3 times as many have malfunction).

It would therefore seem likely that although precursors of disease imply high subsequent risk, onset of disability is dependent on factors additional to the duration of the precursor. Such factors may include interacting variables (see below) and it is speculated that they may often be of a social nature.

If this assessment is true then it follows that the understanding of such factors may provide a potent means of preventing disability.

Disease

Disease is disability caused by mental or somatic malfunction. Disability is failure in performance of a task. This must always include tasks considered essential, might include tasks considered normal and, when more is known, will include tasks that are considered optimal. In applying this, it is necessary to state the level of the biological hierarchy to which it refers. Disease, as defined, is different at the cell, organ, organism, family, community level.

In this volume, we will be concerned mostly with the individual, family, worker group, work institution, and community.

Interacting variables

These are mental, physical, or social factors which alter the action of causative factors arising from a social situation at the psychobiological programme, mechanism, precursor, or disease stage. By 'alter' is meant that they promote or prevent processes that lead to disease. Of course interacting variables may modify the social situation, i.e. the environmental situation to which the subject is exposed. This may be a practical way of preventing ill effects and is embodied in the notion of matching the work conditions, living conditions, etc. to the subjects' psychobiological programme.

But, given a social situation that is ordinarily likely to produce a pathogenic stimulus in a particular person, for example, dismissal from work, interacting variables may:

Intensify or reduce the stimulus (e.g. expected or unexpected; new job available or not available; spouse support or anatagonism; health good or bad);
Intensify or reduce the mechanism (e.g. other problems—for example at home; psychopharmacologicals; social support);
Intensify or reduce precursors of disease (e.g. lack of social support; intensification of work problems; finding a suitable job; provision of medical treatment or a health regime);
Intensify or reduce disease (e.g. non-recognition or failure to treat adequately; availability and utilization of medical services, rehabilitation including social adjustments to make work possible).

The reader will be interested in Susan Gore's study (Cobb and Gore 1970) of 100 men who experienced an unanticipated loss of employment when the 'works closed down'. She found an association between lack of social support and a relative excess of disease or of the mental or physical precursors of disease. The social support measures were: confidence and sympathy from wife, relatives, and friends; participation in the local social network; opportunities to talk about his problems. The mental or physical precursors of disease or disease included; depression; sense of economic deprivation persisting after re-employment; elevated blood cholesterol levels; increased frequency and duration of illness and complaints.

MODEL OF PSYCHOSOCIAL–STRESS –HEALTH SYSTEM

Fig. 2.1 is a model of the concept of the relationship between the factors defined above. It shows that stimuli arising from social situations, acting through the higher nervous processes in individuals or groups with a particular type of psychobiological programme, cause physiological changes which produce or prevent precursors of disease, or disease. Interacting variables, by modifying the psychobiological programme or mechanisms, may enhance or reduce the precursor or disease-forming tendency. Interacting variables may act on the precursors to prevent or enhance disease and may act on the disease process to reduce or enhance it.

Ways in which this model has been applied to a proposed programme for the Laboratory for Clinical Stress Research are indicated in Chapter 42.

SUMMARY

This article links the present volume of *Society, stress and disease* with others in the series. The purpose of the symposium on which this volume was based was to consider whether psychosocial stimuli, arising through social situations common in working life, cause or prevent disease; to recommend health actions on the basis of present knowledge if possible; and to indicate priorities for research.

Terms used by the author and his colleagues in previous volumes to refer to the elements of a model of the psychosocial health system are defined or redefined. The model and its elements are discussed in relation to working life. It has been of use to the author and his colleagues to plan and administer a research programme part of which is described in Chapter 42.

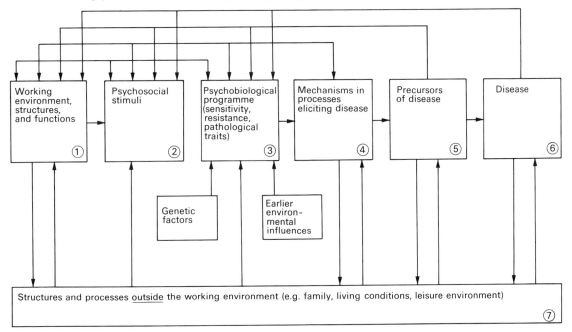

FIG. 2.1. Psychosocial stress–health model.

REFERENCES

COBB, S. and GORE, S. (1970). *Unemployment, social support and health.* American Physiological Association, Montreal.

KAGAN, A. R. and LEVI, L. (1974). Health and environment—psychosocial stimuli: a review. *Soc. Sci. Med.* **8,** 225–41.

3. PSYCHOSOCIAL STRESSORS IN WORKING LIFE: PROBLEMS SPECIFIC TO DEVELOPING COUNTRIES

M. A. EL BATAWI

INTRODUCTION

Many publications are available on the impact of industrialization on health. Studies have also been carried out of the health problems associated with development. Psychosocial factors at work in the developing countries, however, have hardly been investigated. The following account is therefore limited to some of the writer's own observations in these countries.

It would not be totally correct to draw a parallel between stressors encountered by workers during the Industrial Revolution of the eighteenth century and those of workers in developing countries nowadays. There may be similarities with respect to changes in the physical working environment causing occupational diseases, but the Industrial Revolution differed from the present industrial movement in developing countries in that mechanized processes were a gradual development associated with innovation, thereby probably providing a better opportunity for psychosocial adaptation. The rapid introduction of complex work methods and tools in developing countries is associated with psychosocial stress; the main problem is that of adjustment to change.

It may be useful to classify these psychosocial stressors into two main categories; those resulting in health problems of varying magnitude, and those that may contribute positively to workers' mental health.

PSYCHOSOCIAL STRESS AND DISTRESS

To a large extent, workers in the developing countries have managed to adapt to the rather strange psychosocial environment of mechanized labour. They have been required to change from the quiet and more intimate rural life to the noisy speed of factories; from a traditional dependence on natural processes and manual labour to standardized production, precise timing, and dependence on energy; and from the old identification with land and crops to the impersonal environment of machines. They are likely to move away from their friendly work associates, to work with busy strangers, different management, in a different hierarchy. On the other hand, the benefits expected mainly from material rewards may play an important role in motivation to meet such challenges. In many instances however, adaptation may fail, either because of too much stress or of personal susceptibility or both, resulting in desertion of work or in psychological and psychosomatic disorders.

Absenteeism and labour turnover

In many developing countries, absence from work and labour turnover are relatively high. While these may be closely related to economic and employment problems, cases were found in association with failure to adapt to an alien psychosocial environment in relatively large industrial undertakings. When a new steel mill was first established in Burma in 1967, although most of the newly recruited workers were familiar with iron processing as blacksmiths in private shops, the annual turnover exceeded 200 per cent in the first two years, and the mill was forced to slow down on production for months because of labour shortages. The main causative factor was the difficulty in adapting to the style of work, where workers were responsible for only limited parts in a line of production, communication was difficult, and personal identification, despite the rewarding pay, was limited.

Another example which illustrates the impact of a fear of imminent work hazards to health and life is shown in some of the South Korean mining operations. The isolation of mines in remote areas, coupled with reports of irreversible pneumoconiosis and mortality in underground collapses, resulted in almost 300 per cent labour turnover per year, despite such attractions as high pay, housing, free schooling, and free medical care for workers and their families.

Psychological and psychosomatic disorders

These examples illustrate the inevitable breakdown of homeostasis where escape from mounting psychosocial stress was difficult. Naturally, there is a gradual process of psychological disturbance that may appear in various manifestations of discontent and dissatisfaction. In this respect, the experience of the maladjusted or unhappy industrial worker in industrialized societies is not different. But while compensation may be found in these societies in habituation to alcohol or drugs or in behavioural anomalies, this has not been observed so much in industrializing countries, or at least there has been no evidence of serious occurrence. There are also no data on the magnitude or prodromal manifestations of psychological disorder and frank psychosomatic disease. However, the striking nature of the latter led me to observe and partly study psychosocial factors associated with episodes of psychosomatic disorders among workers in rapidly developing societies.

In the early 1960s, the writer was notified of a relatively high prevalence of peptic ulcer in a glass factory. In investigating the problem, it was found that in addition to diet and minor physical stress in the work environment, the main associating factors with what proved to be a significantly high incidence of acute ulcer included faulty management of the payroll and determined provocation in seeking an increased output from individual glass blowers who were the key workers in the factory.

Very recently, the Director of the Industrial Health Unit in Singapore informed the writer of a series of cases of 'epidemic hysteria' which had appeared at a number of work places in that country. The preliminary investigation of the problem, which temporarily caused complete suspension of work in the affected factories, showed that there were several psychosocial stressors relating to age, sex, types of tasks, hours of work, and pay in common among the workers, who also shared a common ethnic origin.

FACTORS WITH POSITIVE HEALTH EFFECTS

The positive effects on health associated with work should not be overlooked in referring to psychosocial stresses of working life. As a matter of fact, it is the impression of the writer that many employers in developing countries are sticking to long-inherited humane traditions. Close and more intimate work relations exist in small work establishments, which employ the major part of the productive manpower in these countries. There is evidence, despite many undesirable physical hazards in these factories, that absenteeism from work is lower and this has been attributed to the comparatively better work relations in the small enterprise.

In many large establishments in developing countries, religious traditions are upheld, and the workers are allowed to go for prayers in the temple or mosque built on the factory premises. There are also examples where the workers themselves have actually introduced changes in complex industrial processes to suit cultural and traditional habits, and that such changes not only have made them happier in what would otherwise be a stressful situation, but have also increased industrial productivity.

NEED FOR INVESTIGATIONS

Systematic studies of psychosocial factors in the work environment in the developing countries are needed and highly recommended, with a view to: (a) putting under control at an early stage of industrial development those factors that may lead to excessive strain thereby avoiding the mistakes of older industrialized countries; and (b) identifying those psychosocial factors that play a role in health promotion and the education of employers and health practitioners in the utilization of such factors for the betterment of health of the working populations in the developing countries.

SUMMARY

One of the main psychosocial problems in working life in developing countries is that associated with change from traditional work methods to mechanization. Observations were made of increased absenteeism from work, labour turnover, and occurrence of psychosomatic disorders in association with psychosocial stressors. In several instances however, there are factors that may contribute to the betterment of health; and in others, the workers succeeded in introducing changes in the work methods to suit their cultural and traditional habits.

4. PSYCHOLOGICAL JOB STRESS AND WORKER HEALTH—A PROGRAMMATIC EFFORT

W. KROES*

INTRODUCTION

For the past three years, our Institute has been conducting a programme of research concerning the relationship between psychological stress at work and the physical and mental health of the worker, and of fostering practices which will either reduce undue job stress or improve an individual's adjustment to it. Except for an additional study of the effect of psychological job stress on a worker's accident potential, our goal three years later remains the same.

In the beginning there were real difficulties in deciding how to attack a problem of truly overwhelming proportions. At what level of analysis were we to concentrate in determining the relationship between job stress and health (i.e., correlational, identifying the exact causal chain at the molar and/or molecular level, etc.)? Should we attack stress in one occupation, albeit a high stress one, or should we look at stressors across the board? Should we attack the problems of stress in an applied, results-oriented manner or should we develop and test theoretical notions about the subject? These were some of the questions we had to wrestle with in the beginning. But if we were ever to meet our overall goal we realized that we had to deal with them in a direct manner. We needed a programmatic approach. The particular programme we adopted and have since followed was a result of answering these questions.

It consists of five distinct problem areas, termed 'Programme aspects' with separate projects planned under each. Some of these projects have begun; others are still to be initiated. The following is an account of the five programme areas.

FIRST PROGRAMME ASPECT—TO ESTABLISH THE NATURE, PREVALENCE, AND SEVERITY OF PSYCHOLOGICAL JOB STRESS PROBLEMS

Our first programme need was to determine if, in fact, psychological job stress was a significant problem. Many a manager and fellow professional had reacted to our concern with comments such as: stress is good for the worker, all you want to do is mollycoddle the worker, they need a strong firm hand, etc. We firmly believed these views to be based on ignorance and established folklore; yet without a graphic display of the extent and health cost of psychological job stress we would have a difficult time convincing others. Facts are the best dispellers of myths, so our first programme efforts were aimed at getting these facts. Three projects were initiated to this end.

Job demands and worker health

The intent of our first project was to establish associations between stressful elements in different jobs and the health difficulties of workers in them. The protocol as developed consisted of three major tasks. The first task involved the selection of at least ten job types, i.e., foremen, middle manager, assembly line worker, etc. which, based on previous literature and/or personal observation, had characteristics which appeared to be psychologically stressful. Some of the psychological stressors that were to be considered in the selection were high levels of responsibility, role conflict, role ambiguity, task overload (both quantitative and qualitative), poor employee–employer interrelationships, changing work hour routines, perceived inequities in pay and job status, and other on-the-job problems. The second task was to draw 900 workers for study from ten or more job-types evidencing high psychological stress components and 100 other workers from job-types which were not considered psychologically stressful. The latter subjects were to serve as controls. Job environments for all workers in the study were to be free of significant physical or chemical agents which might confound the effects of psychological stress. The third major task was to define the level of psychological stress perceived by the subject job-holders via questionnaires and to relate such stress to their physical and mental health status as defined by medical histories and in some cases, physiological measures to be described below.

This study was conducted for NIOSH by the Institute for Social Research (ISR) at the University of Michigan (French *et al.*, unpublished). The results are presented in the publication: *Job demands and worker health*, NIOSH Research Report, April 1975. As it turned out, 23 occupations† were studied and over 2000 male workers surveyed (see Table 4.1). Interestingly, we found it almost impossible to find a matched non-stressed control occupation††. Every group had at least one major stressor.

*Present address: Wilshire Crest Medical Group, 5266 West Olympic Blvd., Los Angeles, California 90036, USA.

†Through consultation with plant personnel/union leaders, it was established that workers tested in the above occupations were not subject to extreme environmental hazards.

††Tool and die makers were conceived of as a good control group, but it was found that decreased production leading to plant lay-offs had increased the stress of job insecurity for this group.

TABLE 4.1

Sample sizes by occupational group

Occupational group	N
White collar†	
Accountant	92
Administrator	254
Air traffic controller	
large airports	82
small airports	43
Engineer	110
Physician, general practice	104
Professor	74
Professor–Administrator	25
Programmer	90
Railroad dispatcher	86
Scientist	118
Supervisor	
of blue collar (foreman)	178
of white collar	42
White/blue collar	
Electronics technician	94
Policeman	111
Blue collar	
Assembly	
machine-paced	79
nonmachine-paced	69
Continuous flow monitor	101
Fork lift driver	47
Delivery service courier	25
Machine tender	34
Tool and die maker	77
Miscellaneous, gathered incidentally	
Assembly, machine paced, varied	27
Product handler, petro-chemical	8
Miscellaneous	49
TOTAL	2019

†The designation of collar colour is approximate

Now let us turn to a few of the findings. These data should be interpreted with caution because they have not been controlled for possible confounding variables such as age and education. The first step in the analyses has been to conduct research on the ecological level. That is, we are looking at the relationships between stress and strain across the occupations rather than across the individuals. Since there are 23 occupations under study, the sample size for this analysis is 23. This type of analysis will give us a first look at whether the occupations which we picked as stressful or non-stressful are indeed that way according to the perceptions of the people who work in them. We also want to know whether these occupations which have high levels of job stress also have high levels of strain. The findings which I would like to present deal with two strains—job satisfaction and somatic complaints.

Fig. 4.1 presents a summary of the correlates of jobs with high job satisfaction. Such occupations tend to be characterized by high job security, highly educated people, good social support, high utilization of abilities, responsibility for the work of others, and relatively high work load. These occupations have a significant amount of complexity in them, involve participation in decision-making, and have little role conflict. The Duncan socio-economic status score of such occupations tends to be relatively high. On the other hand, occupations where the average level of satisfaction is low tend to lack these qualities. Interestingly enough, gross income is not significantly correlated with job satisfaction. Money does not appear to buy job-related happiness, although it may contribute to feelings of well-being in other areas of life.

A stepwise multiple regression produces three significant predictors of job satisfaction out of this set. They are job security, social support from one's superior, and a high level of education. These predictors account for 82 per cent of the variance in job satisfaction

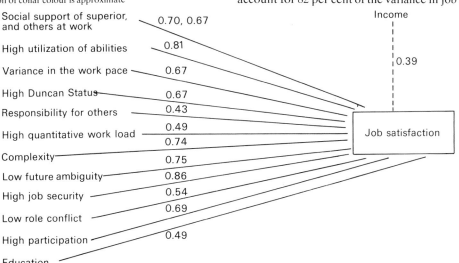

Fig. 4.1. Correlates of occupations with high employee satisfaction. $N = 23$ white and blue collar occupational groups. $r \geq 0.41$, $p < 0.05$, $r \geq 0.53$, $p < 0.01$.

15

when adjustments in R^2 are made for degrees of freedom. These three predictors are apparently most representative of the entire set of correlates of job satisfaction. Consequently, occupations which are characterized by these predictors are also characterized by correlates such as high social support and low role conflict.

Somatic complaints constitute a second measure of strain in this study. Somatic complaints share about 36 per cent common variance with job satisfaction. Occupational groups where dissatisfaction with the work tends to be expressed tend to show evidence of psychosomatic discomforts such as spells of dizziness, feeling short of breath when you are not exercising or working hard, having a loss of appetite, and having trouble sleeping at night.

Fig. 4.2 presents some of the significant correlates of somatic complaints. They are similar to the correlates of low job satisfaction. Lack of job security, low com-

plexity, low utilization of skills and abilities, and low social support are found in occupations in this study characterized by somatic complaints. Of all the correlates, income is only marginally related to somatic complaints.

Use of stepwise multiple regression with the more important correlates of somatic complaints identifies two significant predictors—low social support from the immediate superior and difficulty in finding comparable alternative employment. One might think of the latter as a measure of the extent to which the person is relatively trapped in his job by a lack of other acceptable forms of employment. Later analyses will tell whether this condition exacerbates the effects of job stress on employee health. Together these two predictors account for 76 per cent of the variance in the index of somatic complaints.

Finally, I wish to present some data from this study which deal with specific occupations. In the left half of Fig. 4.3 five occupational groups have been chosen who

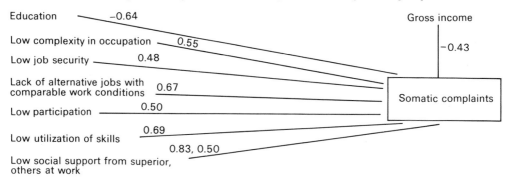

Fig. 4.2. Significant correlates of somatic complaints. $N = 23$ occupational groups. $r \geq 0.41$, $p < 0.05$; $r \geq 0.53$, $p < 0.01$.

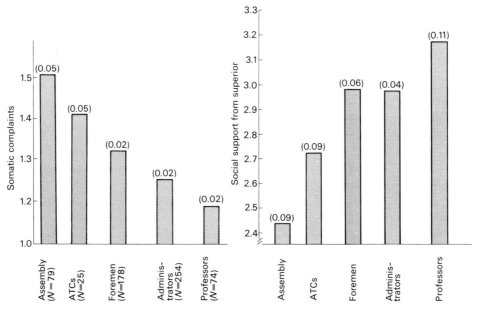

Fig. 4.3. Somatic complaints and social support among five diverse occupational groups. Numbers in parentheses represent the standard error of the mean.

16

differ significantly in their mean levels of somatic complaints. These groups are machine-paced assembly workers, air traffic controllers,[†] blue collar foremen, administrators, and university professors. As you can see, the assembly line workers have the highest level of somatic complaints, followed by air traffic controllers and foremen. Administrators have the next to the lowest of somatic complaints in this group, and university professors seem to have the lowest level of strain of all these groups.

In the right half of the figure these five occupational groups are again presented in the same order. This time the ordinate of the figure represents social support from the immediate superior. Those occupations with the greatest amount of somatic complaints have the lowest support from the supervisor, and vice versa. This finding seems almost ironic. Assembly line workers, who, given the nature of their job, may need all the support they can get, receive very little. On the other hand, university professors who enjoy a large amount of autonomy in their work report that the quality of social support they receive is very good.

These findings are only illustrative. We want to consider the entire array of 23 jobs. Furthermore, the ecological level of analyses leaves unanswered the extent to which the stresses and strains under study will also be related at the individual level. Then too we are concerned with whether our more intensive samples of selected occupations will produce findings which are in line with previous research utilizing national, stratified sampling procedures.

Quality of employment survey

In the first project we specifically sought out high stress jobs. In the second project, a different approach was taken. Here we wanted to know if psychological stress was a factor in health problems across jobs and occupations. Knowing this, would give us more insight into the extent of the problem with which we were dealing. Toward this end we co-sponsored with the Department of Labour's Employment Standards Administration a questionnaire survey which involved a representative national sample of approximately 1500 American workers (Margolis *et al.* 1974). In the survey instrument we included items referencing psychological stress from one's job and aspects of safety and health. Briefly summarizing the results, we found that the correlation between overall job stress and nine of the ten measures used as health and strain indicators were significant. These latter measures listed in descending order of strength of relationship were: job satisfaction, motivation to work, depressed mood, self-esteem, life satisfaction, intention to leave the job, overall physical health, escapist drinking, and absenteeism. The only non-significant strain indicator was frequency of

[†]Mean differences in somatic complaints are non-significant for controllers from high- and low-density airports; their means have been averaged.

suggestions to employer. In general, those who perceived less job stress had fewer health problems. The overall job stress measure had been determined by summing responses connected with six specific job stressors. These were role ambiguity, under-utilization, overload, resource inadequacy, insecurity, and non-participation. One stressor, worker non-participation, appeared to be of special significance, correlating highest among all of the different stressors with eight of the strain measures. This finding would suggest that efforts aimed at job enrichment, participatory management, or humanization of work can be a valuable source of stress reduction.

Data base for psychological job stress

A third project, *Data base for psychological job stress and health,* is aimed at identifying which occupations are actually associated with high levels of psychological stress and resultant health problems. We tend to agree that the air traffic controller's job is one of truly high stress and there is research evidence to verify the health problems coupled with such work. But what of other occupations and jobs?

Hopefully, results from the Data Base project in conjunction with results from the previous two projects will allow us to establish priorities for researching psychologically stressful occupations and enable us to discard the current criterion of the educated guess. Specifically, the Data Base project is the first step in the direction of providing a basis for such a listing by:

(1) Obtaining relevant morbidity data on all major occupations in one state (a major occupation is being operationally defined as one employing more than 1000 workers in that state);

(2) Developing a scheme or rationale for identifying that part of the morbidity data most related to psychological job stress;

(3) Offering a basis for separating health problems related to psychological job stress from health problems predominantly influenced by chemical and physical hazards at the workplace;

(4) Rank-ordering occupations in terms of frequency and severity of health problems associated with psychological job stress.

This project was conducted in the State of Tennessee (Dr. W. Richard, principal investigator). We had chosen that state because of accessibility of data and because the classification of major occupations is representative of the nation as a whole. There are over 200 occupations containing more than 1000 workers each including the categories of professional and technical, managerial, sales, clerical, craftsmen, operatives, service workers, labourers, and farm workers.

SECOND PROGRAMME ASPECT—TO EVALUATE THE NATURE AND EXTENT OF PSYCHOLOGICAL JOB STRESS AND ASSOCIATED HEALTH AND SAFETY PROBLEMS SPECIFIC TO CERTAIN OCCUPATIONAL GROUPS

Preliminary findings do indicate that certain occupations have higher psychological health related problems than other occupations (Colligan *et al.* 1977).

The intent in this programme area is to individually study high stress or accident occupations on an in-depth basis, identifying the stressors therein, and taking measures to present or mitigate their effects. By using this approach we hope to be able to obtain meaningful insights into occupational stress problems that might be overlooked using just the approach taken in the first Programme Aspect. Also, we shall be readily able to tailor our results directly to the specific occupations under study. At this point, two distinct groups are being studied, policemen and underground coal miners, and a follow-up effort to the Data Base study (undertaken under the first Programme Aspect) is planned. Concerning the latter, the two occupations having the highest rate of psychogenic illness will be investigated to identify specific psychological job stress factors and possibilities for stress reduction.

Policemen

As mentioned earlier, an obvious choice of high-stress occupation to study is that of air traffic controller. However, on gathering background data we found several major research efforts aimed at air traffic controllers already underway. Thus, to avoid duplication we began looking for another group to study. The group finally chosen was policemen. This was due to the very 'visible' psychological stress attributes associated with police work, the relatively large size of the work force, and the fact that this occupation is in the 'public eye'.

The first step in the study of policing was to identify the types of psychological job stressors that policemen face. To do this we conducted interviews with 100 patrol car officers from the Cincinnati Police Department (Cincinnati is a city of 500 000 with a police force averaging 1500 officers) (Kroes *et al.* 1974). The police officers were asked (1) to identify conditions that bothered them about their jobs; (2) to comment on a list of specific stressors that several leading police consultants had identified as potentially significant stressors; and (3) to describe an incident (critical incident approach) concerning the last time they felt particularly uncomfortable on the job. The officers were also asked to describe their current health status and effects of their work on their homelife via open-ended questions. The major stressors identified are presented in Table 4.2.

The stress problems of administration, courts, community relations, and equipment seem to be con-

TABLE 4.2

Problems mentioned most frequently by 100 patrol car officers

Category	Definition
Administration	Administration policy and procedures, and administration backing and support of patrol-men.
Courts	Lack of consideration by the courts in scheduling police-men for court appearances, and court leniency to criminals.
Community relations	Public apathy, negative reaction to, and lack of support of policemen.
Equipment	Adequacy and state of repair of equipment.
Changing shift routines	Problems arising around twenty-eight day rotating shift work schedule.
Line of duty/crisis situations	Emergency situations, such as hold-ups or family crises, in which the health and safety of the police officer may be threatened.
Isolation/boredom	Periods of inactivity arising from long spells of quiet and separation from social contacts.

nected by one major thread; all produce a threat to the individual patrolman's self-image and to his sense of *professionalism*.

The remaining stressors (changing shift routines, crisis situations, and isolation/boredom) do not involve a threat to the policeman's sense of professionalism, but are part and parcel of the nature (or at least established culture) of police work. Significantly, as stressful as these appear to be, the patrol car officer accepts them.[†] It is the problem related to the officer's professionalism and self-image that appear to create the greatest stress effect on him.

Given that the police officer is under job stress, we were interested in taking a preliminary look at how he holds up under this stress. That some adjustment must be made to job stress is clear. It is the quality and type of adjustment made that has an effect on the amount and kind of resultant strain. The health data obtained from this study point out that a high proportion of both major and minor health problems are of the kind that have

---

[†]It is significant to note that, despite the fact the police officer is in constant danger of assault, more policemen die annually from suicide than from homocide.

been traditionally considered to be stress related (ulcers, colitis, hypertension, indigestion, and headaches).

It would be desirable to be able to answer the question, 'Does job stress in policemen, indeed, produce a greater health problem than exists for the work force in general?' For a number of reasons, the question cannot be categorically answered by this survey. To begin with, the validity and reliability of self-report health data is often questionable. Therefore, in making comparisons with other groups of workers, the data presented in this study should be considered cautiously.

Indigestion was the most frequently mentioned minor health problem (32 of the 100 officers complained of having it). Until further research is undertaken, the exact causes of the indigestion problem will remain unclear. In all likelihood, however, indigestion arises from either the difficulty of adjusting to the 28-day changing shift routine, and/or the fact that a police officer often has to eat on the run while on duty or completely interrupt his meal because of an emergency situation.

The problem of headaches was the second most frequently mentioned minor health problem. Twenty-four per cent of the officers reported headaches as a health problem. In a 1960–2 nationwide health survey conducted by the American Bureau of Census, approximately 14 per cent of the 3091 males interviewed between the ages of 18 and 79 years reported 'frequent and/or severe headaches' (U.S. National Health Survey 1970). Thus, a significantly greater percentage of patrol car officers indicated that they were bothered by headaches than did the sample selected to represent the United States male population.

It was noted that 22 officers had minor on-duty automobile accidents, i.e., accidents that did not result in an injury to the officer. A surprising number of these accidents (73 accidents for the 22 officers) occurred under non-hazardous conditions, i.e., no chase or high-speed activity involved. Based on recent research into causes of automobile accidents, there is reason to believe that some of the accidents can be attributed to psychological stress (see, for example, Selzer and Vinokur 1973).

Finally, looking at the stress effects on home life, 79 of the 81 married officers indicated that police work negatively affected their home life. Sixteen of the 19 single policemen replied in a similar manner. As an example of some of the problems that occur, I vividly remember the poignant tale of one officer's dilemma whose son had been coming home crying from school. When the officer asked his son what the trouble was, the son replied that the kids teased him in school and said that his father is a pig. As the officer related to us, 'What can I do? I know my son loves me; how can I tell him the kids don't know what they are saying. It eats me up.'

In our study of patrol car officers it became of interest to determine if police administrators and field supervisors experience different stress problems than patrolmen. To answer this question, a separate survey of police administrators was initiated. The results of this survey are as yet unpublished; however, the following are some of our findings. As with the patrol car officers, we found community relations to be a major stressor; also administration, but here the problem arises from higher echelon support of the administrator himself. Many of the problems attributed to administration by the patrol car officers were in fact out of the hands of the administrator and equally frustrating for him. Equipment again appeared as a major stress category but here the major complaint concerned the lack of equipment rather than its condition. Three new categories appeared:

(1) Work overload—more work than could be done in a given period of time;
(2) Work ambiguity—decision-making without sufficient information;
(3) Work conflict—having to please too many bosses.

The stressors discussed above fit under one general phenomenon—the man in the middle. The police administators appears to be caught between his superiors, the community, and other city government officials on the one hand, and his own subordinates on the other. He receives pressure from both ends. Often he must act without sufficient information and is so constricted that his decisions generally please no one.

One additional question asked of the administrators that had not been asked of the patrolmen, was to discuss the last time the administrator felt particularly good in his job. In line with our current view on what motivates a man to work, the two most frequently mentioned positive categories were:

(1) achievement: incidents in which the administrator and his subordinates had done a good job;
(2) recognition: incidents in which the administrator received a compliment or encouragement either from the public or his superior officer.

Are the police really unique in the types of stressors they must undergo? At this point, the intuitive answer would be yes. The policeman, to a large segment of our society, is subject to negative reaction. It is one of the few occupations that carries a stigma affecting the worker's family. Policing is also one of the few occupations where the worker is asked to lay his life on the line for the community and at the same time finds open opposition from members of the same community. The additional pressures arising out of these factors may not have a major direct impact, but it is probable that they do serve to reduce the tolerance for handling the many other stressors associated with police work.

A third study of police, now being completed, has looked at the differential effects of environmental conditions on job stress in policemen. The primary question to be answered by the study is whether police officers working in a transitional socio-economic high crime rate community experience greater psychological job stress (poorer person–environment fit) and thus more health-strain consequences than those working in an affluent low crime rate area. Answering this question

TABLE 4.3

List of areas covered in major police study

Section 1—general job stress and health		Section 2—police specific stress	
Stress	*Strain*	*Stress*	*Strain*
Role conflict	Depression–Anxiety	Courts	Effects on home life
Responsibility for others	Company satisfaction	Administration	Car accidents on duty
Responsibility for equip-	Job satisfaction	Community relations	Stress-coping techniques
ment, budget, projects	Work alienation	Equipment	Training
Workload	Boredom	'Professionalism'	Effects on personality
Utilization	Self-esteem	Line of duty—use of force	Effects on work performance
Role ambiguity		Physical dangers	
Future ambiguity		Crisis situations	
Workhour satisfaction and	*Demographic*	Minority group pressure	
interference		Communication	
Equity	Age	Shift work	
Nonparticipation	Education	Lack of training	
Resource inadequacy	Tenure		
	Work hours		
	Income level		
Health	Social support		
Psychological stress			
symptoms	*Personality*		
Health status			
Smoking	Internal–external control		
Drinking	Type A coronary prone personality		
	Dogmatism		

will hopefully allow us to focus more clearly on the causes of stress for policemen.

These studies are offering some background to a major study of policemen now in progress. Here we will look at police job stress and also take a much closer look at the health consequences in a larger study sample of police departments across the country. The plan is to do an in-depth study of police departments in one major geographic region (the West coast of the United States) and spot sample police departments in five other regions. The sample will be stratified according to type of police force and community (i.e., urban, surburban, and rural police departments). A summary of the factors to be covered in the questionnaire to be administered to policemen and administrators in the various police departments is presented in Table 4.3. The first factor area will be surveyed via the General Job Stress and Health Questionnaire which was designed and tested so that it is applicable to any occupational group.

Underground coal miners
To learn more of miners' attitudes toward utilization of established health and safety procedures, our staff is conducting a survey of miners in 15 high accident and 15 matched low accident mine sites. Two thousand of these miners were asked to fill out the General Job Stress and Health Questionnaire (see section 1 of Table 4.3). Another 1500 interviews of underground miners, foremen, higher management, surface mining personnel,

union stewards, and miner's wives will be undertaken to identify psychological variables which enhance or impede coal miner health and safety consciousness. I can think of no occupational group which is more worthy of our attention from a stress, accident, and disease point of view than the underground coal miner. Coal mining is annually the highest accident industry in America in terms of both frequency and severity of accidents. In terms of health consequences, in the past, 15 to 18 per cent of all miners developed pneumoconiosis (black lung) to some degree before leaving the mining industry. Approximately one-third of these individuals were severely disabled. In addition, underground miners evidence high rates of other health problems such as emphysema. New dust control measures should bring the black lung statistics down to 10 per cent but coal mining by any measure will still be a hazardous occupation. Interestingly, the Federal Coal Mine Health and Safety Act of 1969 provides that the coal miner who shows evidence of development of pneumoconiosis has the option to change to a less dusty job at his place of employment. Despite this provision, the number of eligible coal miners actually switching to a less dusty job environment has been relatively low (about 10 per cent of those eligible). Fears of being blackballed by management or losing high levels of pay, among other reasons, may contribute to the miner's decision not to take advantage of his legal option.

Despite the potentially dire consequences to his health

and safety, the underground miner works on. Some researchers label this 'fatalism'. For a number of reasons, I strongly question this view. For one, it appears that the miners have few other job alternatives. Secondly, is the coal miner so atypical? As the term is defined, aren't we all fatalistic? We know it's unsafe to drive a car and car accident statistics are alarmingly high; yet most of us drive anyway. Are we any less fatalistic than the coal miner who works underground knowing that the accident statistics in mining are high? Lastly, in emergency situations miners act quite cool-headedly and display no so-called 'fatalistic behaviour'.

THIRD PROGRAMME ASPECT—
(1) TO DETERMINE THE IMPORTANCE OF JOB STRESS IN THE AETIOLOGY OF MAJOR HEALTH PROBLEMS AND
(2) TO CONDUCT IN-DEPTH ANALYSIS OF INDIVIDUAL JOB STRESSORS WHICH MAY HAVE SIGNIFICANT HEALTH IMPACT

Stress and coronary heart disease

The first project in this area will look at the relationship between psychological job stress and coronary heart disease. In the United States, cardiovascular disease alone accounts for about 50 per cent of all deaths each year. Coronary heart disease (CHD), the most serious problem, accounts for about one-half of those deaths due to cardiovascular disease. The danger from heart disease is particularly acute among males of working age for whom CHD is the leading cause of death from age 35 on. The direct economic cost to the nation of cardiovascular disease (in terms of medical care and losses of output from members of the labour force) was estimated at $32 billion in 1963 by the President's Commission on Heart Disease, Cancer, and Stroke (Moriyama et al. 1971). This is not to mention the family, community, organizational, and even societal distruption that results from sudden coronary death or disability. To the extent that occupational factors are implicated in its aetiology, coronary disease constitutes perhaps the major occupational health problem. In fact, research over the last 10–15 years has increasingly demonstrated a clear association between psychological job stress and coronary heart disease and its risk factors such as high blood pressure, high cholesterol levels, and heavy smoking (for an excellent review, see House 1974).

However, almost all prior research on psychological job stress and CHD has been cross-sectional or retrospective in design, and therefore fails to address certain key questions. First, is the issue of causality. Although we know there is an association between psychological job stress and CHD, or CHD risk, and although it may be most plausible to assume that stress causes CHD or CHD risk rather than vice versa, only longitudinal research can demonstrate that psychological job stress precedes and potentiates CHD risk and CHD. Many medical and business people will not seriously contemplate new ways of preventing CHD by reducing stress unless such longitudinal evidence is presented.

Second, stress researchers now recognize that stress results from the *interaction* between an individual and a work environment over time. That is, not all people will experience a given job as stressful, nor will a given individual experience all jobs as equally stressful. Rather, stress occurs when the needs and abilities of the person are incongruent with the demands and opportunities of the job environment, i.e., when there is a poor fit between the person and his working environment. The degree of stress experienced is not, however, invariant over time, but changes as the work environment and/or as the person changes. This understanding of the nature of stress emphasizes that psychological job stress can be reduced *only* by (1) preventing the occurrence of bad fits between individuals and jobs or (2) re-establishing a 'good fit' where a bad one exists. This means studying how people get into and get out of stressful jobs or how changes by the organization and/or the person can reduce the amount of stress experienced. These are topics which can be adequately researched only in longitudinal studies. Thus, the major purpose of this research project is to examine how psychologically stressful job situations may affect coronary heart disease risk over time, and to determine how variations in perceived levels of job stress may induce changes in CHD risk. Also to be considered in the context of this research are worker selection and adjustment factors which may moderate or enhance the impact of job stress on CHD risk.

The focus of this project[†] will be three potentially psychologically stressful and CHD-inducing jobs within a single organization. A minimum sample of 400 persons comprised of recent incumbents to the focal stress jobs, persons eligible to accede to the focal job (i.e., the pool from which future incumbents are likely to be drawn), and a subsample of individuals drawn from this second group which the company has identified as most likely to accede to the focal job. All 400 workers will be assessed via questionnaire and physiological testing initially on CHD risk factors and psychological stress variables. At least 200 of these subjects will then be retested at 5-month intervals over a 20 month period. Another 20 workers will be physiologically tested at more frequent intervals. Measurement requirements for assessing coronary heart disease risk factors will include: pulse rate, blood pressure, cholesterol level, smoking behaviour, and blood sugar.

The study population will be drawn from workers in a large company within the aerospace industry employing approximately 20 000 workers, about half of which are professional employees. The three job types to be studied are middle management, liaison engineers, and financial analysts. The middle management personnel

†Principal investigators on this project are Dr. J. Chadwick, Stanford Research Institute; Dr. P. Insel, Stanford University; Dr. R. Rosenmann, Mt. Zion Hospital, and Dr. G. Sevelius from Lockheed Missiles and Space Company.

will be group leaders and supervisors drawn from the Advanced Systems and New Business Group of the subject company. These people experience severe deadline pressures in addition to working in a highly competitive environment. Liaison engineers face the stress of having to work in alien territory (sometimes called crossing organizational boundaries), i.e., co-ordinating between manufacturing and engineering design. Further, they experience high role conflict as they, in effect, must take directions from two different supervisors. The third job type, financial analysts, experience quantitative work overload as well as working in a very formal, rigid organizational environment.

Shift work and stress

A second project in this area, in progress, is examining the stress effects of shift work. Shift work has been a part of industrial life for many years and social and technological trends suggest that it will become increasingly more important in our industrial society in the future. However, there is relatively little knowledge concerning the biological, psychological, and social consequences of shift work. The research that does exist is somewhat fragmentary, often contradictory, and largely atheoretic in nature. It would seem imperative that in order to make the most efficient and beneficial use of our human and industrial resources we examine shift work more thoroughly.

The roots of some of the problems of shift work appear to lie in man's circadian cycle of rest and activity. The human adult through evolution and acculturation has become attuned to a cycle of activity during the hours of daylight and sleep during those of darkness. When the cycle is reversed, the body seems to perform both processes less efficiently. There are at least 50 bodily processes that follow a rhythm (though not necessarily a circadian one). Circadian rhythms are seen in the fluctuation of body temperature, urine flow, renal excretion of sodium, potassium, and phosphates, and cognitive functioning. Though there are demonstrated effects of shift work in altering these rhythmic activities, it is unclear at this time whether these altered activities cause significant physical or mental health problems.

The few studies reported to date have been limited in scope (see Chapter 13 for an excellent review of shift work research). While concentrating on certain, admittedly important effects such as loss in productivity, sleep problems, and ulcer rates, they have neglected other factors which could have a bearing on whether persons can effectively cope with shift work problems. The latter include such factors as self-selection of shift workers, influence of psychological adjustment problems, lack of community facilities for late shift workers, influence of environmental noise on day time sleep, etc. It is the purpose of this planned project to take account of all such factors in a more comprehensive evaluation of shift work.

FOURTH PROGRAMME ASPECT— TO FOSTER PRACTICES THAT WILL EITHER REDUCE JOB STRESS OR IMPROVE AN INDIVIDUAL WORKER'S ADJUSTMENT TO IT

Included here will be efforts aimed at evaluating the relative effectiveness of various stress-reduction techniques (such as sensitivity training, job redesign, transactional analysis, and other organizational development techniques that seem applicable). Once this is accomplished, demonstration programmes will be developed for the more promising techniques. Because we felt it would be best to first learn more of the nature and extent of job stress problems before we tackled possible remedies we have delayed institution of projects in this area.

FIFTH PROGRAMME ASPECT—TO STUDY THE IMPACT OF PSYCHOLOGICAL JOB STRESS ON SAFETY

Questions on accidents in the questionnaire form used in the Survey of Working Conditions study discussed in the first programme aspect yielded an interesting result. Individuals categorized as belonging to a high job stress group reported twice as many work-related accidents as those in low stress group. The implication of these results is that psychological stress arising from the job may increase the likelihood of having an accident. The mechanisms by which this might take place can be quite varied. For example, preoccupation with some stressful situation may lead to lack of attention to the task at hand, or increased use of drugs or alcohol to escape stressful situations may lead to decreased efficiency, etc.

This thought is deserving of further study. We hope in the near future to research aspects of life stress as well as job stress factors in relation to work accidents.

CONCLUSION

With the discussion of the stress and safety area, I bring to a close this presentation of our programmatic attempts to understand, define, and hopefully bring some measure of relief from psychological stress to the American work force.† In reviewing our activities of the past three years, I am aware of the slow course of events. Understandably there is always a time lag between project inception and final product output. We hope the optimistic goals we set for ourselves in the beginning will be realized in the not too distant future. As the findings from each project come forth and become integrated with the results from the other projects within a programme aspect, we will gain some closure on that programme aspect. And by combining the knowledge obtained in each programme aspect, we should establish a solid base from which we hopefully can have an impact on industry, and be able to do some good for the worker who has and will suffer the many inconveniences of our research intrusions.

SUMMARY

The National Institute for Occupational Safety and Health has initiated a programme seeking to identify the impact of psychological job stress on workers' health and safety, and of fostering practices which will either reduce job stress or improve worker adjustment to it. As presently conceived, the programme consists of five distinct aspects which are elaborated in this paper. These are: (1) to establish the nature, prevalence, and severity of psychological job stess; (2) to evaluate job stress and associated health problems specific to certain occupational groups; (3) to determine the importance of job stress in the aetiology of major health problems and to study individual job stressors which may have significant health impact; (4) to develop practices to alleviate job stress; and (5) to study the impact of job stresses on safety.

†One may note the absence of projects on alcoholism and drug abuse in industry. We view these as strain consequences resulting from stress (job or otherwise) and feel that it is best, at least initially, to try to get at the stress or causal factors. Further, there is a National Institute for Alcoholism and Alcohol Abuse, which we hope is beginning to make some in-roads here.

REFERENCES

COBB, S. and ROSE, R. (1973). Hypertension, peptic ulcer, and diabetes in air traffic controllers. *J. Am. med. Assoc.*, **224** (4), 489–91.

COLLIGAN, M., SMITH, M., and HURRELL, J. (1977). Occupational incident rates of mental health disorders. *J. Human Stress*, **33** (3), 34–9.

FRENCH, J. R. P., Jr., COBB, S., CAPLAN, R. D., VAN HARRISON, R., and PINNEAU, R. Unpublished work.

HOUSE, J. S. (1974). The effects of occupational stress on physical health. In *Work and the quality of life* (ed. J. O'Toole). M.I.T. Press, Cambridge, Massachusetts.

KROES, W. (1976). *Society's Victim—the policeman: an analysis of job stress in policing*. C. C. Thomas, Springfield, Illinois.

KROES, W., MARGOLIS, B., and HURRELL, J. (1974). Job stress in policemen. *J. Police Sci. Admin.*, **2** (2), 145–55.

MARGOLIS, B., KROES, W., and QUINN, R. (1974). Job stress: an unlisted occupational hazard. *J. Occup. Med.*, **16** (10), 659–61.

MORIYAMA, I., DROEVEI, D., and STANBE, Jr. (1971). *Cardiovascular disease in the United States*. Harvard University Press, Cambridge, Massachusetts.

QUINN, R. P., SEASHORE, S., KAHN, R. L., MANGIONE, T., CAMPBELL, D., STAINES, G. L., McCULLOUGH, M., OLIKER, N., and SHULMAN, N. (1971). *Survey of working conditions*. U.S. Department of Labor.

SELZER, M. and VINOKUR, A. (1973). Life events, subjective stress and accidents. (Paper presented at the 126th Annual Meeting of the American Psychiatric Association, Honolulu, Hawaii.)

U.S. National Health Survey (1970). *Selected symptoms of psychological stress*. Publication No. 1000, Series 11 (37). Public Health Service.

5. PSYCHOSOCIAL STRESSORS IN THE WORK ENVIRONMENT AND IN NON-WORK SETTINGS: MANAGEMENT'S VIEWPOINTS

NILS MASRELIEZ

Problems of the work environment have been a subject of growing attention in recent years. There are many reasons for this. Increased understanding of the influence of various agents on the human organism allows more possibility of control and safer guidance of preventive work. Changing values have brought with them a desire for self-fulfilment in the working population of today. Satisfaction and security have become more and more prominent. However, it will be found that in the debate on the influence of stress on the individual, the role of the working environment has in fact been emphasized rather one-sidedly, while factors outside work have been neglected. Naturally, it is important that problems of the working environment itself should be debated and scrutinized so that it may be gradually improved. But it seems to me as important to pinpoint various social problems, which may also influence the working capacity and adaptability of the individual, and to try to come to grips with them.

The reaction pattern of the human organism to various stressors is rather stereotyped. Physical as well as mental strain results in symptoms of a relatively uniform kind, regardless of whether the strain emanates from the working environment or from factors outside it. The individual is often incapable of appreciating these origins and of separating them.

STRESSORS OUTSIDE THE WORK SITUATION

Many factors outside work act as stressors. Increasingly rapid urbanization produces rootlessness and loss of identity. Problems of isolation are experienced by single mothers. Immigrants have language difficulties. The double role of mothers who go out to work often produces stress, as do housing problems involving long journeys between home and work or housing problems of shift workers. Rapid changes in socio-political development cause the citizen to feel alienation, insecurity, and impotence. The distance between the citizen and the decision-makers is often felt to be very great.

OCCUPATIONAL STRESSORS

Physical factors

For a few decades now increasing attention has been devoted to the physical environment, and the need for systematic analysis and supervision is becoming increasingly clear to those who wish to achieve optimum working conditions. The occupational health service plays a key role here. The aims of this service are primarily preventative, and it provides a set of guidelines for new offices and factories to be followed at the planning stage. It also carries out inspections of existing places of work and lists potential hazards. The service is completed by a medical assessment of the standard of health among the workers and a survey of how the workers themselves feel about their working conditions. It should be stressed that ideally all three of these methods should be employed.

Psychosocial factors

As regards the psychosocial working environment, this is considerably harder to map. Quite generally, we may say that our methods of measurement are still unreliable and that our knowledge is limited concerning such things as the interplay of different environmental factors. The complexity of the working situation makes it all but impossible to seek a connection between a single factor and its results. If you add to that the experience of the individual outside working hours, the picture becomes even more obscure. The value of experiments where a specific factor is singled out and the reaction of the organism studied is dubious. However, we agreed today that work should contain certain qualities, as self-evident as they are fundamental and which certainly require no research to confirm them.

Job satisfaction

The concept of job satisfaction could, of course, be made a heading for how the individual experiences his total work situation. Seen in a more restricted context it is one of the keystones of good adaptability at work: making the worker sense that his work is meaningful—that what he achieves is useful and essential. We want influence, want to be able to affect our work situation, but at the same time we want others to take an interest in it. As a group we want our own area of responsibility, but at the same time we want to have stimulating contacts and an interplay with other parts of the enterprise and with the surrounding world. We want to develop ourselves and we want to be able to believe in the future and to have a feeling of security when facing it. Since we are different, we have to try to adapt the working task and the concrete manner in which the job is to be done to the physical emotional and psychological qualifications of the individual. In each situation you must work on a number of basic assumptions. Some of them are general—others more concrete. The chance of success depends on knowledge, will, but also on economic resources.

We know that our defence mechanisms against stress are often well adapted to their purpose, and furthermore necessary. Symptoms of ill health can arise only if the influence of stress is too strong, too weak, or wrongly directed. A suitable amount of stress can be positive and stimulating and may increase capacity.

Discrepancy between job demands and the capacity of the worker

What we refer to, generally speaking, as stress at work arises from an imbalance between job requirements and the capacity of the individual. This usually manifests itself in the form of lowered productivity, qualitatively or quantitatively, most often both. At the work place the turnover of staff increases, new employees must be trained, the percentage of rejects increases, and the volume produced goes down. The person under pressure fails and begins to be absent from work, a few days at a time to begin with, and gradually, when manifest illness has become a fact, for longer periods; a sickness develops which may lead to permanent disability and early retirement pension. Those hit most frequently are middle-aged or elderly people with scant margins for mental strain.

Preventive action

What factors may then be considered to be serious environmental risks from the point of view of psycho-socially induced stress and what can be done to prevent them? Let us note here that activities aimed at improving both physical and mental environments are of mutual interest to all parties at the place of work. We must be certain that our efforts to improve the environment achieve the intended results without any unwelcome side-effects. Before taking action we must pose the question to ourselves: is this what is most urgent?

I shall not attempt to list all conceivable stressors at work; I shall try, however, to indicate some examples and various attempts to come to grips with them.

Communication at work

Exchange of information or communication enters into all co-operation between people. In an enterprise where many human beings are to co-operate, information is necessary. Management defines the goals set and the activity and sees to it that the relevant information reaches everyone in the enterprise, not just the top-level ranks. In the intermediate ranks the managers inform their workers of the conditions and content of the work. If you take pains to define the goals set to the employees and to specify the distribution of the roles, this creates clarity and increases the freedom of movement of the individual groups. If you intend to carry through a change of production in an enterprise or to effect a reorganization, this should be preceded by adequate information at the right time—information which features the main points without unimportant

details that may clutter up the overall view. In working life, important information systems, moving upwards as well as downwards, have been established in recent years. Consultation and reference groups are often brought in to discuss the complex of problems before the taking of important decisions. Today we consider it quite natural that management should keep themselves informed of the decisions and views of the employees. An example: Acting on a proposal from the employees concerning the length of meal breaks, the enterprise takes the trouble to send out a questionnaire so that the matter can be discussed with the employees on the basis of the results. A leading personnel officer in Swedish industry recently stated that 'nowadays at least half my working hours are spent in informing various groups within the enterprise of planned measures and in gathering information from the employees before a decision is made'. Thus information should be bilateral, sufficiently enlightening, and occur so early that the problems of adjustment are still 'impersonal'.

Feedback

But the individual has a constant need to know what his position is: stress in this case is often not having too much to do, but not knowing if what one does is sufficient. Have I accomplished the task? Do I meet the requirements of management? If the only information received from management is in the form of a salary slip, this is often felt as frustrating. Not knowing whether you are appreciated causes an uncertainty of conduct and provides further ground for the negative assessment of the manager. It is therefore essential to induce managers to give continuous information on the position. In certain cases this may mean negative information. A good management will recommend the employee for a more suitable occupation if the percentage of unsatisfactory work has grown too high.

Repetitive tasks; piece wages

Are repetitive tasks with short cycles always stressful? The contact opportunities of the individual are no doubt highly important in this connection. In the 'small environment' the punching machine operator finds it easier to evaluate her results and the appreciation she gets, if any. In larger contexts this immediately becomes more difficult.

Is piecework as a wage system a stress factor? No one can possibly deny that piecework has a built-in incentive towards higher performance. Against the background of what has been said above, piecework might then also be part of the required and useful stimulus we are looking for in our work, especially in such tasks which do not themselves offer many interesting aspects. However, this positive effect may be transformed into a harmful strain.

To young and healthy persons, a hectic job situation may be handled without any grave injuries, at least on a short-term basis. For middle-aged and elderly persons with scant margins, it probably entails a certain health hazard. It may be mentioned here that an investigation made by the Swedish Employers' Confederation at 36 enterprises which had switched from piecework rates to fixed wages indicated that neither absenteeism owing to illness nor the turnover of staff showed any changes in this connection. But the complaints which are made against piecework rates as inducing stress may depend on the rates often being fixed unevenly. Thus for instance you may work for 2 hours at a favourable rate and thereafter for 5 hours at an unfavourable one. The unevenness of the rates causes work to lag behind, for which it will be found desirable to compensate. This creates irritation in the employee. The same applies when you have got a much less favourable rate than your comrade at work! It is by no means easy to solve this problem. The parties should jointly aim at achieving secure and just wage systems which at the same time favour production. Stagnation or decline in this respect should be incompatible with the aims of the majority in our country.

Assembly-lines

Technical systems, which chain the individual effort to a certain task and a certain work pace, are found by the majority to be trying. Examples will be found on the assembly-line, at presses, etc. 'I have to do my share' or else the process is stopped. The machine chains the individual to itself. In order to break up this situation the simple measures of creating buffers and stores have been taken. The stores feed the machine and enable the individual to leave it for a while. Or if two machines depend on each other, a buffer can be built up between them: a number of items are stored as a buffer. Both these methods have been tried several times in industry and constitute examples of how a bind can be broken, when the machine is the guiding factor.

Industrial robots

Another solution has been found in the so-called industrial robot, especially useful for restricted series with variations in the assortment. In 1974 robots, which can be programmed, number about 200 in Swedish industry. The prognosis is that there will be about 10 times as many in 1980. These robot systems are probably capable of being highly developed, for instance by combining them with optical reading capability. Thus the industrial robot performs physically heavy and psychologically difficult work while man, standing by, has only to control the system.

Mass production systems

Let us take another example, car manufacturing. Here enormous volumes of material have to flow through. Activities must therefore be mechanized. In all countries, regardless of their political system, a similar work organization is applied: a store is created where the car is built along an assembly-line. The technique means that parts are gradually added and at the end station all parts have found their proper places. At each station must efficient

auxiliary methods can be devised. This is economy. The worker's role in such a system becomes highly specialized and governed to an extreme degree by the assembly-line. This is what all car factories look like all over the world. We know that a human being can feel strained by this type of work organization. If you have been allowed one minute, then the task must be performed within one minute. How then can the constraint be reduced? This was already discussed in the 1950s. Thus for instance you can run two parallel lines, which doubles the length of the work cycle. This would, however, require much more space, a larger storage capacity, etc. However, something must be done to overcome the constraint. Otherwise recruiting difficulties will put an end to all further production.

New approaches to production problems

Within the Swedish car industry a different kind of material handling system and a different kind of car factory have developed. Saab–Scania car engines are now fitted in a new factory in which the assembly-line has been replaced by small wagons. These wagons move around an endless trail and can be shunted into work places where working groups receive and fit the entire car engine. They do it at their own pace and according to their own pattern of work.

At Volvo, a whole new factory has been erected for the assembly of entire cars. Here, too, the assembly-line has been abandoned. The system relies on automobile assembly wagons and working groups are each responsible for a large part of the assembly work, the entire electric system of the car for instance. Also here the groups work at their own pace and according to their own pattern of work. It may be mentioned that development work for the assembly wagon alone has cost several million kronor. This new technique has attracted attention from all over the world and will probably change the working methods of car factories.

Small groups of workers

In the same factory there is another environmental factor which has been considered. It is generally known that the individual feels more at ease in a small group than in a large one. The larger the factory hall, the more desolate it seems, and this reduces the feeling of security in the minds of the employees. This was taken into account when the factory was built. The material is placed at the centre and the people are placed all around in the various angles of the house structure. In this way, it is felt that the better psychological climate of the small factory unit has been combined with the requirements for economic material processing met by the large unit.

In our efforts to ameliorate both the physical and the psychological climate at our work places it is important that we should not lower the requirements set on the employee to a level where the primary risk the employee runs is that of falling asleep. At this type of work place job rotation is therefore applicable.

CONCLUSIONS

Thus we may state today that enterprises, especially the larger ones with better resources, are at great pains to improve the physical environment. This is also to some extent applicable to the psychosocial environment, although here certain doubts over suitable approaches have restricted development. More reliable rules of thumb are also required for the psychological ergonomics. Rules of thumb which are fairly generally applicable would considerably enhance our possibilities of creating safe and secure work places.

6. STRESS AND DISEASE AT WORK FROM THE VIEWPOINT OF A CONFEDERATION OF TRADE UNIONS

ERIK BOLINDER

TECHNOLOGICAL DEVELOPMENT AND ECONOMIC GROWTH

The creation of the welfare state has largely been made possible by the technological advances of the past twenty years. Structural change and improved efficiency in trade and industry have formed the basis for the economic growth that has made it possible to build up national prosperity. The trade union movement has accepted this process of rationalization on the whole, a process which has given us the means of improving the economic and social situation of the wage earners. The economic conditions created by the process of industrial change have also been used to build up a society that guarantees its citizens economic and social security, at the same time as we have been striving to narrow the economic, social, and cultural gulfs that divide different groups in society.

We can distinguish two distinct phases in trade union activities during this process. Up to the 1960s, the trade unions concentrated mainly on improving the economic and social situation of their members by obtaining better wages, fairer principles of income distribution, shorter working hours, increased job security, etc.

Changing priorities

Then in the 1960s, people began to take a new and more sceptical view of some negative consequences of development that were becoming increasingly obvious and alarming. As economic, social, and cultural standards rose very rapidly owing to the industrialization process, new values and new demands began to emerge. A new type of human being was making his voice heard in a democratic society where the individual's opportunities for self-expression, critical analysis, influence on his own situation, freedom of choice, etc. were regarded as vitally important. Greatly expanded education open in principle, to everybody, new technological advances in the field of communications, and so on, also offered hitherto unknown vistas and an opportunity for making comparisons.

All these trends in society combined to create a new view of the conditions of working life, and there was a growing realization of the discrepancies between the values that governed the development of society and those that determined development in trade and industry. People started questioning the ability of society to shoulder responsibility for the consequences to human beings of an economy that was rather one-sidedly governed by purely economic and tecnological con-

siderations. People increasingly questioned the values underlying discussions on economic growth and the measurement of well-being. They started to insist that other environmental and social aspects should be taken into account when making the assessments on which future planning of industry and society were based. The outcome was that from the beginning of the 1960s, questions like job security, environment, and democracy on the job became top priority issues in the trade union movement in Sweden.

As this volume is primarily concerned with questions of the psychosocial conditions in working life, it is fitting to give an account of some investigations carried out in the 1960s and 1970s by the Swedish Trade Union Confederation. The aim of these investigations was to identify the consequences for our members of the developments I have mentioned. All of them are linked to the kind of conditions that ultimately determine whether the employee can enjoy physical, mental, and social well-being and function well at work.

NEW TECHNOLOGIES: CONSEQUENCES FOR THE LABOUR FORCE

The Swedish Trade Union Confederation (1966) presented a study called *The trade unions and technological change*, which presented points of view on the consequences for the labour force of technological development up to that time. It included accounts of a number of enquiries into the situation in various industries, showing how efforts to improve efficiency had entailed radical structural change in practically all areas. New and efficient techniques had resulted in a complete transformation of the structure of certain industries, and meant that a very large number of small companies had been closed down and production concentrated in a few technologically and economically competitive units. The membership of trade unions affected by these changes had been heavily reduced, in some cases by up to 50 per cent. Large groups of members had been forced to take new jobs in their branch of industry or to transfer to other trades, and this had often meant their having to move to another part of the country.

In some industries, forestry for example, the entire occupational structure was changed. New techniques and new production methods demanded a quite new type of worker. The old type of worker had become more or less redundant in a short space of time. A new kind of manpower was needed—well-trained and with specialized skills.

Other studies showed how improvement in efficiency forces industry to adopt new work methods and a new work organization, so that many of the old, freer types of work disappear to be superseded, on the one hand, by high-speed work at the assembly line, and, on the other, by highly specialized work operations demanding training, special skills, etc. This means that jobs for older workers or partially handicapped workers with little training tend to disappear. Figures illustrating the structural change that is taking place are given in Table 6.1. The most striking feature in Table 6.1 is the rapid reduction—typical of the industrialized countries—in the number employed in agriculture and fishing and the dynamic expansion of the service sector, particularly public services, where education, social welfare, and health services are the main areas demanding more and more manpower. But even in the apparently stable sectors, considerable changes are taking place in the structure of industries and companies.

Company closures; urbanization; migration
Another feature characteristic of this structural change is the increase in company closures. Fig. 6.1 shows the growing number of advance notices to the labour market authorities of companies closing down and of production cut-backs in the 1960s and Fig. 6.2 shows the number of employees affected by these notices.

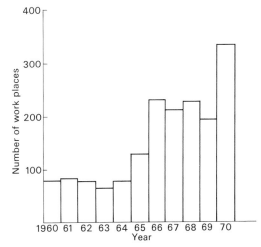

FIG. 6.1. Advance notices of company closures 1960–70, in terms of work places. (Labour Market Board).

In the wake of rationalization comes urbanization. The population is concentrated in larger and more densely populated areas. Table 6.2 shows some regional differences between regions of varying size. Table 6.2 indicates that net immigration, average income, vacancies per unemployed, and participation rate vary greatly from one size of region to another. Sparsely populated regions have a high rate of removals, low average income, few vacancies, and a low participation

TABLE 6.1

Percentage distribution of Swedish manpower by sector, 1950–75 (from Ministry of Finance 1966, 1976)

	1950	1960	1965	1970	1975
Agriculture, forestry, and fishing	20	17	12	9	6
Industry and crafts	32	30	31	30	27
Construction and power stations	9	9	10	10	10
Commerce, transport, and private services	29	31	31	31	32
Public services	10	12	15	20	24

TABLE 6.2

Regional difference in employment and income (from Swedish Government Official Reports 1970)

Regions in order of population base (population in thousands)	Average domestic net immigration 1961–5 (per cent)	Average income per employee 1967 (kronor)	No. of vacancies in relation to number of unemployed 1965 (per cent)	No. of employed per 100 inhabitants 1.11.1965
29–59	−7·0	19 275	1·04	41·4
60–95	−4·0	19 379	1·15	41·4
96–132	−1·4	19 666	2·04	42·6
133–184	+0·4	20 570	1·92	43·8
Göteborg/ Malmö/Lund Hälsingborg/ Landskrona	+6·8	23 751	4·55	45·9
Stockholm/ Södertälje	+6·9	26 681	6·67	47·6

rate. This gives a good picture of both the reasons for, and the effects of, migration. Those who remain in these regions are the older unskilled workers with low incomes; the young people move out in order to get work and make use of their training.

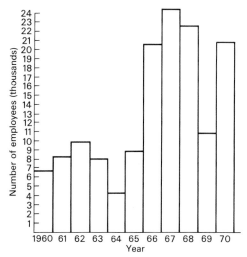

Fig. 6.2. Number of employees affected by notices of closures and production cut-backs, 1960–70 (Labour Market Board).

In this industrial phase, consequences have been negative particularly for certain groups of workers who for various reasons cannot cope with the more specific and harsher requirements of modern working life. Working life has become more and more marked by a process of elimination that has made growing demands on society. To meet these demands increasing efforts are being made within the framework of the national labour market policy, including various kinds of rehabilitation measures for people who find it difficult to get work as well as measures to create new employment opportunities.

UNEMPLOYMENT: FORCED WORK CHANGES

Some idea of the consequences which rationalization and structural change in industry and trade have on people can be obtained from an investigation carried out in connection with the regular manpower studies done by government authorities. These manpower studies are based on a random sample large enough to enable findings to be adjusted upwards to the level of total population. The investigation mentioned here was carried out in May 1972. A summary of some of its findings is given in Table 6.3. In the first three columns we can see the effects of rationalization and structural change on those who were in the labour force at this time and were thus still active job-seekers. On the one-hand, there are those who were unemployed, wanting but unable to get jobs; on the other, people who were engaged in some kind of

TABLE 6.3

Persons who have left—or whose situation had deteriorated on—the open labour market. Analysis by primary reason and by sex. Percentages

	Workers in sheltered employment		Unemployed		Persons in labour market training		Persons outside the labour force		Persons forced to change to work with less pay		Weighted average and total
	Men	Women	Men	Women	Men	Women	Men	Women	Men	Women	
Company closed down	7	21	7	11	2	10	15	13	10	14	11
Production cut-backs	14	5	28	17	7	10	7	4	20	10	12
Reorganization	14	16	4	13	9	10	5	6	11	13	9
Injury at work	12	5	4	4	9	11	1	0	5	5	4
Other injury or illness	17	32	7	9	28	30	38	16	13	10	15
Other	36	21	50	46	45	29	44	61	41	48	49
Total	100	100	100	100	100	100	100	100	100	100	100
Total in absolute figures (thousands)	21·0	7·3	41·5	28·3	15·7	3·5	29·3	144·5	96·0	54·85	442·0

manpower rehabilitation activity arranged by public authorities: sheltered employment, public training, or education schemes for improving workers' competitiveness on the labour market. Table 6.3 illustrates how much efficiency improvement has affected the situation of these people.

The same applies to the group that is outside the labour force. The main element in this latter group consists of young women who have withdrawn from the labour market on account of having small children. Otherwise there are many, particularly among the 30 000 or so men, who have gone through all the stages of failure and hopelessness until they have at last given up the struggle.

It should be observed that these figures do not include any of those who have been granted advance retirement pensions. It is particularly interesting to look more closely at those who have received advance pensions during recent years, as we have adopted new rules in Sweden whereby the employment situation is considered of great importance relative to medical indications. Estimates have been made that, in May 1972, 100 000 people drawing advance pensions had been working after 1960. We can assume that most of these had chosen this alternative because their possibilities of getting work had been considered negligible.

The last column but one in Table 6.3 gives figures on those who reported that at some time during the preceding five years they had been forced to change work and take a job with poorer pay. It appears that about 150 000 people were faced with this situation, and this problem is closely associated with the above-mentioned processes of efficiency improvement and structural change.

Lack of security and power

In my opinion, this investigation illustrates the lack of security and the powerlessness people experience in industrial development, where the rapid and dramatic changes entail consequences that cut deep into a man's way of life and where all he can do is passively to submit to the adjustments that development requires of him. Many groups of people who are not equipped with the qualities required by this process of readjustment cannot cope with their personal situation on their own, but need the help of society. But the resources of society also tend to be overstrained. Many people have to stay in some kind of sheltered activity arranged by the community and can never, no matter what is done, compete successfully for jobs on the labour market.

Some idea of this is given in Table 6.4, which shows the total number of job-finding measures, divided between work on the open market and in sheltered employment, during the period 1951–67 for people who have received rehabilitation training. Table 6.4 shows how it has become increasingly difficult over the years to find work for these people on the open labour market, while the risk of having to remain in public sheltered employment increases.

I should now like to discuss the consequences of efficiency improvement and structural change on the work environment, seen from the physical and psycho-social standpoints. Once again, I shall base the discussion on investigations carried out within the Swedish Trade Union Confederation.

SURVEYS OF WORKER OPINIONS ON WORK CONDITIONS

The purpose of these investigations was to find out the opinions of our members on certain specific questions. The findings thus reflect opinions rather more than facts.

In both cases the method used was a postal questionnaire sent to a selection of Confederation members. Questionnaires were sent to every 500th member in the Confederation's register of about 1·8 million throughout Sweden. This gave us a study material that was to

TABLE 6.4

Total number of employment-finding measures, by work on the open market and in sheltered employment, 1951–67 (from Swedish Government Official Reports 1968)

Placing	Year					
	1951 (per cent)	1955 (per cent)	1960 (per cent)	1964 (per cent)	1966 (per cent)	1967 (per cent)
Work on the open market	96·2	92·8	74·7	52·4	47·3	35·2
Work in sheltered employment	3·8	7·2	25·3	47·6	52·7	64·8
Total employment-finding measures	100	100	100	100	100	100
Total in absolute figures	9860	10 285	14 221	27 667	30 930	34 644

constitute a Confederation in miniature. It was hoped that the answers received would give a representative picture of the situation in the Confederation as a whole. The first investigation was done in 1969 and aimed to get an idea of how Confederation members felt about the hazards present in their work environment as far as ergonomic, physical, and occupational hygiene conditions were concerned.

Subjective reports of environmental hazards
In this investigation, 82 per cent of those asked reported that they were troubled by one or more of the environmental factors specified and 41 per cent replied that they experienced a high degree of discomfort. Fig. 6.3 shows that strains of an ergonomic nature were the main reason given for health hazards. Fifty-one per cent reported that such risks were present in their work places and 19 per cent reported that they were present to a high degree. Then come noise hazards reported by 41 per cent, with 16 per cent of these reporting 'to a high degree'. The third environmental hazard in Fig. 6.3 is draughts, indicated by 40 per cent, 14 per cent 'to a high degree'. If we combine this factor with temperature, which was reported by 29 per cent as a reason for discomfort at work, and humidity indicated by 9 per cent, we get some idea of the problems coming under the heading of climate. It should also be observed that eczema hazards come high up on the list of subjectively experienced health hazards. Twenty-six per cent say that these are present, and 5 per cent indicate the 'high-degree' alternative. These felt risks are well in accordance with the great and increasing quantities of chemical substances being used in industry today.

In addition to these predominant health hazards, there are a number of others with a more widespread distribution, but when taken together, these are a source of worry and anxiety from the health point of view. They include various air pollutants, such as gases, steam, dust, etc. Today we know of a number of long-term effects from this group of pollutants, and it appears that our members are becoming increasingly apprehensive about these effects.

Views on work-related ill health
We also tried to get some idea of how many of the group had contracted diseases which they considered had some connection with their working conditions and their work environment. Twenty per cent replied that they had become ill for reasons they considered were linked with the specified environmental conditions. Fig. 6.4 shows an analysis of such types of ill health.

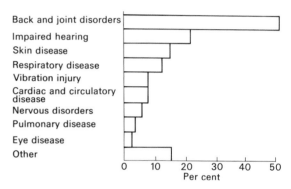

Fig. 6.4. Reported ill health by disease category. Number of participants: 739.

Here, as in so many other inquiries, skeletal and muscular disorders are predominant and these are associated with poor ergonomic conditions at the workplace. Then comes impaired hearing associated with the widespread and high level of noise in industry. A large proportion have various kinds of eczema associated with the great quantities of chemical products.

The primary significance of this questionnaire inquiry for the Confederation was that it directed attention towards the physical quality of the work environment in various respects, and the consequences of industrial development on employees when it comes to determining safety norms in the case of various health hazards connected with ergonomic and hygienic problems. It played an important part in the efforts of the trade unions to get environmental factors taken into account in industrial planning. It was also a very weighty argument in the political debate that led up to more stringent legislation on industrial safety and increased investments in work environment research, company health services, public control and service agencies in the field of work environment, etc.

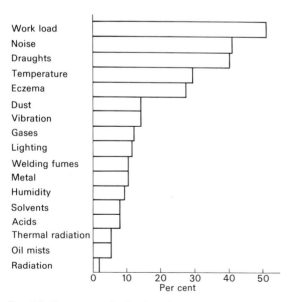

Fig. 6.3. Percentage distribution of subjectively experienced environmental hazards. Number of participants: 3886.

PHYSICAL AND OTHER HAZARDS ACTING AS STRESSORS

The fact that I have given an account of this investigation in this volume on stress at work is primarily due to another aspect I should like to discuss. In my view, poor physical conditions at work and particularly anxiety about the health hazards present in the work environment are also significant factors underlying mental strain. I am also of the opinion that poor physical work environment often interacts with other defective working conditions of a more specifically psychosocial nature.

I should like to illustrate this in more detail by describing another questionnaire enquiry carried out by the Swedish Trade Union Confederation in 1970, using a group of participants representative of the Confederation as a whole. The purpose of this inquiry was to get some idea of our members' experience of mental strains in the work environment and to try to find out what conditions at work were contributory factors.

The questions we used to identify those in the group who experienced mental strains and stress at work are given in Table 6.5. It must be noted that the term 'stress' is used here in its broadest sense and not strictly scientifically. Instead of regarding each question as a separate indicator of feelings of mental strain and tension (stress in popular terminology), we made an index based on replies to questions. This index indicated the degree of felt mental strain for each individual. The figure in brackets at the beginning of each reply alternative indicates the value given to each reply. The value figures for these four questions have been added up for each individual, giving an index number between 4 and 18, with 4 indicating minimum and 18 maximum mental strains.

This gave us four groups varying as to mental strain experienced at work. One group comprised 43 per cent of participants which we later called 'not stressed'; one group of 34 per cent we called 'somewhat stressed'; a group of 14 per cent we called 'fairly stressed'; and finally a group of 9 per cent we called 'very stressed'.

Stressors at work

In one question, participants were asked to state what factors in the work environment they thought caused the stress and mental strain they felt, and to grade the extent to which they thought a particular factor contributed. The replies are summarized in Fig. 6.5. We have calculated the mean for each factor in such a way that the

TABLE 6.5

Questions intended to measure stress at work and replies received in absolute figures and percentages

Do you think your present work is stressful or mentally trying?

	No.	Per cent
(4) Yes, very stressful and mentally trying	343	9
(3) Yes, fairly stressful and mentally trying	870	22
(2) Yes, somewhat stressful and mentally trying	1811	45
(1) No, not at all stressful or mentally trying	939	24
No answer	27	1

Do you usually worry or feel uneasy when you go to work?

	No.	Per cent
(4) Very often	124	3
(3) Quite often	265	7
(2) Sometimes	1605	40
(1) Seldom or never	1984	50
No answer	12	0

If you have been ill in 1970: have you ever been off sick (sick-listed or otherwise absent from work) when the main reason has been tiredness or stress caused by conditions at your work place?

	No.	Per cent
(1) No	3130	78
(3) Yes, once	350	9
(4) Yes, two or three times	169	4
(5) Yes, more than three times	69	2
No answer	272	7

Have you consulted a doctor during 1970 for a disorder you think is connected with mental stress?

	No.	Per cent
(1) No	3458	87
(4) Yes, on one occasion	341	9
(5) Yes, on several occasions	131	3
No answer	60	2

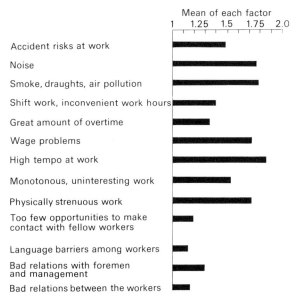

Fig. 6.5. Reported reasons for mental strains at work.

reply 'to a very great degree' has the value 4, 'quite a high degree' the value 3, and so on. The length of the bars thus indicates the mean of each factor for the entire material.

Fig. 6.5 shows that the forced work tempo was, in the aggregate, the factor most often indicated as the reason for stress and uneasiness, followed by smoke, draughts, air pollution, noise, wage problems, and physically strenuous work. A little further down the list came monotonous, uninteresting work and accident risks at work.

We also tried to identify the connection between feelings of mental strain on the one hand, and working conditions measured by other questions on the other, not putting them in direct relation to feelings of stress and mental strain. A variable of this type is the freedom workers have on the job and the qualifications required for the job. By using certain sets of questions we have tried to identify conditions in these respects (Table 6.6).

We see here that 16 per cent of Confederation members consider they have mainly repetitive, monotonous work. Nine per cent cannot leave their work for 10 minutes without being replaced by another worker and 7 per cent must work at a rate that is entirely determined by a machine. We constructed an index in this case as well,

giving us three groups under the following headings; controlled work, somewhat controlled work, and non-controlled work.

In this analysis 4 per cent of participants came under the heading 'controlled work', 47 per cent the inter-mediate group 'somewhat controlled work', and 47 per cent the group 'non-controlled work'. Table 6.7 shows the correlation between the degree of 'control' of work and feelings of stress and mental strain. Twenty per cent of those whose work is controlled experience a feeling of stress, compared to 6 per cent of those whose work is non-controlled.

Industrial democracy is significant in many ways for feelings of mental strain at work. We could not demonstrate the whole of this complicated spectrum in an inquiry of this kind, but we did use one question to try to identify 'the democratic climate' on the job. The question had the following wording:

Which of the following descriptions do you think best describes the atmosphere at your workplace?
1. At my workplace no distinction is made between different groups of employees. Blue-collar workers, white-collar workers and directors are treated in much the same way, irrespective of wage levels.

TABLE 6.6

Questions on freedom at work and qualifications required.
Replies received in absolute figures and percentages

Which of the descriptions below best fits the degree of planning and judgement ability required of you in your work? Put a cross against one of the alternatives'.

		Number	Per cent
(1)	My work is mainly repetitive, monotonous	634	16
(2)	My work requires of me a certain degree of planning and judgement ability	2385	60
(3)	My work requires of me a high degree of planning and judgement ability	914	23
	Total	3933	99

Can you leave your **work for ten minutes** to go to the toilet or the like **without** being replaced and without causing appreciable inconvenience in production?

(1)	Yes, at any time	2193	55
(2)	Yes, mostly	1423	36
(3)	No, I cannot leave my work without being replaced	351	9
	Total	3967	100

Is your rate of working controlled by a conveyor belt or a particular machine?

(1)	Yes, entirely	288	7
(2)	Yes, partly	644	16
(3)	No	3041	76
	Total	3953	99

TABLE 6.7

Mental strain felt by workers according to the degree of control in their jobs

Degree of control	Number	Percentage	Not stressed (per cent)	Somewhat stressed (per cent)	Fairly stressed (per cent)	Very stressed (per cent)	Total (per cent)
Controlled work	159	4	21	28	30	20	99
Somewhat controlled work	1967	47	39	34	15	11	99
Non-controlled work	1997	47	49	32	13	6	100
Total	4123	98					

2. One often feels that distinctions are made between different groups of employees—blue-collar workers are on a somewhat lower level than the others.
3. Definite distinctions are made between different groups of employees at all levels—blue-collar workers are quite definitely treated as second-class citizens.

The analysis of replies is shown in Table 6.8.

Seven per cent felt sharp distinctions were made, 40 per cent constituted an intermediate group, and 52 per cent considered no distinctions were made. Here we see a very strong correlation with feelings of stress and mental strain at work. Among those who considered that the democratic climate was good, only 4 per cent had the highest stress index, whereas among those who considered the democratic climate to be poor, no less than 27 per cent had a high stress index.

The investigation showed that the type of wages has a strong correlation with feelings of stress. This is illustrated in Table 6.9. We see that 17 per cent of those who have straight piece rates come in the category 'very stressed', compared with only 7 per cent of those who have fixed wages. It has also been found that there are connections between feelings of stress and shift work, particularly the two-shift and three-shift systems, and irregular working hours.

Morbidity; absenteeism

Our questionnaire also sought to get information on how often the participants had been on the sicklist or otherwise absent from work on account of ill health during the year. We also asked how many days altogether during the year our informants had been sicklisted or otherwise absent from work on account of ill health. The findings were as follows:

	Per cent
Not absent from work at all in 1970	35
1–3 times absent from work	55
4–6 times absent from work	6
7–10 times absent from work	1
More than 10 times absent from work	2

TABLE 6.8

Mental strain and differences in treatment of various categories of employees

Differences in treatment	Number	Per cent	Not stressed (per cent)	Somewhat stressed (per cent)	Fairly stressed (per cent)	Very stressed (per cent)	Total (per cent)
No distinction made	2210	52	55	29	10	4	98
Distinction often made	1671	40	31	39	17	12	99
Definite distinction made	275	7	15	27	29	27	98
Total	4156	99					

Not one day absent in 1970	31
Less than a week altogether	19
1–2 weeks altogether	18
Between 2 weeks and a month altogether	12
1–2 months altogether	9
More than 2 months altogether	7

This indicates that 30 per cent of Confederation members were probably not absent from work on account of illness for one single day in the course of one year. About 70 per cent account for 100 per cent of sick leave. About 3 per cent of members are away from work on an average of once per month to once every other month. About 7 per cent of members are absent from work on account of illness for a total of at least two months a year.

Earlier we had extracted the percentage distribution of the various stress index groups from the total questionnaire material. We proceeded in the same way with the three groups 'never absent', 'long-term sick-leave', and 'short-term sick-leave', which we could identify on the basis of the above questions detailing the reasons for absence on grounds of ill health. The findings are given in Table 6.10.

We find here that there is a much lower proportion of people with a high level of stress experience in the group that has never been absent from work on account of illness than is the case for the questionnaire participants as a whole. The proportion is much higher in the group 'long-term sick-leave', while in the group 'short-term sick-leave' the proportion of workers with a high level of stress experience at work is nearly three times as high as for the material as a whole.

As in all industrially advanced countries, absence from work on account of ill health has been rising rapidly in Sweden. Between 1950 and 1970 absence from work has risen from about 5 to about 11 per cent. This is a serious problem in production.

Even if it is not possible here to make a thorough analysis of a number of complex correlations relevant to absence from work, it can be maintained that absence from work on account of ill health, both long-term and short-term, could be reduced by improving the work environment in a number of important respects, and by changing the psychological climate in the company and the way work is organized.

Deterioration of the work environment

These two investigations have shown us that the environment in which our members are working has deteriorated in pace with technological progress and the efficiency-improvement process. Mechanization and the development of new techniques motivated by efficiency considerations only enhance the risk of the old well known health hazards, such as air pollution, noise, etc., becoming more widespread. Technical design and work methods, which do not take sufficient account of ergonomic principles in a work organization where human beings have less and less scope to plan and vary their work themselves, increase the risk of physical overloading and this leads to people becoming ill and worn out. The constant influx of new chemical products increases the risk of occupational diseases, which are often difficult to detect in their early stages and take a long time to cure. Modern methods and organization of work in many cases create conditions that engender mental strain—monotony, the feeling that work is meaningless, and alienation. Workers find it increasingly difficult to experience any kind of togetherness and to make contact with their fellow workers.

TABLE 6.9

Mental strain experienced by workers with different wage forms

Wage form	Number	Per cent	Not stressed (per cent)	Somewhat stressed (per cent)	Fairly stressed (per cent)	Very stressed (per cent)	Total (per cent)
Time-studied straight piece-work	340	8	24	38	20	17	99
Time-studied basic + piece rates	171	4	29	36	19	15	99
Non-time-studied piece rates	1172	28	37	36	16	9	98
Fixed wages, time rates	2433	58	49	30	12	7	98
Total	4116	98					

TABLE 6.10

Stress index

	Not stressed (per cent)	Somewhat stressed (per cent)	Fairly stressed (per cent)	Very stressed (per cent)	Total (per cent)
Total sample	43	32	14	9	98
Never absent	55	32	11	2	100
Long-term sick-leave	31	33	17	13	94
Short-term sick-leave	22	29	22	25	98

PROMOTION OF OCCUPATIONAL HEALTH AND INDUSTRIAL DEMOCRACY

The experiences of workers illustrated by these Confederation enquiries have formed the basis of trade union policy since the mid-1960s, and are the main reason why high priority has been given to questions concerning job security, work environment, and industrial democracy.

In recent years these efforts have resulted in a number of specific measures and programmes as regards both legislation and agreements with the employers. Various action programmes have been carried out jointly by the employers and employees, both in the field of work environment and for the promotion of broader and deeper industrial democracy.

An amended Labour Welfare Act came into force in 1974. This primarily aims to give employees real influence over their work environment. Public agencies responsible for control and for providing services to companies in these respects have been expanded considerably. A fund has been built up via employer pension contributions, and this will be used for research, training, and information in the field of work environment. A programme for the expansion of corporate health services has been drawn up jointly by the government and the parties on the labour market and it is intended that these services will be available in all workplaces during the 1980s.

New legislation came into force in 1974 providing guarantees for job security in a number of respects. Dismissals and lay-offs are regulated by law in a way guaranteeing greater job security. Special rules will apply to workers who, on account of age or disability, find it difficult to keep or get work. Rules are laid down concerning co-operation between employees, employers, and public authorities for the purpose of improving facilities for providing these categories with employment and improving their situation in working life. The parties on the labour market have concluded an agreement providing for the expansion of security guarantees of a similar kind.

A trade union programme for industrial democracy is now being implemented via various measures. For some years now, the parties on the labour market have been carrying on joint research on new types of work organization and co-operation, in order to create a higher degree of involvement and sense of responsibility at work. The idea is to get away from the old types of split-up, high-speed serial production and find new patterns for work organization that give groups of workers greater freedom to plan and organize their work themselves.

A review (Swedish Government Official Reports 1975) has been made of legislation concerning terms of employment in order to limit or eliminate the sole right of an employer to lead and organize work. We are moving towards greater equality between the management and the employees when it comes to the organization and management of work, personnel policies and job security. These efforts also embrace demands for worker participation in the long-term planning of companies, where issues such as employment requirements and job security, a good work environment and meaningful and interesting work must be considered on equal terms with economic and efficiency requirements. The trade unions are well aware that new knowledge and new kinds of expertise are necessary if these future goals are to be attained.

Research is needed

An important part of trade union work, particularly in the last few years, has been to press for an expansion of research and education in the field of labour science. The Labour Welfare Fund mentioned earlier has played a leading role here, in so far as it has been able to direct research towards the kind of knowledge that is relevant to working life. It is essential that research findings are applied in practice at the workplaces.

It is thus very gratifying to the trade union movement

that questions concerning the psychosocial conditions of working life are being given such consideration in this volume. We take it as a proof of growing international interest in these questions, which we consider to be of primary importance. We hope that both national and international efforts in this field will result in a new scale of values being applied in future industrial development.

REFERENCES

Ministry of Finance (1966). *Long-term economic surveys, Swedish economy 1966–1970*. The Ministry of Finance, Stockholm.

—— (1976). *Long-term economic surveys, Swedish economy 1971–1975*. LiberFörlag/Allmänna förl., Stockholm.

Swedish Government Official Reports (1968). Report no. 61. Ministry of the Interior, Stockholm.

—— (1970). Report no. 15, p. 7:25. Ministry of the Interior, Stockholm.

—— (1975). *Democracy at the place of work*. Report no. 1. LiberFörlag, Stockholm.

Swedish Trade Union Confederation (1967). *The trade unions and technological change.* (A research report submitted to the 1966 congress of Landsorganisationen i Sverige.) George Allen and Unwin, Ltd., London.

7.   A MODEL OF PERSON–ENVIRONMENT FIT

JOHN R. P. FRENCH, Jr., WILLARD ROGERS, and SIDNEY COBB

During the past seventeen years the Social Environment and Mental Health Program of the Institute for Social Research at the University of Michigan has been conducting research on the effects of the social environment on health and mental health. This interdisciplinary programme in social science and medical science includes persons in social psychology, epidemiology, sociology, biochemistry, psychiatry, clinical psychology, and other disciplines. Members of both the Survey Research Centre and the Research Centre for Group Dynamics contribute their special skills in the methods of survey research and laboratory experiments, but the programme has also used other methods including field experiments in which the experimenter manipulates certain variables while controlling others, natural experiments in which chance introduces certain changes (such as the closing of a factory) which provide the opportunity for a quasi-experimental design, organizational studies, the analysis of existing medical data, and various combinations of these methods. The different disciplines and the two centres have also contributed a variety of theoretical formulations which have been used and tested in the programme. However, the approach has not been eclectic in the usual sense, for there has been a very self-conscious effort to develop a single unified theory and to test it in a programmatically planned series of studies. Our conception of health has avoided a sharp distinction between what we believe are intertwined mental and physical aspects, and we have been just as concerned with positive health as with illness. In our studies, the usual mental illnesses have been conspicuous by their absence because they pose formidable problems of diagnosis and measurement. It seemed wise to avoid such problems in a programme whose central focus is the social and organizational environment. Instead, we have chosen to study measurable psychological variables such as job satisfaction and self-esteem and psychosomatic illnesses such as coronary heart disease.

STRESS AND PERSON–ENVIRONMENT FIT

In the course of our research on the effects of environmental stresses on human well-being, we had many discussions regarding the definition of stress. We eventually concluded that we could talk about the stressful effects of environmental events most fruitfully when we considered the characteristics of the individual in relation to those events. Accordingly, we have turned our attention to the concept of person–environment fit as the immediate predictor of health and well-being, and as the interactive product of relevant properties of individual and situation. In a sense, the concept of person–environment fit is one concept of adjustment.

We have turned from the concept of stress to the concept of person–environment fit in order to meet two goals which we have set for ourselves. First, we wanted to develop a more precise, a more differentiated, and especially a more *quantitative* theory; and second, we wanted to relate the conception of adjustment as person–environment fit to several other apparently unrelated definitions of adjustment (French *et al.* 1974).

The person–environment fit model starts with four basic elements:

(1) The *objective environment* (E_O) refers to the physical, biological, and especially the *social* environment which exists outside the individual and independent of the person's perceptions of it.
(2) The *subjective environment* (E_S) refers to perceptions and cognitions of those aspects of the objective environment which impinge upon the person.
(3) The *objective person* (P_O) refers to all those objectively demonstrable characteristics of the person such as physical characteristics, traits, and abilities.
(4) The *subjective person* (P_S) consists of the self concept of self-identity corresponding to the properties of the objective person.

Using these four elements, we can define two types of person–environment fit: *objective person–environment fit* (F_O) is the goodness of fit between the objective person and his objective environment; *subjective person–environment fit* (F_S) is the corresponding goodness of fit between the subjective person and his subjective environment. Within each type we can distinguish two further types: the most fundamental is the degree to which *motives* in the person are satisfied by *supplies* for these motives in the environment; for example, the degree to which hunger in the person is matched by food in the environment; a second type of fit is the degree to which *demands* emanating from the environment, such as job requirements, are matched by *abilities* in the person.

How can one quantify goodness of fit? Kurt Lewin (1951; p. 37) has provided the general answer to this question.

(1) Only those entities which have the same conceptual dimension can be compared as to their magnitude.
(2) Everything which has the same conceptual dimension can be compared quantitatively; its magnitude can be measured, in principle, with the same yardstick (units of measurement). . . .

So the key to the problem is *to conceptualize both the person and his or her environment along the same dimensions* and then to develop measures, using the same units of measurement, along these commensurate dimensions. For example, we might measure a person's need for food along the dimension of *calories per day*, and we might measure that person's environment along the commensurate dimension of *available calories per day* of food. Then we can compare these two magnitudes quantitatively and calculate the number of calories of deficiency or excess as one measure of goodness of fit between the person and the environment.

Given such commensurate dimensions, we can write the equations for the two main forms of fit between motives and supplies:

(1) Objective person–environment fit = Objective environment minus objective person.
(2) Subjective person–environment fit = Subjective environment minus subjective person.

In both equations a positive difference indicates an excess of supplies for motives and a negative difference indicates a deficiency of supplies for motives.

The two equations for the goodness of fit between environmental demands and abilities can most conveniently be written:

(3) Objective person–environment fit = objective person minus objective environment.
(4) Subjective person–environment fit = subjective person minus subjective environment.

As for eqns (1) and (2), a positive difference indicates an excess and a negative difference a deficiency, but now the deficiency refers to abilities in the person. For all four equations we expect that a deficiency will be stressful for the person. The measure of fit will also be an indicator of the amount of adjustment the person must make to reach perfect person–environment fit.

We turn now to the question of how these equations are related to each other and to other conceptions of adjustment or mental health. Let us examine this question by taking an example of motives and supplies (eqns (1) and (2)) but keeping in mind that the other cases of eqns (3) and (4) are parallel. We choose as an example the motive to participate, which is defined as the desire to influence decisions which affect one and to control the conditions of work. This motive is both a need and a value; people want more participation and they also have values prescribing how much participation they legitimately ought to have (French *et al.* 1960). The amount of subjective participation accorded to a person is one of the strongest environmental variables affecting job satisfaction, job-related threat, self-esteem, relations with other people, and job performance (French and Caplan 1973). So it is a strong hypothesis that goodness of fit with respect to participation should be strongly related to these variables. Table 7.1 presents the case of an employee whose objective environment provides very little participation (only $1 \cdot 0$ units on a 5-point scale) while the person actually desires a very high level of participation (5.0 units on the same scale). Consequently, this person suffers a deficiency of $-4 \cdot 0$. In order to decrease this bad objective fit, this person uses denial to distort the subjective environment, thus perceiving two units of participation where there is only one. Furthermore, this employee uses a 'sour grapes mechanism' to minimize desires for participation. Together these two defence mechanisms reduce objective misfit from –4 to a subjective fit of –2. The third

TABLE 7.1

An example of person–environment fit with respect to participation. Notation given in parentheses

	Objective	Subjective	Accuracy
Environment: e.g., amount of participation accorded	$1 \cdot 0$ (E_O)	$2 \cdot 0$ (E_S)	'Contact with reality' $-1 \cdot 0$ ($R = E_O - E_S$)
Person: e.g., the amount of participation desired	$5 \cdot 0$ (P_O)	$4 \cdot 0$ (P_S)	'Accessibility of the self' $1 \cdot 0$ ($A = P_O - P_S$)
Person–environment fit	$-4 \cdot 0$ ($F_O = E_O - P_O$)	-2 ($F_S = E_S - P_S$)	

column of Table 7.1 shows at what cost: The employee has impaired both contact with reality and accuracy of self-perception (accessibility of self) by one unit each. In this model the *amount* of improvement in subjective fit achieved by defensive distortion will always be offset by an *equal amount* of decrease in the two other criteria of mental health, i.e., contact with reality and accessibility of the self.

However, a person might use *coping* rather than defence to improve fit. One might change the objective environment by securing more participation (a form of environmental mastery); and this change, assuming it was accurately perceived, would improve both objective fit and subjective fit without decreasing contact with reality.

FOUR CONCEPTIONS OF MENTAL HEALTH

To summarize, the model in Table 7.1 defines quantitatively four important conceptions of mental health (objective fit, subjective fit, contact with reality, and accessibility of the self) and it specifies the static relations among them. It provides the basis for a dynamic model which predicts how coping and defence of various forms (that is, a change in one or more of the four basic elements of construction) will change these four measures of mental health.

We have already suggested that any deficiency, either in the supplies to satisfy the persons' motives or in their abilities to satisfy the demands of their jobs, will produce strain within the persons. Now let us try to specify these predictions from our model. The model requires that we distinguish between objective fit and subjective fit. It further specifies that the relation between these two types of fit will affect, in predictable ways, the level of contact with reality and accessibility of the self. Some of the literature (e.g., Mechanic 1962; Hamburg *et al.* 1953; Friedman *et al.* (1963) suggests that such defensive distortion may reduce strain. So it is not possible to make predictions about the effects of any one type of fit without specifying these other conditions. Let us start, therefore, with the simple case where variations in objective fit are always veridically perceived and accuracy is perfect. Fig. 7.1(a) presents the example of the relation between goodness of fit between ability and work load, and cholesterol. Our finding that a given stress does not affect all strains in the same way (French and Caplan 1973; Caplan 1971) warns us that different strains will probably behave differently in response to misfit, but we have no good basis for making these differential predictions, so cholesterol here exemplifies any strain.

Fig. 7.1(a) shows that the more excessive the work load, the higher the level of cholesterol (the right-hand side of the solid curve). But what are the effects of *too little* work? One simple assumption (the rest of the solid curve) is that variations in the level of work load make no difference so long as the demands are less than the person's ability.

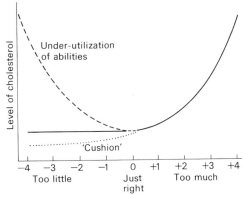

FIG. 7.1(a). The hypothesized effect on cholesterol level of congruent objective and subjective person–environment fit with respect to work load demanded on the job and abilities in the person.

A slightly more sophisticated hypothesis takes account of the future as well as the present (the dotted extension of the solid curve). It assumes that persons will be under less strain if they have a little 'cushion' against possible future fatigue or fluctuations in demand. We have noticed, for example, that piece workers who earned tickets for every piece produced, and who were supposed to turn in their tickets at the end of each day so that their pay could be figured, often developed the habit of 'saving tickets'. They would turn in most of their tickets, but they would save out a few so that they could use them to meet the quota on a day when they felt tired or had more difficult work to do. Evidently, they felt more comfortable when they did not always have to work up to capacity, especially when someone else was setting the quota. Fundamentally the threat which motivates the 'cushion' and which also causes the strain when there is a deficiency in ability and performance, is the threat that others will cut off the supplies to meet one's needs; either positive rewards such as pay, promotion, and approval will be withdrawn or else negative sanctions like punishment or discharge will be applied. It is in this sense that the misfit between motives and supplies is always fundamental, even in cases where the measured discrepancy is between demands and abilities.

This brings us to the third interpretation of insufficient work load, namely that quite other motives than the avoidance of fatigue and effort may become involved. Underload can be stressful (Vickers 1974) because two important motives are threatened. First, under the threat of a general reduction in the work force, those who have the least work to do may be most likely to lose their jobs; second, an underload, especially a qualitative underload, can frustrate a person's needs for self-utilization and achievement. Both of these threats would predict that the curve of cholesterol should rise with increasing underload, thus following the dashed line in Fig. 7.1(a).

41

How will *subjective* person–environment fit affect strain? Remembering that other examples are likely to differ, we again examine in Fig. 7.1(b) the case of work load and cholesterol. Now we must distinguish between the realists who accurately perceive themselves and their environments, and the defenders who, like the person in Table 7.1, distort both their self concepts and their subjective environments in such a way as to reduce subjective misfit. The realists we have already discussed in Fig. 7.1(a), for their subjective fit is always equal to their objective fit. So from among the three possibilities presented in Fig. 7.1(a) we choose to illustrate in Fig. 7.1(b) the same U-shaped curve.

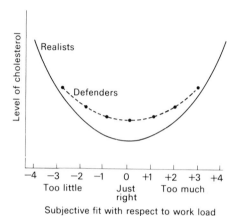

FIG. 7.1(b). The hypothesized effect on cholesterol level of subjective person–environment fit with respect to work load demanded on the job and abilities in the person.

But how will the defenders respond? One prediction is clear and certain; there will be no cases reporting an extreme misfit of −4 or +4, and there will be a piling up of cases near the middle of the distribution; for all defenders will, by definition, report a better subjective fit than the objective fit. Some may distort from an objective deficiency of −4 to a subjective deficiency of −3, while others may move as far as −2 or −1. Similarly, persons with an objective fit of −2 might distort to −1 or to 0. It is difficult to predict the exact level of cholesterol for these various kinds of defenders because we would expect their defences to succeed in reducing strain in some cases but to fail under other circumstances. Let us assume, somewhat arbitrarily, that the mild defences encountered in our samples of relatively well adjusted men are generally partially successful in reducing strain (as measured by cholesterol level). Then each defender in Fig. 7.1(b) would have a level of cholesterol which is lower than we would predict from his objective fit but higher than we would predict from his reported subjective fit (and therefore also higher than for realists who have the same subjective fit). Under this assumption the curve for defenders will be higher than the curve for realists at all points. The exact form of this curve will

depend on how the degree of distortion is distributed along the dimension of fit. In Fig. 7.1(b) we illustrate a flatter curve for defenders which is based on the reasonable assumption that those who have a greater objective misfit will distort more. Of course, other assumptions would generate other curves. The main point of the figure is to illustrate that these important distinctions between realists and defenders cannot be made where we have only subjective measures of person–environment fit. If only measures of subjective fit are available, then we cannot make precise predictions of strain. Generally speaking, the relation between subjective fit and strain should be curvilinear, but if the amount of defensive distortion is both large and widespread, then the curvilinearity should be greatly reduced. Even so, measures of subjective person–environment fit should account for additional variations in strain over and above what we can account for by the main effects of their component measures of the person and of the environment. In short, we should expect to find significant interaction effects.

RELATION OF PERSON–ENVIRONMENT FIT TO HEALTH

Having illustrated our model or person–environment fit, we are now in a position to relate this model to our basic schema of the relationship of fit to health. This model is presented in Fig. 7.2.

The effects of the objective environment on responses are mediated by the intervening subjective environment (arrows 2 and 3). Similarly the objective person influences the subjective person (arrow 9) which in turn influences responses (arrow 6). These responses in turn influence morbidity and mortality from coronary heart disease (arrow 8).

The dashed lines represent discrepancy scores, and the arrows running from them show how these discrepancies affect responses. Thus arrow 7 signifies that objective fit, either a deficiency or an excess, will influence the person's responses. In this case it may be either a deficiency (or excess) of abilities to meet job demands or else a deficiency (or excess) of supplies (such as money) to satisfy one's motives for working. Similarly, arrow 5 shows the effect of subjective person–environment fit on responses. It is implied that the effects of objective fit are often mediated by subjective fit as an intervening variable.

We conceive of the person and his environment as an open cybernetic system (see Chapter 29) with feedback mechanisms which, for purposes of simplification, have been omitted from Fig. 7.2. Two feedback loops are especially important. First, the behavioural responses of the person to job stresses may include such coping behaviours as requesting an assistant to help with an overload or asking for a pay rise; and these behavioural responses may actually change the objective environment. Second, if the job stresses eventuate in a heart

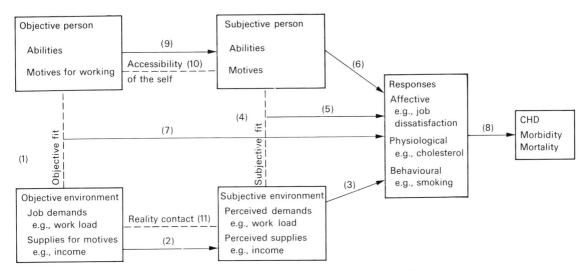

Fɪɢ. 7.2. A hypothesized relationship between person–environment fit and coronary heart disease.

attack, then the influence of factors from outside the system depicted in Fig. 7.2 (for example, the intervention of a physician) may change both the person and his environment. Thus the model deals not only with the static relations among objective fit, subjective fit, contact with reality, and accessibility of the self; but it also includes the dynamic changes over time in those relationships (French *et al.* 1974).

Although our model is abstract enough to encompass all aspects of a person's environment, most of our empirical research has focused on the work environment. Accordingly, we have been interested in such dimensions as fit as: the person's motive for participation and the amount of participation accorded to him in his job, the need for achievement, and the supplies for this need, the need for pay and the income received, the demand of a heavy work load and the ability to meet this demand, the amount of role ambiguity and the amount of ambiguity a person would like to have in his job, the amount of responsibility for other people and the desired amount of responsibility. Most of our studies have measured only subjective fit, and these studies have typically shown that subjective fit, on many dimensions, is related to affective strains such as job dissatisfaction and job-related threat (Caplan 1971; French and Caplan 1973; French 1973; Vickers 1974). Better fit is associated with lower affective strain. However, we have not usually found parallel relations between subjective fit and physiological strain.

In only one study have we dealt with objective person–environment fit. In this laboratory experiment (Sales 1969) persons were given either *more* or *less* mental work (solving anagrams) than they were able to accomplish. In general, overload produced more psychological strain and higher pulse rates than underload. More pertinent to the present discussion, those subjects who had a good fit between the experimental task and their motives and abilities showed a decrease in cholesterol during the experimental hour, whereas those subjects who had a poor fit showed no such decrease in cholesterol.

A key question about this theoretical model is: Can the measure of person–environment fit account for additional variance in strain over and above the variance accounted for by its two component measures? If the additive effects of the component measures of the environment and of the person can account for as much variance, then the concept of fit is of dubious value. The question has been examined extensively in a large study of employed men (Caplan *et al.* 1975) and in two other studies summarized by Harrison (1978). The results of all these studies are in general agreement: first, the predicted asymptotic and U-shaped curves do occur for the relationships between many dimensions of fit and many psychological strains; second, careful analyses of the data demonstrate that measures of person–environment fit can account for additional variance in strain which cannot be predicted by linear relationships with the E or P components, either singly or in additive combination.

REFERENCES

Cᴀᴘʟᴀɴ, R. D. (1971) Organizational stress and individual strain: A social–psychological study of risk factors in coronary heart disease among administrators, engineers, and scientists. University Microfilms No. 72–14822. Institute for Social Research, Ann Arbor, Mich.
——, Cᴏʙʙ, S., Fʀᴇɴᴄʜ, J. R. P., Jr., Hᴀʀʀɪsᴏɴ, R. V.,

and Pɪɴɴᴇᴀᴜ, S. R. (1975). *Job demands and worker health: Main effects and occupational differences.* U.S. Government Printing Office, Washington, D.C.
Fʀᴇɴᴄʜ, J. R. P., Jr. (1973). Person role fit. *Occup. ment. Health,* **3,** 15–20.
——, and Cᴀᴘʟᴀɴ, R. D. (1973). Organizational stress and

individual strain. In *The failure of success* (ed. A. J. Marrow) AMACOM, New York.

——, ISRAEL, J., and AAS, D. (1960). An experiment in participation in a Norwegian factory. *Human Relat.,* **13,** 3–19.

——, RODGERS, W. L., and COBB, S. (1974). Adjustment as person–environment fit. In *Coping and adaptation* (ed. G. Coelho, D. Hamburg, and J. Adams). Basic Books, New York.

FRIEDMAN, S. B., MASON, J. W., and HAMBURG, D. A. (1963). Urinary 17-hydroxycorticosteroid levels in parents of children with neoplastic disease: A study of chronic psychological stress. *Psychosom. Med.,* **25,** 364–76.

HAMBURG, D. A., HAMBURG, B., and DeGOZA, S. (1953). Adaptive problems and mechanisms in severely burned patients. *Psychiat.,* **16,** 1–20.

HARRISON, R. B. (1978). Person–environment fit and job stress. In *Stress at work* (ed. C. L. Cooper and R. Payne). John Wiley, New York.

LEWIN, K. (1951). *Field theory in social science* (ed. D. Cartwright). Harper, New York.

MECHANIC, D. (1962). *Students under stress.* Free Press, New York.

SALES, S. M. (1969). Differences among individuals in affective, behavioral, biochemical, and physiological responses to variations in work load. Doctoral dissertation, University of Michigan.

VICKERS, R. (1974). Job stress, coping, and risk factors in coronary heart disease. Doctoral dissertation, University of Michigan.

8. THE ILO AND SOME PSYCHOSOCIAL ASPECTS OF WORKING LIFE IN INDUSTRIAL SOCIETY

E. MASTROMATTEO and N. GAVRILESCU

Contemporary industrial society as well as the industrialized sectors of developing countries have recorded important economic and social changes in recent years. The rapidity of the technical evolution and the progress made in the use of machines on a large scale in production have produced great benefits which have permitted a dramatic increase in the standard of living in the entire society.

BENEFITS AND COSTS

Technical progress has caused the disappearance of a large number of heavy manual jobs and hazardous work but it has replaced these with other jobs which, in many cases, are no less hazardous. Monotony and the emotional stress inherent in modern work organizations exert a marked influence on the physical and mental health of workers and on their social well-being.

Continued technological progress has at the same time paved the way towards some discontent among workers. Many of them, in particular unskilled and semi-skilled industrial workers, seem less and less satisfied with their work. Too many jobs have been rationalized to the limit, requiring the worker to accomplish simple, repetitive, and monotonous tasks that would better suit a robot than a human being.

In our industrial society one encounters more and more situations in which work organization is based on the functioning of machines, which restricts the operations of the worker within very narrow limits.

Utilization of mental abilities
On this subject Friedman (1946) made a pertinent remark: 'Human intelligence seems little by little to be withdrawing from production operations, to concentrate on design, conception, machine construction, and on Taylor-type office studies.'

A large number of workers are at present required to accomplish tasks which are well below their training and their mental ability. This situation produces a feeling of frustration and dissatisfaction.

Dehumanization of work: some consequences
The dehumanization of work, through nervous tension, is one of the most characteristic sources of stress in our industrial society. This phenomenon can produce important social, economic, and political consequences as well as disturbance of the physical and mental health of the workers.

In the last few years in many industrial plants, an increased absenteeism and increased labour turnover, especially among young workers, has been recorded along with greather apathy or indifference to work, a decrease in work quality, and an increase in 'wildcat' strikes. Considering the consequences of the dehumanization of work as they affect the physical and mental well-being of the workers, one might also speak of excessive fatigue, increase in certain psychosomatic diseases, work accidents, etc. The increase in alcoholism and the abuse of drugs might also be attributed in large measure to this general feeling of dissatisfaction, produced by the conditions of work in modern industrial society.

ILO STUDIES AND ACTIVITIES

At the Second ILO Regional European Conference the Director-General of the ILO in his report on *Human values and social policy* (ILO 1974) has underlined the necessity of intensifying international action to guard against the physical and mental well-being of man being unnecessarily compromised by the increase in industrialization and technological progress. For its part, the ILO will continue to direct its efforts towards broad co-operation among all interests involved in this field: government, employer and worker. The main objective of its activities is to promote constructive dialogue among all those who may contribute towards valid solutions.

Although a large number of aspects of this vast problem are outside the competence of the ILO, two aspects are relevant; namely the promotion of greater job satisfaction through changes in the organization of work and the improvement of social relations at plant level.

In its long-term plan of action, the ILO proposes, first of all, in industrialized countries in particular, to promote a greater awareness of the extent and the importance of the problem in order to understand the causes and to introduce new methods and practical means for humanizing work and promoting job satisfaction as well as the physical, mental, and social well-being of the workers.

In this regard, the following priorities will be taken into consideration:

(a) *The organization of work*, for example, the definition of tasks and the establishment of production standards;
(b) *The conditions under which work is done*, in par-

ticular, the physical and psychological characteristics of the work environment and the conditions of employment (wages, promotion, work hours, etc.);

(c) *Social relations in the plant,* especially its social organization, the psychological climate, and the mechanism for consultation and participation in the plant's affairs;

(d) *External plant factors,* in particular, training, education, vocational guidance, leisure, transportation, housing, etc.

Diverse activities are currently under way or in preparation at the ILO as well as at the International Institute for Social Services in Geneva and at the International Centre for Advanced Technical and Vocational Training which are aimed at elaborating appropriate measures to help ILO member states fight effectively against the unfavourable consequences of work dehumanization. As an example, the ILO programme concerning general conditions of work for the period 1974–5 plans to examine the contribution which ergonomics may make to job satisfaction and to humanization of work and the practical possibilities which if offers for adapting equipment, processes, and the working environment to the normal levels of physical and mental response of the human being. The main object in this field is to examine how recent advances can best be utilized to reduce on-the-job stress, which is detrimental to the worker's health and general well-being as well as to his capacity for work.

A number of studies will be made on certain aspects of wages and work conditions which influence work humanization, in particular the wage structure and the pay system in industrialized countries, harmonization of work conditions of manual and non-manual workers, and the adaptation of working hours. In the planning and promotion of employment programmes, studies will be devoted to the evolution of industry's need for workers, which may result in a general change of production methods with a progressive abandonment of the conveyor belt in favour of autonomous production teams. As regards labour legislation and industrial relations, stress will be laid on studies relating to worker participation in decisions which influence their employment.

All these activities and studies are aimed at facilitating a wide exchange of views, at the national as well as the international level, concerning problems of work humanization in modern industry and thereby leading to a better world-wide co-operation for the improvement of working conditions.

SUMMARY

With technical progress, many heavy manual and hazardous jobs have disappeared but modern organization of work multiplies repetitive and monotonous tasks which are well below the training and mental ability of the workers. This leads to feelings of frustration, dissatisfaction, nervous tension, and mental stress, which can be related to such questions as increased absenteeism and labour turnover, apathy and decrease in work quality, even alcoholism and drug abuse.

The ILO is concerned to promote the physical and mental health of the workers as well as their well-being and greater job satisfaction. The causes of the problem should be analysed and a constructive dialogue opened among all those concerned. Factors such as organization of work (including ergonomics), conditions of work (including wages and pay system, hours of work, etc.), and social relations in the plant (including participation of the workers) should be studied so that solutions may be found and humanization of work promoted.

REFERENCES

FRIEDMAN, G. (1946) *Problèmes humains du machinism industriel,* p. 168. Gallimard, Paris.

ILO (1974) *Human values in social policy.* (Report of the Director-General of the ILO to the Second European Regional Conference, Geneva, January 1974).

SESSION 2

Potentially pathogenic psychosocial stressors in modern working life

9. CHANGING CONCEPTS OF WORK

ALAN A. McLEAN

Long before the advent of our present technological society, the concept of work was more or less a way for man to explain the cruel world to himself. In biblical history, man is expelled from a state of bliss for having tasted the knowledge of good and evil, and is faced with a life of constant strife between himself and nature. This story explains man's travail: work is a necessary evil placed upon him because of his fall from grace. Recall the lines from Genesis, uttered at the fall: 'Cursed is the ground because of you; in toil you shall eat of it. . . .'

A recent popular Broadway musical presentation 'Don't bother me, I can't cope' included a delightful song, 'Time brings about a change'. The rapidity of social change is highlighted by lines which (paraphrased) say that, if a man called a Negro 'black' ten years ago he would 'punch him'; if he called a black a 'Negro' today he would 'punch him'. The meaning of words associated with work may not alter so fast, but change does seem to come with increasing rapidity.

This chapter will briefly highlight a few historical considerations of work's meaning—both from Western and Eastern perspectives—and consider such activity today.

HISTORICAL CONSIDERATIONS

Contemporary examples of primitive hunting and gathering societies may be seen among peoples in central Australia and Africa. They have in common the fact that simply securing a means of existence is so pressing that everyone in the tribal grouping is expected to 'work', even comparatively small children. Under these conditions it is unlikely that the concept of work as a sphere of behaviour was able to acquire a specific meaning.

Where the labours of procuring the means of existence are so all-pervasive that everyone must participate and where need is so pressing that such labours may be virtually continuous, they may not be perceived as separate activities at all. The hunting and gathering tribes apparently display almost nothing resembling a division of labour except between man and woman. Males are more heavily engaged in activities related to hunting and fishing and women are primarily engaged in the gathering of natural products, the fabrication of clothing and 'household' implements, and the processing of foods for consumption.

Language provides indirect but impressive evidence of the diffuseness of work in these societies, confirming that among the most primitive peoples life is much more of a totality than it is for Western man today. In many cases there is not even a word for work. If one were to talk about work in a primitive society we should find ourselves unrealistically limited to our own ideas of the nature of work as a special area within our own contemporary Western societal activity or else we would be forced to speak of something as broad and indefinite as the very incentive to live.

Neff (1968) points out that one began to see differentiation of work (that is beyond male–female) as the evolution into an agricultural and pastoral society gradually came about. Occupations developed which were clearly degrading and of low esteem and others developed which were acceptable or even noble. The differentiation was not always connected to the difficulty or monotony involved. For example the contemporary nomadic Bedouin in central Arabia and north Africa are willing to labour very arduously in breeding and training camels, which are their primary source of wealth and power, but they will not soil their hands with agriculture or the fabrication of weapons and equipment. To procure these necessities they use slaves or serfs, secure the needed products by raids on sedentary villages, or engage in trade.

This differentiation became more clear as a consequence of the early development of large-scale agriculture and the institution of slavery. The original objective of a military raid may have been loot, but it soon became clear that conquered peoples could be compelled to be a continuous source of food and labour.

In most civilized times, men have distinguished between 'labour' and 'work'. Arendt (1958) uses the term *animal laborens* to describe the kinds of work which repetitiously produce the essential consumable goods necessary for the maintenance of life. On the other hand she used the term *homo faber* for the production of craftsmen or artisans. Above these classes, the mature citizen of Greece and the prosperous Roman found his life divested of all need to labour through the possession of slaves. He could thus devote all of his time to the activities of politics, the management of human relations, and war.

As we move into *anno Domini* we begin to confront the Protestant ethic and what can also be considered an essential element in Roman Catholic doctrine. As early as the sixth century A.D. many new ideas about the meaning of work were confined to members of the monastic brotherhoods and tended to lose their force as monastic orders became increasingly rich and powerful.

49

Luther declared that the monks had become idle and parasitic, living off the labour of the peasant just as the landlord did.

By this time, however, the agrarian feudalism of the early middle ages had already undergone marked changes. Cities were in the process of reestablishing their sway over the countryside as centers for trade and fabrication. . . . The idea that work was ennobling began to pass from the monastic orders to these new men in the late Middle Ages—merchants, artisans and traders—who wanted to find merit in their own persuits. (Neff 1968).

The idea that work was a path to salvation had its roots in religious controversies but was also congenial to the new citizens of the growing towns and cities where merchants and artisans became enthusiastic supporters of the Protestant reforms and saw work as a path to *individual* salvation.

And here it was that Calvinist concepts arose from grounds well fertilized by the merchants and artisans and the new religious content of ideas about work and their secular application emerged. Calvinist doctrine apparently is not explicit in stating that an industrious life is a prerequisite to salvation. In fact, the concepts of original sin and predestination imply that salvation is a matter of God's will and the elect are chosen in advance of their lives on earth.

Although 'work' was increasingly seen as 'good', the rapidly developing division of labour in the new manufacturing society invented additional subtleties of meaning. Distinctions arose between mental and manual labour, between the skilled and the unskilled and between the labour of the manager and the labour of the hands. While all labour was perceived as good, there were emerging degrees of goodness.

In the United States the concept of work has strongly influenced its history. From the beginnings of colonial America, work was persistently glorified as intrinsically good. The reasons are clear and rest in the special history of the settlement of North America. Activity has always been considered a national characteristic. Americans have always been interested in making new things, changing, taking advantage of opportunities, exploring new frontiers. Justice Oliver Wendell Holmes asserted that the main purpose of life is 'to function', and on another occasion said that 'life is action—the use of one's powers.'

An oriental view
In the Orient the traditions are vastly different. Many Eastern philosophies give work as such little special meaning. Work derives meaning only in relating to one's philosophy of life and in harmonizing the being of the individual with the totality of nature. Lao-tsaze and Buddha were prophets of this world. They did not contemplate the next world. Nor did they teach about the afterlife. The primary thrust of Buddha's concepts of work is simple: 'I teach only two things,' he said, 'the fact

of suffering and the possibility of escape from suffering' (Siu 1971).

From Buddha's standpoint, the minimizing of suffering rather than the maximizing of happiness constitutes the good of living. If work is to have the best of meanings it must contribute to decreasing misery, grief, anguish, or pain. Increased suffering on the part of one person cannot be justified as a desirable trade-off for augmented happiness on the part of another. Furthermore, since suffering can only be experienced by individual persons and not by organizations, suffering to individuals cannot be justified by gains to an organization—whether it be in terms of enlarged profits for a corporation, increased converts for a church, or enhanced power for a nation.

An organization is often interested in decreasing suffering or mental anguish on the part of its members, because in so doing it is able to achieve its organizational objectives more effectively. But this does not alter the fact that the minimizing of suffering *per se* is seldom the immediate objective of an organization. The first practical purpose of an organization is to survive and the second is to grow.

The contrasting polarities of the individual and the organizations are always present. Somehow, both must be brought into the workings of life as a totality. In attempting this assimilation, the Taoist first senses the kind of continuum which is necessary for serenity over his lifespan. This continuum must not be broken by work. If a person's behaviour at work disrupts this continuum of feeling, then one will not be able to retain his sense of wholeness and tranquility when he retires from work. This is a most important point of reference (Siu 1971).

An opposite oriental observation about life is that a person emerges from the womb alone and he dies alone. He lives alone during many days of his childhood and lives alone during many days of his old age. Not quite alone—but alone with the world of nature, as shared by the child in his wonderment at the birds and insects and trees and animals and people. It is from this totality that he came when he was born and it is into this totality to which he must return when he dies. If he is able to retain the joy of living alone throughout his life—that is, with nature—then he would be able to realize the harmony of his self. Neither retirement nor death would be a burden. He should never let work jeopardize this state. The most important single meaning of work, then, is a negative one. Work must not pre-empt one's natural ease of living alone, of living without work and its derivative values.

This does not mean that an individual should not work at all and lead the life of a hobo or a so-called useless member of society. There is a reasonableness about everything in the Easterner's orientation. This is what the *yin–yang* concept is all about. So the Taoist would advise: 'Certainly work, by all means. And do a good job while you're at it. Enjoy the rewards. But do not be attached to them. When you hold an office, do not let the office hold you' (Siu 1971).

Work defined

Quite recently attempts have been made to gather greater empirical evidence on the definition of 'work'. Friedmann and Havighurst (1954), for example, used interviews and questionnaires among steel workers, miners, sales people, printers, and physicians. Each subject was asked what 'work' meant to him. In this instance lower socio-economic groups viewed work as simply concerned with making a living. Kahn and Weiss (1960) asked 'In your opinion, what makes the difference between something you call work and something you would not call work?' Here more educated workers felt that 'work was a necessary evil' and less educated workers answered 'pay'. Very nearly half their sample suggested the word 'work' meant or was equated with 'not enjoyed'.

More recently Mangione (1973) differentiated work, job, and occupation. Subjects were asked for differentiation among these terms. Both 'work' and 'occupation' were characterized by one definition: 'Work' was 'not enjoyed' and 'occupation' was 'something you were paid for'. 'Job' on the other hand, was *not* clearly characterized by a single definition but rather combined elements of displeasure, remuneration, and requirement.

Work then is somewhat more than just a synonym for 'job' and often carries quite negative connotations. 'Occupation' on the other hand, carries positive connotations that are not to be found in the term 'work' such as the exercise of skill and resultant satisfaction—which are found to some degree in concepts of 'job'.

Such studies as these designed to determine the meaning of words related to work suggest that considerable care must be exercised in matters of language when framing questions which deal with the meaning of work or with the satisfaction gained from one's vocation. The terms 'work', 'job', and 'occupation' are clearly not interchangeable and different connotations introduce biases which make it extremely difficult to compare data collected in different studies. These few examples are drawn from the literature of but one country, the United States. Efforts to develop a communality of meaning in other countries which use the English language as a mother tongue become more difficult. And in non-English speaking societies the matter (for those of us who use English) is even more complex.

From here on I will consider work as the process (be it a job or an occupation) which is productive of sustenance.

WORK IN THE WEST TODAY

Today we live more than twice as long as we did a little over 100 years ago (in 1850 the average life expectancy of the factory worker was only 32 years) and work three times as long. As a result of increasingly complex technologies and greater specialization, the process of personal identification with work has undergone startling change..Composition of work groups and tasks has been dramatically altered. Skills are made rapidly obsolete. In some cases (teaching and nursing, for example) job status has diminished. The larger ratio of service industries to production industries is beginning to make profound changes in the entire sphere of labour. Both labourers and professional employees are demanding greater job satisfaction and fulfilment, and the exigencies of the post-industrial society have brought about an increasing number of 'non-work' roles.

Yet much of industry still appears to operate under the anachronistic concept of work as a means of exorcising guilt. The typical supervisor will express in many ways his feelings that work is 'good' for you, pointing to the example he sets with long hours, few avocations, and dedication to his company. He tends to be highly critical of those who won't or can't emulate *his* work ethic. He points to today's higher salaries, shorter hours, and greater benefits and does not hide his impatience at the 'ingratitude' of the younger worker who does not demonstrate his appreciation.

The inability of some managements to adapt to changing values lies partly in the fact that during times we may consider 'stressful' (such as dealing with current problems of inflation, the energy crisis, etc.) work organizations as well as individuals regress to earlier modes of behaviour that served them well in the past. This sort of regression can be dangerous. Work organizations that fail to recognize the realities inherent in the changing nature of work will have less chance for survival than those that do.

Workers increasingly expect work to provide satisfaction. Professionals are increasingly challenged to be relevant. Much of this stems from the fact that the work force in Western society is both better educated and more affluent than prior generations. Workers generally recognize that society will not let them starve. There are increasing numbers of non-work roles which can be assumed such as welfare dependency, prolonged education, and early retirement. Other non-work roles are absenteeism and disability. It is not uncommon for someone to have become disabled and to find that he, consciously or unconsciously, gains great satisfaction from his dependent state, finding little motivation to return to the monotonous routine of a job which fosters more alienation than stimulation.

The values and ethics of youth in American society have now graduated to the work force and younger workers are bringing new perspectives. In routine assignments they often have considerable difficulty in adjusting and are restless, mobile, changeable, and demanding. In the automobile industry one-third of the employees are now thirty or younger. Absenteeism has doubled in the past decade. In 1970 there was an absentee rate of 5 per cent midweek and 10 per cent on Mondays and Fridays (Gooding 1970). In 1969 Walter Reuther, then president of the United Auto Workers (UAW), focused on the problem of young workers. These men, he said, feel they are not master of their own destiny on the job and are going to escape from it whenever they have an opportunity. Younger workers are interested in a sense of fulfilment as human beings. The lack of involvement at work, Reuther said, is a major contributing factor to absenteeism and poor work performance (Gooding 1970).

The landmark settlement between the auto workers and their industry in 1973 overcame the traditional focus of labour contracts on wages, monetary benefits, and mechanical working conditions. The contract between the UAW and Chrysler Corporation in September of that year gave emphasis to a worker's freedom of choice as to how he would spend his time after the regular eight-hour work day. From Chrysler's point of view, the issue involved cherished management prerogative: the right to require men to work longer than their regular shifts if necessary to meet the demands of production.

During the settlement UAW president Leonard Woodcock said, 'We are challenging, in effect, whether human beings exist for the sake of production and profit, or whether we are engaged in production for the sake of human beings.'

William Stevens (1973) commenting in the *New York Times* said, 'For the first time, a major industrial union had achieved contractual guarantees aimed at improving the quality of a worker's life, rather than simply fattening his wallet.'

Other factors in the landmark automobile industry agreement gave union members a voice on questions of health and safety conditions in plants. With regard to reducing boredom on the assembly line, the union won the right to participate in experimental projects. As an example, union members were given quite autonomous responsibility for techniques for manufacturing engines. They organized the job themselves as they saw fit, supervised themselves, and worked at their own pace. They were held accountable only for delivering the finished product at the right time.

The many research studies in the behavioural sciences which have clearly demonstrated the value of employee participation in programmes of job enrichment are well documented in the report of the task force of the Secretary of Health, Education, and Welfare (1973). This study group *Work in America* concluded that programmes which stimulate employee involvement in the definition and activities of their own work not only enhance job satisfaction and mental health variables but stimulate greater productivity. Similarly, work frustrations, job alienation, boredom, and monotony were shown to adversely affect employee health, reduce productivity, and adversely affect major satisfaction.

Contributing to the change in the world of work are both rapidly evolving technology and the obsolescing of skills. On both counts it is the pace of change which is increasing. Not only has technology restructured many jobs, but the change outside of work in society at large also has an impact on the job. As the then United States Secretary of Labour William Wirtz said in 1967: 'Over the years the changing nature of work has been the cause of the greatest continuing restructuring of American lives of any major force in our history.'

American philosopher, Donald Schon (1971), confronts the issues of the rapidly accelerating change that is undermining the stability of our society in his book *Beyond the stable state*. He points out that we live in a time of loss of the stable state—a period in which stable views of occupational, religious, and organizational value systems have been eroded. He clearly demonstrates how our established institutions normally respond to change: 'Faced with challenges they cannot meet, they respond with "dynamic conservatism"—they fight to remain the same.'

But change, and adaptation to it, is inevitable. The only question is how it will come about. Schon maintains that work organizations must become learning systems—maintaining the flexibility to adapt to situations as they arise, decentralizing control, and organizing themselves not around products but around functions.

THE FUTURE

Compared with a scant 25 or 30 years ago, work in many larger organizations today seems for many to be less fun. Back in those 'good old days' there was more challenge, there was stimulation, there was mobility. People worked hard not only because of the Protestant ethic but because they were personally involved in what they did. There was great competitiveness but also an excitement about risk-taking and a feeling that if you were really able you could be picked out by the president and lifted from down 'here' to up 'there'. But as organizations grew in size, they grew in complexity, and the personal, human element suffered. By now everyone has begun to look like everyone else. People are rewarded for conforming. If you get an idea, instead of having the opportunity to try your luck, it seems as though you meet all sorts of corporate barriers in the form of 'studying the problem': Is the market ready for it? Are we using the right technology? Even when an idea is realized, there have been so many departments, divisions, and auxiliary services involved in it (just a little piece each) that no one really feels a personal identification with the original concept. There is a great deal of wheel spinning and company politicking. Moreover, much work—the sort of work that involves moving things or transforming them—can be performed better by machines than by people.

The service economy we are moving into offers an opportunity to make work more involving and fun. If industrialization tends to alienate a worker from his job, service industries give employees a chance to relate more closely to their work; often these employees render a highly personalized service that provides ample scope for the development and exercise of personal skills.

But Western society thinks in terms of units—pricing, pounds, lengths, weights, all those physical elements that are better handled by machines. We are so accustomed to using figures to describe production activities that we tend to use figures to describe people too—beyond the point where these data have any real significance. If we cannot find new ways of measuring in a service economy, we will continue to be trapped in this 'thingness', the very thingness that is so abhorrent to many workers and that perpetuates the assembly-line kind of orientation so inappropriate in a service economy. Services can't be mechanized in the way products can.

In the future it will be more important than ever for work to provide satisfaction for each individual. This is the challenge to the employer, and the pressure for him to meet that challenge is beginning to mount.

It is not unreasonable to consider any organization as an entity with its own demands for survival, its own personality and nature, and its own peculiar demands upon its individual members. These demands may at times be at cross purposes with the needs of the individuals and thus can produce severe emotional reactions. Many psychiatrists might consider that those individuals who are unable to adapt to the organization are 'ill' (McLean and DeCarlo 1972).

But maybe madness lies the other way. Can we really expect people to adapt to situations that are harmful to their own personal development? When we consider the relationships and the differences between the collective organization that is the personality, and the collective personality that is the organization, and when we look at the changes in the meaning of work to the individual, we may realize that it is the organization that must adapt more. At least, it must adapt more fully to the individual than has been the case in the past.

REFERENCES

ARENDT, H. (1958). *The human condition*. Chicago, Illinois.

FRIEDMANN, F. A. and HAVIGHURST, R. J. (1954). *The meaning of work in retirement*. Chicago, Illinois.

GOODING, J. (1970), Blue collar blues on the assembly line. *Fortune*, 32 (3), 132–5, 158, 162, 167, 168.

KAHN, R. and WEISS, R. (1960). Definitions of work and occupation. *Social problems* 8, 142–51.

MANGIONE, T. H. (1973). The meaning of 'work': a matter of language. In Quinn, R. P. and Mangione, T. W. *The 1969–1970 survey of working conditions* (ed. R. P. Quinn and T. W. Mangione), Chapter 7. University of Michigan, Ann Arbor.

MCLEAN, A. A. and DECARLO, C. (1972). The changing concept of work. *Innovation*, 38–49.

NEFF, W. S. (1968). *Work and human behavior*. New York.

SCHON, D. (1971). *Beyond the stable state*. New York.

SECRETARY OF HEALTH, Education, and Welfare, Report of a Special Task Force to (1973). *Work in America*. Cambridge, Mass.

SIU G. H. (1971). Work and serenity. *Occup. Ment. Hlth*, 1 (1).

STEVENS, W. (1973). *New York Times*. September 23.

10. SOME THOUGHTS ABOUT STRESS AND THE WORK SITUATION

R. S. LAZARUS

In previous volumes of *Society, stress, and disease* and elsewhere, I have presented a theoretical approach which views stress emotions as products of particular kinds of adaptational commerce between a person and his environment. When an individual appraises such commerce as harmful or threatening to his well-being one of a variety of stressful emotional reactions follows (see, for example, Lazarus 1966; Lazarus *et al.,* 1970). Depending on the pattern of motivation and belief systems of the person, any situation can be appraised as damaging, threatening, challenging, productive of gratification, or as irrelevant to his well-being. Although some environmental contexts are more likely than others to be seen by most people as threatening or damaging, or at least highly involving (Thaler-Singer 1974), and we tend to speak of these contexts as stressors, it must never be forgotten that it takes both a demanding environmental situation *and* a susceptible person to produce a stress reaction.

The present volume concerns work as a source of stress or a stressor, so to speak. Work does indeed create the *potential* for many forms of gratification, harm, challenge, and threat. Indeed, it occupies a major part of most people's lives, both in the percentage of time taken up, and in the importance for our well-being of the events that take place in our working lives. It is not surprising, therefore, that many of the major stresses to which we must adapt occur in the work setting, though this does not mean that work is necessarily stressful at all times, for everyone, or for the same reasons in different individuals and subgroups within the society or in different societies.

POTENTIAL STRESSORS IN THE WORK SITUATION

In thinking about psychological stress in the work setting it might be useful to identify some of the most important potential sources of stress in such settings. In this brief essay, I have attempted below to list some of these and to comment briefly on them. I have identified eight below: evaluation, affiliation, meaninglessness, pay, boredom and overload, authority relations, change, and ageing and retirement. There are undoubtedly others.

Evaluation
A nearly universal stressor that is usually found within the work context is being evaluated. Evaluation serves both as an opportunity or barrier to advancement and a test of one's adequacy compared with others. In competitive societies, which means all those industrialized countries with which I am familiar, the child begins his experience with evaluation threats in the form of examinations at a very early age and certainly by the time he gets very far along in school. Marked anxiety about examinations has been observed in several field studies, the most notable of which is that of Mechanic (1962) with graduate students who were taking comprehensive examinations for the doctorate. Examination anxiety is so widespread and serious in the school setting that a number of major research programmes have been directed at it (I. G. Sarason 1972; Phillips *et al.* 1972; S. B. Sarason, 1972). In all such studies there is evidence of marked distress experienced by many of those anticipating upcoming examinations, and often severe psychosomatic and behavioural disturbances associated with the apprehension. In all such studies too, individuals varied greatly in the severity of the disturbance, and in the adequacy with which they coped with the problem. Little attention has been directed at the consequences of success and failure, that is, at what happened afterwards. Evaluations do not occur merely once in a person's life, but they are apt to be experienced again and again, thus giving examinations, or the evaluation experience, the quality of a chronic or repeated stressor. Many of the research observations about examinations in school, or evaluation in general, can be applied also to the work setting, where evaluations are a common experience, especially at the higher occupational levels.

As was noted earlier, not all individuals are equally vulnerable to the potential stress of evaluation, and determining the personality or personal history variables that are relevant is an important theoretical and research task. Some individuals are not greatly disturbed by evaluation because their definition of themselves as persons is out of keeping with the terms of the evaluation; this can, in short, be treated as a motivational question, with some people having strong needs to achieve or to be positively regarded and others minimal needs of this sort. Moreover, even if the person accepts the premises of the evaluation, some seem to have great confidence in their abilities and are not easily threatened by evaluation, while others are very fragile in the context of evaluation and react to any possibility of evaluation with marked apprehension and doubts about their ability to meet their own or others' standards. In addition, while some receive great pressure from friends and relatives to achieve at a standard beyond their ability, others obtain support, acceptance, and understanding of their position. And at the environmental end of things, evaluation situations differ among themselves, some being particularly destructive and punitive especially in the event of limited performance, while others are far more supportive and less threatening or damaging both to the person's self-esteem and in regard to the actual consequences of failure. In sum, for some the work setting is almost constantly threatening because of its evaluative implications, while for others evaluation is a negligible source of psychological stress; such variations stem either from differences in the personalities of the persons involved and/or in the situational parameters, such as the manner in which evaluation is conducted and the outcomes that are connected with it.

Affiliation
Work for most people is a social experience and over and above its achievement-centred role one of its major potentials for gratification and threat are interpersonal relationships. Work settings have important sociometric features. For example, one finds social isolates as well as those who seek and establish close interpersonal ties with many other people. Some persons are rejected; others are accepted, and even sought after and influential. As such, there are constant potentials in the work context for social treat and gratification.

As in the arena of evaluation, here too personal ways of handling such needs, and belief systems about others and one's relationships with them, vary from individual to individual, making one person more vulnerable to threat (say, because of strong or insatiable needs to be liked and accepted by others), and others little if at all engaged by the social pressures of human interaction and affiliation. As those interested in organizational sources of stress have observed, (e.g., Kahn *et al.* 1964), certain types of settings tend to facilitate positive interpersonal relationships while others thwart them. The late anthropologist, Ruth Benedict (as cited by Maslow 1964), has even suggested that societies organized in such a way that individual persons simultaneously contribute to the group's welfare by the same acts which benefit themselves (Benedict referred to this as high synergy) tend to be less aggressive and warlike than those organized in a competitive fashion where one sacrifices himself when he contributes to the group. Thus, if there is little room for advancement in a school, industrial, or business setting, distrust and lack of co-operation among persons are encouraged because anything that helps advance another person may defeat the individual's own hopes of moving ahead.

Meaninglessness and meaningfulness
When achievement, prestige, responsibility, and creativity are pretty much outside the realm of possibility for large groups of persons in the industrialized work setting, work may offer little involvement or meaning and become merely a necessary means to survive. A person in such a work setting may do what is necessary, but also make every effort to escape work and achieve other kinds of gratification, and orient his thought entirely outside the work setting in which he spends most of his time. Much has been written by sociologists about work alienation and the disappearance of pride and artisanship in one's work in the modern industrial society, and there is no need to repeat this well known theme again here. The propaganda of women's lib which equates home-making with uselessness and boredom and promotes a career orientation as a means of self-expression and commitment has possibly created new sources of stress in women. One is that there are relatively few types of jobs capable of providing truly meaningful and involving work, so that an emphasis solely on careers for women (or for that matter, men too) may, of necessity, result in as much thwarting and stress for the largest proportion of women as the emerging negative attitude on the part of women toward the work roles of wife and mother. Studies by Wilensky (1964) suggest, for example, that a relatively small proportion of men, whose role has been fixed in the work world, feel challenged by and involved in their work. And to make things even more difficult for both men and women, the work ethic as a basis of self-satisfaction may be dying in the Western industrialized world. On the other hand, there are probably great individual differences in the extent to which lack of meaningfulness in work poses a serious problem.

Income and the good life
Large numbers of persons in the Western industrialized world work for a very marginal income, and this very marginality, especially in an inflationary time, can be a constant source of stress in work extending to the home and family. Such jobs provide only barely what their families need, or what they are constantly led to expect or hope for in a relatively affluent society whose mass media constantly bombard every one with propaganda about the joys of the material and good life. There may be the constant threat of being laid off, of having to participate in costly strikes that barely if at all permit keeping up with the cost of living, of economically devastating illness or accidents, and of facing old age with little or no retirement income when productive work is no longer possible, and so on. In addition to the stresses associated with economic marginality, for many individuals, the size of one's pay-packet has symbolic value, communicating one's worth in a competitive society. Thus, in addition to the economic pressures, marginal income may have implications also for a person's sense of personal worth.

Boredom versus overload
Work that is uninvolving produces boredom unless other interests, for example, interpersonal ones, can be found, and lack of involvement sometimes leads to alienation and depression. Work that is too demanding, requiring too many responsibilities and decisions that cannot all be met, creates a different kind of stress, that of overload. Clearly, some working persons face the former problem,

others the latter. To some extent this is a matter of self-selection. For example, the ambitious person is apt to face the latter. This is similar to the graduate students studied by Mechanic who face threatening examinations; they volunteered themselves into competitive situations which made heavy demands on their skills and capacities, exposing them to overload and evaluative situations. Often the problem for such persons is to keep the commitments to which they address themselves at a level compatible with their energies and capacities, and this is often difficult to do because of personality characteristics (such as 'high drive') which they bring with them into the work context. Perhaps this is the same as the A-type persons studied by Friedman and Rosenman (1974) who seemed to be very prone to coronary disease because of their hard driving, time-pressured pattern of life. Personality-centred research on stress and bodily disease of this sort strongly suggests that overload is not merely imposed from the outside but is, in large measure, a self-generated phenomenon.

Authority relationships
Still another work-centred source of stress which may be found in other contexts too is the difficulty that many persons have in dealing with authority and power. Most work situations have some authority-based chains of command, of which the military organization is probably the most obvious example. The stress of the work situation is then based on the turmoil generated by having a supervisor or boss, or, at the other end of the scale, by having to exercise authority over another person in a subordinate role.

Work changes or changes in the organizational arrangements
A very common source of psychological stress in the work setting consists of changes in the mode of operation of an organization, or in the procedures acquired and used over a long past period. One supervisor is lost and another takes his place. One process is abandoned and another put in its stead. An industry suffers an economic depression and one must take a job in another. Such a change can be regarded as a challenge or as a threat and, when it is necessary, the individual who is habitually insecure or lacks resources or adaptability to change may suffer greatly psychologically and physically. As in previous examples, the problem lies in both the nature of the external demands to which the person must respond and in the person himself whose personal resources and characteristics may make him especially vulnerable or enable him to weather the changes and even grow from them.

Ageing and retirement
There are a number of developmentally-centred sources of psychological stress operating in the work-setting, and one obvious example is the problem of ageing and retirement. The prospects of ageing and retirement face the person with a struggle between engagement and disengagement in the life process. Disengagement threatens the person with loss of significance, a sort of psychological death. The problem is often anticipated long before it happens in the gradual movement toward this period of life, and loss of potency is signalled in many ways, say by the attitude of management, or of one's peers, or by the inability to function as well as previously in the job. As with all the other psychosocial sources of stress mentioned above, this one is not restricted to the work context, but it may have its clearest and most poignant expression at the job.

Miscellaneous stressors
This category consists of potential stressors in the work setting which this writer regards as either less widespread and important, or simply of less general interest, although they may include some sources of stress which others would regard as basic. In any event, the use of this category allows me to list some additional potential sources of stress in the work setting without elaborating greatly upon them.

a. *Conflict between needs for affiliation and achievement as generated by role changes.* I have in mind here the situation of the shop worker who is suddenly promoted to foreman. As a foreman he is regarded by his ex-peers as no longer one of them, and yet he is on the lowest management rung without significant power or influence, a man-in-the-middle, so to speak. Such a person may have to accept thwarting of his wish for warm supportive interpersonal relationships and acceptance in the interests of achievement desires. The problems of stress created in this kind of organizational situation are sometimes discussed under the rubric of *role conflicts*, and perhaps even *role ambiguity* since it is not always clear how the new role is to be played.

b. *Existence of institutional patterns that block vital modes of coping.* Since coping processes are, I believe, crucial in the successful management of stress-emotions, and individuals differ greatly in the kinds of coping that are serviceable for them, any institutional pattern which blocks use of such forms of coping in its explicit norms and value systems, will increase the stress load for that individual. This is a subcategory within the larger rubric of conflict between an individual and an institution, and one that has been little examined. There are many possible examples. For example, if drugs or homosexual encounters are effectively proscribed in prisons, long-term inmates may be deprived of one of the important ways in which they make their imprisonment more tolerable; or if a husband who uses alcohol to ease his problems or to break down crippling social inhibitions is pressured about this by a wife who cannot abide drinking, he too may be impaired in his efforts to function within the limits of his own coping resources. Consider too the shy and introverted person who has difficulties in social situations, but who is pressured by management practices or institutional custom to participate in frequent social situations. The rule here is that institutional practices often interfere with the individual's idiosyncratic ways of coping, and as such, such practices add stress by impairing the individual's ability to manage his life effectively by means of the coping devices on which he depends.

c. *Institutional practices which violate the personal standards of the individual.* What does a person do who finds himself working for a company which manufactures napalm and who thinks that this is immoral, or for a company which requires him to contribute to political institutions which he abhors, and so on? It is easy to say that he ought to give up his job, but this is a solution which may create its own economic and social stressors. For most people, the personal values involved are not important enough for this to be a serious problem, and besides, a little bit of mental legerdemain (e.g. rationalization, denial, etc.) often neutralizes the issue (see Sanford and Comstock 1971). On the other hand, there are probably many instances in the daily work setting in which the person is called upon to take part in activities which violate standards of conduct which are important to him. For such persons, much stress can probably be produced by the conflict between institutional practices and personal values.

We must be very wary of assuming that any of the above sources of stress will reach serious proportions in any individual case, or that their mere presence alone determines the psychological or somatic outcome. Elsewhere (Lazarus 1973) I have emphasized the importance of *coping processes* in the regulation of stress-emotional states. Stress may be coped with effectively, and when stress emotions result in serious psychological disturbances (such as severe anxiety or depression) or stress diseases, we can say there has been a failure of coping. Stress is a universal in human life. However, individuals vary greatly in the extent to which they can cope with any given stressor. Moreover, when things get out of hand, there are often ways of helping the person to cope more effectively. By the same token, some work settings are more stressful or more destructive of coping processes than others, and such settings can be altered with the purpose of decreasing the stressful load on personnel, or facilitating effective coping processes. The possibilities inherent in the above are, indeed, one of the major reasons for studying the mechanisms of psychological stress, coping, and disease in any setting, including that of work. Knowledge of such mechanisms could help us ultimately to suggest the kinds of institutional settings which are most productive of stress and disease, and to assist individuals to cope better.

We must never forget that although the above partial list of sources of psychological stress in the work setting consists of some of those which are widely shared by groups and subgroups of people, their impact depends very much on what individuals bring with them into the work situation, based on their patterns of motives or commitments, on their belief systems about themselves and about how their lives are shaped, and on the kinds of coping processes of which they are capable. We must look to the individual as well as to the external environment in which persons function. The stress emotions arise out of patterns of *commerce* between a person and his environment. The type of relationship between the person and his environment over the long run determines whether there will be stress and disease, and what things might be done in the way of intervention to alleviate problems.

WORK AS A REFUGE OR FORM OF COPING

In the discussion thus far I have emphasized some of the components of the work setting that are potential sources of stress-emotion, and hence of stress disorder. I have also pointed out that the capacity of these components to generate stress depends on properties of persons which make them vulnerable to stress, and on the coping resources that the person can muster when there is some type of stressful commerce. However, there is another side to work that must not be overlooked. For many persons, work is a vital part of the processes of coping with life stress. This idea has two aspects: First, without work the potential for boredom and meaninglessness is immeasurably increased for many, perhaps most persons. This is implied in Freud's epigrammatic definition of psychological health as involving the capacity to love and work. Work is often the main means by which the person feels useful in life, and through which a significant sense of personal identity is established. Erikson (1963) has suggested, in fact, that the young adult must find a useful and meaningful place for himself in the society, and only in this way does a man or woman develop a firm sense of 'ego-identity'. Erikson cites the character of Biff in Arthur Miller's play, *Death of a salesman*, as suffering from ego-diffusion because he cannot take hold and find a productive and useful place for himself in the world. This does not necessarily imply work in the career sense, or work within the industrial or business world of the social system, but work in the sense of being useful and producing. Such a concept could apply equally to those who do not work for pay, but who raise children and help take care of households or others in the family or society at large, or who donate their efforts to what they believe to be constructive enterprises, regardless of whether or not this produces income.

Second, work is often a form of coping and a refuge. Consider, for example, the frequent use of work by people who are grieving. Many report that instead of work being a burden, in the process of 'mourning' and reorienting their lives after major loss, they are grateful for work as the best refuge against continuing high levels of distress and depression. One speaks here of 'burying oneself in work'. Work may provide a psychological haven against problems that otherwise would be insurmountable, or against loneliness and depression. For such people, not to work is to be deprived of the only viable means of coping with non-work-related stresses.

Thus, although traditionally we tend to focus attention on the *demands* or pressures of the work situation, we need to realize that the work setting can often fruitfully be regarded as a psychological *resource* rather than a source of stressful demands. My colleague, Reuvan Gal, in an unpublished study, adds the provocative observation that perhaps only certain kinds of persons are able to use work as a coping resource. Among Israeli Navy personnel in whom seasickness is a problem, even though suffering from severe levels of objective distress, some persons manage to do their work aboard ship quite well, while others cannot function at all. Those who functioned despite being sick were identified through personality testing as copers, that is, oriented toward attacking problems, productive effort, and vigilance, in contrast to others who were avoiders or deniers in outlook and style. Perhaps the most interesting point Gal makes is that among the former (copers), pursuing shipboard duties seems to minimize their subjective distress and makes them feel better. In short, for such persons work can be regarded as a resource rather than a demand or pressure; they use work not only to preserve a given image of themselves and certain value commitments, but as a way of coping with a distressing problem coincident with their work obligations. If we are to understand stress and work, we must recognize this two-sided nature of work, that it is *both* a resource for self-actualization and coping and a psychosocial source of stress. Which it is undoubtedly depends on the nature of the work setting, the non-work stressors facing the person, and his personality characteristics.

REFERENCES

ERIKSON, E. H. (1963), *Childhood and society* (second ed.). W. W. Norton, New York.

FRIEDMAN, M. and ROSENMAN, R. H. (1974). *Type A behavior and your heart*. Knopf, New York.

KAHN, R. L., WOLFE, D. M., QUINN, R. P., SNOEK, J. D., and ROSENTHAL, R. A. (1964). *Organizational stress: studies in role conflict and ambiguity*. John Wiley and Sons, New York.

LAZARUS, R. S. (1966). *Psychological stress and the coping process*. McGraw-Hill, New York.

—— (1973). The self-regulation of emotion. Paper given at symposium entitled *Parameters of emotion*, Stockholm, Sweden. [Organized by L. Levi.]

——, AVERILL, J. R., and OPTON, E. M. Jr. (1970). Towards a cognitive theory of emotion. In *Feelings and emotions* (ed. M. Arnold), Academic Press, New York.

MASLOW, A. H. (1964). Synergy in the society and in the individual. *J. Ind. Psychol.*, **20**, 153–64.

MECHANIC, D. (1962). *Students under stress*, The Free Press of Glencoe, New York.

PHILLIPS, B. N., MARTIN, R. P., and MEYERS, J. (1972). Interventions in relation to anxiety in school. In *Anxiety: current trends in theory and research*, Vol. II (ed. C. O. Spielberger), pp. 410–64. Academic Press, New York.

SANFORD, N. and COMSTOCK, C. (1971). *Sanctions for evil*. Hossey-Bass, San Francisco.

SARASON, I. G. (1972). Experimental approaches to test anxiety: attention and the uses of information. In *Anxiety: current trends in theory and research*, Vol. II (ed. C. D. Spielberger), pp. 383–403. Academic Press, New York.

SARASON, S. B. (1972). Anxiety, intervention, and the culture of the school. In *Anxiety: current trends in theory and research*, Vol. II (ed. C. D. Spielberger), pp. 470–8. Academic Press, New York.

THALER-SINGER, M. (1974). Engagement-involvement: A central phenomenon in psychophysiological research. *Psychosom. Med.*, **36**, 1–17.

WILENSKY, H. L. (1964). Varieties of work experience. *Man in a world at work* (ed. H. Borow), pp. 125–54. Houghton Mifflin, Boston, Massachusetts.

11. MODELS OF MOTIVATION AND THEIR IMPLICATION FOR OCCUPATIONAL STRESS

H. LEVINSON

DISTANCE BETWEEN EGO IDEAL AND SELF-IMAGE

The core occupational stress is the increase in the distance between the ego ideal and the self image

$$\frac{1}{\text{Self-esteem}} = \text{ego ideal} - \text{self image}$$

The greater the gap, the less a person thinks of himself and the more angry he becomes with himself (Levinson 1972). This increase in self-directed anger, a product of feelings of guilt and inadequacy, in turn produces depression. Depression is the most pervasive of all emotional illnesses and frequently precipitates physiological symptoms. The depression and physiological symptoms following experiences of loss, and the history of coronaries also following such loss, are both examples. There is a long history of animal studies which indicates that animals lower in the pecking order within a given flock, pack, or other unit have a significantly higher incidence of death and withdrawal than do victors (Mazur 1973). Defeated male mice cling to the corners of their cages for their bodily functions as contrasted to the victors who may extrude body products anywhere in their cages. Defeated male cockroaches die at significantly higher frequencies than those who are victorious (Ewing 1967). Among men, there is an inverse relationship between position in the hierarchy of the organization and the incidence and prevalence of both physical and mental illness (Kornhauser 1965). Loss of self-esteem and lower self-esteem give psychological weight and importance to the loss of a job, of a family member, or of a familiar community support.

THEORETICAL MODEL OF MOTIVATION

With this statement as a criterion, I propose to review the major theoretical models of motivation in business and industry to indicate the implications of their assumptions for occupational stress. These models should be viewed against their historical mainstreams for it is within those that the fundamental assumptions about motivation lie.

Environmental and nativistic conceptions

Two major conceptions of man dominated psychological thinking in the nineteenth and twentieth centuries. One conception, with a tradition stemming from Locke through Watson to Skinner, is an 'outside' or environment theory of motivation. It views man's motivation and behaviour as shaped primarily by forces outside himself. It is largely an empirical theory which leads to research focused on forces and factors external to the person, and is correspondingly less preoccupied with such internal factors as thinking, feeling, and subjective experiences.

The second conception is a nativistic or 'inside' theory of motivation. In its more modern form it stems from Kant, and its two most widely known contemporary exponents are Freud and Piaget. Nativistic conceptions view man as unfolding and developing physiologically and psychologically from biologically based givens. The focus is on the development and refinement of internal capacities, primarily emotional and cognitive, which give rise to certain feelings, wishes, fantasies, perceptions, attitudes, and thoughts.

Research and practice based on environmental theories tend to be concerned with the *control* of behaviour, implicitly assuming someone is controlled and someone else is controlling. Referring to work motivation, the question usually is asked, 'How can the employee *be* motivated?' Often the implication is that by doing something to the person or his environment, he can be made by someone else to do what is either desired or expected of him.

Research and practice based on nativistic theories tend to be concerned with *understanding* behaviour, and often with freeing a person to behave more nearly in keeping with his wishes or with opening a wider range of choices from which he presumably may choose alternative courses. Managerial practice based on nativistic theory related to work motivation seeks to understand the person's own motivations and to create conditions under which these can flower in the work situation to meet both the person's and the organization's needs.

Each of these major orientations leads to certain ways of organizing work, work relationships, policies and procedures, organizational structure, and managerial practice. Each in turn also has implications for the nature and degree of psychological stress experienced in the work role.

ENVIRONMENTAL APPROACH: CONSEQUENCES AND IMPLICATIONS

The environmental point of view sees man as rational

and economic in his outlook and therefore to be motivated by money or other extrinsic rewards. In the work organization man exists to serve the needs of the organization and is rewarded to the extent to which he does so. Traditionally his work process is designed for him in a highly rationalized manner, the underlying rationale of which is industrial or organizational efficiency. Such a mechanical conception operates most congenially in a bureaucratic structure in which one person is presumably interchangeable with another. In such an orientation, a person's feelings, if considered at all, are viewed as a troublesome interference in an otherwise rational, organized, controlled system. The dominant mode of motivation is to appeal to reason, on grounds presumed to be obvious, backed up by 'carrot-and-stick'. The greater wisdom of superiors in the hierarchy is taken for granted and a person's economic fate is dependent on their greater knowledge and power. In such a system a person's value is related to his position in the organizational hierarchy. In the Western world, particularly in the United States, there is intense competition for position in the hierarchy, stimulated and fostered by higher management. Thus a population is developed which includes not only winners, but also proportionately greater numbers of losers. Those who cannot enter the hierarchy at all in a context which values power and position are the most helpless and, therefore, by definition, defeated.

Some organizations and some managements, in an effort to cope with the more and more blatantly impersonal aspects of such assumptions and organization structures, seek to obtain loyalty and commitment from employees on the basis of paternalism, an echo of the ancient feudal conception of *noblesse oblige*.

Most industrial sociology and organizational theory is concerned with describing bureaucratic structure, assuming that structure to be given and further, assuming a reward–punishment model of individual motivation. Much industrial psychology, with its emphasis on testing, selection, placement, rewards, supervision, morale, and motivation, is heavily environmental in its underlying motivational assumptions.

Competition; defeat; alienation. A number of stresses are precipitated by this conception and orientation. The first of these is obviously that many people who lose out in the competitive struggle for position or authority feel themselves defeated. Others who feel themselves to be engineered into a work process as the equivalent of pieces of machinery, particularly those who are doing monotonous and repetitive tasks, view themselves as being relatively powerless to cope with the fragmentation of work and the impersonality of the work organization; this in turn alienates them from each other, and from gratification in the work process, and lowers their self-image.

Furthermore the erratic ups and downs of levels of employment in such highly rationalized industries, a phenomenon over which the employee has little control,

serve further to create a sense of inadequacy and passive helplessness which, for the same reason, magnify and intensify feelings of self-directed anger.

When employees rebel against this view of them and against being manipulated by others, they usually do so in the form of strikes, sabotage, resistance, and other forms of hostility. Thus, anger and often guilt are mobilized. These, together with economic losses, constitute further stresses.

In such a manipulative context it is difficult to evolve an identification with the organization. This inability undermines social relationships at work.

Thus the reward–punishment motivational thesis built on an environmental psychology which views man as an object to be controlled and modified, and personality as the product of such 'learning' bears within it the potential for being even more destructive to the mental health of individuals.

Interpersonal relations

The second major orientation arose largely from the work of Elton Mayo and his colleagues (Mayo 1933). This, too, is an environmental theory, often coupled with reward and punishment assumptions, but calling into question the economic man model. That is, he thought people worked primarily because of the social relationships on the job and not primarily because of the money they could earn there. Mayo called attention to the need for human contact, group relationships, group control of their work effort, and the essence of relatedness within the organization. In fact, he saw interpersonal relationships as primary and work as secondary. His work stimulated interest in supervisor–supervisee relationships and work group interaction and gave impetus to the human relations movement in industry. It also led to criticism of the ennui of much factory work, followed by efforts at job enlargement, concern with making the workplace more congenial, and, sometimes, to paternalism.

Mayo laid heavy emphasis on group membership and thus in turn on people's need for affiliation with their work groups. He recognized that such affiliation and interdependence provided mutual support and group cohesion which enhanced self-esteem by providing affective bolstering of the self-image and simultaneously increased his power by giving one as a member of a group greater influence over what went on in the work process.

In many ways, Mayo's assumptions and the practices based on them were much more supportive of the mental health of individuals and work groups than the classical reward–punishment model, which pitted men against each other. Nevertheless there are certain consequences of operating with such assumptions.

Group pressure. If group membership, group cohesion, and interpersonal relationships are primary, there is great pressure on the individual to sacrifice his individuality as the price of getting along. It is an old story that some work groups are preoccupied with feather-bedding or stretching out the work to occupy the time available. Other groups are concerned with limiting production, still others with engaging in hostilities with managements, and yet others in fighting off innovation. Many devote themselves to sustaining guildlike protective devices which result in increasing obsolescence of competence or skill. Such practices ultimately result in fewer jobs in the marketplace. In the United States such overprotection has happened among coal miners, among those in construction craft work, and even among airline navigators, thus compelling unnecessary redundancy and forcing managements to turn to other possible avenues of achieving those same goals by circumventing those groups which are regarded as obstructionistic.

The goals of the group, often political in nature, may deviate from those of the individual, thus increasing the anger, guilt, inadequacy, and hostility of the individual. The individual may be made so dependent on the group, as frequently happens in American unions, that he dare not act according to his conscience. Furthermore, preoccupation with in-group and out-group matters tends to divide the world into a 'we' and 'they' or warring factions of management and labour. Often there is an uneasy truce between such factions with frequent labour disturbances resulting in hostilities, sabotage, and other destructive acts, some of which may tear apart whole communities.

The employee pays for the degree of cohesion and support he gets in the form of being controlled by others. Except by organized bargaining methods, he has little control over his own fate. In the United States, even the most highly unionized plant can be closed down. Frequently the employee is caught in the middle, torn by dual loyalties which may be magnified by official differences, as between labour leaders and managements, with which he has little identification.

Aspiration increase through cognitive means
Another environmentally based conception of motivation is that of David McClelland (1967). He contends that people can be taught to aspire to higher levels of achievement by cognitive means, defining and meeting their own levels of aspiration and setting goals for themselves. I have serious doubts about such a theory because, as McClelland himself points out, such a motive 'induced' in adulthood requires continued group support to sustain it. It seems to me unrealistic to assume that by brief teaching, exercises, and games one can evolve and sustain a powerful drive to achievement over a long period of time even if that achievement feeds on itself, that is, that success breeds more success. Many who are subjected to such training may well feel disappointed in themselves for failing.

Expectancy theory neglects underlying psychological issues
Some industrial psychologists like Lawler, Hall, and Porter offer what they speak of as expectancy theory (Lawler 1973). That is, people are motivated to achieve those ends which are likely to meet their expectations. However, this orientation is without substantive content. It has no underlying theory of motivation except a reward–punishment one. It is difficult to define consistent expectations except in personality terms. This theory is therefore descriptive but not explanatory.

The mental health consequence is that it may well lead to manipulative efforts to determine expectancies by asking questions and getting conscious answers. Thus managements can respond to what people say they expect without ever dealing with underlying psychological issues. For example, employees who feel alienated, alone, powerless and otherwise inadequate, may respond to questionnaires about pay by saying they want higher pay. Raising pay however will not deal with their underlying feelings of alienation. In fact a rise may contribute to their feelings of not being understood at all in the same way that a parent who substitutes gifts for understanding may anger his child. Thus they may feel even more unrelated to the major forces which have an effect on their lives and therefore more helpless as pawns in other people's manipulations. The same general criticism is true of Vroom's (1964) goal-path theory. The problem lies not in describing the path but in adequately and accurately understanding the nature of the underlying internal motive which gives a goal meaning.

SATISFACTION OF NEEDS

Most of the work on nativistic theory revolves around defining people's needs which, in turn, lead to motivations and then again, when those needs are fulfilled, to satisfaction or gratification. Much of this work is based largely on the tension reduction theories of Kurt Lewin (Marrow 1969) and Abraham Maslow (1954). Lewin's is largely descriptive; Maslow's in categorical.

Maslow defined a hierarchy of normative needs, that is, needs which are distributed across the population of human beings. Maslow classified human needs on five levels. In ascending order these are: physiological needs, safety needs, needs for belonging and love, needs for esteem, and need for self-actualization. When a lower order need is fulfilled the next higher level order need becomes prepotent and therefore motivating.

Maslow based his self-actualization conception on the work of Kurt Goldstein (1939). Working with brain-injured soldiers in the First World War, Goldstein noted that when a part of the brain was injured the remainder of the brain tried to compensate and to operate as a whole. By simple extrapolation Maslow concluded that there is a tendency in the organism toward fulfilling its own potential, thus for actualizing itself.

While superficially valid, closer inspection discloses that this simple extrapolation has many shortcomings. As a matter of fact, people do not strive to fulfil their potential. Many people are quite contented operating at an intellectual or cultural level quite different from that for which they might be ideally competent. There is no clinical or experimental evidence to indicate that failure to achieve self-fulfilment in the sense of fulfilling potential precipitates neurosis. I know of no study which delineates what people are fully capable of achieving, then contrasts that with what they have achieved, and demonstrates that the gap produces stress. There are a number of studies which indicate that people are less satisfied with the degree of autonomy they have at work than that which they would like to have. However, we do not know whether the stated wish for autonomy is: (1) the same as self-actualization; (2) whether it is a mask for denying underlying dependency needs; (3) a means by which people have rationalized the fact that they have not attained greater autonomy; (4) whether it is merely a reflection of hostility to anybody else who has greater power than they have; or (5) whether they are using a conscious statement referring to greater objective freedom as a metaphor to speak of the constrictions of their own consciences which they unconsciously feel. It is difficult if not impossible to ascertain for any given individual, let along a group of individuals, what constitutes self-actualization. Many may be led to frustration in pursuit of a psychological ghost.

On the other hand, while it is not an easy task, it is possible to define the approximate nature of the ego ideal for individuals and groups of individuals, and to contrast that with well-defined self-images. It is also possible to measure intensity of disappointment, with accompanying anger toward oneself, as well as degree of self-esteem, and to relate those feelings to the incidence and prevalence of symptoms.

Thus the Maslow conception is not only inaccurate when it comes to dealing with specific individuals and groups, but it can also contribute to the intensity of stress. When people are told that they should actualize their potential but they have no way of ascertaining their potential and cast about in random fashion in an effort to do so, then their frustration is increased. When autonomy is equated with self-actualization, and there is a failure to explore the underlying psychology of that wish, one may try to give greater autonomy to work groups which are happily dependent. Then, despite their wish as expressed in words, they may well panic when asked to make their own decisions. Furthermore, the heavy emphasis on autonomy often leads to greater participation in decision-making. Naïve participatory management efforts often result in emasculating leadership or in abdication of leadership. The absence of leadership leads to greater chaos, lack of direction, lack of cohesion, and falling back on group defences and group norms as people try to control the anomalous situations in which they find themselves.

As indicated in the earlier discussion of the difficulties with the Mayo thesis, groups too can produce destructive stresses and tensions. While on the one hand it may be possible for some few people, particularly in managerial ranks, to have higher self-images because of greater autonomy, there may be other products of the theory

and its applications which have destructive effects. The theory and its applications are never examined for these implications.

In all fairness it must be said that the proponents of self-actualizing man sees him as spontaneous, creative, and seeking self-expression. They seek to free the working man and the manager from the constraints of bureaucracy and unilateral power. They continue to view work as a necessity but contend that it need not be psychologically destructive to the worker. Furthermore, they point out that what seemed efficient to the bureaucratic model of economic man is really less efficient, because control by hierarchical relationships and industrial engineering not only dehumanizes man but requires him to defend himself against such control by passive resistance and reluctance to be involved in the system. In fact, between the lines of conceptions of self-actualizing man is the notion that organizations exist to serve man rather than vice versa.

Those who have built on Maslow have sought to reduce power differentials in bureaucratic structures. Their work has given rise to such conceptions as participation in decision-making, more adequate support from higher level management, and responsible involvement in the work itself and in decisions about how it is to be done. They have raised questions about organizational structure. The group dynamics movement brought into vogue emphasis on communication, partnership with respect to task accomplishment, and the reduction of psychological barriers to co-operation.

However, there is an inherent contradiction between many of these efforts and the continued acceptance of a reward–punishment psychology. None of these theorists has a systematic theory of personality on which to base conceptions of need. They often implicitly see man as having limited motivational dimensions and frequently try to force nativistic conceptions into organizations which are based fundamentally on reward–punishment assumptions.

MASLOW-BASED THEORIES ABOUT WORK

Examination of a few of the more prominent theories about work motivation based on the Maslow conceptions will help to clarify some of the mental health problems they pose.

The work of Frederick Herzberg (1966) on motivation through the work itself emphasizes job enrichment. Herzberg conceives of satisfiers and dissatisfiers. Satisfiers are achievement, recognition, the work itself, responsiblity, advancement, and growth. Dissatisfiers include company policy and administration, supervision, working conditions, interpersonal relationships (with superiors, subordinates, and peers), salary, status, job security, and personal life. Satisfiers are motivating; dissatisfiers cannot motivate people to work but can counteract motivation. In Herzberg's conception they are *hygienic* factors which can contaminate the psychological environment. Herzberg urges management to increase the challenging aspects of the job to make it more self-fulfilling, achievement-motivated, and self-actualizing. Although Herzberg does not follow the model of economic man, he assumes that *higher management* should enrich the jobs of lower level people. He raises few questions about organizational structure, controls or power relationships, and minimizes interpersonal relationships as significant motivating forces. Work must be given meaning largely by expanding responsibility and extending recognition, and from the intrinsic satisfaction the person derives from it.

McGregor's (1960) position is largely nativistic, holding that man's needs are primarily social and egoistic. He holds work to be a natural expenditure of energy, and derives commitment from esteem and self-actualization. Commitment frees people to be imaginative, self-disciplined, responsible, and co-operative. He envisaged the possibility of integrating individual and organizational goals, and emphasized interpersonal relationships and flexibility of organizational structure.

Argyris (1964), too, seeks to integrate individual and organizational needs. He sees bureaucratic structure as inhibiting the fulfilment of individual needs, particularly those for a sense of personal value, self-esteem, and independence. Like Herzberg and McGregor, he views individuals as self-motivated rather than motivated by forces outside themselves. Both McGregor and Argyris advocated sensitivity training as a medium for obtaining openness, co-operation and commitment, although Argyris and Schon (1974) have since de-emphasized sensitivity training.

Likert (1961) advocates a group-type organization structure rather than the traditional bureaucratic model. He sees the optimum organization as a mosaic of interacting and overlapping groups, connected by 'linking pins', persons who are members of two groups within the organization. He gives heavy emphasis to small group interaction, and that between superiors and subordinates. He advocates group accountability, consensus decision-making and group goal-setting. His major theme is the principle of supportive relationships as basic to a sense of personal worth and importance.

Blake and Mouton (1978), too, see no necessary conflict between individual and organizational objectives. They emphasize managerial style as the major device for counteracting bureaucracy, and their *Grid*, a set of projects, exercises, and tasks done with others, is a way of providing managers with insight into their own behaviour, with heavy emphasis on interpersonal relationships.

Herzberg's work is heavily based on the method he used to obtain his results. For many people money is indeed of primary importance. Furthermore, almost all of the research on supervision and leadership as well as role stress indicates that the key relationship between superior and subordinate has significant impact on the behaviour of individuals. Herzberg's work denies these relationships as well as the underlying problem of dependency. Furthermore job enrichment and job enlargement have turned out not to be as widely useful as Herzberg's theory would suggest because many people prefer not to have more complex jobs. Increasing challenge may make for increasing stress.

Criticism of the four theories
None of these four theorists take significantly into account individual variability or other significant factors. As Bennis (1972) points out, these theories place a heavy burden of responsibility on the boss without taking into acount his needs. They do not allow for anger, destructiveness, inconsistency, playfulness, loners, weaklings, liars, villains, or those who don't want to be helped or nurtured. Furthermore because they do not differentiate among individuals and groups, they prescribe for an environmental void. There are indeed extremely powerful external forces in management situations, Bennis notes.

In essence, these theories have introduced a certain naïvety which may lead to managerial abdication and failure to differentiate the psychological needs of one person or group from those of another. Many who are involved in participative management find that activity to be chaos unless managers are well trained and understand the complexities of the dimensions they are working with. In Likert's conception, the whole idea of supportive relationships is very important for mental health. But in all these conceptions there is a total lack of emphasis on creative leadership without which there can be no effective organizations.

PSYCHOLOGICAL MAN

In contrast to the humanistic, self-actualizing theories of motivation, which are derived largely from academic conceptions of personality, there are the considerably more complex theories of motivation derived from insights originally based on clinical practice with individuals, largely by clinical psychologists and psychiatrists. These theories, which might be categorized under the rubric of 'psychological man', are heavily nativistic in that they place strong emphasis on the conception that man is continuously balancing his sexual and aggressive drives, the pressures and demands of his super ego or conscience, and the realities of his world in an effort to master himself and it. This view is also environmentalistic because the focus is not on man alone or on the organization alone but, significantly, the man–organization relationship. Major theorists of this point of view are Elliot Jaques, Abraham Zaleznik, and myself.

Jaques (1970) is concerned with two areas: superior–subordinate relationships, modes through which employees can express their power constructively with respect to policies, and practices of salary administration, which enable employees to compare their level of pay with that of other groups whom they judge to be carrying equivalent levels of responsibility. Jaques seeks to cope with the employee's sense of insecurity and the stirring of his unconscious anxieties when contemporary threats and problems reawaken repressed childhood conflicts that then lead to irrational behaviour.

Zaleznik and Kets de Vries (1975) direct most of their attention to the special psychological problems facing people who become organizational leaders and to the psychological forces that compel people to invent systems of organizing work that then influence society and thereby affect other people. Zaleznik and his students have investigated the ways in which the unconscious motives of individuals affect decision-making. In addition, he has emphasized the capacity of the individual to mould his own life, both at work and at home. That emphasis on what the individual can do to act responsibly to control his own destiny contrasts with the humanists' appeal to enlightened management.

Three classes of needs

My own conception is built around an ego psychology model. I have defined the three broad classes of needs to be met as (1) ministration needs—for care and support from others; (2) maturation needs—for growth and development; and (3) mastery needs—for control of one's fate—allowing considerable variation in the definition of such needs for different individuals and groups of people (Levinson 1968).

As indicated in the introduction, my fundamental thesis is that the most powerful motivating force for any human being is his wish to attain his ego ideal. In the course of growing up, out of our identifications with our parents, out of our wish to emulate them, out of the encouragement and affection of our teachers and other people who are important to us, out of the refinements of our skills and competencies, we evolve a picture for ourselves of how we should be at our ideal best. When

we work toward our ideal best we like ourselves; when we come close, we are elated. When we do not, we become extremely angry with ourselves.

Meeting the demands of one's ego ideal

Therefore I view a person's relationship to his work and work organization as part of his generalized effort to meet the demands of his ego ideal and, as a result, to be significantly related both to his emotional health and his motivation at work. The kind of work he does and the nature of his relationship to the organization either supports his personality structure and enables him to use himself psychologically as he would like to do, thereby enhancing both his motivation and his health, or it impairs both.

Thus I do not see bureaucracy as either good or bad by definition, for some tasks require bureaucratic structure and some people need more structured organizational support than others to satisfy their dependency needs. I take seriously the psychological interaction of the person and his organization and the psychological usefulness of organizational structure.

I am particularly interested in the leadership role, which I consider to be more complex and active than do most of the other theorists. If all organizations in any society are essentially recapitulations of the family structure in that society, then the leader is psychologically in a parent-like role (that is, he or she encounters unconscious expectations that he behave in the modal way a parent behaves in this culture). He must understand and act upon that role to ensure the perpetuation of the organization.

I believe the theories of psychological man to have a greater promise for contributing to the mental health of individuals. I think they also have significant potential for contributing to the organization, structure, and leadership of all kinds of institutions in such a way as to increase the capacity of people to adapt more effectively to their rapidly changing environments.

REFERENCES

ARGYRIS, C. (1964). *Integrating the individual and the organization.* New York.
ARGYRIS, C. and SCHON, D. A. (1974). *Theory in practice: increasing professional effectiveness.* San Francisco, California.
BENNIS, W. (1972). Chairman Mao in perspective. *Harvard Bus. Rev.*, **50**, (4), 140.
BLAKE, R. and MOUTON, J. (1978). *The new managerial grid.* Houston, Texas.
EWING, L. (1967). Fighting and stress from death in a cockroach. *Science*, **155**, 1035–6.
GOLDSTEIN, K. (1939). *The organism.* New York.
HERZBERG, F. (1966). *Work and the nature of man.* Cleveland, Ohio.
JAQUES, E. (1970). *Work, creativity and mental health.* New York.
KORNHAUSER, A. (1965). *Mental health of the industrial worker.* New York.

LAWLER, E. (1973). *Motivation in work organizations.* Monterey, California.
LEVINSON, H. (1968). *The exceptional executive.* Cambridge, Massachusetts.
—— (1972). *Executive stress.* New York.
LIKERT, R. (1961). *New patterns in management.* New York.
MCCLELLAND, D. (1975). *Power.* New York.
MCGREGOR, D. (1960). *The human side of enterprise.* New York.
MARROW, A. (1969). *The practical theorist.* New York.
MASLOW, A. (1954). *Motivation and personality.* New York.
MAYO, E. (1933). *The human problems of an industrial civilization.* New York.
MAZUR, A (1973). A cross species comparison of status in small established groups. *Amer. Soc. Rev.*, **38**, 513–530.
VROOM, V. (1964). *Work and motivation.* New York.
ZALEZNIK, A. and KETS DE VRIES, M. F. R. (1975). *Power and the corporate mind.* Boston.

12. PSYCHOSOCIAL ASPECTS OF INDUSTRIAL PRODUCT METHODS

BERTIL GARDELL

DEFINITIONS

The psychosocial problems of working life may be structured in many different ways depending upon the purpose of the analysis. Individual rewards and strains in the job world are obviously affected by various factors relating both to society's and the job world's macro aspects, the design of the leadership system, to social and physical micro aspects in the working environment, as well as to circumstances away from work. This chapter does not intend fully to portray this whole problem complex but will restrict its focus to production technology, as expressed in the organization and content of work, and its effects on man from the psychosocial viewpoint. This delimitation is mainly justified with reference to the present state of knowledge in behavioural science which emphasizes the central importance of industrial technology, both for the institutions and life-style offered by industrial society and for the more immediate working conditions typical of large-scale industrial manufacture. It should also be observed that principles taken from the area of goods production are being applied today both to administrative work and to the organization of various types of service work.

There are great similarities among the industrial systems in countries which otherwise differ from one another culturally and politically. Research on the human condition in industrial work shows that man's problems and stresses in industrialized production are very similar from country to country. However, this is not to suggest that one need surrender to technological determinism: if anything, existing conditions point to the necessity of subordinating technico-economic values to a welfare objective, one that allows for what we know about man as a biological and social being. Thus yet another motive for limiting the discussion given here is the conviction that production technology is not only one of the main issues in the working environment but that it can also be affected by social and humanistic values and the knowledge that research, anchored in these values, can provide. In this perspective it becomes important to try to isolate the effects of technology on man and society, because this research will provide us with a scientific basis for concrete discussions on how to shape and organize technology with reference to values other than short-term efficiency. It stands to reason that other factors also affect man's situation at work, but these intervening factors must not be permitted to divert attention away from the work itself, its organization and content, and the importance this has for the human condition in the industrial society.

ORGANIZATION AND CONTENT OF WORK: A SUMMARY OF BEHAVIOURAL SCIENCE KNOWLEDGE

In the past few decades, much of the psychological research dealing with the human condition at work has focused on the organization and content of work and the significance of this for different aspects of the individual's status, rewards, and effort costs in the modern, highly industrialized, goods production sector. This research is using criterion variables (dependent variables) from many disciplines, among them physiology, medicine, and psychiatry, clinical psychology, social psychology, and family and political sociology. The experimental (independent) variables comprise different measurements and descriptions of the nature, conditions, and organization of work.

A great deal of interest has been devoted to the psychosocial consequences flowing from a far-reaching fragmentation of work and a control of work pace and work methods through detailed preplanning and through the machine system. Much attention has been called to the relation between working conditions of this kind and feelings of monotony, social isolation, lack of freedom, time-pressure, and mental strain. The connections between these perceptions and the individual's behaviour on the labour market, his health, his democratic participation, and his use of leisure have also been studied, but to a lesser extent. Examples from the investigations referred to are given in the following sections.

Theoretically, a large part of this research proceeds from assumptions concerning the general structures of basic human needs, which should be understood as something quite apart from the demands and aspirations created in a specific situation at a specific time. Much of the analysis has concerned the ability of the mechanized and bureaucratized job world to satisfy these basic needs. Although this research is, of course, aware that people are different, it believes that a perspective which looks at basic similarities between people rather than the dissimilarities and states of adaption is better able to yield the generalized knowledge that is needed to underpin a discussion about the effects of production technology on working men and women and on society. Over and above matters of material survival and security, this research has attached particularly great weight to those technological or organizational factors in work which have central bearing upon the individual:

1. Influence in the job world and self-determination over work pace and working methods;
2. Overview and meaningfulness in the working role;
3. Co-operation and fellowship with other people.

These three factors seem to be at the core of work motivation and enjoyment of work. Shortcomings in the satisfaction of these ego-needs are often described in terms of alienation or in terms of time pressure, fatigue, and physical and mental illness. The effects of these working conditions on the individual's interest in decision-making at the work place have lately also been subjects of public debate and of research on industrial democracy.

Some of the problems concerning the organization and content of work may also be regarded in terms of overstimulation and understimulation, e.g. the question of how repetitive and one-sided jobs or mechanically controlled work pace affect the individual. Social psychology has shown that workers tend to react to these jobs as being monotonous and associated with mental pressure, but it is not known whether these work characteristics also lead to physiological stress reactions and, if so, whether subjective and objective reactions occur at the same time as effects of the given situation. However, research on psychophysiological stress has shown under laboratory conditions that efficiency and well-being are maximal with moderate stimulation and diminish both in extremely stimulus-poor situations and in cases of excessive stimulation. Experiments have also shown that the subjective interpretation of a situation is of critical importance for physiological stress reactions and that this interpretation may be influenced by increased personal control over the work situation.

In this way, this experimental laboratory research closely ties into the more practically oriented discussion of job design. The desirability of letting the individual exercise greater influence over work planning and performance is, of course, chiefly motivated on general ideological and sociological grounds, but it can also be justified on biological grounds by virtue of this research.

Studies have been carried out in various industrialized countries which seek to explain as exactly as possible which characteristics of work organization and job design describe central prerequisites for satisfying ego-relevant needs in the job world, and which may conceivably explain the perceptions of monotony, time pressure, feelings of indifference to work, etc., which so many people experience in the industrial society. If one looks to the whole international field it may be contended by way of summary that psychological and sociological research has furnished ample evidence to prove that the following factors are incompatible with sound working conditions:

(1) Authoritarian and detailed leadership;
(2) Tasks which seriously curtail the individual's opportunities to make all-round use of his resources;
(3) Working conditions which indicate that the production system asks little contribution from the individual in terms of knowledge, responsibility, and initiative;
(4) Working conditions which afford the individual little scope for exercising influence over work planning and layout;
(5) Tasks which prevent the individual from deciding work pace and working methods for himself;
(6) Tasks which afford few or no human contacts on the job.

Results of this nature have been obtained in many investigations, performed with different methods and under varying political and economic conditions in the larger society. In so far as research reports are available from industrialized countries with socialistic economies, they seem to show that the problem complex bound up with large-scale manufacturing work is more or less the same as in the Western world. Further, the results have been shown to hold valid for groups of different ages, sex, education, and income even though, of course, severe criticism is more often to be found among young people and among those of good educational attainment.

The effects of these working conditions will, of course, vary depending on the method and the groups studied. The following effects have repeatedly been observed:

(1) *Feelings* in the individual, e.g. of monotony, social isolation, strain, fatigue, powerlessness, apathy;
(2) *Active behaviour* such as grievances, suggestions for changes, in some instances go-slows and strikes, employee turnover, and reluctance to take on certain jobs;
(3) *Passive behaviour* such as resignation, low motivation, indifference to product quality, absence from work;
(4) *Social spillover effects*, e.g. lower life satisfaction, lower political and cultural activity;
(5) *Repercussions on individual health and well-being*, e.g. lower self-esteem; more symptoms of anguish and anxiety, such as depression, sleep disorders, and mental fatigue; greater propensity for psychosomatic symptoms, such as hypertension and cardio-vascular disease, gastro-intestinal disturbances, and various aches in the head, back, joints, and muscles which are not readily explainable on physiological grounds alone.

Obviously, these results are to be understood as reflecting dominant tendencies in the populations studied; there will always be considerable individual differences in the reaction to any one environment. In spite of long psychological research on these issues it has not been possible, however, to show what types of individual characteristics make people more vulnerable or resistant to repetitive and constrained tasks—except such 'characteristics' as age, sex, and education, which are readily interpreted in terms of bargaining power on the labour market or in terms of values held by these people as a result of educational processes related to the larger society. In addition, we have to consider the effects caused by different types of selection mechanisms. Their impact is unclear, however, and in many cases it may well be that the effects of a particular environment on the individual are *disguised* rather than explained by these selection mechanisms. Even if we have to take into account a considerable area of uncertainty, the principal results arrived at by all these investigations seem clear enough: namely, certain, identifiable characteristics of job design give rise in most people to certain types of reactions which are harmful to the individual as a biological and social being and thus are of profound importance for him personally as well as for the whole of industrialized society.

ORGANIZATION AND CONTENT OF WORK: EXAMPLES OF RESEARCH RESULTS ON PSYCHOSOCIAL EFFECTS

To support the overview given above, examples will be given here of results which are typical of the research under consideration. Preference will go to citing Swedish investigations, but some outstanding international research, which has greatly influenced Scandinavian research, should first be mentioned.

One of the best-known socio-psychological studies of man's working conditions ever made was done in the late 1940s in an American car-manufacturing plant (Walker and Guest 1952). Above all, this study shows how the assembly-line—with its mechanical work pace and rigidly fragmented tasks—leads to serious discontent, stress, and alienation among the workers. Those who could adapt to this kind of work were reported to be a minority of about 10 per cent. A high wage level tied the workers to their jobs but did not promote an acceptable psychological adjustment. Since accounts of this seminal project have appeared in several publications, it need not be described at greater length in the present context. None the less it may be of interest to mention that the guide-lines for restructuring of work in the form of job enrichment, increased autonomy, etc., which are now being discussed so animatedly in most industrialized countries sprang full-fledged from a study that was published nearly 25 years ago! Not only that, but one of its authors, Robert Guest, did a renewed study more than 20 years later in which he observed that no major changes had taken place in work layout or in the workers' reactions (Guest 1973). Perhaps it could be inferred from this follow-up study that criticism had

become even more accentuated, especially among the younger workers, and had found its chief expression in high rates of absenteeism and staff turnover.

Of other well-known investigations mention may be made of Kornhauser's *Mental health of the industrial worker* (Kornhauser 1965) and Blauner's *Alienation and freedom* (Blauner 1964). Kornhauser notes that different signs of low mental health were systematically more widespread among workers assigned to distinctively repetitive jobs with one-sided or low skill requirements. An extensive control of the individual's background and family origins led Kornhauser to conclude that such jobs tend directly to affect man's mental health unfavourably. Blauner's investigation primarily demonstrates the importance that production technology has for the individual's feeling of alienation at work and in society. That feeling is chiefly induced by mass production technology with its fragmented tasks, machine-paced work systems, and isolating social organization. Reference to these investigations will be made at various places in the text.

The present author conducted a series of Swedish studies concerned with the relation between job design, individual perceptions of work, and mental health during the years 1964 to 1975. The central document, *Produktionsteknik och arbetsglädje* (Technology, alienation and mental health), which summarizes the whole project, was published in 1971 (Gardell 1971). The studies show the following results, among others:

(a) Feelings of monotony, mental strain, and social isolation are much more common in relation to tasks objectively marked by serious curtailments of autonomy, skill requirements, and social interaction. These results persist after allowance is made for age, sex, education, income, type of supervision, and satisfaction with earnings, and they stand out with particular clarity in the mass production industry. A measure of ambivalence was found for the continuous flow/process industry, showing that the more skilled and autonomous jobs in this industry are simultaneously perceived to be more interesting and more strenuous mentally compared with the less skilled jobs. These main results tally pretty well with those of other studies, including the ones by Blauner, Kornhauser, and Walker and Guest referred to above.

(b) There are considerable individual differences in subjective perceptions of jobs that are objectively similar. About one-fourth of the group doing jobs with low discretion and low skill requirements perceive their work to be sufficiently interesting. In both types of industry, persons over 50 years of age are strongly overrepresented in these groups. In the mass production industry, furthermore, the groups who are satisfied with repetitive work contain an overrepresentation of women. Also, there are some relatively young and well-educated people in skilled tasks who perceive their jobs as monotonous. By and large these variations may be explained in terms of bargaining power on the labour market and aspiration associated with formal training.

(c) The breakdown by *age* shows that young people react especially negatively to the monotony and lack of freedom associated with narrowly defined, machine-paced, short-cycle jobs. Younger persons also perceive their work to be more strenuous mentally than older persons. But if the younger manpower is assigned to skilled jobs with a high degree of autonomy these generational differences tend to disappear. This reaction among younger workers doing repetitive tasks has also been referred to in several other investigations (Sheppard and Herrick 1971).

(d) The research population evinces a marked selection by *sex* towards different types of jobs, indicating a relatively larger proportion of women in repetitive, low-paying work. For purposes of sex comparison, therefore, the nature and content of work has been kept under control. It then turns out that the difference between men and women, both as regards work motivation and absenteeism, tends to disappear when both men and women are placed in equivalent jobs with *high* skill requirements and *high* autonomy. The women workers in this type of job also show higher aspirations and greater self-esteem. Comparisons of men and women doing equivalent jobs with *low* skill requirements produce an irregular picture, but usually show that women are less critically disposed than men towards repetitive work. This is interpreted as a function of lower aspirations among women associated with their weaker status on the labour market (Gardell *et al.* 1968).

(e) There is a substantial difference, *between* entry-level non-manual and manual workers in the general attitude to work, with the former less inclined to regard work solely instrumentally, i.e. from the earnings aspect. Moreover, far fewer non-manual workers perceive their jobs to be monotonous, mentally strenuous, and as isolating them from workmates (Gardell 1967). As to differences *within* the non-manual group, these go in the same direction as within the manual groups, i.e. the lower the degree of autonomy and the lower the skills required by the job, the more it is perceived to be dull and hectic. This finding holds irrespective of age group and for both men and women. Similar results have been obtained by Bradley (1970) in a study of women bank employees as well as in non-Scandinavian studies. In summary, it should be observed that when the work of non-manuals is organized along the same lines as manufacturing work, then the perception of work and the general attitude to work will ressemble that of the manual production worker.

(f) The combination of 'authoritarian' supervisor and one-sided work is associated with distinctive feelings of monotony, stress, and lack of freedom in both types of industry. This is also the most usual combination in the mass production industry. On the other hand, it would appear that an immediate superior is often in a good position to compensate for those constraints on discretionary behaviour and skilled conduct which are created by the production technology. This is in line with the notion of 'social support' as a buffering factor between job demands and worker health (Kahn 1973).

(g) A concurrent breakdown by work content and income shows that feelings of monotony and strain are not affected by size of income. Obviously, this does not mean that income is immaterial to the evaluation of a job, but income differentials are apparently unable to explain the differences of monotony and mental strain which prevail in jobs of varying content and design.

(h) The connections between work's socio-technical and economic conditions and different criteria of mental health show that persons doing one-sided jobs and/or having low pay consistently exhibit a lower life satisfaction and lower self-esteem, and they also report various mental and somatic complaints to a higher degree. This result accords well with the findings of Kornhauser's extensive studies in the United States. If at the same time allowance is made for work perception, the Swedish studies make the added observation that the ones who primarily show different signs of lower mental health are the alienated workers. According to a special study from the forest industry, job satisfaction and different criteria of mental health correlate with doctor-diagnosed symptoms from head and back and with gastro-intestinal complaints (Gardell 1969). A later investigation of the saw-mill industry shows that workers, whose jobs are simultaneously characterized by extremely short operating cycles, machine-controlled work pace, and high standards of judgement-making, report feelings of monotony and strain to a much higher degree than other workers, in addition to which they show drastically higher absenteeism and many more psychosomatic symptoms such as nervous complaints, sleep disorders, and gastro-intestinal symptoms. In some cases they even report trance-like, 'psychedelic' reactions resembling those that have been found in experiments with extremely one-sided stimulation or in isolation experiments. It should be observed that these sawmill workers are highly skilled, have high pay, and are carefully chosen by management (Frankenhaeuser and Gardell 1976; Johansson *et al.* 1978).

INVESTIGATIONS CONCERNED WITH POSSIBLE SPILLOVER EFFECTS FROM WORK ON CONDITIONS OUTSIDE WORK

Studies which more directly concern themselves with the relation between qualitative aspects of work and the individual's circumstances away from work are very rare. The Swedish studies cited above indicate that jobs of low autonomy and low skill requirements have a low needs-satisfying value for the individual. This state of affairs is accompanied by lower self-esteem, lower general life satisfaction, and an increased number of nervous complaints. In some American studies it has been found that individuals who are strongly alienated from their work generally show lower political activity, i.e. they take less part in activities and proceedings of the kind that might affect their own living conditions (Sheppard and Herrick 1971).

The Swedish Low Incomes Investigation have shown some results of interest in this connection. First, employed workers who suffer from physical handicaps of different kinds, such as impaired vision, hearing, and locomotion, are found to take less part in leisure activities than those without these physical handicaps. The same holds for those groups whose mental health is considered to be greatly impaired. All these groups are also isolated from relatives and friends to a greater extent than non-handicapped persons, and isolation correlates in its turn with less involvement in leisure activities. Second, the studies show that employees doing heavy and fatiguing work take much less part in various leisure activities than persons who do not have such jobs. This finding may be said to hold with particular force for cultural and intellectual activities of the kind which require active participation and communication with the surrounding world (Lundahl 1971).

In a secondary analysis made on these data the joint effects on 'political participation' of varying job demands and worker control were analysed (Karasek 1979). It was shown that in jobs with a low workload and low control ('passive jobs') are the ones with the least varied leisure and the lowest political efficacy. In following up changes in working conditions for the same population between 1968 and 1974 Karasek is able to demonstrate that those whose jobs have changed in the direction of increased skill-demands and increased control are also more active *off the job* in 1974 than they were in 1968 and vice versa. Similar effects have also been demonstrated in follow-up studies of experiments in Norway and Sweden with autonomous groups (Elden 1977; Andersson 1976).

According to a Canadian investigation, work can be organized and designed either to support or hinder the individual from developing and maintaining knowledge and skills which will help him to take initiatives, to take an active part in decision-making, and to improve his social relations. When the exercise of discretion is curtailled by spatial, temporal, or technical restrictions built into the work process, the individual's ability to develop active relations during his spare time will diminish (Meissner 1971). These investigations show that persons whose jobs entail serious constraints on autonomy and skill requirements, and/or have slight direct contact with other people in their work, take far less part in organized and goal-oriented activities outside work with high standards of planning and of co-operation with other people, i.e. in activities of the kind which are ordinarily regarded as expressing the integration of people with the larger society.

Education for leisure is widely seen to be a central issue. The idea is that it ought to be easier for better-educated persons to find an active and self-realizing relation to the world about them in their leisure hours, even if they are doing relatively routine work which asks little in the way of initiative, co-operation, and decision-making. However, British studies have shown that the character of work tends to 'kill' the effects of education, i.e. work does more to determine the character of leisure than education does. This relation would seem to apply both to lowly educated and highly educated persons (Parker 1972).

The tentative conclusion to which these investigations lead is that working conditions not only affect the individual's rewards and effort costs on the job but also that these effects may spill over into his activities and relationships off the job. Strains and adjustment costs incurred during working hours act to limit the individual's participation and activity during non-working hours. The idea that job strains and inadequate work content can be fully made good in leisure hours, provided only there are enough of them, seems to be very much oversimplified. Thus the investigations reported can be seen as advancing yet another argument for a change in working life in the direction of increased worker participation and a restructuring of work in order to make better use of the whole man, his intellectual, social, and manual resources.

REMUNERATION SYSTEM

A central issue is whether stress effects and perceptions of time pressure can be related to different methods of wage payment and whether these reactions might also have some connection with prolonged states of fatigue and with ill health. In discussing existing scientific material and the results of practical experiments with wage payment methods it should be observed that one has to deal with a complicated reality, which makes it very hard to isolate the effects of piecework from other factors that affect the individual's feelings and behaviour at the same time. To take an example, work content and the remuneration system are intimately bound up with one another. More or less by definition, the piece-rated jobs are those in which different operations lend themselves to measurement. As a rule this also mean a rather narrow and repetitive job. More elusive and complicated jobs, e.g. of an administrative nature, are rarely paid for by the piece. It should also be paid out in this context that the adoption of, say, monthly salaries in many cases may well bring other types of managerial control instruments in their wake, such as close supervision, centralized computer-based planning, and the like, whose significance from the standpoint of stress is unknown.

With these reservations in mind we can look at some of the evidence that does exist. Studies from the building industry show that group piece rates may go together with heavy strains on the individual and also lead to the expulsion of members who are unable to meet the group's performance standards (Åstrand et al. 1966). In Swedish and Danish surveys of representative samples of LO-affiliated manual workers a correlation has been found between wage-system and self-reported stress reactions. In both studies were shown that straight piece-rates were associated with intense stress reactions, but none of these studies allow for other possible influences operating at the same time (Bolinder and Ohlström 1971; Arbejdsmiljögruppen 1975).

Attempts have been made to study the differences in perception of monotony and mental strain between workers paid by the piece and by the hour, with work content, kind of work, and income level held constant (Gardell 1971). These investigations show, *first*, that piece-rates in themselves are perceived as stress factors and, *second*, that repetitive tasks are felt to be more monotonous and mentally strenuous if they are also paid by the piece. The income level does not affect these parameters. These results may be interpreted to mean that if one wants to get at the problems of stress in industrial work, then the question of remuneration system and job design will have to be tackled in parallel.

A possible connection between the remuneration system and accident rates has been widely discussed. In Sweden several practical experiments from various industries introducing fixed salaries have been evaluated from this point of view. In a large state-owned mining company the introduction of fixed salaries has been followed by an independent research team (1-year follow-up) as well as by the company itself (3-years follow-up). Both studies show a steep decline in severe accidents (cases requiring more than 90 days sick-leave), a smaller decline in medium severe cases (7–90 days sick-leave), and a rise in minor accidents. In both studies the conclusion is drawn that fixed wages signifies less stress and less risk-taking. In the independent study the rise in minor accidents is explained by referring to the possibilities for workers under fixed wages to attend to minor accidents without loss of income. The company study also points out an overall loss in productivity of 10 per cent in the mining operation and no decline in productivity in the more automated benefication plants

(Kronlund *et al.* 1974; Kjellgren *et al.* 1975). In Swedish forest industries one-year follow ups of the introduction of fixed wages in logging have been published. By and large, these companies report a decline in severe accidents. In one case the total number of accidents decreased by 10 per cent but days lost through accidents were cut 50 per cent (Domänverket 1975). Both companies report a productivity loss of about 10–15 per cent but at the same time increased quality of work (SCA-Tidningen 1975).

In a one-year follow-up made by the present author and associates in highly mechanized saw-mill, the intro-duction of fixed wages led to no decrease in productivity (Aronsson 1976; Gardell 1976.) At the same time the workers reported greater security, improved relations at the workplace, and a smoother working rhythm. To a certain extent, work was reported less hectic, but mental strain and monotony were not very much affected by the change in wage system. This is explained by the fact that no changes were made in pace or production methods, a result well in line with our previous findings.

In summary, all these findings points to piece-rate being a factor with several negative aspects from the point of view of health and safety. Above all piece-rates seem to induce an intensified working rhythm, increased risk-taking, and competition between individuals or teams (Pöyhönen 1975). Obviously piece-rates may lead to increased productivity but at a cost carried by the worker and the larger society.

PSYCHOSOCIAL ASPECTS OF ADVANCED TECHNOLOGY

One factor that is highly instrumental in changing work organization and job content is technological develop-ment. As was shown earlier, we now have a sub-stantial and comparatively clear understanding of the psychological import of the rationalization and mechani-zation programmes implemented to date. This develop-ment may be described as the step from low to medium level of mechanization. By contrast, the psychological import of tasks done in plants with a high degree of mechanization is very incompletely understood, even though 'automation' and its social consequences have attracted great attention. Internationally there is a well-developed body of psychological research oriented to problems of perception, learning, vigilance, and the like, which is utilized in the design of control rooms and instrumentation (Crossman 1960). On the other hand, stress related to uncertainty and risks, as well as the impact of various socio-psychological factors such as social isolation, fatigue and tension, monotony, and job satisfaction, are more poorly understood. Besides, the investigations that exist present a rather contradictory picture. Different summaries of this research have been made (Sadler 1968; Wedderburn 1972).

Several studies have discussed the psychological meaning of mechanization, proceeding from the assumption of a U-shaped correlation between mechanization level and job satisfaction. The rationale for this assumption is that the exercise of discretion as well as skill requirements will, in the case of high mechanization level, be restored to values resembling those customarily associated with craft types of production, even though the tasks are otherwise of a highly different character, e.g. with respect to job content, skills required, level of abstraction, etc. From the psychological aspect it has been assumed that these manifest differences between craft types of production and jobs of operating highly automated process industries are less important compared to the relatively similar determinants of discretionary and skilled behaviour.

Within the framework of the Swedish investigations referred to earlier (Gardell 1971), ratings made by technical experts show that a raft of different, psychologically relevant work requirements course through this U-shaped curve; i.e. the technological determinants of job satisfaction are relatively high both in craft-type jobs and in the monitoring of highly automated process plants. These characteristics of work are also accompanied by a higher degree of job satisfaction and better mental health. Similar results have also been shown in other studies (Blauner 1964; Sheppard 1970; Wedderburn 1972).

However, the results also show that certain characteristics of job design continue to be psychologically unfavourable when mechanization is carried to great lengths; indeed, in some respects, such as control over work methods, a deterioration has supervened in relation to the assembly-line jobs. An important observation: when processes are highly automated, personal control over work performance may be low, at the same time as a great deal is asked of the worker in assuming responsibility, paying attention, comprehending production interrelationships etc., in some instances even more than in jobs of medium mechanization. This ambiguity in the work role may lead to tension, anxiety, and signs of mental strain as shown in studies of automated plants (Mann and Hoffman 1960) as well as in other areas of work (Kahn 1973).

It is often claimed that advanced technology through use of computers, industrial robots, etc. may take over tedious and dangerous jobs. To what extent this is going to happen seems to be dependent on the goals and values that are guiding the application of new technology (Gardell 1978). In a widely known analysis (Braverman 1974) it has been shown that computer technology—both in industrial and office work—means a transfer of skill and control from man to the machine-system, according to the same basic principles inherent in earlier phases of mechanization. It is quite possible that the U-shaped relationship between mechanization and skill requirements referred to earlier represents only an intermediate stage and that systems development in the long run means less skill and control for those operating the machine systems. Obviously there are many instances in which monotony, social isolation, and increased machine-control have been the result of computer installation (Johansson and Gardell 1978). It may be argued, however, that there is no such thing as technological determinism and that the consequences of advanced technology for man depends on the efforts made to create a sound interface between man and the machine-system. Cases may be found where computers have been deliberately introduced as advanced tools for skilled workers and where these workers report great pride and satisfaction in operating such systems (Johansson and Gardell 1978). From the point of view of worker health and satisfaction there may be an optimum degree of mechanization, when the critical variables are defined in terms of skill and control. In competitive economic systems the realization of such a strategy for the use of computers in industry, if at all possible, probably presupposes that a strong organized opinion on these matters can be expressed in legislation and/or collective bargaining; and that these values are also introduced as guiding principles for technical research and development in this area.†

CONCLUSION ON JOB DESIGN

In my opinion, the research performed to date is sufficiently comprehensive and clear-cut to support the conclusion that certain characteristics of industrial work are bound up with psychosocial problems so serious that they should be avoided in the future. These characteristics are above all the following:

> Mechanically controlled work pace;
> Standardized motion patterns;
> Detailed predetermination of working methods and tools;
> Constant repetition of short-cycle operations;
> Requirements of high superficial attention, especially in combination with systems-controlled work pace;
> Utilization solely or primarily of motor functions in the individual;
> Combination of the foregoing work characteristics with payment by results;
> Inadequate opportunities for social interaction in the course of work;
> Authoritarian supervision of work.

Several investigations have also demonstrated that these work characteristics are often positively correlated, i.e. they appear together. Particularly deserving of attention are the severe working conditions that arise when repetitive short-cycle and machine-controlled tasks are

†A special problem bound up with technological advance is posed by the increased capital investment, which intensifies demands to keep the plants ticking round the clock. Substantial medical, psychological, and social drawbacks may attach to shift work, since this usually reinforces the difficulties of reconciling the work role with other life roles (Chadwick-Jones 1969); Mott et al. 1965; NIOSH 1976; Magnusson and Nilsson 1979.)

combined with high demands on attention, skilled evaluation, and decision-making (Johansson *et al.* 1978; Broadbent 1979). The fact that a few people feel no discomfort or malaise in jobs with these characteristics can hardly be taken to justify their acceptability on psychosocial grounds. In the first place, these groups are usually small compared with those who report various signs of discomfort or ill health. Second, there is no clear evidence to prove why tasks with these characteristics are acceptable to certain persons. We have no clear descriptions, suitable for use in recruitment, of those people who can stand working conditions of this kind without damage. Third, there are no indications to suggest that people would find it harder to adjust, except perhaps temporarily, if the work characteristics mentioned were removed. Individualized job design may be seen as an ideal, but it seems unrealistic today other than for certain groups of, say, older and handicapped persons. An overly strong emphasis on individual needs and differences may lead to failure to see the bigger problem, namely that large and probably increasing segments of the labour force do not enjoy psychosocially acceptable working conditions. The quest to improve the psychosocial environment for the vast majority by resort to general interventions in the organization of work does not conflict, however, with a more individualized philosophy dedicated to meeting the special needs of certain groups.

EXPERIMENTS WITH AUTONOMOUS GROUPS AND SOCIO-TECHNICALLY BASED JOB DESIGN

Some of the criticism levelled at the industrial production system by social scientists and others has in many Western countries been taken up by both the trade unions and the employers. In Sweden the 1966 congress of LO (the Swedish Confederation of Trade Unions) discussed, on the basis of various research reports and special investigations, the whole battery of social, psychological, and medical consequences and risks flowing from the technological development (Anderman 1967). Management, for whom increased absenteeism, increased labour turnover, and increased recruitment difficulties had begun to pose growing problems during the 1960s, saw these reactions partly as consequences of repetitive and constrained work. Both industrial relations parties agreed that it would be necessary to change the organization of work to permit the increased exercise of employee influence and to provide more varied and skilled tasks. Even though their interests diverged on the issue of participatory management, the parties managed to agree on a programme of change aiming both at increased productivity and increased job satisfaction. On that basis it became possible to form a joint committee (the Development Council for Collaboration Questions), mandated to sponsor a series of research-based development projects

concerned with improving work organization and job design. Counterpart bodies were also formed in the public administration sector (DEFF) and within the state-owned enterprises (the Industrial Democracy Delegation). However, both LO and TCO (the Swedish Central Organization of Salaried Employees) stressed the industrial democracy aspects and saw the development of self-determination at the shop-floor level mainly as part of the broader quest to 'increase worker influence at different levels in the firms'. The firms, on the other hand, primarily saw a change in job design as an instrument to make the jobs more interesting and attractive, and thus better adapted to the demands made by the younger generation. In this way managements hoped that a socio-psychologically more reasonable job design could contribute towards increased productivity, improved product quality, and lowered costs of absenteeism and labour turnover.

All of the joint committees have now been terminated, largely because management did not allow worker influence to grow into participation at the higher levels of the company. The workers then asked for a legal change of the industrial relation system intended to give equal rights to labour and capital in all questions related to the operations of the firm. This has resulted in a new set of laws: the law of co-determination, made effective on 1 January 1977, is especially important in relation to work organization. However, it has not been possible to reach central agreements based on this law outside the public sector, and it is still too early to say anything about the effectiveness of this strategy of government intervention in the field of industrial democracy.

Swedish management, however, has kept and further developed an interest in work re-organization at the shop-floor level. Some of its attempts in this field are internationally well known, such as group assembly at Volvo and Saab–Scania (Augurén *et al.* 1976: Forslin and Söderlund 1977). There are today several hundred other examples of efforts to create more challenging tasks and somewhat greater individual freedom at work, in order to decrease boredom and mental pressure (SAF 1974). This development has also been supported by the Swedish Employers' Confederation, which set up a special department for assisting and stimulating local developments and publicizing results considered to be of more general interest. Unfortunately it has been part of employer policy not to identify these efforts as scientific research or to call in social scientists to assist in field experiments. Possibly as a result of this policy it is difficult for outsiders to make independent evaluations of what has been achieved. Nevertheless, available evidence indicates that this employer-initiated development has also been of great interest from a more general human point of view and it represents no doubt a most important answer to some of the problems discussed in this paper.

At the same time, however, it is also quite clear that this management approach to problems in working life is conceptualized within too narrow a frame of reference.

With a few exceptions most experiments have very little to do with industrial democracy in a sense which includes forms for worker influence on larger economic and technological decisions. By and large, these cases—important as they may be—represent only new ways to increased productivity through increased motivation to work. This means that this approach is not answering all the relevant problems involved—such as worker claims for a broader base in decision-making—and it also means that its potential is not fully utilized, as it has been shown that autonomous groups and more skilled tasks lead workers to develop aspirations to increased participation in and increased responsibility for overall planning and control since they have come to a better understanding of how such functions affect the immediate job (Gardell 1977). As a rule such an expansion of worker influence has not been accepted by management and this has led to frustration and feelings of powerlessness on the part of the workers.

VIEWPOINTS ON LEGISLATION CONCERNING PSYCHOSOCIAL ASPECTS OF THE PRODUCTION SYSTEM

My purpose in this chapter has been to show that the industrial production system can be organized in a manner incompatible with a broadened concept of occupational health and safety.

First, certain production systems or characteristics of work organization and layout can lead a man to react with stress in the psychological and physiological sense and with different signs of ill health. As a matter of course this syndrome will be affected by individual factors as well as by the individual's other life circumstances, but I think it has been sufficiently clarified that working conditions of the kind here in question also correlate directly with different signs of stress, impaired function, and ill health. Reference has been made above (*Conclusions on job design*) to particularly critical characteristics of work organization and content.

Second, man tends to develop mechanisms for adapting to technological restrictions on his exercise of skill and control which are characterized by passivity, non-participation, and a holding back of human resources. Although these adjustment mechanisms may be combined with symptoms of ill health, they need not be. On the other hand, they appear to conflict with desired values in the community relating to active participation in the democratic processes both on and off the job.

I have also tried briefly to indicate that repetitive and constrained tasks can under certain circumstances lead to absenteeism, labour turnover, and recruitment difficulties, especially among young workers. Many firms have responded by stepping up their efforts to bring about production systems which are better suited to man's demands and mode of operation. Even though some firms have come a long way in rethinking their production technology and have apparently managed to improve their working conditions, it cannot be satisfactory to let the necessary change process rest solely on the economic judgements that are made within the firms. I therefore think it would be desirable to introduce certain statutory provisions, directives, or regulations that would be generally applied to the layout of production and the design of work tasks.

These rules should be broadly formulated in order to give guide-lines for a desired direction of change. Based on the research in this paper the following psychosocial guide-lines for work organization and job design may be formulated.

> Work should be arranged in a way which allows the individual worker to influence his own work situation, working methods, and pace.
> Work should be arranged in a way which allows for an overview and understanding of the work process as a whole.
> Work should be arranged in a way which gives the individual worker possibilities to use and develop all his human resources.
> Work should be arranged in a way that allows for human contacts and co-operation in the course of work.
> Work should be arranged in a way which makes it possible for the individual worker to satisfy time claims from roles and obligations outside work, e.g. family, social, and political commitments, etc.

By having such criteria included in a Work Environment Act, political sanction is given to the direction in which working conditions should be developed. This expression of political will could then be used *both* by the labour inspectorate, by the safety committees and safety stewards or other arrangements in the plants related to safety work, *and* by the trade union in collective bargaining over working conditions (Gardell and Gustavsen 1979).

These criteria may also be expressed, albeit roughly, in rating instruments with quantitative values attached to them, which could be used both in trade-offs between economic, technological, and psychosocial requirements or new equipment and methods *and* in the evaluation of existing plants from the psychosocial aspect. Provision for the worker to call in outside experts to help in these assessments could also be arranged as part of the resources society is investing in a better working environment. As a matter of course, criteria of this kind should also be used by engineers and others in the process of technological research and development.

Over and above the foregoing provision for general psychosocial criteria, it should be feasible to introduce some more precise regulations to define certain minimum levels of acceptability. Their purpose would be to ensure that at least the most extremely negative situations could be avoided in the future. No minimum level should be applied except in cases where manifest economic risks or technical restrictions interpose obstacles to more sweeping changes. In cases where such minimum levels are applied, provisions should also be made for some form of job rotation aimed at introducing more variation and reducing lopsided load on the individual. As examples, we can mention the length of the operating cycle, machine-controlled work pace, and the removal of barriers to human contacts in the course of work. The length of the operating cycle— supplemented by data on variations within the cycles— gives simple expression to a craft of interrelated, negative, psychosocial aspects of work organization, such as monotony-variation, physical constraint, machine-paced work, skill requirements, etc. It would presumably have a great impact if work tasks were not permitted to be broken down into shorter cycles than, say, 3 minutes. Precisely worded regulations of this kind should also make it feasible to prevent rigidly detailed specifications of machine-controlled work pace and motion patterns and cutting off the worker from human contacts on the job.

Taken together, these two catagories of measures— general psychosocial recommendations and precisely worded regulations—should provide a good foundation for working conditions which are substantially improved from the psychosocial aspect. The scope of rules which entitle the employees to make prior examination of drawings and other documentation on capital expenditure should be extended to obligate management to account for detailed manpower planning in terms that will permit physical and psychosocial assessments of job demands on the individual. Obviously, such measures do not cover more than some parts of the psychosocial problem complex, but in my opinion they bear down upon extremely important conditions in the working environment.

EPILOGUE

Since this paper was written, both Sweden and Norway have introduced new Work Environment Acts. Both these acts deal with the working conditions discussed in this paper. Special emphasis is laid on the arrangements of work in a way which make it possible for the individual worker to influence his own work situation, thereby also making it possible to counteract repetitive, machine-paced, and socially isolating jobs. The state has also provided for various resources in implementing these acts. Among these resources, research funds in which workers have decisive influence may be of special interest in this context. It is however, far too early to say anything more substantial about the effectiveness of the new act and its remedies on the psychosocial conditions in work. Obviously, there will be many difficulties of an economic and technological nature. To what extent these will be possible to overcome—well, that is another story.

REFERENCES

ANDERMAN, S. D. (Ed.) (1967). *Trade unions and technological change.* George Allen and Unwin, London.

ANDERSSON, A. (1976). *Företagsdemokrati vid tobaksfabriken i Arvika* [Industrial democracy at the tobacco plant at Arvika. An evaluation]. Mimeograph. Department of Industry, Stockholm.

ARBEJDSMILJÖGRUPPEN (1975). Rapport No. 3 *Arbejdsmiljö* [Work environment]. Arbejdsmiljögruppen of 1972, Köpenhamn.

ARONSSON, G. (1976). *Från ackord til fast lön—utvärdering av en löneformsförändring i högmekaniserat arbete* [From piece-rate to fixed wages. An evaluation]. Psykologiska institutionen, Rapport No. 14, Stockholm.

ÅSTRAND, I., GARDELL, B., PAULSSON, G., and FRISK, E. (1966). *Arbetsanpassning hos byggnadsarbetare* [Adjustment to work in the building industry], pp. 40–50. Institute for Industrial Medicine, Labour Research Foundation of the Building Industry, Stockholm.

AUGURÉN, S., HANSSON, R., and KARLSSON, K. G. (1976). *Volvo–Kalmarverken. Erfarenheter av nya arbetsformer* [Volvo–Kalmar Plant. Experience of group assembly]. Rationaliseringsrådet, SAF-LO, Stockholm.

BLAUNER, R. (1964). *Alienation and freedom.* Chicago University Press, Chicago.

BOLINDER, E. and OHLOSTRÖM, B. (1971). *Stress pa svenska arbetsplatser* [Stress in working life]. Prisma, Stockholm.

BRADLEY, G. (1970). *Arbetsattityder och befordringsintresse hos kvinnliga bankanställda* [Attitudes to job and career among female bank-employees]. PA-Council, Stockholm.

BRAVERMAN, H. (1974). *Labour and monopoly capital.* Monthly Review Press, New York/London.

BROADBENT, D. (1979). Chronic effects from the physical nature of work. In *Man and working life. A social science contribution to work reforms.* (Ed. B. Gardell and G. Johansson). Wiley, London. (In press).

CHADWICK-JONES, J. K. (1969). *Automation and behaviour* John Wiley & Sons, New York.

CROSSMAN, E. R. F. W. (1960). *Automation and skill.* D.S.I.R. Problems of progress in industry. No. 9. Her Majesty's Stationery Office, London.

DAHLSTRÖM, E., GARDELL, B. *et al.* (1966). Teknisk förändring och arbetsanpassning [Technological change and worker satisfaction]. Prisma, Stockholm.

DOMÄNVERKET (1975). *Ettårsrapport: Månadslöneförsöket. Korpilombolo revir* [One-year report on experiment with monthly salaries in logging]. Mimeograph 13.11.75. Domänverket, Stockholm.

ELDEN, M. (1977). *Political efficacy at work.* Mimeograph. I.F.I.M. Norwegian Technical University, Trondheim.

FORSLIN, J. and SÖDERLUND, J. (1977). *Automation and work organization. A case study from the automotive industry.* Mimeograph, Stockholm.

FRANKENHAEUSER, M. and GARDELL, B. (1976), Underload and overload in working life: outline at a multidisciplinary approach. *J. Human Stress,* **2,** (3), 35–46.

GARDELL, B. (1967). *Upplevelse av arbetet* [Job satisfaction among insurance workers]. From Samarbete och arbete. Folksam, Stockholm.

—— (1969). *Skogsarbetares arbetsanpassning* [Job satisfaction and mental health among forest workers]. PA-Council, Stockholm.

—— (1971). *Produktionsteknik och arbetsglädje* [Technology, alienation and mental health. A socio-psychological study of industrial work]. PA-Council, Stockholm.

FOR ENGLISH SUMMARY see Levi, L. (Ed.) (1971). *Society, Stress and Disease*, Vol. 1, Ch. 16. Oxford University Press, London.

—— (1976). *Arbetsinnehåll och livskvalitet* [Job content and quality of life] Prisma, Stockholm.

—— (1977). Autonomy and participation at work. *Human Relat.*, **30** (6), 515–33.

—— (1978). *Produktionsteknik och arbetsvillkor* [Technology and conditions of work]. Ur: Attityder till tekniken. Riksbankens Jubileumsfond. R. J. 1978:6, Stockholm.

—— and WESTLANDER, G. (1968). *Om industriarbete och mental hälsa* [On industrial work and mental health]. PA-Council, Stockholm.

—— BANERYD, K. *et al.* (1968). *Arbetsupplevelse och könsroller* [Job satisfaction and sex-roles]. PA-Council, Stockholm.

—— and GUSTAVSEN, B. (1979). Work environment research and social change—current developments in Scandinavia. *J. Occup. Behav.* (In press.)

GUEST, R. H. (1973). *The man on the assembly line: A generation later. Tuck to-day.* Dartmouth College.

JOHANSSON, G. and GARDELL, B. (1978). *Psykosociala aspekter på process-operatörens arbete* [Psychosocial aspects of process-monitoring], Rapport No. 22. Psykologiska institutionen, Stockholm.

——, ARONSSON, G., and LINDSTRÖM, B. O. (1978). Social psychological and neuroendocrine stress. Reactions in highly mechanized work. *Ergonomics*, **21** (8), 583–99.

KAHN, R. L. (1973). Conflict, ambiguity and overload: three elements in job stress. *Occup. Ment. Hlth*, **3** (1), 2–9.

KARASEK, R. (1979). Job socialization and job strain. The implications of two related psychosocial mechanisms for job design. In: Gardell, B., Johansson, G. (Eds.): *Man and working life. A social science contribution to work reforms* (ed. B. Gardell and G. Johansson). Wiley, London. (In press.)

KJELLGREN, O. (1975). *Löneadministrativa utredningen.* [Wage administrative study]. LKAB, Stockholm.

KORNHAUSER, A. (1965). *Mental health of the industrial worker.* Wiley, New York.

KRONLUND, J. (1974). *Demokrati utan makt* [Democracy without power]. Prisma, Stockholm.

LUNDAHL, A. (1971). *Fritid och rekreation* [Leisure and recreation]. Allmänna Förlaget, Stockholm.

MANN, F. C. and HOFFMANN, L. R. (1960). *A study of social change in power plants.* New York.

MAGNUSSON, M. and NILSSON, C. (1979). *Att arbeta pa obekväm arbetstid* [To work at inconvenient working hours]. Prisma, Stockholm. (In press.)

MEISSNER, M. (1971). The long arm of the job. A study of work and leisure. *Indust. Relat.*, **10** (3), 238–60.

MOTT, P. E., MANN, F. C., McLOUGHLIN, Q., and WARWICK, D. P. (1965). *Shift work. The social, psychological and physical advantages,* Michigan University Press.

NIOSH (1976). *Shift work and health.* U.S. Department of Health, Education, and Welfare, Washington D.C.

PARKER, S. (1972). *The future of work and leisure,* pp. 108–9. Paladin, London.

PÖYHÖNEN, M. (1975). *Urakkapalkka ja stressi* [Piece-rates and stress]. Rapport 115. Institutet för Arbetshygien, Helsingfors.

SADLER, P. (1968). *Social research on automation.* Social Science Research Council. Heinemann, London.

SAF (1974). *Nya arbetsformer* [New trends in job design. A report on 500 experiments]. Swedish Employers' Confederation, Stockholm.

SCA-TIDNINGEN (1975). *Manadslön i skogen* [Monthly salaries in logging]. SCA-Tidningen, No. 10, 26.11.75

SHEPARD, J. M. (1970). Functional specialization, alienation and job satisfaction. *Indust. Labour Relat. Rev.* **23**, 207–19.

SHEPPARD, H. and HERRICK, N. (1971). *Where have all the robots gone?* Free Press, New York.

WALKER, C. R. and GUEST, R. H. (1952). *Man on the assembly line.* Harvard University Press, Boston.

WEDDERBURN, D. (1972). *Workers' attitudes and technology.* Cambridge University Press, Cambridge.

13. NIGHT AND SHIFT WORK EFFECTS ON HEALTH AND WELL-BEING

TORBJÖRN ÅKERSTEDT AND JAN E. FRÖBERG

The importance of working hours for the work environment is increasing. The working week and working day have been shortened in Western societies but there are still people for whom working hours constitute a problem, not because of their length so much as their placement or irregularity.

Shift work, in the narrow sense, is a problem for only a few per cent of the working population, i.e. mainly workers in process industries. But if the definition is extended to include other irregular shift-like schedules, a very significant proportion of the population is involved. Table 13.1 summarizes a study of the distribution of working hours in the Swedish working population. The results show that shift work appears to encompass at least one-fifth of the working population, while no more than three-fifths enjoy the traditional daytime hours (SCB 1974).

TABLE 13.1

Relative frequency of main types of work hours.
$N = 56 \cdot 000$

	Per cent
Permanent day work (07–18)	67·0
Permanent work at least partly outside (07–18)	11·0
Two-shift work	2·9
Three-shift work	1·6
Other rotating schedule	7·5
Irregular	8·0
Other	2·0

The shift workers are found in process industries but also in transportation, hospital care, and service occupations, where work is done at least partly outside the 'normal' daytime hours, with or without rotation, with regular or irregular schedules, etc. For all these people, the distribution of working hours may constitute a problem—a social problem because it may not allow them to participate in important activities, a physiological and psychological problem because the pattern of bodily functions may be disturbed, and a health problem because these disturbances may constitute stressors which in the long run may cause psychosomatic symptoms and disease. This paper reviews results from research on relations between the distribution of working hours and measures of health, well-being and performance. For other recent reviews see also Maurice (1975) and Åkerstedt and Froberg (1976).

SHIFT WORK EFFECTS

Health and well-being

A most important aspect of shiftwork is the question of sleep and sleep disturbances. The amount of sleep after night shifts has been reported to average around 6 hours and problems concerning sleep have been suggested as one of the main reasons for leaving shift work (Aanonsen 1964; Bruusgaard 1949; Åkerstedt 1976).

Although housing conditions seem to play an important role for the duration of sleep, it has also been shown that shift workers who were isolated from environmental disturbances during their sleep hours still had problems with their daytime sleep (Van Loon 1958). Similar conclusions were reached by Aanonsen (1964). The consequences of partial sleep deprivation for health and performance are unclear, and frequently night- and shiftworkers are seen to compensate for their deficit by sleeping more when on dayshifts (Browne 1949; Lille 1967; Smith and Vernon 1928; Åkerstedt et al. 1977).

Electrophysiological recordings of shift workers' day sleep show a deficit of REM sleep, excess of other stages (1 and delta), and a decrease of stage 4 (Dervillee and Lazarini 1957; Kripke et al. 1971). The temporal organization of night workers' sleep has also been shown to differ from that of day workers' in that the periods and amplitudes of ultradian (approximately 90-min) cycles are more unstable (Globus et al. 1972). These results have been interpreted tentatively as indicating less desirable qualities of sleep. There is, however, no indication of relationships between sleep disturbances and pathological processes.

Sickness absence has been reported to be lower in shift workers than in their day-working colleagues (Aanonsen 1964; Taylor 1967). The same is true of mortality rates, which were lower for shift workers (Thiis-Evensen 1949) or did not differ at all between day and shift workers.

In the case of specific illnesses or symptoms, those most studied seem to be *gastrointestinal dysfunctions*, which in a number of studies have been shown to be more frequent in shift workers than in day-working control groups (Wyatt and Marriott 1953; Andlauer 1960; Andersen 1970; Bonnevie 1953; Bruusgaard 1949; Ensing 1969; Wesseldijk 1961; Åkerstedt et al. 1977). However, others have not been able to detect any differences between such groups (Loskant 1957, 1970; Graf et al. 1958; Bjerner et al. 1948).

Nervous symptoms were found to be more frequent among shift workers than among day workers in some studies (Andersen 1970; Bruusgaard 1949; Bolinder et al. 1969) while no differences in this respect have been obtained by others (Aanonsen 1964). A Swedish investigation showed that there was a relation between self-rated 'stress' at work on the one hand and the placement of working hours on the other (Bolinder and Ohlström 1971). Those who regarded shift work or irregular work hours as a stressor had more psychosomatic symptoms than those who did not.

In all, there is today no firm answer to the question of shift work being a hazard to health. Some researchers in the field say yes (Wyatt and Marriott 1953), others definitely no (Raffle 1967; Vernon 1940).

Social effects

Absenteeism has been reported by some researchers to be higher among shift workers (Smith and Vernon 1928; Wyatt 1945; Masterton 1965; Brandt 1969), by others lower (Aanonsen 1964; Taylor 1967; Wade 1955; Taylor *et al.* 1972a). Taylor and co-workers concluded from their studies (Taylor *et al.* 1972b; Shepherd and Walker 1958; Taylor 1967) that there are very significant differences between day and shift workers in that the latter often function in smaller work groups where the absence of one member of the team gives rise to a heavier load on his co-workers than it would do in a day work group. Taylor also claims that job satisfaction and identification are higher in shift workers. These factors may be part of the explanation for the lower rate of absenteeism that is sometimes reported for shift work.

Chadwick-Jones (1967), in a study of a company which changed from a traditional production system to an automatized, continuous system, found that shift work induced certain changes in *social patterns*. The employees complained that the new working hours interferred with their social activities outside work, especially their contacts with workmates and their commitment to associations and unions, etc. But the new leisure pattern yielded more time for family life, and the wives' attitudes were for this reason positive.

In another of the few studies in this area (Mott *et al.* 1965) it was concluded that shift work may produce difficulties for the husband's role as a father and participant in housework, as well as sexual disturbances. Similar results have been obtained in a few other investigations (Andersen 1970; Brown 1959; Banks 1956; Mann and Hoffmann 1960; Gardell *et al.* 1968; Åkerstedt and Torsvall 1978).

Performance

In many studies on shift workers no differences in performance or productivity have been obtained between day and night shifts (Health of Munition Workers Committee 1917; Osborne 1919; Wyatt 1944; De la Mare and Walker 1967; Makowiec-Dabrowska *et al.* 1967; Oginski 1966; Högger 1958). Some studies have shown, however, a tendency towards worse performance during the night shift (Wyatt and Marriott 1953; Pradhan 1969; Grandjean and Wotzka 1972; Browne 1949; Bjerner *et al.* 1955; Pafnote 1967;

Gavrilescu 1966; Rzepecki and Wojtczak 1969). It has also been reported that the maintenance of a high performance may exact a higher physiological 'cost' from the individual (Makowiec-Dabrowska *et al.* 1967).

The expectation that night work would carry more accidents than day work has not been confirmed, although tendencies in this direction have been reported in some studies (Wyatt and Marriott 1953; Wanat 1962; Pradhan 1969; Kojima and Niiyama 1965). On the other hand, it has been suggested that night accidents tend to be more serious than those during day work (Andlauer 1960; Oginski 1966; Newbold 1926).

COMMENTS ON THE REVIEW

As a whole, then, the research reviewed above has only to a limited degree been able to support the common feeling that shift work is a hazard to health and well-being. Only results concerning social problems and sleep seem to be conclusive. Many results might even be considered paradoxical in the sense that shift workers in various indices seem to be a favoured group compared to day workers. The inconclusive results probably stem from the complexity of the problem. Considerable resources of an interdisciplinary kind are required to cover all the aspects involved in an understanding of such a complex problem. Also, much of the work reviewed has been limited to transverse approaches, often of the questionnaire type, where the distribution of working hours has been related to frequencies of certain diseases or problems. With this approach a great deal of important material is lost through the selection into and away from shift work. Thus, many of those who in fact encounter problems in shift work often do not show up in their proper category in the analyses because they transfer to day work, thus biasing the interpretations in favour of shift workers. Also, in the initial process of choosing work, there is a certain positive selection in the sense that individuals with health problems are often advised to refrain from shift work. This is, of course, a good thing in its own right, but it does not transverse studies less powerful tools in revealing relations between shift work and health. Recently, two experimental studies have been published which clearly indicate the pronounced effects on health and well-being of shift work (Åkerstedt and Torsvall 1978; Meers *et al.* 1978). We also feel that the search for mechanisms must be a main objective in all approaches to the investigation of problems in shift work. This leads into the field of biological rhythms research. This field has expanded rapidly in the last 15 years and it appears to offer great opportunities for building and testing theories about the mechanisms involved in the adaptation to shift work.

BIOLOGICAL RHYTHMS AND SHIFT WORK

Circadian rhythms

Basically, cyclic change over time is a property of all

organic life and as such is of great evolutionary importance. (For reviews see e.g., Aschoff 1967 or Pittendrigh 1961). A special case of this rhythmicity is the circadian (*circa dies* = about 24 hours) rhythm.

Generally the circadian rhythms have their maxima during the active part of the 24 hours and minima during the inactive part (e.g. Mills 1966). Practically all physiological and many psychological functions have been shown to exhibit circadian rhythms, e.g. heart rate, metabolism, skin conductance, body temperature, cortical and medullary production of adrenal hormones, problem-solving performance, reaction time, mood, etc. (for reviews see e.g. Halberg 1960; Pittendrigh 1961; Sollberger 1965; Conroy and Mills 1970; Colquhoun 1971, 1972; Wever 1979).

An aspect of particular importance for adjustment to shift work is the endogenous nature of many rhythms. A person shielded from all time cues in the environment and left to lead his own life will, for instance, retain the cyclical behaviour of bodily and psychical functions— except that the period will exceed 24 hours (Aschoff 1969). However, these endogenous rhythms are subject to alterations when influenced by synchronizers. These are important environmental time cues which influence the position of the phase and length of the period. The most powerful synchronizers for humans are probably social factors like distribution of working hours, but also factors like lighting schedules, and times for meals and sleep. Furthermore, the change takes time; about a week is needed for most physiological and psychological functions to change 180°, i.e. from day to night activity (see Aschoff *et al.* 1975). The ability to adjust to changes of the synchronizers also differs considerably between functions. Psychological variables, for instance, generally change more easily than physiological (Conroy and Mills 1970).

Short-term implications for shift work

The 'acute' reduction of well-being in connection with shift work probably depends on the lack of agreement between environmental demands and a rhythm-related ability to cope (see Aschoff 1978). When an individual takes up night work he is exposed to a considerable phase-shift. The environment demands that he, during work hours, be fit to work even though his bodily functions are set to rest. On returning home from a night of work, he expects to sleep. However, his bodily functions are still running according to the old day-active schedule and have already begun to prepare for the habitual activity during the day. Under these conditions it seems obvious that sleep, general well-being, and performance will suffer, at least during the period before adaptation to night work is accomplished (if this ever occurs).

The difficulty of adapting depends to a considerable degree on the strength of the synchronizers. When these are strong and homogeneous, adaptation is swift, as is the case for the person who, say, makes an inter-continental flight half-way round the earth (equivalent to a change from day to night activity). All temporal cues at the site of arrival then jointly strive to re-phase the traveller. This is contrary to the position of the night worker, who has to battle the strongly opposing synchronizers in the surrounding day-oriented society. For him adaptation often proves difficult. If the changes between day and night work occur frequently (e.g. rotating shift work) and the process of adaptation has to be met several times each month, it appears that the difficulties of adaptation to night shift will increase still further. Thus some authors have found tendencies towards an inversion of the body temperature rhythm in subjects working night shifts for some time (Gibson 1905; Sharp 1961; Toulouse and Pieron 1907), some only a minor phase shift (Teleky 1943; Bonjer 1960) or a flattening of the circadian curve. Several studies, however, have shown that no change at all occurs in the temperature rhythm (Migeon *et al.* 1956; Pawlowska-Skyba 1968; Rutenfranz 1967; Rutenfranz *et al.* 1969; Knauth *et al.* 1978).

Investigations which include other bodily functions than temperature are very sparse. Conroy *et al.* (1970b) showed that the 11-OHCS rhythms were phase-shifted in continuous night work, while workers on rotating shifts did not differ from day workers, or, in some cases, displayed no circadian variation at all. In another study, the same authors (1970a) found that the excretion of potassium was lowest during sleep irrespective of working hours, while the diuresis was often high when a night worker slept during the day. Lack of adjustment to rotating shift work but fair adjustment to permanent night work has also been found for adrenalin excretion (Fröberg *et al.* 1972; Åkerstedt *et al.* 1977; Pátkai *et al.* 1977).

Incidentally, these problems of adaptation to frequent phase-shifts initially made researchers recommend long spells on night shift in order to give enough time for adaptation. However, today social considerations have in many fields of work practically ruled out long spells on night shift.

Long-term implications for shift work

As noted above, the acute effects of phase shifts are disturbances of circadian rhythms in e.g. hormone production, body temperature, metabolism, alertness, performance, mood, etc. Over time these disturbances may be the cause of increased tiredness, uneasiness, nervousness, decreased performance, etc. Also, wrong timing of activity can reduce the resistance to noxious stimuli, as susceptibility has been shown to exhibit clear circadian patterns (e.g. Halberg *et al.* 1959; Reinberg 1967). The disturbance of rhythms through e.g. shift work may accordingly expose the individual to noxious influences when resistance is low (Shilov and Kozar 1967). The same idea of mismatch between activity and physiological 24-h rhythms can be traced in some of the explanations for gastro-intestinal and sleep disturbances in shift workers. Other implications of disturbed rhythms have been suggested by Stroebel (1969). He showed that intense stress caused strong desynchronization of certain rhythms in monkeys. He also found a strong relationship between desynchronization and psychotic behaviour.

The most outstanding characteristic of shift work is, of course, its disturbance of various temporal patterns. These disturbances are coped with through adaptation and this adaptation has to be performed repeatedly. We know little of the effects of the frequent adaptation that is required in shift work but the long-term effects of repeated adaptation in general have begun to engage researchers' interest. Some work in this area suggests that the costs of repeated adaptation are cumulative and may gradually leave the individual with less means to handle the pressure of subsequent demands. These ideas were put forward originally by Selye (e.g. in 1950; 1956). New empirical support for them has been presented by some authors. Thus, repeated adjustment to life-changes seems to add up, bringing individuals into the risk zone for myocardial infarction (Rahe 1972). Theorell *et al.* (1972) have provided support for this notion by showing a notable relationship between adrenalin and extent of life change. Theorell (1970) showed that individuals with a high secretion of adrenalin belong to the high risk group. A bit more far-fetched in this context are the results of Aschoff (1971), who showed that flies which are exposed to rapidly changing synchronizers led a 20 per cent shorter life than flies under 'normal' conditions. Harker (1960, 1964) showed that cockroaches started to grow brain tumours when they received brain tissue from another cockroach which had led a life 180° out of phase with the recipients. Cockroaches in phase did not develop tumours.

However, it must be remembered that there is still no *proof* of direct causal relations between disturbance of circadian rhythms on the one hand and health and well-being on the other. The relations indicated above are still merely suggestions, inferred from research on other types of adaptation or other organisms than the human. Much more research is obviously needed.

CONCLUDING COMMENTS

Many experts and laymen today harbour the suspicion that shift work may strongly disagree with sizeable parts of the working population. We know that round-the-clock production of goods and services will employ an increasing number of people. In spite of this, we have few empirical facts to support our suspicions. The problem is obviously complex, but we have earlier in this paper touched upon some points of importance for future research. Thus, *first*, we would like to emphasize the necessity of broad interdisciplinary approaches. In this type of psychological–sociological–medical research, stimulus and response may more often than not be found in different territories of science. *Second*, the problem of selection into and out of shift work must be dealt with. A way to check this influence may be through careful experimentation in natural settings or simply through close and longitudinal monitoring of shift workers who have never been exposed to shift work before. *Third*, research efforts should be concentrated on uncovering the mechanisms of the pathogenic processes. These efforts should, whenever possible, be focused less on purely associative studies and more on hypothesis testing through experimentation—in natural as well as laboratory settings. *Fourth*, the field of biological rhythm research appears to offer an abundance of testable hypotheses or mechanisms.

REFERENCES

AANONSEN, A. (1964). *Shift work and health*. Norwegian Monographs on Medical Science, Oslo.

ÅKERSTEDT, T. (1976). Interindividual differences in adjustment to shift work. In *Proceedings of the 6th Congress of the International Ergonomics Association 1976*. Human Factors Society, Santa Monica, California.

—— and TORSVALL, L. (1978). Experimental changes in shift schedules—their effects on well-being. *Ergonomics*, **21**, 849–56.

—— and FRÖBERG, J. E. (1976). Shift work and health—inter-disciplinary aspects. In *Shift work and health—a symposium* (ed. P. G. Rentos and R. D. Shepherd). HEW Publication No. 76–203.

——, ——, LEVI, L., TORSVALL, L., and ZAMORE, K. (1977). *Shift work and well-being*. Reports from the Laboratory for Clinical Stress Research, 63b, Stockholm.

——, PÁTKAI, P. and PETTERSSON, K. (1977). Field studies of shift work: II. Temporal patterns in psycho-physiological activation in workers alternating between night and day work. *Ergonomics*, **20**, 621–31.

—— (1970). Three-shift work—a sociomedical study. Social-forskningsinstituttet, Copenhagen.

ANDLAUER, F. (1960). The effect of shift working on the worker's health. European Productivity Agency, *T U Information Bulletin*, **29**.

ASCHOFF, J. (1967). Adaptive cycles: their significance for environmental hazards. *Int. J. Biometeorol.*, **11** (3), 255–78.

—— (1969). Desynchronization and resynchronization of human circadian rhythms. *Aerospace Med.* **40** (8), 844–9.

—— (1971). Die Lebensdauer von Fliegen unter dem Einfluss von Zeitverschiebungen. *Naturwiss.* **58**, 574.

—— (1978). Features of circadian rhythms relevant for the design of shift schedules. *Ergonomics*, **21**, 739–54.

——, HOFFMAN, K., POHL, H., and WEVER, R. (1975). Re-entrainment of circadian rhythms after phase-shifts of the Zeitgeber. *Chronobiol.*, **2**, 23–78.

BANKS, O. (1956). Continuous shift work: The attitudes of wives. *Occup. Psychol.*, **30**, 69–84.

BJERNER, B., HOLM, Å., and SWENSSON, Å. (1948). Om Natt- och Skiftarbete [On night and shift work]. Statens

Offentliga Utredningar, 1948:51.

——, ——, and —— (1955). Diurnal variation in mental performance—a study of three-shift workers. *Brit. J. indust. Med.*, **12**, 103–10.

BOLINDER, E., MAGNUSSON, E., and NYRÉN, L. (1969). *LO-medlemmars subjektiva uppfattning om arbetsplatsens hälsorisker.* Landsorganisationen i Sverige.

—— and OHLSTRÖM, B. (1971). *Stress på Svenska Arbetsplaster.* Prisma, Stockholm.

BONJER, F. H. (1960). Physiological aspects of shiftwork. *Proc. Intern. Cong. occup. Health*, **13**, 848–9.

BONNEVIE, P. (1953). Gesundheitliche Schäden durch Nachtarbeit. Ergebnisse einer dänischen Untersuchung. *Ärztl. Prax.*, **5** (46), 10.

BRANDT, A. (1969). On the influence of various shift systems on the health of the workers. *XVI Intern. Cong. Occup. Health.*

BROWN, H. G. (1959). Some effects of shift work on social and domestic life. *Yorkshire Bull. econom. soc. Res.*, Occasional paper, **2**.

BROWNE, R. C. (1949). The day and night performance of teleprinter switchboard operators. *Occup. Psychol.*, **23**, 1–6.

BRUUSGAARD, A. (1949). Shiftworkers, *recommendations on the shortening of working hours in certain occupations.* Ministry of Local Government and Labour, Oslo.

CHADWICK-JONES, J. (1967). Shift-working: physiological effects and social behaviour. *Brit. J. Ind. Relat.* **5**, 237–43.

COLQUHOUN, W. P. (Ed.) (1971). Biological rhythms and human performance. Academic Press, London and New York.

—— (Ed.) (1972). *Aspects of human efficiency.* The English Universities Press, London.

——, FOLKARD, S., KNAUTH, P., RUTENFRANZ, J. (Eds.) (1975). *Experimental studies of shift work.* Westdeutscher Verlag, Opladen.

CONROY. R. T. W. L. and MILLS, J. N. (1970) *Human circadian rhythms.* J. and A. Churchill, London.

——, ELLIOTT, A. L., and MILLS, J. N. (1970a). Circadian rhythms in plasma concentration of 11-hydroxycorticosteroids in men working on night shift and in permanent night workers. *Brit. J. indust. Med.*, 170–74.

——, ——, and —— (1970b). Circadian excretory rhythms in night workers. *Brit. J. indust. Med.*, **27**, 356–63.

DE LA DARE, G. and WALKER, J. (1967). Stress on the shifts. *Management Today.*

DERVILLEE, P. and LAZARINI, H. J. (1957). Considérations sur le travail par roulement et ses répercussions sur la santé. *12e Cong. int. méd. trav.*, **III**, 128–30.

ESING, H. (1969). Occupational aspects of peptic ulcer. *T. Soc. Geneesk.* **47** (6), 78–86.

FRÖBERG, J. E., KARLSSON, C.-G., and LEVI, L. (1972). Shift work: a study of catecholamine excretion, self-ratings and attitudes. In *Night and shift work* (ed. Å. Swensson), pp. 10–20. Studia Laboris et Salutis, Report No. 11.

GARDELL, B., BANERYD, K., GOMBRII, B., and LUNDQVIST, L. (1968). *Arbetsupplevelse och Könsroller.* PA-rådet, Stockholm.

GAVRILESCU, N. (1966). Control board shiftwork turning every two days. *Proc. XV Intern. Cong. Occup. Health.*

GIBSON, R. B. (1905). The effects of transposition of the daily routine on the rhythm of temperature variation. *Amer. J. med. Sci.*, **129**, 1048–59.

GLOBUS, G. G., PHOEBUS, E. C., and BOYD, R. (1972). Temporal organization of night workers' sleep. *Aerospace Med.*, **43** (3), 266–8.

GRAF, O., PIETKIEN, R., RUTENFRANZ, J., and

ULICH, E. (1958). Nervöse *Belastung im Betrieb. I. Teil. Nachtarbeit and nervöse Belastung.* Forschungsberichte d. Witrschafts- u. Verkehrsministeriums Nordrhein-Westfalen, **530**, 1–51.

GRANDJEAN, E. and WOTZKA, G. (1972). *Fatigue related to day-time and night-time and to the duration of work hours in air traffic controllers.* (Unpublished)

HALBERG, F. (1960). The 24 h scale: A time dimension on adaptive functional organization. *Perspectives Biol. Med.*, **3**, 491–527.

——, HAUS, E., and STEPHENS, A. (1959). Susceptibility to ouabain and physiologic 24 hour periodicity. *Federation Proc.*, **18**, 63.

HARKER, J. E. (1960). Internal factors controlling the subesophageal ganglion neurosecretory cycle in periplaneta americana. *J. exp. Biol.*, **37** (1), 164–70.

—— (1964). Diurnal rhythms and homeostatic mechanisms. *Symposia of the Society for Experimental Biology*, **18**, 283–300.

HEALTH OF MUNITION WORKERS' COMMITTEE (1917). Industrial efficiency and fatigue. Cd 8511, HMSO, Interim report, London.

HÖGGER, D. (1958). Nachtarbeit und Leistung. *Schweiz. med. Wschr.*, 408–10.

KNAUTH, P., RUTENFRANZ, J., HERRMANN, G., and PÖPPEL, S. J. (1978). Re-entrainment of body temperature inexperimental shift work studies. *Ergonomics*, **21**, 775–86.

KOJIMA, A. and NIIYAMA, Y. (1965). Diurnal variations of 17-ketogenic steroid and catecholamine excretion in adolescent and middle-aged shift workers with special reference to adaptability to night work. *Ind. Health*, **3**, 9–19.

KRIPKE, D. F., COOK, B. and LEWIS, O. F. (1971). Sleep of night workers: EEG recordings. *Psychophysiol.* **7** (3), 377–83.

LEVI, L. (1972). Stress and distress in response to psychosocial stimuli. *Acta med. scand.*, **191**, Suppl. 528.

LILLE, F. (1967). Le sommeil de jour d'un groupe de travailleurs de nùit. *Le Travail Humain*, **30** (1–2), 85–97.

LOSKANT, H. (1957). Erfahrungen über der gesundheitlichen Einfluss verschiedener Schichtformen in einem Werk der Chemischen Industrie. *Proc. XII Intern. Cong. Occup. Health.*

—— (1970). Der Einfluss verschiedener Schichtformen auf die Gesundheit und das Wohlbefinden des Wechselschichtsarbeiters. *Zentralblatt Arbeitsmed. Arbeitsschutz.*, **20** (5), 133–44.

MAKOWIEC-DABROWSKA, T., WOJTCZAK-JAROSZOWA, J., and BRYKALSKI, D. (1967). Night work and alternate shift working—pulmonary ventilation, oxygen consumption and energy expenditure at rest and at work at various times of the day. *Medycyna pracy*, **18**(4), 340–9.

MANN, F. C., and HOFFMAN, R. R. (1960). *Automation and the worker, a study of social change in power plants.* New York.

MASTERTON, J. P. (1965). *Patterns of sleep.* In *The physiology of human survival* (ed. G. Edholm and A. L. Bacharach). Academic Press, London.

MAURICE, M. (1975). *Shift work.* ILO Publications, Geneva.

MEERS, A., MAASEN, A., and VERHAEGEN, P. (1978). Subjective health after six months and after four years of shift work. *Ergonomics*, **21**, 857–60.

MIGEON, C. J., TYLER, F. H., MAHONEY, J. P., FLORENTIN, A. A., CASTLE, H., BLISS, E. L., and SAMUELS, L. T. (1956). The diurnal variation of plasma levels and urinary excretion of 17-hydroxycorticosteroids in normal subjects, night workers and blind subjects. *J. clin.*

Endocrin., **16** (1) 622–33.

MILLS, J. N. (1966). Human circadian rhythms. *Physiol. Rev.*, **46** (1), 128–71.

MOTT, P. E., MANN, F. C., McLOUGHLIN, Q., and WARWICK, D. P. (1965). *Shift work.* University of Michigan Press, Michigan.

NEWBOLD, E. M. (1926). A contribution to the study of the human factor in the causation of accidents. IFRB, **34**, HMSO, London.

OGINSKI, A. (1966). Comparative research on three-shift work: morning, afternoon and night. *Proc. XV Int. Cong. Occup. Health.*

OSBORNE, E. E. (1919). The output of women workers in relation to hours of work in shell-making. IFRB, **2**, HMSO, London.

PAFNOTE, M. (1967). Some aspects of human adaptation to weekly turning of working shifts. *IIIrd Cong. on Ergonomics.*

PÁTKAI, P., ÅKERSTEDT, T., and PETTERSSON, K. (1977). Temporal patterns in psychophysiological activation in workers with permanent night work. *Ergonomics*, **20**, 611–19.

PAWLOWSKA-SKYBA, K. (1968). Night work and shift work III, effect of three shift work systems on the body physiological activity. *Medycyna Pracy*, **19** (4), 321–32.

PITTENDRIGH, C. (1961). On temporal organization in living systems. *Harvey Lectures*, **56**, 93–125.

PRADHAN, S. M. (1969). *Reaction of workers on night shift.* Society for the Study of Ind. Med., Bombay.

RAFFLE, P. A. B. (1967). Automation—another change in working environment. *Abstr. world Med.*, **41** (9), 657–70.

RAHE, R. H. (1972). Subjects' recent life changes and their near-future illness susceptibility. *Advan. Psychosom. Med.* **8**, 2–19.

REINBERG, A. (1967). The hours of changing responsiveness or susceptibility. *Perspect. Biol. Med.* **11** (1), 111–28.

RUTENFRANZ, J. (1967). Arbeitsphysiologische Aspekte der Nacht und Schichtarbeit. *Arbeitsmedizin–Sozial-medizin–Arbeitshygiene*, **2** (1), 17–23.

——, MANN, H., and ASCHOFF, J. (1969). Circadian-rhytmik physischer und psychischer Funktionen bei 4-stundigem Wachwechsel auf einem Schiff. *Studia Laboris et Salutis*, **4**, 31–41.

RZEPECKI, H. and WOJTCZAK, J. J. (1969). Night work and shiftwork: IV. Changes in the performance of psychological tests during work in various hours of the day. *Madycyna Pracy*, **20** (1), 40–9.

SCB. (1974). *Oregelbundna och Obekväma Arbetstider.* Statistiska Centralbyrån, Stockholm.

SELYE, H. (1950). *Stress.* Acta inc. Montreal.

—— (1956). *The stress of life.* McGraw-Hill, New York.

SHARP, G. W. G. (1961). Reversal of diurnal temperature rhythms in man. *Nature* (*London*), **190**, 146–8.

SHEPHERD, R. D. and WALKER, J. (1958). Absence from work in relation to wage level and family responsibility. *Brit. J. indust. Med.*, **15**, 52–61.

SHILOV, V. M. and KOZAR, M. I. (1967). [Changes in the immunological reactivity of man exposed to various day schedules in a sealed chamber.] *Biologicheskiye ritmyi*

voprosy razrabotki rezhimov truda i otdykha [Biological rhythms and construction of work-rest schedules], pp. 71–2. Materialy, Moscow.

SMITH, M. and VERNON, M. D. (1928). A study of the two shift systems in certain factories. IFRB, **47**, HMSO, London.

SOLLBERGER, A. (1965). *Biological rhythm research.* Elsevier Publishing Company, Amsterdam, London and New York.

STROEBEL, C. F. (1969). Biologic rhythm correlates of disturbed behaviour in the Rhesus monkey. In *Circadian rhythms in nonhuman primates* (ed. F. H. Rholes), pp. 91–105. Karger, New York and Basel.

TAYLOR, P. J. (1967). Shift and day work: a comparison of sickness absence, lateness, and other absence behaviour at an oil refinery from 1962 to 1965. *Brit. J. indust. Med.*, **24** (2), 93–102.

——, POCOCK, S. J., and SERGEAN, R. (1972a). Absenteeism of shift and day workers: A study of six types of shift system in 29 organizations. *Brit. J. indust. Med.*, **29**, 208–213.

——, ——, and —— (1972b). Shift and dayworkers' absence in relationship with some terms and conditions of service. *Brit. J. indust. Med.*, **29**, 338–40.

TELEKY, L. (1943). Problems of night work. Influences on health and efficiency. *Indust. Med., indust. Health, occup. Diseases traumatic Surg.*, **12**, 758.

THEORELL, T. (1970). Psychosocial factors in relation to the onset of myocardial infarction and to some metabolic variables—a pilot study. Doctoral dissertation, Department of Medicine, *Seraphimer* Hospital, Stockholm.

——, LIND, E., FRÖBERG, J., KARLSSON, C.-G., and LEVI, L. (1972). A longitudinal study of 21 subjects with coronary heart disease: Life changes, catecholamine excretion and related biochemical reactions. *Psychosom. Med.*, **34** (6), 505–16.

THIIS-EVENSEN, E. (1949). *Skiftarbeid og Helse.* Eidanger Salpeterfabriker, Porsgrunn, Norway.

TOULOUSE, E. and PIERON, H. (1907). Le méchanisme de l'inversion chez l'homme du rhythme nycthémeral de la temperature. *J. Physiol. Path. gén.*, **9**, 425–40.

VAN LOON, J. H. (1958). Enkele psychologische aspecten von ploegenarbeid. *Mens en Ondern.*, **12**, 357–65.

VERNON, H. M. (1940). Sickness and accidents amongst munition workers. *Ind. Welf. Pers. Manag.*

WADE, L. (1955). *Arch. ind. Health*, **12**, 592.

WANAT, J. (1962). Accident incidence in various periods in pits. *Prace Glo. Inst. Gorn., Ser. A*, Kom 285.

WESSELDIJK, A. T. G. (1961). The influences of shiftwork on health. *Ergonomics*, **4**, 281–2.

WEVER, R. (1979). *The circadian system of man.* Springer, New York.

WYATT, S. (1944). *A study of variations in output.* Med. Res. Council, Ind. Health Res. Board.

—— (1945). *A study of certified sickness absence among women in industry.* Industrial Health Research Board, 86, HMSO., London.

—— and MARRIOTT, R. (1953). Night work and shift changes. *Brit. J. indust. Med.*, **10**, 164–72.

14. ON THE PSYCHOPHYSIOLOGICAL CONSEQUENCES OF UNDERSTIMULATION AND OVERSTIMULATION

MARIANNE FRANKENHAEUSER and GUNN JOHANSSON

In the technologically advanced countries the interaction of man and environment is characterized by growing maladjustment on the *psychological level*. With the abatement of material poverty, new expectations and needs have come into focus and psychological problems tend to dominate the lives of an increasing number of people. Many of the demands now being made on human adjustment concérn various forms of psychological under- or overstimulation. This new type of problem calls for greater consideration of human needs, adaptability, and tolerance limits.

Research on human stress and coping is concerned with the dynamics of person–environment transactions (see Lazarus 1977). The biological approach is centred on adaptive processes and asks the following questions: How adaptable is the human organism; how far can the tolerance limits be stretched; what happens if they are exceeded? Can adaptability be measured; can the limits be predicted and hence the harmful effects prevented? These questions have high priority in experimental, clinical and epidemiological stress research.

This chapter outlines problems connected with understimulation and overstimulation, emphasis being placed on experimental contributions relevant to working life. Examples are also given from an ongoing project which combined psychophysiological and social psychological approaches to studying the impact of modern technology on workers' health and satisfaction (Frankenhaeuser 1976a, 1979b; Frankenhaeuser and Gardell 1976; Johnson *et al.* 1978).

THE AROUSAL CONTINUUM

Human beings living in a 'normal' environment are aware of only a fraction of the multitude of stimuli to which they are exposed. However, if the inflow of impulses fall below a critical level, disturbances in brain function and behaviour ensue. Under the opposing conditions, i.e., when the stimulus flow exceeds a certain level, adequate functioning is also threatened.

The concept of arousal (or activation) is central to theories dealing with phenomena related to under- and overstimulation. When stated in terms of behaviour, arousal refers to an intensity dimension ranging from unconsciousness and sleep through drowsiness, quiet awakening, and excitement to disorganized behaviour.

Neurophysiological research has identified the reticular activating system (RAS) of the lower brain stem as a key mechanism for regulating arousal level, 'a kind of barometer for both input and output level, a structure serving as a homeostat regulating or adjusting input–output relations' (Lindsley 1961). Through the ascending part of the RAS, stimulation reaches the cerebral cortex and creates a level of arousal necessary for effective cognition and learning. The RAS is controlled not only by sensory stimulation from below, but also by cortical stimulation from above. In other words, the RAS may be activated both by cognition and by sensation. For arousal to be maintained, stimulation must be variable. When stimulation is perfectly constant, the RAS habituates, the percept 'blanks out' and cortical arousal assumes a pattern resembling that of no stimulation.

According to the arousal theory advanced by Hebb (1955), stimulation from any source has two functions: a 'cue function' guiding behaviour, and an 'arousal or vigilance function'. While a foundation of arousal is a prerequisite for an adequate cue function, high arousal is detrimental. The relationship postulated by Hebb between the arousal function and the cue function (effectiveness of discrimination and learning) is shown in Fig. 14.1. Other investigators (e.g., Duffy 1962; Malmo 1959; Schlosberg 1954; Freeman 1948) have related arousal to physiological indicators of emotion such as the EEG, the EMG, and the GSR as well as cardiovascular and respiratory measures.

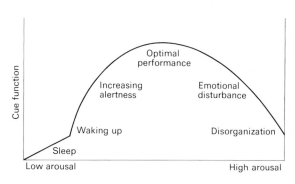

There is general agreement between activation theorists in postulating an inverted- U relationship between mental efficiency and arousal. At low arousal levels the organism may be inattentive and easily distracted, and poor performance is probably associated with a slowing down of cortical processes. At somewhat higher arousal levels, the organism's resources are mobilized, full attention is given to the task, and it performs to the best of its abilities. Still higher arousal levels are associated with excessive tension and intense emotions: the decline in performance probably reflects impaired cortical control or selectivity of responses.

The *optimal level of arousal* differs for mental functions varying in complexity, and it is generally assumed that the arousal required for maximum performance is higher for simple than for complex tasks. Fig. 14.2 (from Bindra 1959) shows hypothetical curves for three kinds of tasks: weight lifting, typewriting, and drawing. In each case the subject will be 'too excited' above the upper limit of the optimal range and 'not warmed up' below the lower limit of the optimal range (Bindra 1959, p. 247).

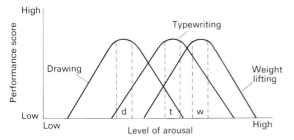

The *range* of the optimal arousal level may also differ between tasks. The width of the region within which maximally effective performance can occur is probably related to the difficulty of the task. While good performance in a simple task may be possible within a wide range of arousal, maximum effectiveness in a difficult task probably occurs only within a narrow arousal zone.

A difficult task can be defined as one with several necessary conditions for successful performance. Thus success on a intellectual task may require the possession of certain skills and knowledge gained from prior experience, certain innate capacities, an appropriate orientation of motivation, and appropriate activation level. In this connection, success refers to the close approximation of the individual's actual performance to his potential performance, that is, to the extent to which he does as well as he can (Fiske and Maddi 1961, p. 33).

Zuckerman (1969) has attempted to tie together the various hypotheses concerning arousal level and mental functioning in a theory of an optimal level of stimulation. The key proposition in this theory is that every individual has a characteristic optimal level of stimulation and arousal for cognitive and motor activity and for subjective well-being. Thus, individuals differ with regard to their *stimulus need* and *tolerance*.

The obvious evidence of these differences are all around us. Consider the individual who needs absolute quiet for cognitive activity and the person who can work only with the din of music and voices around him. Consider persons who manage their lives so that every event is repeated, regular and predictable, and those whose lives are in continual uproar because of their need to vary their stimulation and maintain a high level of excitement (Zuckerman 1969, p. 429).

According to Zuckerman, optimal levels of stimulation vary with a number of factors such as constitutional characteristics, age, learning experience, recent levels of stimulation, and diurnal cycle. Complex cognitive mechanisms like attitudes also influence the optimal level.

UNDERSTIMULATION

Research in social psychology has identified monotony and repetitiveness as factors affecting the worker's experience of his job and his feelings and attitudes towards the job (Gardell 1971). In essence, the empirical evidence shows that repetitive, monotonous tasks tend to be accompanied not only by low job satisfaction and low utilization of personal talent, but also by low self-esteem and low life satisfaction in general as well as by disturbances in mental health and social adjustment (e.g. Kornhauser 1965). The scale of these problems is evident from survey data showing that large groups of workers in an advanced industrial society find their jobs monotonous, demanding little in the way of planning and judgement (e.g. Gardell 1976).

Experimental research concerning effects of monotonous environments has been carried out along essentially two lines. One approach has dealt with *restricted environments*, emphasis being placed on varying the degree of sensory input and studying physiological and psychological effects. In these experiments the individual is typically passive most of the time. The other approach, *vigilance studies*, is concerned with performance in attention-demanding tasks under monotonous conditions. These two approaches will be illustrated by examples.

Restricted stimulation

The first large-scale laboratory investigations on humans carried out in this field were initiated in 1951 by D. O. Hebb and his associates at McGill university (reported by Bexton *et al.* 1954). Their aim was to study the mechanisms underlying 'brain washing' as well as fluctuations in attention during monotonous work. The results of the experiments were startling. Subjects who were required to spend their time lying unoccupied in a sound-proof room developed severe symptoms already after a few hours: anxiety, hallucinations, and delusion. Objective test data indicated impairment in perceptual and cognitive functions. The practical implications of these dramatic effects were evident, and the McGill experiments became the starting point for intense research activities in laboratories in different parts of the world. For an overview of research in this area the reader is referred to a volume edited by J. P. Zubek (1969), *Sensory deprivation: fifteen years of research*.

There are four main techniques for reducing environmental influences in laboratory experiments with human subjects: sensory deprivation, perceptual deprivation, perceptual monotony, and social isolation.

Sensory deprivation involves reducing sensory stimulaton to a very low level. This is usually accomplished by having the subject lie more or less motionless in a dark, sound-proof room, with arms and hands encased in gloves and cuffs. A variant of this method is to restrict the inflow from only one sense modality, usually vision or hearing. A more drastic procedure, infrequently used, is the so-called water-immersion technique: the subject (wearing a mask) is instructed to remain motionless while suspended in a tank of slowly circulating tepid water.

Perceptual deprivation refers to a procedure which aims at reducing the patterning and meaningful organization of sensory input, while maintaining a more or less normal level of stimulation. Typically, the subject, wearing gloves and translucent goggles, lies in a cubicle. The goggles permit diffuse light to enter the eyes, but eliminate all pattern vision. A masking noise is applied via earphones.

Perceptual monotony represents a less common variant of perceptual deprivation. The subject is exposed to a highly restricted sensory environment which is characterized mainly by monotony. An example of this technique is provided by experiments in which subjects have been confined to tank respirators for poliomyelitis patients and exposed to the blank walls of a screen and the repetitive drone of a motor.

All these methods can be combined with a more or less severe *social isolation*, which means that subjects, either alone or in small groups, are cut off from contact with other people. When the social-isolation technique is applied by itself, no attempt is made to restrict the level or patterning of stimulus input. All kinds of confinements, of either single individuals or small groups, are associated with some degree of perceptual monotony.

The methods outlined above have been used to study effects on physiological as well as perceptual, cognitive, and emotional functions. Inter-individual differences in resistance to the harmful effects of understimulation have also been investigated, as have relations between tolerance level and personality characteristics. The results from different studies may appear somewhat contradictory but a closer analysis often relates the discrepancies to the type of understimulation employed. Perceptual deprivation, for instance, is more effective than sensory deprivation in impairing cognitive and perceptual functions. The picture presented by the pioneer group at McGill has been revised in certain respects. A critical analysis has shown, for instance, that the visual phenomena associated with restricted stimulation should be classified as visual distortions, fantasies, and hypnagogic states rather than as hallucinations.

Studies of effects on physiological functions point to effects on the central and peripheral nervous system as well as the endocrine system. Zubek *et al.* (1963) showed that after 14 days of perceptual deprivation the EEG pattern had changed markedly, alpha activity decreasing and remaining low (though recovering) seven days after the end of isolation. These changes in brain activity were accompanied by a sharp drop in motivation. Together with these signs of subdued cortical activity there were changes indicating increased autonomic arousal, e.g., a continuous decrease in skin resistance. Moreover, the secretion of adrenal hormones (catecholamines and corticosteroids) increased markedly under deprivation periods of less than 24 hours (Zubek 1969). The overall picture of physiological changes during severe under-stimulation thus suggests a dissociation between autonomic and cortical arousal.

Psychomotor and *perceptual functions* are sensitive to various forms of restricted stimulation. Performance is impaired, for instance, in tests requiring eye–hand-co-ordination, whereas stereoscopic vision and the perception of size are not affected. It is noteworthy that some of the reported changes represent functional improvements, e.g. lower thresholds for pain and olfaction as well as for two-point discrimination (Zubek 1969).

The picture of *cognitive functions* is incomplete and contradictory, partly because the sensitivity of different types of function varies with the method for restricted stimulation. Difficulty in concentrating is a common symptom and there is sometimes pronounced intellec-tual ineffectiveness. In some cases, however, improved performance has been demonstrated.

Large interindividual differences have been found in *limits to tolerance* of various kinds of understimulation. Some individuals can endure several days of isolation, others no more than a few hours. Results from a number of laboratories indicate that roughly one-third of volunteer subjects interrupt their isolation during the first three days. Attempts to predict the tolerance of individual subjects from physiological data have shown that those with a relatively low pre-experimental excretion of adrenalin under basal conditions have a comparatively low tolerance (Zubek and Schutte 1966). A search for methods to raise the tolerance of isolation has shown that under certain circumstances, physical activity (e.g. exercises) can counteract the functional impairments associated with prolonged deprivation (Schultz 1965). Conversely, sensory deprivation always induces more severe effects when combined with restricted movement. The tolerance level is also related to the attitudes and expectations induced in the subjects before the experiment starts, and information about the coming discomfort may raise tolerance. The fact that many subjects cope with deprivation experiments with-out any appreciable discomfort reflects the selection processes influencing voluntary participation in studies of this kind.

Monotonous work
The combination of a monotonous situation and demands for sustained mental preparedness imposes severe demands on the worker. During the Second World War attention was drawn to the work conditions of personnel in radar stations, submarines, and aircraft. Soon, however, highly automated monitoring tasks

became a common characteristic of industrial and military systems. These systems have tended to become both more complex and more automatic, and man's function has changed from that of an 'active operator and controller to that of a passive overseer of automated equipment whose job is to detect changes in the system output' (McGrath 1963, p. 3). However, man is a poor monitor, and observers required to maintain attentive watch for prolonged periods typically show a decline in detection efficiency as the watch progresses. Experimental efforts have been mainly directed towards identifying the factors associated with vigilance decrement and with maintenance of performance. The practical implications are obvious, and the laboratory research on vigilance has generally been conducted in close connection with applied problems. For overviews of the experimental aspects of this field the reader should consult Broadbent (1958, 1971) and Buckner and McGrath (1963) and for applied aspects Edwards and Lees (1974).

The starting point for *experimental vigilance research* was a series of studies by Mackworth (1950), who devised a 'clock' test for simulating the task of radar watch. The subject is required to watch a clock pointer which moves in steps and to report any occasion on which the pointer moves twice the usual distance. Typically, the number of signals (double steps) reported declines within a period of 30 min. A similar performance decrement is generally found in other vigilance situations as, for example, when the subject is required to detect small, irregularly occurring changes in repetitive signals, either in the loudness of an intermittent sound or in the brightness of an intermittent light (McGrath 1963).

The performance decrement can be prevented by inserting rest pauses, by providing knowledge of results when a signal is either missed or correctly detected, and by intake of stimulant drugs. It can also be counteracted by using signals that are not transient but remain available over a prolonged period.

Theoretical approaches to vigilance phenomena have emphasized 'filter' mechanisms (Broadbent 1958) as well as processes of inhibition (McCormach 1962) and activation (McGrath 1963). Fiske (1961) in his analysis of features common to monotonous conditions and restricted stimulation, notes that:

In both types of experiment, the most marked effects are found in conditions with the greatest reduction in temporally varying stimulation. Conversely, any external stimulation that varies over time will reduce the probability of occurrence of performance decrements or disturbances of normal functions.

It is also proposed that subjects exposed to either of these conditions attempt to increase the *impact of stimulation*, especially the amount of variation. Some subjects are successful and manage to adapt by providing themselves with stimulation having an 'appropriate degree of inpact', thereby maintaining an appropriate level of activation.

Vigilance has come to play a key role in job stress with the transition to completely automated production systems, which is a dominant trend in current technological development (see Bainbridge 1979; Frankenhaeuser 1979a, b; Johansson, in preparation). On the one hand, automation eliminates detrimental influences related to repetitiveness and restriction of movement and social interaction; instead, it provides the worker with supervisory, controlling, and comparatively qualified tasks. On the other hand, automation introduces new stress components that may be still more detrimental. These are most clearly seen in the control rooms of large-scale plants. Monitoring a process calls for acute attention and readiness to act throughout a monotonous period of duty. But the brain needs an inflow of impulses in order for optimal alertness to be maintained. Moreover, the process operator works in shifts, which means that he has to perform his tasks also when, due to the circadian rhythm, his adrenalin output is low and his ability to concentrate reduced (e.g., Fröberg *et al.* 1975).

Another critical aspect concerns the abstract nature of the work, the fact that the operator deals with symbols and signals and is never in touch with the actual products of his work. These problems are given high priority in an ongoing study of workers in the Swedish steel industry (Johansson, in preparation).

OVERSTIMULATION

Conditions of excessive stimulation

A state of overload is induced when stimulation exceeds the receiver's capacity to process stimuli. In principle, overload can be counteracted both by reducing the input and by increasing the receiver's capacity to handle the incoming signals. The symbolic value or 'meaning' of the incoming stimuli constitutes the major determinant of their impact on the individual. However, even apparently meaningless sensory stimuli may evoke personally meaningful associations. Therefore sensory stimulation may be regarded as a variation of information input (cf. Lipowski 1973).

An important distinction is that between quantitative and qualitative overstimulation. The quantitative aspects refer to, for example, intensity, duration, frequency, and rate of stimulation, while the qualitative aspects involve novelty, complexity, incongruity, and ambiguity (Berlyne 1966). In his analysis of occupational stress and the role concept, Kahn (1973) distinguishes between quantitative and qualitative aspects of work load, the former representing a continuum from 'having too little to do' to 'having too much to do', the latter a continuum from 'having work to do that is too easy' to 'having work to do that is too difficult'. It is interesting that whereas both kinds of work were found to be associated with psychophysiological stress reactions, they differed with regard to the threat to self-esteem experienced by different occupational groups. Thus, among professors, in contrast to administrators, self-esteem was not threatened by mere quantity, but only by qualitative overload.

Laboratory investigations of overstimulation fall into two major categories, both of which deal with significant aspects of real life conditions. In one type of study, the subject remains passive while exposed to sensory stimulation, in the other type he is required to cope actively with the incoming signals.

Subjects who *passively endure* intense visual or auditory stimulation, e.g., coloured lights or white noise, generally experience feelings of unpleasantness, discomfort, and arousal. Within a few hours, severe disturbances such as 'psychedelic' experiences may occur in healthy volunteers (Ludwig 1971). Subjects exposed to a situation designed so as to induce an experience of 'being surrounded by a total environment of colour and sound' (Gottschalk *et al.* 1972) showed evidence of cognitive impairment as well as increased social alienation and personal disorganization. Physiological reactions to this kind of sensory overstimulation have not been examined systematically in human subjects, but data from animal studies suggest that marked changes may occur. For example, rats exposed to intense light, sound, and motion stimuli developed hypertension, hypertrophy of the left ventricle, and hyperfunction of the adrenal cortex.

Experiments in which the subject is *actively engaged* in dealing with incoming signals are more similar to realistic work situations. Overload can be induced either by the task itself (Frankenhaeuser and Johansson 1976; Broadbent 1979) or by external factors, such as noise, interfering with the task (Frankenhaeuser and Lundberg 1977; Lundberg and Frankenhaeuser 1978). In one study (Ettema and Zielhuis 1971), mental load was varied systematically by a binary-choice task. The results showed that the amount of information handled per time unit correlated positively with increases in heart rate, blood pressure, and respiration rate.

Sympathetic-adrenal medullary activity, as measured by adrenalin and noradrenalin excretion, is also a sensitive indicator of overload induced by psychosocial conditions such as novelty, rush, choice, and conflict (see reviews by Frankenhaeuser 1971, 1975a, b, 1979a, b; Johansson and Lundberg 1978; Levi 1972). In one experiment Frankenhaeuser *et al.* 1971) a complex sensori-motor task and a monotonous vigilance-type task were both shown to increase subjective and physiological arousal. However, performance was superior in high-adrenalin subjects during understimulation and in low-adrenalin subjects during overstimulation. These results may be interpreted in terms of the inverted-U relationship between arousal and performance. Another illustration of the sensitivity of the adrenal medulla to different work loads is provided by a field study (Levi 1972) showing that a change from salary to piece-work wages was accompanied by an increase of about 40 per cent in adrenalin excretion.

Studies involving measures of physiological and subjective functions at different levels of stimulus input permit the assessment of 'the cost of adaptation' to conditons of overstimulation. One significant finding is that stress reactions such as adrenalin secretion can be counteracted by increasing the subject's own control over the situation (e.g., Frankenhaeuser and Rissler 1970). This has also been demonstrated in comparisons between workers engaged in machine-paced vs. self-paced work (Johansson *et al.* 1978).

Additional information can be obtained by studying the temporal pattern of arousal in reaction to temporary overload. The assumption underlying this approach is that the biological cost is higher when the arousal level remains high after cessation of the stimulus than when there is a rapid return to baseline level. In other words, individuals who take a long time to 'unwind' pay a higher price. It is interesting that interindividual differences in the temporal pattern of adrenalin output appear to reflect fundamental aspects of individual adjustment to environmental demands (Johansson 1976; Johansson and Frankenhaeuser 1973; Rissler 1977).

When assessing after-effects of overstimulation it is important to note that the time pattern of maximum susceptibility varies between functions. Thus, subjective stress reactions tend to decline more rapidly than physiological reactions (Frankenhaeuser and Lundberg 1974). This discrepancy in the pattern for subjective versus physiological arousal reactions may lead to an underestimation of harmful consequences. The problem was emphasized by Glass and Singer (1972) in their study of urban stress which showed that noise exposure during mental work induced performance decrements, but not until after the noise had ended.

Related studies dealing with overstimulation induced by *crowding* (Henry *et al.* 1967; Henry and Stephens 1970) have shown that mice placed in a box system designed to maximize social stimulation develop hypertension as well as a number of biochemical changes, including increased adrenalin and noradrenalin content in the adrenal medulla. It is interesting that studies of humans suggest that cognitive factors, including the relationships between the people in the crowd, play an important part in modifying the physiologial reactions to crowding. This view is supported by recent experiments on endocrine and subjective arousal reactions of train commuters in Sweden (Lundberg 1976; Singer *et al.* 1978).

Surfeit of attractive stimuli: theory and implications
The brief survey presented above illustrates the variety of contexts in which problems relating to overstimulation have been studied. On the whole, the approach to overstimulation has been much less systematic than that to understimulation. However, thanks to Lipowski's (1971, 1973) efforts to integrate data from seemingly unrelated studies of overload, a conceptual framework has emerged as well as a theory of 'attractive stimulus overload', also called the 'surfeit theory'. The core idea is that an affluent technological society is characterized by a surfeit of attractive stimuli which all incite consump-

tion. Commercial forces, advertising, and mass communication interact in building up expectations and demands in all areas of life. The consumer is exposed to a multitude of material and symbolic goals, including educational opportunities, leisure activities, travel, social contacts, life styles. The pressure to consume is reinforced by the prevailing ideology of growth and achievement, by the striving for 'recognition as a successful, joyful consumer of abundant opportunities'. Due to his inherent restrictions, economic limitations and to lack of time, man can only take advantage of part of the offer. Different groups in society are affected differently. The poor are exposed to the same offers as the rich, but their freedom of choice is severely restricted. To be excluded from the opportunities presented so stridently may generate feelings of frustration, failure, or anger.

The economically well situated face a purely psychological problem, a choice between equally attractive but mutually exclusive alternatives. Those who fail to cope with the decision stress find themselves in the position of Buridan's ass between two stacks of hay, unable to decide which one of them to approach. While Lipowski issues a warning against generalization and oversimplification, he nevertheless expresses the belief that his theory may contribute to our understanding of the expressions of discontent, apathy, unrest, and violence in affluent societies.

Exposure to a surfeit of attractive stimuli elicits a need for *coping strategies*. Some persons try to cope by selectively ignoring a large part of the impinging stimuli, whereas others adopt the reverse strategy of maximizing consumption by approaching as many goals as possible. Other strategies involve reducing the number of impinging stimuli by avoidance or withdrawal, by the intake of pharmacological agents which restrict the perceptual field, by devotion to a cause, or by avoiding commitment (Lipowski 1971). When the coping strategies fail, there is a risk that the individual will come to harm. Since overstimulation is closely linked with ways of life emanating from technological advances, the problems are likely to grow and to spread over many areas of life. This leads to heavier demands on man's adaptive capacity.

Implications for health and disease of a development along these lines are attracting increased attention. This is manifested, for example, in studies concerned with relationships between *life-change events* and vulnerability to disease (for a review see Rahe 1972). Whether or not adjustment to change will lead to disease depends on complex interactions between the individual's constitutional characteristics and his past and present experiences. However, even under conditions where the threat to health is not imminent, long-term risks may be involved, since change, at least when associated with novelty and unpredictability, evokes psychophysiological arousal reactions. Repeated exposure to change therefore adds to the wear-and-tear of the organism.

Recent developments within communication technology impose new, apparently unforeseen problems, which relate closely to the theory of attractive stimulus overload (Frankenhaeuser 1976b). The characteristic feature of advances in communication technology is increased flexibility, which brings greater possibilities to choose more differentiated information, adapted to suit individual preferences. Such possibilities of choice create conditions which favour the well-educated groups in society.

The most serious long-term consequences of straining human tolerance limits probably relate to the *emotional level*, to the process of habituation that is our most effective means of coping with overstimulation. When we are bombarded with too many, too strong, or too frequent stimuli, the response of the nervous system gradually weakens—the stimuli lose their impact and the reactions diminish. The physiological stress effects become less intense and feelings of distress and discomfort fade. But so do feelings such as involvement, engagement, and sympathy and concern. This wear of our feelings tends to be a hidden process, not preceded by warning signals, because the mechanism of habituation involves desensitization, a reduction of receptiveness and reactivity. Therefore, overstimulation may form part of a general process of passivization.

Emotional satiety has a counterpart on the cognitive level, in man's limited capacity to process information. The rapidity with which a state of cognitive satiety may develop is strikingly illustrated in experimental studies showing that *decision-making* tends to deteriorate with an increase in the number of information units on which the decision is based (Nystedt and Magnusson, 1972).

CONCLUDING COMMENTS

Most empirical data concerning psychophysiological effects of under- and overstimulation can be interpreted in terms of a homeostatic model, and Lindsley's (1961) postulate of a central mechanism mediated by the reticular formation has become widely accepted.

It is interesting to speculate further about common factors in under- and overstimulation and to link these to 'altered states of consciousness', e.g., dream states, hypnotic states, and drug-induced states (e.g., Tart 1975). Typical of all these states, including those induced by extreme under- and overstimulation, are symptoms such as hallucinatory and delusory visual sensations and fantasies, altered time experience, and an altered mode of cognition (impaired logical reasoning, increased imaginative and associative thinking). Ornstein (1972) has suggested that 'ordinary' and 'altered' states of consciousness differ with respect to the balance between activity in the two brain hemispheres. There is evidence suggesting that the left hemisphere is involved in analytical thinking, whereas the mode of operation of the right hemisphere is 'holistic' and diffuse (Sperry *et al.*; Ornstein 1972). Following this line of reasoning, it may be hypothesized that the right hemisphere 'takes over' under conditions of extreme stimulation, when the input to the brain is either too weak, too diffuse or too intense to suit the 'left-hemisphere thinking'. Such a change in balance between the two hemispheres could explain the feeling of lack of cognitive control which commonly occurs in subjects exposed to severe under- and overstimulation.

The part played by cognitive factors in regulating the physiological reactions to under- and overstimulation has been emphasized throughout this chapter. The activating effect, the impact of stimulation, depends upon its symbolic value or subjective meaning. In other words, it is not the quantity of the stimulation as measured in physical terms that determines its effects on the organism, but the psychological significance of the stimulation.

Novelty, or variation, is also a major source of impact: the effectiveness of a stimulus is largely determined by the amount of *change* that it provides. Thus, the extent to which a stimulus differs from the one preceding it, or from the whole range of previously experienced stimuli, plays a decisive role. This means that the degree of unexpectedness of a stimulus—its deviation from the pattern built up by the previous stimulation—will contribute significantly to its impact (see Frankenhaeuser 1975a). In this connection it should be noted that stimuli occurring in the early childhood environment are particularly potent in shaping response and coping patterns of the adult individual as well as his expectations with regard to the quality and quantity of psychosocial stimulation.

In conclusion, the psychophysiological impact of the environment is determined by a dynamic process of transactions in which the resources of the individual are matched against the demands of the environment. Adaptive behaviour is directed toward increasing or decreasing the impact of stimulation to the end of maintaining an optimal level of arousal.

REFERENCES

BAINBRIDGE, L. (1979). The process controller. In *The study of real skill* (ed. W. T. Singleton). London. (In press).

BERLYNE, D. E. (1966). Curiosity and exploration. *Science*, **153**, 25–33.

BEXTON, W. H., HERON, W., and SCOTT, T. H. (1954). Effects of decreased variation in sensory environment. *Can. J. Psychol.*, **8**, 70–6.

BINDRA, D. (1959) *Motivation: a systematic reinterpretation.* New York.

BROADBENT, D. E. (1958). *Perception and communication.* New York.

—— (1971). *Decision and stress.* London.

—— (1979). Chronic effects from the physical nature of work. In *Man and working life* (ed. B. Gardell and G. Johansson). New York. (In press.)

BUCKNER, D. N. and McGRATH, J. J. (Ed.) (1963). Vigilance: a symposium. New York.

DUFFY, E. (1962). *Activation and behavior.* New York.

EDWARDS, E. and LEES, F. P. (Ed.) (1974). *The human operator in process control.* London.

ETTEMA, J. H. and ZIELHUIZ, R. L. (1971). Physiological parameters of mental load. *Ergonomics*, **14**, 137–44.

FISKE, D. W. (1961). Effects of monotonous and restricted stimulation. In *Functions of varied experience.* (ed. D. W. Fiske, and S. R. Maddi), pp. 106–44. Homewood, Illinois.

—— and MADDI, S. R. (Ed.) (1961). *Functions of varied experience.* Homewood, Illinois.

FRANKENHAEUSER, M. (1971). Behavior and circulating catecholamines. (Review article). *Brain Res.*, **31**, 241–62.

—— (1975a). Experimental approaches to the study of catecholamines and emotion. In *Emotions—their parameters of measurement* (ed. L. Levi.), pp. 209–34. New York.

—— (1975b). Sympathetic-adrenal medullary activity, behaviour, and the psychosocial environment. In *Research in psychophysiology* (ed. P. Venables and M. Christie), pp. 71–94. London.

—— (1976a). The role of peripheral catecholamines in adaptation to understimulation and overstimulation. In *Psychopathology of human adaptation* (ed. G. Serban), pp. 173–91. New York.

—— (1976b). Our capacity to receive information. In *The role of new communications systems*, Chapter 6, pp. 31–5. Canadian Broadcasting Corporation, Ottawa and International Broadcast Institute, London.

—— (1979a). Psychoneuroendocrine approaches to the study of emotion as related to stress and coping. In *Nebraska symposium on motivation 1978* (ed. H. E. Howe and R. A. Dienstbier). Lincoln. (In press.)

—— (1979b). Coping with job stress—a psychobiological approach. In *Man and working life* (ed. B. Gardell and G. Johansson). New York. (In press.)

—— and GARDELL, B. (1976). Underload and overload in working life: Outline of a multidisciplinary approach. *J. Hum. Stress*, **2**, 35–46.

—— and JOHANSSON, G. (1976). Task demand as reflected in catecholamine excretion and heart rate. *J. Hum. Stress*, **2**, 15–23.

—— and LUNDBERG, U, (1974). Immediate and delayed effects of noise on performance and arousal. *Biol. Psychol.*, **2**, 127–33.

—— and —— (1977). The influence of cognitive set on performance and arousal under different noise loads. *Motivation and Emotion*, **1**, 139–49.

——, NORDHEDEN, B., MYRSTEN, A.-L., and POST, B. (1971). Psychophysiological reactions to understimulation and overstimulation. *Acta Psychol.*, **35**, 298–308.

—— and RISSLER, A. (1970). Effects of punishment on catecholamine release and efficiency of performance. *Psychopharmacologia*, **17**, 378–90.

FREEMAN, G. L. (1948). *The energetics of human behavior.* Ithaca, New York.

FRÖBERG, J. E., KARLSSON, C.-G., LEVI, L., and LIDBERG, L. (1975). Circadian rhythms of catecholamine excretion, shooting range performance and self-ratings of fatigue during sleep deprivation. *Biol. Psychol.*, **2**, 175–88.

GARDELL, B. (1971). Alienation and mental health in the modern industrial environment. In *Society, stress and disease* (ed. L. Levi), Vol. I., London.

—— (1976). Technology, alienation and mental health. Summary of a social psychological research programme on technology and the worker. *Acta Sociol.*, **19**, 83–94.

GLASS, D. C. and SINGER, J. E. (1972). *Urban stress.* New York.

GOTTCHALK, L. A., HAER, J. L., and BATES, D. E. (1972). Changes in social alienation—personal disorganization and cognitive intellectual impairment produced by sensory overload, *Arch. Gen. Psychiat.*, **27**, 451–7.

HERB, D. O. (1955). Drives and the C.N.S. (Conceptual nervous system). *Psychol. Rev.*, **62**, 243–54.

HENRY, J. P., MEEHAN, J. P., and STEPHENS, P. M. (1967). The use of psychosocial stimuli to induce prolonged systolic hypertension in mice. *Psychosom. Med.*, **29**, 408–32.

—— and STEPHENS, P. M. (1970). Changes in enzymes involved in the biosynthesis and metabolism of noradrenalin and adrenalin after psychosocial stimulation. *Nature*, **225**, 1959–60.

JOHANSSON, G. (1976). Subjective wellbeing and temporal patterns of sympathetic-adrenal medullary activity. *Biol. Psychol.*, **4**, 157–72.

—— Stress perspective on the psychosocial factors in process control. (In preparation.)

——, ARONSSON, G. and LINDSTRÖM, B. O. (1978). Social psychological and neuroendocrine stress reactions in highly mechanized work. *Ergonomics*, **21**, 583–99.

—— and LUNDBERG, U. (1978). Psychophysiological aspects of stress and adaptation in technological society. In *Human behaviour and adaptation* (ed. N. Blurton Jones and V. Reynolds). London.

—— and FRANKENHAEUSER, M. (1937). Temporal factors in sympatho-adrenomedullary activity following acute behavioral activation, *Biol. Psychol.*, **1**, 67–77.

KAHN, R. L. (1973). Conflict, ambiguity, and overload: Three elements in job stress. *Occup. ment. Health*, **3**, 2–9.

KORNHAUSER, A. (1965). *Mental health of the industrial worker.* New York.

LAZARUS, R. S. (1977). Psychological stress and coping in adaptation and illness. In *Psychosomatic medicine: Current trends and clinical applications* (ed. Z. J. Lipowski, D. R. Lipsitt, and P. C. Whybrow), pp. 14–26. New York.

LEVI, L. (Ed.) (1972). Stress and distress in response to psychosocial stimuli. *Acta Med. scand.*, **191**, Suppl. 528.

LINDSLEY, D. B. (1961). Common factors in sensory deprivation, sensory distortion, and sensory overload. In *Sensory deprivation* (ed. P. Solomon, P. H. Kubzansky, J. H. Leiderman, J. H. Mendelson, and D. Wexler). Cambridge, Mass.

LIPOWSKI, Z. J. (1971). Surfeit of attractive information inputs: A hallmark of our environment. *Behav. Sci.*, **16**, 467–71.

—— (1973). Affluence, information inputs and health. *Soc. Sci. Med.*, **7**, 517–29.

LUDWIG, A. M. (1971). Self-regulation of the sensory environment. *Arch. Gen. Psychiat.*, **25**, 413–8.

LUNDBERG, U. (1976). Urban commuting: Crowdedness and catecholamine excretion. *J. Hum. Stress*, **2**, 26–32.

—— and FRANKENHAEUSER, M. (1978). Psychophysiological reactions to noise as modified by personal control over noise intensity. *Biol. Psychol.*, **6**, 51–9.

MACKWORTH, N. H. (1950). Researches in the measurement of human performance. *Medical Research Council Special Report Series* No. 268. H. M. Stationery Office, London.

MALMO, R. B. (1959). Activation: a neurophysiological dimension. *Psychol. rev.*, **66**, 367–86.

McCORMACH, P. D. (1962). A two-factor theory of vigilance. *Brit. J. Psychol.*, **53**, 357–64.

McGRATH, J. J. (1963). Irrelevant stimulation and vigilance performance. In *Vigilance: a symposium* (ed. D. N. Buckner and J. J. McGrath). New York.

NYSTEDT, L. and MAGNUSSON, D. (1972). Predictive efficiency as a function of amount of information. *Multivariate Behav. Res.*, **7**, 441–50.

ORNSTEIN, R. E. (1972). *The psychology of consciousness.* San Francisco, California.

RAHE, R. H. (1972). Subjects' recent life changes and their near-future illness susceptibility. In *Psychosocial aspects of physical illness. Advances in psychosomatic medicine* (ed. Z. J. Lipowski), Vol. III. Basel.

RISSLER, A. (1977). Stress reactions at work and after work during a period of quantitative overload. *Ergonomics*, **20**, 13–16.

SCHLOSBERG, H. (1954). Three dimensions of emotion, *Psychol. Rev.*, **61**, 81–8.

SCHULTZ, D. P. (1965). *Sensory restriction. Effects on behavior.* New York.

SINGER, J. E. LUNDBERG, U., and FRANKEN-HAEUSER, M. (1978). Stress on the train: a study of urban commuting. In *Advances in environmental psychology* (ed. A. Baum, J. E. Singer, and S. Valins), Vol. 1. Hillsdale.

SPERRY, R. W., GAZZANIGA, M. S., and BOGEN, J. E. (1969). Interhemispheric relationships; the neocortical commissures; syndromes of hemisphere disconnection. In *Handbook of clinical neurology* (ed. P. S. Wilden and G. W. Bryn), Vol. 4, pp. 273–90. Amsterdam.

TART, C. T. (1975). *States of consciousness.* New York.

—— and LUNDBERG, U. (1978). Psychophysiological aspects of stress and adaptation in technological society. In *Human behaviour and adaptation* (ed. N. Blurton Jones and V. Reynolds). London.

ZUBEK, J. P. (Ed.) (1969). *Sensory deprivation. Fifteen years of research.* New York.

—— and SCHUTTE, W. (1966). Urinary excretion of adrenalin and noradrenalin during prolonged perceptual deprivation, *J. abnorm. Psychol.*, **71**, 328–34.

——, WELCH, G., and SAUNDERS, M. G. (1963). Electroencephalographic changes during and after 14 days of perceptual deprivation. *Science*, **139**, 490–2.

ZUCKERMAN, M. (1969). Theoretical formulations. In *Sensory deprivation. Fifteen years of research* (ed. J. P. Zubek). New York.

15. A HIGH RISK GROUP: THE MIDDLE-AGED AND ELDERLY WORKER

S. FORSSMAN

THE AGEING WORKER AND HIS WORK

Ageing changes several physiological functions, mainly in such a way that performance capacity rises to a maximum at a certain age and is then gradually reduced. Different functions have a different 'timetable' of ageing as the peak occurs at different ages for different functions and the slope of the downward curve varies from function to function. Some functions of the eye and ear decrease from the age of 10 onwards. The maximum physical capacity for heavy work is at 25 years and declines to 60 per cent at the age of 60. The capacity to carry out precision movements lasts for a very long time but may decrease after 60 or 70 years. There is a considerable individual variation in physiological functioning which increases with age, and there are more individual physiological differences between people in the higher age groups. One factor which is important in connection with working capacity is the gradual reduction of muscular strength with age, as well as reduced perception and decreased ability to receive information and relate it to earlier experience. Short-term memory is also gradually reduced. Learning changes with age, more time being needed for learning at higher ages. The capacity of biochemical defence mechanisms to combat toxic substance is reduced with age and this may increase individual sensitivity to exposure to toxic chemicals (for literature on physiological ageing and working capacity, see Birren 1959; Forssman 1963; Forssman et al. 1969, Welford 1958, 1971).

With increasing age, the incidence of some diseases, such as cardiovascular and degenerative diseases affecting the joints and muscles increases. These diseases which usually increase after the age of 45, influence the working capacity and are the main clinical causes of disability.

The average maximum working capacity of the older worker is thus lower than that of younger men and this is caused both by physiological ageing and by disease. However, ordinary work seldom absorbs the maximum working capacity. The work demand usually needs only a minor part, about 20–30 per cent, except for peak loads. According to studies in work physiology, only up to 40 per cent of the maximum working capacity should be used at continuous work in order to avoid excessive fatigue (Åstrand 1960). The ageing worker has a reduced reserve capacity compared to younger workers. Any extra work load such as peak loads, or any temporary impairment as a result of disease or fatigue may easily disturb the balance between work demand and working capacity.

Consequently, there are several negative aspects to the performance of the elderly worker, such as reduced capacity to work at a continuously high speed, reduced capacity to adjust to changes in the working environment, reduced ability to learn new working methods, and reduced muscular strength. However, there are many compensatory positive aspects that are not known or emphasized to the same extent, such as experience, sense of responsibility, capacity for precision work, low labour turnover, and low short-term absence (less than one week; see Table 15.1).

In order to promote the adjustment of the elderly

TABLE 15.1

The elderly at work (after Forssman et al. *1969)*

Disadvantages	Advantages
Reduced capacity to work at high speed	Work experience that may compensate for many negative aspects
Impaired short-term memory, Reduced near vision (may be compensated by spectacles)	Sense of responsibility Loyalty
Increased need for illumination, More difficult to adjust to changes Longer time needed for learning Reduced muscle strength, etc.	Accuracy and precision at work Low labour turnover, etc.

worker to his work and to preserve a balance between work demand and working capacity, three measures should be emphasized:

(1) *Ergonomics*: this means the adjustment of work to the older man, which often will call for a redesign of jobs for the elderly;

(2) *Individual placement*: work demand and the changed working capacity of the elderly should be taken into account.

The elderly worker should as far as possible be kept on his ordinary job although it may be modified or redesigned so that the work demand is reduced (for examples, see Table 15.1). If a change of job is necessary, proper information should be provided before the worker is transferred, for instance from high-speed to low-speed work, or from piece-work to a monthly wage system. However, the social implications of a change of job should be taken into account as prestige is very important for the elderly worker.

(3) *An efficient occupational health service*: this should provide preventive health services, regular health examinations, and easily available medical care.

These preventive measures are well known and many conferences and studies in several countries have been devoted to them (see, for instance, Bengtsson *et al.* 1960; Forssman 1957, 1963; Forssman *et al.* 1968; Griew 1965; OECD 1967). One of the most recent conferences was devoted to the redesign of jobs for the elderly and was organized by a working group of the Wenner-Gren Centre for Research in Sweden.

The adjustment of the elderly worker to the working environment is, however, not only a physiological or a medical problem. During the last few years, there have been several interdisciplinary studies on the medical, psychological, and sociological adjustment of the elderly worker to his work and in society. It is important to consider the elderly worker as a human being and not only concentrate studies on a few physiological or psychological functions.

It is interesting to notice that there is a trend, increasing with age, for men to overestimate their own health and working capacity, although the industrial physician will notice a definite impairment.

A recent medical, psychological, and sociological study of older workers in Sweden has produced interesting information on the situation of the middle-aged and elderly worker. It was found that health and working capacity gradually decreased with age and the incidence of disability increased, mainly as a result of cardiovascular diseases and diseases of the organs of locomotion. Psychological tests showed a decrease with age of performance standards and of accuracy and increased slowness. The degree of severity and the onset of the

TABLE 15.2

Work adjustment of the elderly (after Forssman et al. *1969)*

Problems of the elderly worker	Preventive measures
Reduced vision	Better illumination and contrast
Impaired near vision	Spectacles adjusted to the work distance
Difficulty in adapting to change between near and distant vision	Consistent work, avoiding changes in distance
Difficulty in adjusting to changes between darkness and light	Consistent light intensity
Reduced hearing	Distinct signals and hearing information
Impaired short-term memory	Less demand on memory, introduce memory in machines, adjust training methods
Difficulty in absorbing information on several channels simultaneously	Simplify work process
Impaired intuition, logic, evaluation, decision-making ability	Introduce work routines
Less able to cope with paced work, assembly line work	Adjust speed, introduce buffer stores, make provision for making up lost time
Reduced strength and physical capacity	Avoid peak loads, and the combination of heavy work, standing, and exposure to heat
Reduced mobility	Avoid uneven floors, situations where moving around is difficult, and transport of heavy or awkward goods
Sensitivity to heat and cold	Provide comfortable climate without great changes
Discomfort caused by exposure of hands to vibration	Reduce vibration and protect hands
Increased need for rest	More pauses and micropauses
Resistance to change	Careful information

decline varied for different functions. Concerning accuracy, a decrease with age was generally found in problem-solving tests, but accuracy did not change or even slightly increased with age in a psychomotor test. Social adjustment did not vary in the same way as physical and mental health but seemed to improve in higher age groups (Forssman 1969; Forssman et al. 1968; Granath and Helander 1966; Helander 1967).

This study was followed up ten years later on the same individuals. Those in whom an objective reduction of health and working capacity was recorded during the first study, were classified in the same way in 1972. Those who had only a subjective impairment of their health and working capacity in 1962 showed impaired adjustment to work ten years later. Those who had an objective impairment of health in 1962 had a higher sickness absence than the average during the following ten-year period. The dominating causes of the sickness absence were back disorders, gastrointestinal diseases, and cardio-vascular diseases. It was found that the work demand had increased for many people during the ten years and there was an impaired balance between work demand and working capacity, especially concerning climate, demands on back and legs, as well as physical endurance. There may also be a maladjustment concerning speed, learning new methods, co-operation with others, and psychological endurance.

This study was also concerned with those who, for health or other reasons, leave employment. This 'drop-out' group was, however, fairly small in this study. It was found that those with impaired health and working capacity usually stayed on as far as possible at the same employment, and those who after the ten years were found in jobs in other factories were those with good health and working capacity who could manage to take on new jobs (Åstrand et al. 1976).

THE PLACE OF THE OLDER WORKER IN AN INDUSTRIALIZED SOCIETY

The preventive measures mentioned above, designed to promote the adjustment of the older worker to his work, are well known and have been applied in a number of places of employment, but in many industrialized countries conditions on the whole do not favour the elderly. Two main factors must be considered. With increasing expectation of life there are more and more older people in the working population of the industrialized countries. At the same time, technological development, creating new working processes in industry or other places of employment, is creating jobs mainly suited to young people. These jobs require high speed, perception, or the ability to absorb large amounts of information. The required skills can usually be acquired in a fairly short time, especially for jobs with short work cycles, such as assembly line jobs. Technological development thus not only creates new jobs

most suited to young people but the skills required for them also emphasize the handicaps of the elderly, such as their reduced capacity to work at high speed and their reduced capacity for perception. The positive characteristics of the elderly, such as long-term experience of work, are of less value in many modern mechanized industries, as new working methods or processes are introduced or the old processes are modified every few years. The workers will consequently have to learn new methods from time to time and adjust to new working conditions. The ten to twenty years of experience formerly needed to become a skilled carpenter, glass blower, or foundry worker are of less value and may sometimes even be a handicap. Industrialized society does usually not appreciate the experience, judgement, and wisdom of the elderly but is more concerned with the physical strength, speed, and efficiency of younger people. It seems that the elderly worker cannot fully compete on the labour market with younger age-groups, although management, unions, and employment services are usually well aware of the need to find jobs for and protect the older worker. Younger workers often get the best jobs, and the elderly are often found doing heavy physical work for less pay.

The consequences for the elderly of technological development are serious. Mechanization reduces manpower requirements in many industries. This results in no new workers being taken on for many years and the average age of the working population rises. In many factories in Sweden, especially in the textile industry and in the foundries and quarries, more than 50 per cent of the workers are over 45 years of age. This creates often difficult and costly problems of adjusting the working process to these older people or of redesigning jobs. In other industries, new, sometimes complicated working processes may be introduced and young people employed and trained for the new jobs. Experts on mechanization and rationalization gradually cut out many jobs which are traditionally given to older or handicapped workers. Studies of the age distribution of the registered unemployed have shown that the higher age groups dominate, especially among those who have been unemployed for more than two months. Many older people have difficulty in continuing in their old jobs or in finding new jobs and have to be found new jobs within the same factory, or sometimes even need to be retrained, or to retire earlier than normal.

Structural changes in industry may also increase the difficulties of the older employee. In many industrial countries, small factories are being closed down or merged into large companies. Larger units or factories will gradually be created and, at the same time, the urbanization process will continue as people move from villages to cities. The trend is for people to be employed more and more in large units in large communities.

The elderly worker, at least in Sweden, usually has close ties with the small community where he has lived for many years. He may have built a small house of his own and is not inclined to move to another place to be trained for a new job. The situation in Sweden and in many other industrialized countries will be that the elderly labour force will be available in smaller communities while the main need for manpower will be in the large factories in the cities.

CONCLUSIONS

The measures to protect the elderly worker such as ergonomics, individual placement, and occupational health services are effective, and when they are well applied, it has proved possible to find jobs for the elderly, satisfactory from the health point of view, even in the highly mechanized machine industry (Heijbel 1963). This may not be enough, however, as in many industrialized countries the older members of the labour force are still in a difficult situation.

With the continuous changes in industry, there will be a great need to replace and retrain older workers. Unskilled older workers will then be in a most difficult situation. On a long-term basis, broad professional training and education as well as job rotation will put the elderly worker in a better position if he has to face a change of job.

Redesign of jobs for the elderly can be improved. In order to keep a balance between the work demand and the changing working capacity of the elderly, it is important gradually to reduce the work demand with regard to speed, perception, and responsibility. When the work load of the elderly worker is reduced, it is important to consider the social prestige of the new job as it seems to be of increasing importance with increasing age to have a meaningful job and feel the importance of one's own performance. Measures to protect and promote the health of the elderly worker have been applied, but only in a very limited number of factories. Further development in this direction is not only a problem of information and education. A major change of attitude among managers, foremen, workers, unions, employment service personnel, and government authorities is needed if they are to appreciate the qualities of the elderly worker which can be utilized in a modern industrialized society.

This is important also because many ageing workers prefer to carry on working rather than retire early. In this connexion, it should be stressed that physical and mental activity promotes and preserves health, especially in the higher age groups. Like everyone else, the elderly worker should have the right to work if he wants to do so.

The preservation of existing small factories and the creation of new ones in small communities, thus counteracting the enormous urbanization and industrialization process that is going on all over the world, will obviously protect and promote the physical, mental, and social well-being of the older worker. Most countries have so far failed to apply this measure.

It will be very important to consider the older worker's problems in planning industry and society for the future.

REFERENCES

ÅSTRAND, I. (1960). Aerobic work capacity in men and women with special reference to age. *Acta physiol. scand.* *Suppl. 169.*

BENGTSSON, S. F., EDGREN, G., HYDÉN, S., LUNDGREN, I., and SVENSSON, I. (1960). *Medelålders och äldre arbetskraft.* [The middle-aged and elderly labour force]. Betänkande avgivet av en arbetsgrupp tillsatt av AMS, SAF, LO och TCO, Stockholm. (In Swedish.)

BIRREN, J. E. (1959). *Handbook of aging and the individual.* The University of Chicago Press, Chicago.

FORSSMAN, S. (1957). *Äldre i industrin* [The health problems of the older worker—a study in Swedish industry]. Publikationer från Svenska Arbetsgivareföreningen, Stockholm. (In Swedish.)

—— (1963). Die Arbeit und der alternde Mensch. *Handbuch der gesamten Arbeitsmedizin, IV. 1* [Work and the ageing man]. Urban & Schwarzenberg, Munich (In German.)

—— (1969). Medical, psychological and sociological studies of middle-aged and older personnel in Swedish industry. *Interdiscipl. Top. Gerontol.*, **4**, 48–56.

——, GRANATH, S., HELANDER, J., and OLHAGEN, G. (1968). 30 år i arbetet [Thirty years at work]. *PA-rådet Med.*, No. 53. (In Swedish.)

——, GRANATH, S., GUSTAVSSON, B., HEIJBEL, C.A., and LUNDGREN, N. (1969). *Arbetskrav och arbetsförmåga hos äldre.* [Work demand and working capacity of the ageing man.] Arbetsmedicinska Institutet, Stockholm. (In Swedish.)

——, HELANDER, J., OLHAGEN, G., and ÅSTRAND, N.E. (1976). *40 år i arbetet.* [Forty years at work]. Arbetarskyddsfonden, Stockholm. (In Swedish, with extensive English summary.)

GRANATH, S. and HELANDER, J. (1966). On some interdisciplinary factors in Gerontology, 7th Int. Congr. Gerontol., Vienna.

GRIEW, S. (1965). Job redesign. *Employment of older workers series.* OECD. Paris.

HELANDER, J. (1967). On age and mental test behaviour. *Acta psychol. Gothoburgensia. VII*: Gothenburg, 1–159.

HEIJBEL, C. A. (1963). Medelålders och äldre arbetskrafts anpassning till högmekaniserat arbete [Middle-aged and elderly workers' adjustment to highly mechanized work]. Ur 'För gammal?' En SNS-konferens om de medelålders och äldre i samhälle och arbetsliv. *Studier och debatt*, **3–4**, 93–106. (In Swedish.)

OECD SOCIAL AFFAIRS DIVISION (1967). Promoting the placement of older job seekers: a guide to methods. *Employment of older workers series.* OECD, Paris.

WELFORD, A. T. (1958). *Ageing and human skill.* Oxford University Press for the Nuffield Foundation.

—— (1971). *Fundamentals of skill.* Methuen and Co. Ltd., London.

16. THE ASSOCIATION BETWEEN INDICATORS OF PERCEIVED STRESS AND PERCEIVED HEALTH FOR WORKERS AND WORK OF DIFFERENT CHARACTER

BENGT EDGREN and GÖRAN OLHAGEN

OBJECTIVES

The purpose of the study reported in this chapter is to analyse the relationship between some indicators of perceived stress and aspects of subjectively perceived health under different conditions. This issue has been chosen because of its relevance in general for occupational health. In Sweden today it is estimated that one-third of the patients who consult a doctor complain about symptoms that are attributable to stress reactions. The more specific aim of this study was an attempt to identify potential risk groups, implying a probability of developing disease, using the individual's own ratings of his degree of stress and ill health.

THEORETICAL BACKGROUND

On the basis of the Selye-Stress concept it has been hypothesized that exposure to stressors implies strain on the organism. If this exposure is long-term, the state of the organism will be impaired and precursors of disease or even disease itself will develop. These ideas have been summarized by Levi (1972) in a model that takes into account the characteristics of the stimulus situation, the psychobiological programme of the individual, and interacting variables. These factors can be conceived as independent variables. Fig. 16.1 shows how the independent variables are related to each other and to the stress mechanisms, the precursors of disease, and disease, which can be considered as dependent variables.

According to theoretical assumptions (Levi 1972) the relation between an individual's perception of stimulation and the stress response (Selye-Stress) is not linear but U-shaped, implying the strongest stress reactions at the two extremes of the stimulation continuum and the lowest stress level in between (Fig. 16.2).

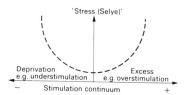

FIG. 16.2. Theoretical model regarding the relation between physiological stress as defined by Selye and various levels of stimulation. According to this hypothesis, deprivation of stimuli as well as excess is accompanied by an increase in 'Selye-Stress.'

AN APPROACH TO THE STUDY OF STRESS AND HEALTH

The strategy behind a series of studies carried out at the Laboratory for Clinical Stress Research can be described briefly in six steps as follows:

1. The identification of drawbacks in the job situation (job dissatisfaction, preceived psychic and physical strain, etc.);
2. The study of the relationship between these drawbacks on the one side and data on health, illness, and absenteeism on the other;
3. The identification of environmental factors in and outside the job in addition to individual factors which could have an influence on the above-mentioned relationship;
4. Multivariate analysis based on steps 2 and 3;
5. Longitudinal studies of the subjects with respect to:

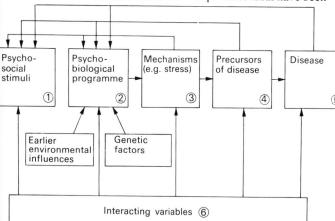

FIG. 16.1. A theoretical model for psychosocially mediated disease. The combined effect of psychosocial stimuli (1) and the psychobiological programme (2) determines the psychological and physiological reactions (mechanisms (3), e.g. stress) of each individual. These may, under certain circumstances, lead to precursors of disease (4) and to disease itself (5). This sequence of events can be promoted or counteracted by interacting variables (6). The sequence is not a one-way process but constitutes part of a cybernetic system with continuous feedback. (From Levi 1972.)

(a) The situation in and outside the job;
(b) The individual's reactions to the situation;
(c) Data on health indicators, all aiming at the identification of hypothetical causal factors;

6. Field experiments to establish the relationship between cause and effect.

The present analysis, which should be regarded as a pilot, represents step 4 above.

Groups studied
Two contrasting subsamples—high and low skilled male workers—were drawn from a larger sample of metal workers in the Stockholm area all aged above 25 years. The number of subjects were as follows: High skilled workers, $N = 273$; low skilled workers, $N = 197$.

Variables
The variables being correlated can be referred to reactions of the individual, i.e. dependent variables according to Fig. 16.1. However, in the present analysis the indicators of stress have been treated as independent variables and perceived ill health as a dependent variable. The term 'control variable' refers to work and worker characteristics.

Independent variables = indicators of stress
From a battery of attitude scales concerning job satisfaction a selection of stress items was made. The scales have been used earlier in a series of studies of Swedish employees by Gardell (1971). The stress indicators selected were:

(a) A measure of an aspect of alienation consisting of a set of items constituting an index of monotony at work and job engagement;
(b) Perceived physical strain in the job situation (single item);
(c) Perceived mental strain in the job situation (single item).

All items included in measures (a)–(c) were to be answered on a 5-point scale, where 1 stands for the most negative and 5 for the most positive attitude and 3 represents the neutral point. The mean values (M) and the standard deviations ($S.D.$) for the high skilled workers were:

	M	$S.D.$
(a) Monotony	3·42	± 0·90;
(b) Physical strain	3·44	± 1·20;
(c) Mental strain	2·70	± 1·19.

The corresponding values for the low skilled workers were:

	M	$S.D.$
(a) Monotony	3·05	± 0·89;
(b) Physical strain	2·48	± 0·18;
(c) Mental strain	1·98	± 0·99.

A comparison of the two contrasting groups shows that the highly skilled workers had a more positive attitude for all of the independent variables. The differences between the means were highly ($p \leq 0.001$) significant. The difference between the groups as to the levels of the independent variables should be kept in mind in interpreting the data.

Dependent variable = measure of perceived ill-health
The measure of subjectively perceived ill health consisted of the following 7 items:

1. Do you easily catch a cold?
2. Do you often suffer from gastric catarrh?
3. Do you often suffer from diarrhoea?
4. Are you often constipated?
5. Do you often suffer from prolonged pain in shoulders and neck?
6. Do you often suffer from prolonged pain in your back?
7. Do you often suffer from headache?

The answer to give to these questions were 'yes' or 'no'. The subjects have been categorized according to the number of 'yes' answers. The distribution of the number of reported symptoms in the two groups is given in Table 16.1

A test for independence gave a non-significant value of chi-square, and a t-test gave no significant difference between the means (M) of the groups. However, there was a tendency to more symptoms in the low skilled group.

The information of a health index based on an unweighted summation of subjective symptoms regardless

Table 16.1

	Number of symptoms							
	0	1	2	3	4	5	Total	$M \pm S.D.$
High skilled workers	138	71	42	15	5	2	230	0·84 ± 1·07
Low skilled workers	87	52	35	13	8	2	203	1←03 ± 1·19

of their qualities has been done with reference to the Selye-Stress concept. This concept implies that prolonged stress may result in non-specific reactions, which in turn may lead to different kinds of symptoms or ultimately disease.

Control variables = environmental and worker characteristics

One worker characteristic has already been considered in the selection of the groups. Other control variables are type of wage, level of income, and level of total job satisfaction.

Two different types of wages were included: fixed salary and individual piece wage. The level of income was dichotomized into a high and low income group, as close as possible to the median in the actual group. Total job satisfaction (TJS), dichotomized in the same way, was measured as the mean of four attitude scales, dealing with:

1. Job engagement;
2. Physical and mental strain;
3. Control over own job;
4. Social interaction in job.

The total number of items in TJS is 23.

The breakdowns of the high and low skilled groups are shown in Figs 16.3 and 16.4, which also give the numbers of subjects in each subgroup.

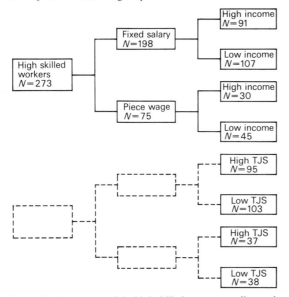

FIG. 16.3. Breakdown of the high skilled group according to the control variables. TJS = total job satisfaction; N = number of subjects.

Statistical procedures

Through analysis the independent, dependent, and relevant control variables have been dichotomized as close as possible to the median for each subgroup. Thus, the independent and dependent variables are cross-tabulated in 2 × 2 tables of frequencies.

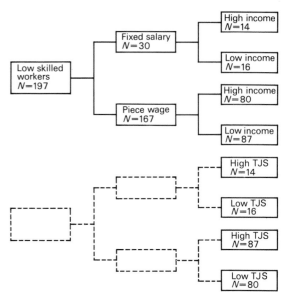

FIG. 16.4. Breakdown of the low skilled group according to the control variables. TJS = total job satisfaction; N = number of subjects.

Yule's Q value (Yule and Kendall 1950) which has properties similar to those of a correlation coefficient, has been adopted as a measure of the strength of the association between the independent and dependent variables. The standard error of Q is related to the number of observations in the 2 × 2 table, i.e. a rather high Q-value in a small group may be of no significance, whereas a small Q-value in a large group can be highly significant. In order to facilitate an assessment of the results in this respect, the level of tendencies in Q has been denoted in addition to significant values. The following levels of tendency and significance have been used:

Tendency: $p \leq 0.20$ is denoted °
$p \leq 0.10$ is denoted °°
Significance: $p \leq 0.05$ is denoted *, in text 'significant'
$p \leq 0.01$ is denoted **, in text 'rather highly significant'
$p \leq 0.001$ is denoted ***, in text 'highly significant'

A *positive sign* of Q indicates a correspondence between the independent and dependent variables in the same direction; i.e. if monotony, physical, or mental strain increase, this is accompanied by an increase in number of symptoms. A *negative sign* of Q indicates the opposite direction.

RESULTS

Data are presented in Figs 16.5–16.15, showing each dichotomy made according to the control variables. Each figure deals with all three independent variables. In each figure, Yule's Q is a measure of association between stress indicators and symptoms. The calculations are based on dichotomized distributions of the independent and dependent variables.

In Fig. 16.5, the total group ($N = 470$) is analysed and the variation between high and low skilled workers considered. *Monotony* showed no relation to symptoms for the total group. The same was the case for the high and low skilled groups but the Q-values were of different signs—negative for the high and positive for the low skilled group. *Physical strain* showed a high, positive significant relation to symptoms for the total group. This significance was reduced to a tendency for the high skilled but remained high for the low skilled group. *Mental strain* was significantly related in the positive direction to symptoms for the total group. This relation disappeared for the high skilled workers but remained for the low skilled.

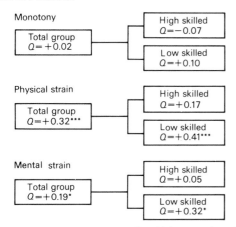

FIG. 16.5. The total group ($N = 470$): high versus low skilled workers.

In Fig. 16.6, the high skilled workers are analysed and the variation between those with fixed salary and those on a piece wage considered. *Monotony* showed no relation to symptoms. For both groups the sign of Q was negative in the same way as for the total group. *Physical strain* showed no association with symptoms for the fixed salary group. Q had a positive value. For piece wage the same positive tendency was obtained as found for the total group. *Mental strain* for the fixed salary group gave a Q-value of O. The piece wage group showed a tendency to a positive relationship, i.e. a strengthened Q-value compared with the total group.

In Fig. 16.7, the high skilled workers with fixed salary are analysed and the variation between those with high and low incomes is considered. *Monotony* showed no relation to symptoms. The negative sign obtained for the fixed salary group was retained in the high income groups. The Q-value for the low income group was about zero. *Physical strain* showed no relation to symptoms. Both Q-values were positive. *Mental strain* showed no relation to symptoms. In the high income group the sign

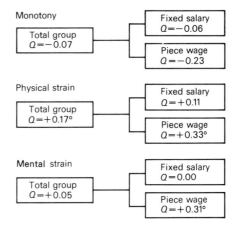

FIG. 16.6. The high skilled workers: fixed salary versus piece wage.

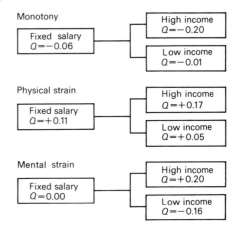

FIG. 16.7. The high skilled workers: with fixed salary: high versus low income.

of the Q-value was positive, compared to a negative sign in the low income group. It is noteworthy that the sum of these results gave a Q-value of zero in the fixed salary group.

In Fig. 16.8, the high skilled workers with piece wage are analysed and the variation between those with high and low incomes is considered. *Monotony* showed a tendency to a negative relation to symptoms in the high income group. For the low income group a significant, negative relation to symptoms was found. *Physical strain* showed a tendency to a positive relation for the low income group. The Q-values were positive in both groups, in the same way as for the piece wage group. *Mental strain* showed no relation to symptoms. A positive Q-value for the high income group and a negative for the low were obtained. Thus, the same shift in signs appeared as for the fixed salary group (Fig. 6.7).

In Fig. 6.9, the high skilled workers with fixed salary are analysed and the variation between those with high and low TJS (total job satisfaction) is considered. *Monotony* showed no relation to symptoms in any

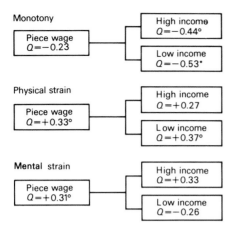

FIG. 16.8. The high skilled workers with piece wage: high versus low income.

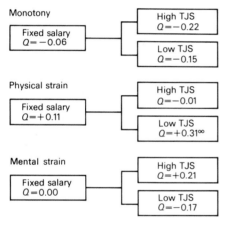

FIG. 16.9. The high skilled workers with fixed salary: high versus low TJS (total job satisfaction).

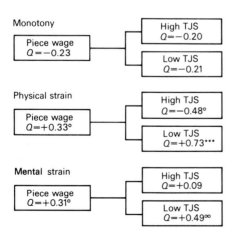

FIG. 16.10. The high skilled workers with piece wage: high versus low TJS (total job satisfaction).

group. The *Q*-values were negative. *Physical strain* in the high TJS group gave a *Q*-value of about zero. In the low TJS group a tendency to a positive *Q*-value was found. *Mental strain* gave *Q*-values, which were positive in the high TJS group and negative in the low, i.e. a similar result to that for high and low income (Figs. 6.7 and 6.8).

In Fig. 6.10, the high skilled workers with piece wage are analysed and the variation between those with high and low TJS is considered. *Monotony* showed no relation to symptoms. *Q* had negative signs for both groups, in the same way as in the piece wage group. *Physical strain* showed a tendency to a negative relation to symptoms in the high TJS group. In the low TJS group there was a highly significant position relation. The *Q*-value of 0·73 was the highest obtained in the whole material. *Mental strain* showed no relation to symptoms in the high TJS group. *Q* had a positive sign. In the low TJS group there was a tendency to a positive relation, which was more pronounced than in the piece wage group.

In Fig. 6.11, the low skilled workers are analysed and the variation between those with fixed salary and those on a piece wage is considered. *Monotony* showed no relation to symptoms. The sign of *Q* was negative in the fixed salary and positive in the piece wage group. *Physical strain* showed no relation to symptoms for the fixed salary group but a highly significant, positive relation in the piece wage group. The sign of *Q* was negative in the fixed salary group. *Mental strain* showed positive *Q*-values in both groups, most pronounced piece wage.

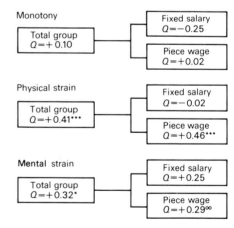

FIG. 16.11. The low skilled workers: fixed salary versus piece wage.

In Fig. 6.12, the low skilled workers with fixed salary are analysed and the variation between those with high and low incomes is considered. *Monotony* showed no relation to symptoms for the level of income. The sign of *Q* was negative for high and positive for low income. *Physical strain* showed no relation to the income level. The *Q*-values were positive. *Mental strain* gave a

98

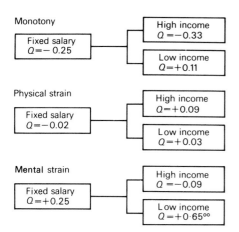

FIG. 16.12. The low skilled workers with fixed salary: high versus low income.

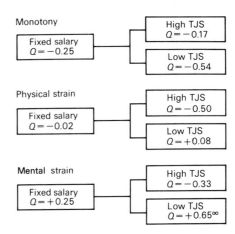

FIG. 16.14. The low income skilled workers with fixed salary: high versus low TJS (total job satisfaction).

tendency to a positive Q-value for the low income group. The Q-value was negative in the high income group.

In Fig. 6.13, the low skilled workers with piece wage are analysed and the variation between those with high and low income is considered. *Monotony* showed no relation to symptoms. It is of interest that the Q-value of about zero in the piece wage group changed to a positive and a negative value after the breakdown according to income level. *Physical strain* showed a rather high positive significance in the high income group. A positive tendency was found in the low income group. *Mental strain* gave, as mentioned, a tendency to a positive relation in the total piece wage group. For the high income group this relation was strengthened to a rather high significance, but for the low income group the relation disappeared.

and low TJS is considered. *Monotony* showed no relation to symptoms. Both Q-values were negative. *Physical strain* showed no relation to symptoms. The Q-value was negative in the high and positive in the low TJS group. *Mental strain* gave a tendency to a positive Q-value for the low TJS group. The Q-value was negative in the high TJS group.

In Fig. 6.15, the low skilled workers with piece wage are analysed and the variation between those with high and low TJS is considered. *Monotony* gave a tendency to a negative relation for the low TJS group. The Q-value was positive in the high TJS group. Again an original zero-correlation changed to a positive and a negative. *Physical strain* showed a high, positive significance in the high TJS group. The sign of Q was positive in the low TJS group. *Mental strain* gave a tendency to a positive relation in the high TJS group. The Q-value was also positive in the low TJS group.

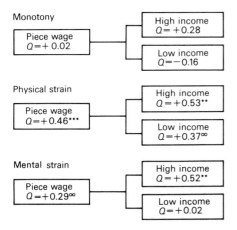

FIG. 16.13. The low skilled workers with piece wage: high versus low income.

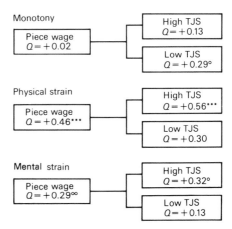

FIG. 16.15. The low skilled workers with piece wage: high versus low TJS (total job satisfaction).

In Fig. 6.14, the low skilled workers with fixed salary are analysed and the variation between those with high

The pattern of the association between the stress indicators and perceived ill health

Monotony. In general, monotony showed no association with symptoms. However, in most cases the coefficients were negative, especially for the high skilled workers. In this group all 11 signs were negative, but one was very close to zero. In the subgroup characterized by piece wage and a low income, the negative relation was significant. For the low skilled workers, 6 out of 11 Q-values were negative. All Q-values were non-significant in this group.

Physical strain. In the high skilled group, physical strain showed no association with symptoms in all groups except one, namely the piece wage group with low TJS. This group showed a highly significant, positive association, $Q = + 0.73$. Most of the coefficients, 9 out of 11, had a positive sign.

For the low skilled group a highly significant, positive association was found between physical strain and symptoms. This association disappeared in the groups with fixed salary. For the total piece wage group as well as the group with high TJS in addition to piece wage, the highly significant association remained. For the group characterized by high income and piece wage, there was a rather high significance in the positive direction. The positive signs dominated, 9 out of 11 were obtained, which was the same distribution of signs as in the high skilled group.

Mental strain. In general, mental strain showed no association with symptoms, but the positive coefficients were in a majority. This holds especially for the low skilled workers, for whom 9 out of 11 Q-values were positive, compared to 7 out of 11 for the high skilled workers. The latter group showed no significant coefficients.

For the total low skilled group the relation between mental strain and symptoms was positively significant All coefficients were positive in the piece wage groups and a rather high, positive significance was observed for the subgroup of piece wage combined with high income.

DISCUSSION

As has been pointed out in the adopted frame of reference, a positive association between stress indicators and perceived ill health is expected. The effect of a breakdown can be well illustrated by considering the total group, consisting of all the high and low skilled workers. The postulated relationship was statistically significant for physical and mental strain (Fig. 16.5). The strength of the association, however is low; only 4 to 6 per cent of the variance in number of symptoms can be explained by these stress indicators. The monotony variable showed no association. After breaking down the total group into the two main groups, high and low skilled workers, no changes were found for monotony, but the original relationship as to physical strain was strengthened in the low skilled group. About 17 per cent

of the variance in number of symptoms can be explained by physical strain. In the high skilled group the original relation was weakened to a positive tendency. For mental strain the relationship remained only in the low skilled group.

In contrast to the hypothesized expectations, monotony showed no positive relationship to symptoms in any case. Rather the results indicate a negative association in the high skilled group. In the low skilled group the positive and negative signs of the Q-values were more balanced. According to the U-shaped curve in Fig. 16.2, there are two explanations for the outcome. Either the degree of monotony is 'normal and just right' or the outcome is the sum of the results from subgroups characterized by over- and understimulation, respectively. The fact that all associations for the high skilled group were negative points to a dominance for the overstimulated groups. For an overstimulated person the theory indicates that an increasing degree of monotony would lead to reduced stress. For the low skilled workers the over- and understimulated subgroups seem to be more in balance, if the degree of monotony was not 'just right'. The hypothesis about over- and understimulated subgroups in balance could be tested by applying control variables relevant for this particular issue.

Physical strain showed, as expected and previously mentioned, a highly significant, positive association with the number of symptoms for the low skilled group. All subgroups with fixed salary showed no association. The lack of association in this fixed salary group and many of the high skilled groups can be explained in terms of over- and underload in physical terms, in analogy with the discussion above for monotony.

The dominance of associations with positive signs for mental strain was most pronounced in the low skilled group, but on the whole the outcome presented a fairly diffuse picture. If there is no true variance between the independent and dependent variables in a main group, the outcome of positive and negative signs of Q should be randomly distributed in the subgroups. If no true variance exists for the high skilled workers, the signs of Q in the main group are caused only by an error variance, and the signs in the subgroups will be a random effect.

The distribution of 10 negative signs out of 10 found for monotony in the subgroups of high skilled workers will appear by chance with a probability of 0.001. The distribution of 8 positive signs out of 10 for physical strain in the same subgroups will appear by chance with a probability of 0.04, and finally the distribution of 6 positive signs out of 10 for psychic strain will appear by chance with a probability of 0.21. Consequently, at least for monotony and physical strain, the negative and the positive sign, respectively, in the main group indicates an association. These associations can either be very low and of no significance for the individual's health, or they can be the sum of strong associations in different directions. The distribution of negative and positive signs in monotony for the low skilled workers could have appeared by chance ($p \leq 0.25$), if there was no true association in the main group.

The only clear-cut results in the whole analysis were found in physical strain for the low skilled workers and in one case for the high skilled. As mentioned above, the first breakdown for the low skilled into fixed salary and piece wage revealed that the original association could exclusively be ascribed to the piece wage group. The following two alternative breakdowns gave associations for the high income and high TJS groups. With these latter breakdowns, the variance in number of symptoms explained by physical strain increased to 28 and 31 per cent, respectively. An interesting finding is that the higher the job satisfaction, the stronger was the positive association between physical strain and perceived ill health for the low skilled. A tentative explanation could be that the characteristics of the job satisfy the individual's needs and expectations at the cost of a high risk that perceived stress is concordant with perceived ill health. The pattern of the significances indicates that an overstimulation was present. Piece wage *per se* is a stimulating agent and, if the piece wage results in a high income, this can be a stimulating factor as well.

A trend toward a positive association between physical strain and symptoms for piece wage *per se* and piece wage combined with a high income or a high job satisfaction could also be observed in monotony and mental strain for the low skilled workers and in mental strain for the high skilled. For the low skilled workers with piece wage the relationship between physical strain and symptoms in the groups with high job satisfaction was independent of the income level. Thus job satisfaction level seems to be a determining factor. See Fig. 16.16.

In the high skilled group, physical strain showed mainly positive non-significant associations. However, after two breakdowns a very strong association appeared in the group characterized by piece wage and low TJS. A Q-value amounting to $+0.73$ was highly significant and explained 53 per cent of the variance in the number of symptoms. A tentative explanation could be made in terms of frustration, which implies that the individual's needs and expectations are not fulfilled. This seems plausible as a piece wage job implies work with lower qualifications than a high skilled worker aspires to. The negative tendency found for the high TJS group and the positive tendency found for the low income group with piece wage support this reasoning.

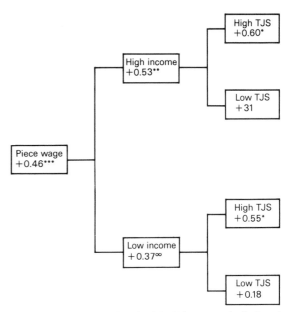

FIG. 16.16. The association (Yule's Q) between physical strain and subjective symptoms for all low skilled workers with piece wage ($N = 167$) and this group divided successively into income and total job satisfaction levels.

It should be noted that the result for physical strain is the outcome of the answers on a *single* item. Had a more reliable measure been used, e.g. an attitude index, the predictive strength would probably have increased.

The difference in outcome for the two main groups, high and low skilled workers, draws attention to the need for a continued multivariate analysis with further efforts to obtain more homogenous groups than was possible in the present study. The analysis has revealed some work and worker characteristics, which connect stress to perceived ill health. The kind of stress was *perceived physical strain*, and the characteristics were:

(a) Low skilfulness;
(b) Low skilfulness combined with piece wage;
(c) Low skilfulness combined with piece wage and high income;
(d) Low skilfulness combined with piece wage and high job satisfaction;
(e) High skilfulness combined with piece wage and low job satisfaction.

REFERENCES

GARDELL, B. (1971). *Produktionsteknik och arbetsglädje.* PA-rådet, Stockholm.
LEVI, L. (1972). Stress and distress in response to psychosocial stimuli. *Acta Med. Scand., Suppl.* **528**.
YULE, G. U. and KENDALL, M. G. (1950). *An introduction to the theory of statistics.* Griffin, London.

17. FIT BETWEEN EXPECTATIONS OF THE WORKERS AND CONDITIONS IN AN AUTOMOTIVE INDUSTRY

JAN FORSLIN

INTRODUCTION

Being a psychologist, I am here going to concentrate on the psychological aspect of the process of human adaptation to work and vice versa. I would like to present a model for studying the psychological process of work adjustment. The model will be illustrated by results from a study on the situation of workers and supervisors in one automotive factory in Sweden.

Hopefully, this approach will contribute to research within the world of work also from the point of view of other disciplines than psychology. I also hope that the data to be presented here will give new insights into the situation which is shared by workers and other employees.

A MODEL OF THE PSYCHOLOGICAL PROCESS OF WORK ADJUSTMENT

The basic belief behind the model used for this work has been that work adjustment is the result of the joint contributions of the individual worker and the work itself. The implicit demands of the worker and the demands of the work always have to be matched. This matching process can be called work adjustment and it involves varying degrees of strain and stress for the individual. The result can also be of varying quality. We know that man's capacity for adaptation to new circumstances, including work, is considerable. Man is flexible, man can learn, he can be compensated for dull work by more money—although this is seldom done. This view of man as an adapting animal has led to a technological determinism; that is, technology is regarded as a constant factor which cannot be changed and thus one-sidedly determines the qualities of the work situation.

A process-related model

First a few words about the need for a process-related model. There are many instances when we want to study reactions of the individual to changes in his working conditions, e.g. technical or organizational changes. We would also like to know how the young worker changes over his first years of employment or what the effects are of recurrent training in terms of changes in the individual's outlook on work.

The traditional attitude indices or measures of job satisfaction, calculated after troublesome factor analyses and other sophisticated procedures, are not very sensitive to changes and give few cues how to interpret the differences we observe; nor are they well suited for the follow-up design required by the study of change.

As an alternative, this model concentrates on the psychology of the individual and gives a fairly detailed description of his conditions of work. The model implies that we—man—react to our situation according to rational decision-making—rational from our point of view, that is. Knowing the inputs to the individual's cognitions, we also understand his behaviour. We can also present to him a picture in which he recognizes himself. And this is a very important aspect of psychological research—to provide the individual with a mirror in which he can see himself and his situation. Then we can also use the individual in the research process for verification of our interpretation of the data.

Informed participation by the individual workers in the research

This is far from common practice in psychological research. You could even say that it has been against the rule to involve the subject in the research process. Ideally, according to our experimental traditions, he should be naïve and ignorant about the design etc.

Usually, you go to the workers and say: 'Hello there, I am your friend. I would like to ask you some questions about your work for scientific reasons. I have checked with the union. They say it is O.K. You may answer my questions.' Then you say: 'Here are some questions about your work place, your supervisor, the company, the hours, etc.' But that is not true, for what you are really after, is to see if the workers are alienated, have an instrumental attitude, have adjusted to work, and the like. And this you do not tell the workers, so five years later when the data analysis is carried out, the worker finds in the newspaper that he is alienated or suffers from stress or is understimulated. Furthermore, they are going to change his job to make him more motivated. And I do not think he recognizes himself or feels that he has participated in the decisions of change.

The point here is that the investigator, with the best of intentions, is trying to improve the worker's conditions without checking the relevance to the worker of his research approach. Are we asking the right questions, is our theoretical frame of reference of any relevance to the worker?

The minimum requirements for participation of the worker in the research is that the model you use is understandable or can be communicated in a comprehensible way and that the measures you use explicitly measure what you are investigating. A few modest steps in that direction have been taken by clearly stating what we are asking for and by arranging the questions in a logically reasonable way as steps in a decision-making process.

The relationship between size of reward and its probability

The psychological model is based on an assumed relationship between the size of rewards and their probability of occurrence. You could say that in working life—and elsewhere for that matter—rewards are scarce products. That is, in general, the more we want of something good, the smaller is the probability of attaining it. Chase the moon and you will reach the tree-tops. The relationship is assumed to look roughly as illustrated in Fig. 17.1.

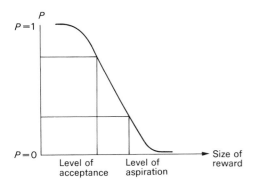

FIG. 17.1. Relationship between size of reward and its probability.

Along the x-axis we have the size of a reward—which can be material as well as immaterial. Along the y-axis we find the corresponding probabilities. If we plot the probability for increasing degrees of reward, we will obtain this S-shaped curve. Unfortunately, it is a backward S, which means that the probabilities for obtaining very small rewards is very high, but with increasing size of rewards the probabilities will decline until finally we reach a level very close to zero. The model implies that this is not only a sound way of describing the situation of human beings, it is also the way the individual—also the worker—perceives his situation, or at least learns to perceive it—from childhood on. The slope of the curve and the level where it approaches zero probabilities vary between individuals and from time to time.

Another basic feature of this approach is that the individual lays identifiable claims for the size of the rewards he obtains in every situation in exchange for the effort he manifests. I am here operating with two levels of claims. The first one you could call level of aspiration, which is the level you are striving to obtain, and the nature of which is that it will never be obtained, except momentarily, because then the aspirations are raised

again. That level is represented in Fig. 17.1, by the solid line cutting the curve at the low probability part.

The second level of claims is the size you do not want your rewards to fall below, the lowest level of rewards you are willing to accept as reasonable. Consequently, this level is named level of acceptance, and is marked with the second solid line cutting the curve at the high probability part. To be satisfactory, the rewards should be between these two levels in every situation.

The model uses some ten concepts in total for describing the situation of the individual. Almost all concepts have been deduced from this simple curvilinear relationship between rewards and their probabilities, and they are all variants of probabilities or size of rewards. I am not going to enumerate them all now; they will be introduced as the results are accounted for.

METHOD OF RESEARCH

This particular study was made in a factory in the Swedish automotive industry; 300 workers and some 100 supervisors participated. The workers were drawn from all parts of the factory. The interviews were carried out in large groups with paper and pencil.

According to the original design, the workers were sampled from three different age groups with equal-sized samples—about one hundred persons. The groups were up to 24 years, 25 to 34 years, and 35 to 44 years of age. The supervisors were on the average a little older than the oldest group of workers. Differences in age reflect among other things differences in length of service.

The interviewees made ratings of each of ten job facets on scales with nine numerical points representing 'very little' up to 'very much' or something similar depending on the aspects rated. The ratings were made according to ten different cognitive dimensions like the ones just mentioned—either probabilities or levels of rewards. The ratings were made of all facets for each dimension in sequence.

For every combination of job facet and cognitive dimension, the mean was calculated. A statistical test of differences between groups in the sample was made by means of multivariate one-way analysis of variance. This test shows if the whole dimension is systematically rated higher by any of the groups. It also gives the relative contribution of each job facet to the difference. As the method takes into account the correlations between job facets, it gives some protection against mass significance. I am not going to bother you with statistical figures, but restrict myself to graphic representations of the results based on means of the ratings.

RESULTS

First we will introduce the ten job facets for which the corresponding rewards were rated. The workers also rated the importance of each facet and the results are shown in the Fig. 17.2. The ten facets are: job security; level of promotion; relationship to comrades; pay; independence; level of training; possibilities of personal development; variety; working conditions; meaningfulness of work. The facets you choose are somewhat arbitrary and the choice should rest on the sample you investigate or your theoretical frame of reference.

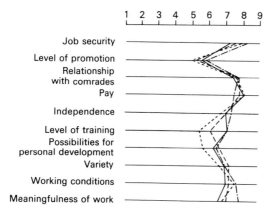

FIG. 17.2. Comparison of importance of ten job facets for: (————) workers aged 17–24 years; (— — —) workers aged 25–34 years; (----) workers aged 35–44 years; and (–·–·–) supervisors.

There is, on the whole, good agreement between the groups and, in general, all facets are judged as important aspects of work. The main deviation is the lower rating of the older workers for two facets concerning training and possibilities of personal development. It should be noted that the supervisors hold the same values as the workers.

The next dimension I would like to mention is the closest to what are traditionally used as measures of job satisfaction. The interviewees rates their satisfaction with each of the job aspects (Fig. 17.3). The ratings do not discriminate systematically between the workers.

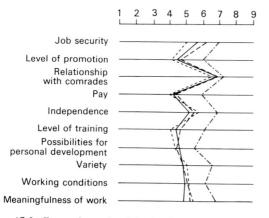

FIG. 17.3. Comparison of satisfaction for: (————) workers aged 17–24 years; (— — —) workers aged 25–34; (----) workers aged 35–44; and (–·–·–) supervisors.

There are differences between the groups for some job facets, but by and large the ratings are very similar. The supervisors, on the other hand, have substantially higher ratings. They are systematically more satisfied than the workers with all facets except with their fellow workers, where the ratings coincide. All groups have given identical ratings of the friendship.

Typically, the workers' ratings lie in the middle of the scale which on a verbal scale like that of Likert would correspond to neither satisfied nor dissatisfied. Thus, this gives us very little information, apart from supervisors being more satisfied than workers, and workers not being terribly dissatisfied. Let us now look at the more detailed description of the work situation of these four groups.

Present job satisfaction and expected future job satisfaction

We shall then start by seeing how reality fits with the aspirations of the participants. Fig. 17.4 shows the ratings of the youngest group. As in the following figures, the solid line to the right shows the aspirations—the level you aspire to reach. The solid line to the left gives the level of acceptance—that is, the level of reward you do not want to go below. According to the model, the aspirations should be rated higher than the level of acceptance, which is done consistently. So far, the data support the model.

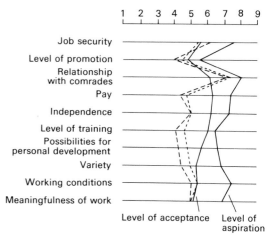

FIG. 17.4. Present outcome (— — —), and expected fulfilment of demands in the next six months (----) for young workers aged 17–24 years.

What about reality then? The broken line represents the perceived outcome of today. The dotted line shows how it is anticipated to be in six months. Obviously, the present situation is not good enough. For every facet except relations with peers and to some extent job security there is a very poor fit between the least you expect to get from the job and how it actually is.

As a small hope we can notify that for all facets with one exception the situation is expected to improve. As this group has a short length of service, they may expect their situation to be even better—maybe satisfactory—in the long run. The answer to that expectation is to be found from the ratings by the older groups, who have long experience with the company.

The ratings of the middle group, aged between 25 and 34, are shown in Fig. 17.5. In most respects, the picture is very similar to the one given by the youngest group. The relationship with comrades is the only aspect of work that gives a satisfactory outcome. If we turn to expectations for the immediate future, the picture points towards a change. For some facets the situation is expected to get worse.

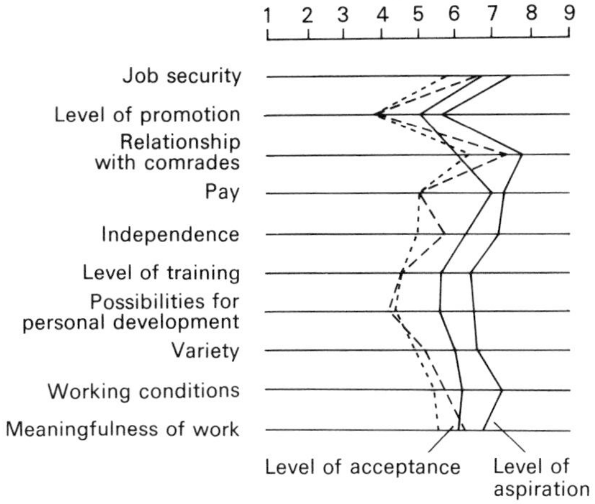

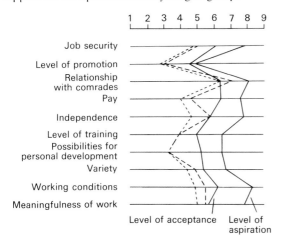

FIG. 17.5. Level of aspiration, level of acceptance, present outcome (— — —), and expected outcome in the next six months (----) for the workers aged 25–34 years.

The oldest group also shows a very similar pattern for the present situation (Fig. 17.6). But here *all* expectations are for the worse. So they give very little support for the optimism of the youngest group.

FIG. 17.6. Level of aspiration, level of acceptance, present outcome (— — —), and expected outcome in the next six months (----) for the oldest workers aged 35–44.

I would like to make a short summary here. For all workers irrespective of age, the present situation is unsatisfactory. The present outcome falls below even the lowest claims. The young workers expect the situation to improve somewhat in the immediate future, but far from enough. With increasing age, the pessimism of the workers grows, and the oldest group expects the situation to become worse than it is today.

At this point, I asked myself if the data were biased. Was there something wrong with the model and/or the method as, all the time, I obtained this incongruity between claims and possibilities? One test of this is to look at the supervisors' ratings. We know that their work situation differs in many important aspects from that of the workers. We also know that they are more satisfied.

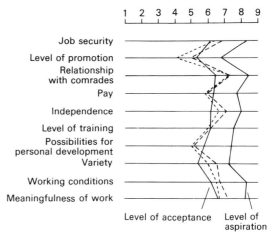

FIG. 17.7. Level of aspiration, level of acceptance, present outcome (— — —), and expected outcome in the next six months (----) for the supervisors.

As Fig. 17.7 shows, the situation for this group is rated as being more favourable. Only three facets have outcomes lower than the smallest claims, nor is the deficit as big as for the workers. But like the oldest workers, the supervisors are pessimistic about the future. They anticipate lower outcomes for all ten job facets.

Personally, I took the supervisors' response as support for method and model. I also thought that deviations from the pattern in the ratings of comradeship supported the validity of the results. I was now very anxious to see how the situation I had pictured could be handled; what the alternatives were for these persons.

Possible responses to a non-rewarding situation
As we have seen, the situation for the workers is unsatisfactory. Well in line with these results is the way different groups perceive their possibilities to realize their aspirations (Fig. 17.8). The older workers are more pessimistic than the others and supervisors are more optimistic.

Lowering of levels of acceptance and aspirations. With these bad prospects people could be expected to lower

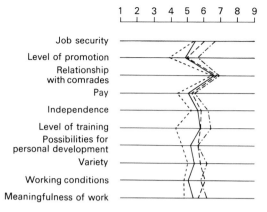

FIG. 17.8. Comparison of probability for attaining the aspirations as perceived by: (———) workers aged 17–24 years; (— — —) workers aged 25–34 years; (----) workers aged 35–44 years; (–·–·–·) supervisors.

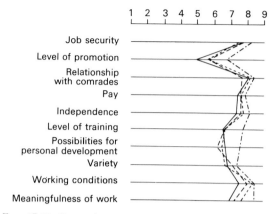

FIG. 17.10 Comparison of level of aspiration of: (———) workers aged 17–24 years; (— — —) workers aged 25–34 years; (- - - -) workers aged 35–44 years; (-·····) supervisors.

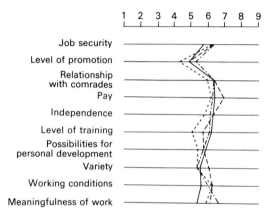

FIG. 17.9. Comparison of level of acceptance of: (———) workers aged 17–24 years; (— — —) workers aged 25–34 years; (----) workers aged 35–44 years; (–·–·–·) supervisors.

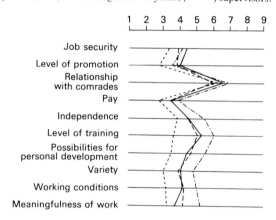

FIG. 17.11. Comparison of possibility to influence as perceived by: (———) workers aged 17–24 years; (— — —) workers aged 25–34 years; (----) workers aged 35–44 years; (–·–·–·) supervisors.

their claims to make the fit to reality more endurable. But, at least so far, none of the groups has lowered its claims—at least not to such an extent as to make reality acceptable. Fig. 17.9 shows the level of acceptance for all four groups. The oldest workers tend to have a lower limit. However, on the whole, the differences are small.

The differences between the workers are even smaller when we compare their level of aspirations (Fig. 17.10). The supervisors, however, have systematically higher aspirations than the workers.

Improvement of working conditions. An active way of handling an unsatisfactory situation is to change the present conditions. The participants were asked to rate their possibility of influencing their situation in the company in a favourable direction. The results can be seen in Fig. 17.11.

Generally, the possibility of improving one's conditions is rated low by the workers. In particular the oldest group is very pessimistic. The supervisors, on the

other hand, have a more optimistic view of their possibilities. Again we find the high degree of agreement concerning comradeship. There is also relatively higher agreement in the low rating for pay, which is largely laid down by centralized negotiations. The more optimistic view of the supervisors is most distinct for facets which are directly related to their own work, which the supervisors usually have more freedom to manipulate.

Changing jobs. The ultimate action in a non-rewarding situation which you cannot change, is to leave it if you have a better alternative. In Fig. 17.12 we get a very vivid picture of the outlook of these four groups on their possibilities of finding a better job on the labour market.

The answers are now polarized. Those of the young and middle groups coincide on a moderately optimistic level with little variation between job facets, whereas the ratings of both supervisors and the oldest group of workers lie on a very pessimistic level. These two groups share a very low estimate of their possibilities. And it

106

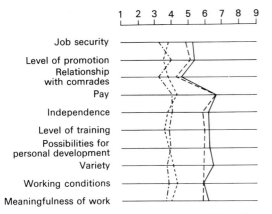

FIG. 17.12. Comparison of the possibility of obtaining a better job as perceived by: (———) workers aged 17–24 years; (— — —) workers aged 25–34 years; (----) workers aged 35–44 years; (–·–·–·) supervisors.

should be stressed that the oldest group of workers is in the age span 35–44 years—men in the prime of life.

So much for psychology and philosophy, but what do the workers actually do? According to our results, *all* workers, irrespective of age, have equally good reasons to look for another job—outside the automotive industry. The only element of satisfaction has to do with

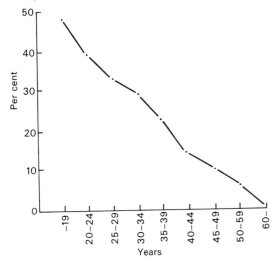

FIG. 17.13. Relative numbers of people leaving their jobs (separations) during the year of investigation.

the fellow workers, other aspects of the work being less than acceptable. We also know that with increasing age you become more and more pessimistic about your opportunities, which would lead to a lower rate of separations. Let us now look at the statistical records of the company under investigation.

Fig. 17.13 shows the relative rate of separations within consecutive age groups. The percentages are calculated on the number of employees at the beginning of the year, plus the number of people employed during the year, i.e. the number of potential leavers. Turnover statistics can be calculated in many ways, but usually you get the same clear trend as here. The majority of separations are attributable to young workers. Above the age of forty few leavers are found.

IMPROVED CONDITIONS IN THE AUTOMOTIVE INDUSTRY

Finally a few words in behalf of the automotive industry. The picture of the working conditions that is mirrored here by the perception of the workers is not very flattering for this branch of industry. However, the investigation was made some years ago, and this company, as well as the other Swedish automotive industry, were then and still are to some extent plagued by difficulties in recruiting labour. Furthermore, once people are hired, they quit—mostly after just a few months. The size of the flow of people through the companies has been grotesque. Evidently, something had to be done if any cars are to be produced in the future.

So, at about the same time as this investigation was carried out, the now well known Scania and Volvo experiments on humanization of work started with the object of improving working conditions. Let me stress that there is *no* causal connection between the research and the subsequent democratization of work. On the other hand, it would have been a good idea to study the effect of such changes in the organization of work by following the changes in perception of work to see if the aspirations of the workers for more responsibility, more qualified and meaningful work could be raised by such changes, to find out if the new work corresponds better to the needs and claims of the workers.

18. THE WORKING ENVIRONMENT OF HOSPITAL AND PUBLIC HEALTH WORKERS

INGRID WAHLUND

THE WORKING ENVIRONMENT—AN EXTENDED CONCEPT

The concept of the working environment has in recent years acquired an extended meaning. Previously the working environment was taken to mean primarily various physical factors in work such as noise, air pollution, heavy loads, various chemical and physical conditions, etc. for example. The detrimental effects of these environmental factors on health and well-being are also relatively well known. Efforts to improve the working environment have therefore been primarily geared to these physical factors.

In recent years, however, attention has been directed not only toward the work experience but also to the fact that physical and mental health is very much dependent on various organizational conditions. By this we mean the organizational structure of the place of work, with its functional divisions, information routines and contact channels, decision-making routines, and means and routines for directing and controlling activities. These factors are of great importance to the individual's work situation and determine to a great extent the individual's opportunity of influencing and controlling his/her work and of using and developing his/her knowledge and ability in a versatile manner. The same applies to the individual's ability to view his/her job as meaningful and important and to experience contact and communion with his/her colleagues.

Extensive research has shown that inadequacies in the organizational working environment cause mental strain and tiredness necessitating long periods of recuperation after work is finished. They also create an estrangement from work resulting in a low level of interest and involvement in the job and the place of work. It has also been found that there is a link between inadequacies in the organization working environment and a deterioration in health and an increase in the frequency of psychosomatic symptoms. Surveys have also shown that working conditions entailing few opportunities of influencing one's own work situation can create passive leisure time with a low level of participation in, for example, political and trade union activities, etc. The concept of the working environment today therefore includes both physical and organizational working conditions.

These views are again reflected in a number of activities in the field of the working environment in recent years. The International Labour Organization (ILO) and the World Health Organization (WHO) have launched programmes in the field of work and health. In 1974 the Council of Nordic Ministers initiated Scandinavian co-operation in the field of 'Stress in the working environment' and the Council's Scandinavian research group is at present, together with the Joint Organization for Scandinavian Trade Unions (NFS), conducting a research project on the organizational working environment of workers and of salaried employees. Together with colleagues from Denmark, Norway, and Finland I am myself co-operating with the Scandinavian Union of Teachers (NLS) within the NFS on a survey into the working conditions of Scandinavian elementary school teachers.

In Sweden the new occupational injuries insurance includes cover for occupational injuries resulting from mental strain at work. The new Swedish Working Environment Act which enters into force on 1 July 1978 also stipulates that 'the working environment must be satisfactory with regard to the nature of the work and social and technical developments in society. Working conditions must be adapted to the individual's physical and mental prerequisites.' This Act and the agreements reached in this field, and primarily the Co-determination Act, which stipulates negotiations on all issues involving employees' working conditions, therefore give the employees the opportunity, through their trade unions, of themselves determining the formulation of their physical and organizational working environment.

TCOs (the Swedish Central Organization of Salaried Employees) activities in the field of the working environment have also been stimulated by the broader view of environmental issues. Relatively little has been known, however, about the working environment of the salaried employee. The surveys which have indicated link-ups between various factors in the working environment and work experience and health have often comprised survey groups provided by the employers. Thus in many instances the salaried employees have not had sufficient bases for the formulation of their views on various environmental issues. In 1975 therefore TCO asked the work Environmental Fund for money to conduct a broad survey on the working environment of salaried employees. The aim of the project is to investigate to what extent various groups of salaried employees have jobs and working conditions which give them job satisfaction and involvement in their work, or jobs and working conditions which involve mental strain. The survey is also studying which factors contribute toward involvement and strain in work. The project will also investigate whether there is any connection between work experience, medical problems, and absenteeism.

The survey was conducted as a mail questionnaire sent to a random selection of TCO members. The questionnaire included some 100 questions dealing with various working conditions, work experience, general health, and absence from work. As stated above, the survey group comprised a random selection of TCO members. The number of interviewees, *circa* 12 000, was motivated by the large spread of the interviewees with regard to occupation and working conditions. Participants included professional nurses, industrial salaried employees, supervisors, teachers, policemen, armed forces personnel, etc. Response was 87 per cent or 10 000 replies. This is a very high level of response which we interpret as an expression of great interest in the working environment on the part of TCO members.

The project's first report *The salaried employee's working environment: work, health, wellbeing* (Wahlund and Nerell 1976), gave a broad description of the working conditions of various groups of salaried employees. The report contained results referring to work organizational conditions among various groups of employees and associations, and their connection with job satisfaction, stress experienced at work, general health, and absence from work. The report also contained results referring to the physical working environment of different groups.

TCO and the associations have in various ways used the results of this report in their union work. In TCOs reply to the proposal for a new working environment act in 1976, for example, reference is made to the report's results regarding the stress experienced at work. The same applies to TCOs reply to the proposal for a new occupational injuries insurance. Results are also cited in various surveys, e.g. the company health survey. The results have also been used in various negotiations on working conditions and in discussions on work demands and work evaluation in respect of the jobs of various groups.

THE WORKING ENVIRONMENT OF HOSPITAL AND PUBLIC HEALTH WORKERS

Further processing of the survey material within the framework of the Salaried Employees' Working Environment Project has mainly dealt with conditions which are essential parts of the working environment of all categories of salaried employees. One of the reasons for especially studying the working conditions of hospital and public health workers is the central importance of medical care to society's qualitative standard of living. The nursing environment of the patient and the working environment of the medical personnel are closely linked, since the quality of the treatment provided is very much dependent on the working situation of the staff. In order to prevent any deterioration in the quality of treatment

in connection with the strong expansion in medical care, we require good knowledge of various conditions in this field.

Another important reason for studying the working environment of hospital and public health workers in more detail is that this category's daily work is so much governed by the inner structure of the work with its clearly defined functional division, work division, stipulated decision-making routines, work methods, and work routines. By charting the working environment of the personnel we are providing an opportunity of illustrating to what extent job involvement, experienced stress in work, and deterioration in health are connected with the organization of the work. This naturally applies to all employees. The link is more apparent, however, in the case of hospital and public health workers since the content of the job and the division of labour and responsibility between various groups at the place of work are more clearly defined in the case of hospital and public health workers than in most other groups.

The working conditions of hospital and public health workers are also more obviously influenced by political decisions, surveys, and regulations formulated outside their own place of work than is the case with most other groups. By providing a review of how political decisions concerning medical care are reached and by examining the main aspects of the decision-making process which leads to the organization of work at individual places of work, we can also provide a means of understanding the working conditions of medical staff, the quality of the medical care, etc. in a greater social perspective. We can also show that certain improved measures at individual places of work are connected with and require changes outside the own place of work.

In this chapter I have elected to present survey results which show connections between various conditions in the organization of medical care, mental strain in work, and medical problems, since these conditions have not previously attracted much interest. I have also considered it important in this context to examine more closely the physical working environment of hospital and public health workers, the inadequacies of which are more apparent than is the case with most other groups of salaried employees and which involve serious consequences with regard to the health of the personnel.

Survey results dealing with the following aspects will therefore be presented:

The connection between the organization of medical care and experienced stress in work, and the link between stress in work and general health;
The physical working environment of hospital and public health workers.

In connection with the presentation of these survey results, SHSTFs (the Swedish Federation of Salaried Employees in the Hospital and Public Health Services) views and demands regarding the conditions discussed will also be presented.

ORGANIZATION OF WORK AND EXPERIENCED STRESS IN WORK

As I mentioned, some of the survey's main aims are the following:

To chart the extent to which hospital and public health workers feel mental stress in their jobs;
To obtain an idea of which factors in work contribute to stress;
To provide bases for suggestions for improvement of various work organizational conditions.

Replying to a direct question asking how often it was felt that work involved mental strain, about one-third of the hospital and public health workers answered that their jobs often involved strain, while barely one-twentieth considered that it rarely or never did so. As Table 18.1 shows, a somewhat greater proportion of hospital and public health workers—compared with the whole survey group—felt that work often involved mental strain.

In order to answer the second main question in the survey, namely what conditions characterize jobs which involve strain, the survey group was divided into two sub-groups, namely;

Respondents who found work *very* or *fairly often* involved *mental strain*	35 per cent of all the hospital and public health workers (*N* = 245)
Respondents who found work *seldom* or *never* involved *mental strain*	18 per cent of all the hospital and public health workers (*N* = 126)

The groups' replies to a number of questions on various working conditions were then compared. This provided an idea of what is typical of jobs which often involve mental strain. The basic task in this context has been to chart to what extent and in what way the two groups' jobs differ with regard to scope for influence and control over the layout and implementation of work. An examination was also made of whether there are any differences with regard to work demands and work loads in the two groups. As mentioned, previous research has shown that the opportunity of influencing one's own working situation and of regulating and controlling work demands and work loads oneself is of decided importance to stress both in work and general health.

The groups' working conditions were therefore analysed in the following dimensions.
Influence and control over own work. Conditions connected with the *nature of the work* e.g.:

Demands and expectations on the part of people not employed at the place of work, e.g. patients and/or the general public.

Conditions connected with *work organization and which facilitate/hamper one's own control over work* e.g.:

Possibility of deciding oneself on the planning and implementation of work;
Routines, organization, etc. at the place of work;
Access to information;
Work routines at place of work, permanent instructions, etc.;
Access to equipment, material, etc.;
Restriction to job and place of work.

Work demands and work load. Conditions connected with the *nature of the work* e.g.:

Demands and expectations from people not employed at the place of work e.g. patients and general public†;
Responsibility, e.g. patient responsibility;
Demand for attention and concentration.

Conditions connected with *work organization* e.g.:

TABLE 18.1

Proportion of respondents among hospital and public health workers in the TCO Project's survey group, whose work involves mental strain

	Very or fairly often mental strain (per cent)	Sometimes mental strain (per cent)	Seldom or never mental strain (per cent)
Hospital and public health workers (*N* = 700)	35	47	18
All respondents (*N* = 9964)	32	44	24

110

Responsibility e.g. supervisory responsibility, economic responsibility†;
Demand for attention and concentration††;
Difficulty level of job;
Work load.

Influence and control over own work

Demands and expectations in work on the part of patients and/or the general public, for example. In the previous analysis of the survey material, contact between patients and their relatives has proved to be one of the factors which contribute very greatly toward hospital and public health workers feeling involvement in their work. In some cases, however, these conditions can involve demands and expectations which reduce the scope for influence and the exercise of one's own control over the work.

TABLE 18.2

Expectations and demands in work on the part of patients and/or the general public and mental strain in work

	Work governed too much by expectations and demands from patients and/or general public (per cent)
Often mental strain in work ($N = 238$)	35
Seldom or never mental strain in work ($N = 124$)	8

As the Table 18.2 indicates, there are strong links between experienced mental strain in work and work situations where work is governed too much by expectations and demands. About four times as many of those for whom work often involves mental strain stated that work was governed too much by expectations and demands from patients and/or the general public than was the case with the other group.

† In the summary given above the condition 'demand and expectations from patients and/or general public' is defined as an influence/own control factor and as a factor connected with work demands and work load. This is connected with the fact that these demands can involve a restriction in the opportunities for determining oneself the implementation of the work at the same time as the demands can also in certain circumstances constitute a work load which to a certain extent makes the work more difficult.

†† The work demand 'responsibility' and 'demand for attention and concentration' have been listed as being dependent on the nature of the job and on the work organization. This is connected with the fact that work demands are in certain cases a direct consequence of the nature of the work, as e.g. in the case of patient responsibility, but sometimes are a consequence of work organization, as e.g. in the case of supervisory responsibility, economic responsibility, etc.

Possibility of oneself determining the planning and implementation of work. The possibility of oneself determining the planning and implementation of work is closely connected with work organization. As mentioned, functional division, access to information, work routines, permanent instructions, etc. largely determined what influence the individual has over his/her own work situation (Table 18.3).

TABLE 18.3

Influence on daily work and mental strain in work

	Work governed too much (per cent)
Often mental strain in work ($N = 238$)	58
Seldom or never mental strain in work ($N = 123$)	24

More than twice as many of those for whom work often involved mental strain have work tasks which are governed too much by one or more of the conditions mentioned above than is the case with those for whom work seldom or never involved mental strain.

Opportunity for own initiative and decisions. The opportunity for using one's own initiative and decisions in work, which is also largely dependent on work organization at the place of work, the formulation of the work tasks, etc. has in previous surveys proved to be connected with job satisfaction. Table 18.4 compares work tasks for the respondents whose jobs often involved mental strain with those of the other group with regard to opportunity for independence in work.

TABLE 18.4

Often opportunity for own initiative and decisions in work and mental strain in work

	Often opportunity for own initiative and decisions (per cent)
Often mental strain ($N = 242$)	40
Seldom or never mental strain ($N = 124$)	55

As Table 18.4 shows, there is a link between the positive work condition 'opportunity for own initiative and decisions' and often experienced strain in work. We could possibly refer here to what is sometimes known as 'over-simulation', which means that work tasks can exceed an optimum level in respect of opinion-forming. Work tasks which allow good opportunity for own initiative and decisions probably often involve a great deal of responsibility and demand for attention and concentration—conditions which together can create 'over-stimulation' and experienced strain in work.

Access to information on issues concerning work. The possibilities of obtaining sufficient information on issues which concern work are highly dependent on information routines and contact channels at the place of work. To have access to information is also a deciding factor with regard to opportunity of independently planning and implementing work tasks and to the feeling of work involvement and meaning in work.

Table 18.5 shows the replies to a question about whether work was made more difficult by inadequate information on issues concerning work, as given by respondents for whom work often and seldom or never respectively involved mental strain. As Table 18.5 shows, work is made more difficult by insufficient information almost five times more often in the case of respondents whose work often involves mental strain than in the case of the others; almost twice as many in the first group receive insufficient information as compared to the other group.

Routines and organization, etc. at the place of work. The routines and organization, etc. at the place of work can in certain respects make exercising one's own control over the work easier and more difficult, respectively. Table 18.6 shows that failings in routines and organization, etc. which make work more difficult also exhibit connections with mental strain in work.

Table 18.6 shows that such failings in routines, organization, etc. as make the implementation of work more difficult occur three times more often among those whose work often involves mental strain than among members of the other group.

Access to equipment, material, etc. for work. Access to

TABLE 18.5

Insufficient information on issues concerning work and mental strain in work

	Work made more difficult by inadequate information (per cent)		
	Often	Sometimes	Seldom or never
Often mental strain in work ($N = 234$)	19	45	36
Seldom or never mental strain in work ($N = 121$)	4	24	72

TABLE 18.6

Failings in routines and organization, etc. at the place of work and mental strain in work

	Work is made more difficult by failings in routines and organization, etc. (per cent)		
	Often	Sometimes	Seldom or never
Often mental strain in work ($N = 234$)	12	42	46
Seldom or never mental strain in work ($N = (119)$)	4	16	80

equipment and material for work also affects the possibility of working independently and exercising control over one's own work. We also find differences between insufficient equipment and material and mental strain in work. The Table 18.7 shows that in the case of the respondents whose work involved mental strain, work was made more difficult by insufficient material equipment, etc. four times more often than in the case of the other group.

Restriction to work. The possibility of being able to leave a task, of being able to do an errand outside the place of work during working hours, and the possibility of being able at short notice to take a half day or a day off, may be said to be a measure of the level of confinement to work and the possibility of oneself being able to control and regulate time utilization in work.

As Table 18.8 shows there is a strong link between the three measures of restriction to work and mental strain in work. Almost twice as many of the respondents whose work often involved mental strain cannot leave work for 5–10 min. than is the case with the other group. Considerably more of the first group cannot leave work for ½–1 hour or take a half day or day off at short notice than is the case with the other group.

Work demands and work load

Demands and expectations from patients and/or the general public. As mentioned previously, the work condition 'demands and expectations from patients and/or the general public' can be defined as an influence/own control factor and as a factor connected with work demands and work load. This is connected with the fact that these demands can sometimes involve a restriction in the possibility of oneself determining the implementation of the work and can in certain cases constitute a hindrance to work, making work more difficult.

That work can be governed too much by various expectations and demands has been shown in a previous section. Four times as many of those whose work often involves mental strain consider daily work to be governed far too much by demands and expectations from e.g. patients and students and/or the general public than is the case with the other group. Table 18.9 shows that these demands can at the same time constitute a work load and that this is more common among respondents whose work involves mental strain than among the others.

Responsibility in work. The work demand 'respon-

TABLE 18.7

Insufficient material, equipment, etc. and mental strain in work

	Work made more difficult by insufficient material, equipment, etc. (per cent)		
	Often	Sometimes	Seldom or never
Often mental strain in work (N = 236)	16	30	54
Seldom or never mental strain in work (N = 123)	4	20	6

TABLE 18.8

Restriction to work and mental strain in work

	No possibility of leaving work 5–10 min (per cent)	No possibility of leaving work ½–1 h (per cent)	No possibility of taking ½–1 day off (per cent)
Often mental strain in work (N = 237, 239, 236, respectively)	27	74	76
Seldom or never mental strain in work (N = 126, 124, 125, respectively)	15	46	46

113

TABLE 18.9

Expectations and demands in work from e.g. patients, students, and/or the general public as a hindrance to work and mental strain in work

	Work made more difficult by demands and expectations from patients, students and/or the general public (per cent)		
	Often	Sometimes	Seldom or never
Often mental strain in work (N = 238)	32	43	25
Seldom or never mental strain in work (N = 122)	6	25	69

sibility' was previously said to be connected with the nature of the work tasks and with the work organization, since responsibility in work is in certain cases a direct consequence of the nature of the work as in patient responsibility, and sometimes a consequence of work organization, as in supervisory or economic responsibility.

Previous surveys have shown us that responsibility in work is one of the factors which contribute toward creating involvement in work. Table 18.10 below compares the replies of those whose work often involves mental strain with the replies of those in the other group as regards work responsibility. As Table 18.10 shows, there is a link between the position condition 'responsibility in work' and often experienced mental strain in work. As in the case of possibilities of own initiative and decisions in work, we could possibly in this context refer to what is sometimes known as 'over-stimulation' which means that work tasks can sometimes exceed an optimum level with regard to responsibility and opinion-forming. It is also likely that considerable responsibility in work is often to be equated with severe demands on

TABLE 18.10

Often considerable responsibility in work and mental strain in work

	Often considerable responsibility (per cent)
Often mental strain in work (N = 241)	95
Seldom or never mental strain in work (N = 123)	72

concentration and attention—conditions which together can create 'over-stimulation' and strain in work.

Demand for attention and concentration in work. Demands for attention and concentration in work were mentioned in the previous section as a factor which can be connected with experienced strain in work. Table 18.11 compares the replies given by the two groups with regard to demands for attention and concentration.

TABLE 18.11

Often considerable demands for concentration and attention and mental strain in work

	Often considerable demands for concentration and attention (per cent)
Often mental strain in work (N = 240)	93
Seldom or never mental strain in work (N = 123)	83

As Table 18.11 indicates, demands for attention and concentration are considerable in both groups. In the case of respondents whose work often involves strain, however, considerable demands for concentration and attention are somewhat more common than in the case of the other group.

Work load. Far too much to do at work and lack of time to carry out tasks are often factors connected with strain in work. The large work load imposed on hospital and public health workers has also often been emphasized in discussions about the working environment of hospital and public health workers.

114

TABLE 18.12

Work load and mental strain in work

	Often too much to do at work (per cent)	Often lack of time to carry out tasks (per cent)
Often mental strain in work (N = 241 and 240 respectively)	62	49
Seldom or never mental strain in work (N = 121 and 122 respectively)	16	3

Table 18.12 compares the replies submitted by the two groups with regard to work load and the time allotted to carry out work tasks. As Table 18.12 shows, there are very strong ties between work load and mental strain in work. Four times as many of those whose work often involves strain feel that they often have too much to do, as compared to the other group. The differences between the groups are even greater with regard to having too little time to carry out tasks. Sixteen times as many responents in the first group have too little time compared to the other group when it comes to carrying out work tasks.

Replies to a question regarding whether there are sufficient personnel to carry out tasks in the ward, place of work, etc. also show that the work load imposed on respondents whose work often involves strain is greater than in the case of the other group. As Table 18.13 indicates, almost three times as many of those whose work often involves strain feel that there is not sufficient staff than is the case with the other group.

Level of difficulty in work. Level of difficulty in work, far too difficult or far too easy tasks, which are dependent on work organization, division of labour, training opportunities, etc. have in previous research proved to be connected with the mental strain experienced. Table 18.14 compares the replies given by

TABLE 18.13

Personnel status and mental strain in work

	Not sufficient personnel in relation to work tasks in ward, place of work, etc. (per cent)
Often mental strain in work (N = 241)	59
Seldom or never mental strain in work (N = 124)	18

TABLE 18.14

Level of difficulty in work and mental strain in work

	Tasks too difficult (per cent)		
	Often	Sometimes	Seldom or never
Often mental strain in work (N = 234)	6	45	49
Seldom or never mental strain in work (N = 121)	0	12	88

the two groups to the question of whether work tasks are far too difficult. The Table 18.14 shows that it is considerably more common for tasks to be considered far too difficult by respondents whose work often involves strain than by members of the other group. In reply to a question regarding whether tasks are far too easy, very few respondents answered yes. There were no differences between the two groups.

Connection between experienced mental strain and anxiety or uninterest in work, tiredness after work, and plans for changing jobs. Previous research has shown that there is a link between mental strain experienced in work and anxiety and uninterest about going to work, difficulties in relaxing and not thinking about work during leisure time, and tiredness after work. Tables 18.15, 18.16, 18.17, and 18.18 show the replies given to a number of questions relating to these factors.

TABLE 18.15

Anxiety or uninterest about going to work and mental strain in work

	Anxiety or uninterest about going to work (per cent)		
	Often	Sometimes	Seldom or never
Often mental strain in work (N = 243)	10	46	44
Seldom or never mental strain in work (N = 126)	0	11	89

TABLE 18.16

Difficulty in not thinking about work during leisure time and mental strain in work

	Difficulty in not thinking about work during leisure time (per cent)		
	Often	Sometimes	Seldom or never
Often mental strain in work (N = 243)	32	45	23
Seldom or never mental strain in work (N = 126)	6	33	61

TABLE 18.17

Tiredness after work and mental strain in work

	Far too tired after work to do anything (per cent)		
	Often	Sometimes	Seldom or never
Often mental strain in work (N = 243)	60	35	5
Seldom or never mental strain in work (N = 126)	21	45	34

116

TABLE 18.18

Plans for changing jobs and mental strain in work

	Seriously considered changing jobs (per cent)
Often mental strain in work (N = 240)	47
Seldom or never mental strain in work (N = 125)	17

As Table 18.15 shows, the respondents whose work often involves mental strain gave essentially different replies to the questions than the members of the other group. One-tenth and one-half, respectively, of the first group replied that they often or sometimes felt anxiety or uninterest about going to work as opposed to only a few of those whose work seldom or never involved strain.

In Table 18.16 there also are considerable differences in the replies given by the two groups. Five times as many of those whose work often involves mental strain often have difficulty in not thinking about work during their leisure time, as compared to the other group. The replies given by the two groups also differed when they were asked whether they sometimes found it difficult to stop thinking about work when they came home.

As Table 18.18 shows, the replies given by the two groups are very different. Three times as many of those whose work often involves mental strain have seriously considered changing jobs than is the case with the other group.

Medical problems and mental strain in work
One of the aims of the survey into the working environment of hospital and public health workers is, as has been mentioned, to study whether there is any connection between mental strain in work and medical problems. In the following sections I will present survey results relating to differences in the frequency of stomach complaints and nervous disorders among

respondents whose work often and seldom or never respectively involves mental strain.

Stomach complaints. In order to obtain a measure of the frequency of stomach complaints among respondents in the survey group, the questionnaire included questions regarding whether the respondents had in the past 12 months experienced:

Acidy eructations, discomfort or ache in upper part of stomach (pit of the stomach);
Gases, stomach cramps, and/or diarrhoea.

The first of the two questions dealing with stomach complaints concerns symptoms relating to the stomach and the duodenum. Such complaints are common in the case of catarrh of the stomach and gastric ulcers. The other question concerns symptoms relating to the colon which can occur in the case of intestinal catarrhs, intestinal ulcers, and other intestinal disorders. Both stomach and intestinal disorders are often psychosomatically induced, i.e. are often connected with mental strain.

Table 18.19 shows summarized measures of the frequency of disorders among respondents whose work often and seldom or never involves mental strain. As Table 18.19 shows there is a link between stomach complaints and mental strain in work. A high and average frequency of stomach complaints is more common among those whose work often involves mental strain than among those whose work seldom or never does so.

TABLE 18.19

Stomach complaints and mental strain in work

	Stomach complaints (per cent)		
	High	Average	Low frequency
Often mental strain in work (N = 238)	9	24	67
Seldom or never mental strain in work (N = 127)	2	14	84

Nervous disorders. In order to obtain a measure of the occurrence of nervous disorders among the respondents in the survey, the questionnaire included questions regarding whether the respondents had during the past 12 months:

Felt miserable and depressed;
Had difficulty sleeping;
Felt more tired than previously;
Felt ill at ease and restless.

Table 18.20 shows summarized measures of frequency of disorders among respondents whose work often and seldom or never respectively involves mental strain. As Table 18.20 shows, the links between mental strain in work and nervous disorders are even stronger than the links between strain and stomach complaints. A high or average frequency is considerably more common among those whose work often involves mental strain than among those whose work seldom or never does so.

SHSTF's DEMANDS WITH REGARDS TO CONDITIONS CONNECTED WITH WORK ORGANIZATION

In the light of own experience and the survey results, *SHSTF demands the following:*

That work organization be so formulated that the work team has the opportunity of working in a satisfactory physical and psychosocial working environment;
That employers assist in research and experiments with various organizational models, including group care;
That personnel strength be adjusted to the nature of the activity involved so that adequate care can be provided;
That medical legislation be adapted so that the intentions of the Co-determination Act can be realized in hospital and public health work;
That employers inform hospital and public health personnel of planned changes which may affect their work situation;
That hospital and public health workers be given a real opportunity of participating in decision-making;

That information and proposals for improved measures initiated by hospital and public health workers be given serious consideration by employers;
That all hospital and public health workers be given functionally targeted training;
That training be adapted to the constant changes in working life, involving *inter alia* shifts in occupational roles and occupational functions;
That newly employed hospital and public health personnel be entitled to introductory training and familiarization to such an extent that a newly employed person can feel secure at his/her new place of work;
That a well planned continuous programme of further training for occupationally trained personnel already employed be created;
That such further training be common to various personnel categories with a view to promoting team work and understanding for one another's functions;
That supervisors be given further training adapted to modern requirements;
That employers provide training during working hours for employees with trade union assignments which involve participation in work groups, committees, etc.

PHYSICAL WORKING ENVIRONMENT

As mentioned previously, hospital and public health workers' work involves considerable environmental risk, as indicated by Table 18.21.

TABLE 18.21

Physical hazards in the working environment (N = 614)

Hazard	Per cent
Contagious substances	72
Heavy loads	57
Risk of accidents	29
Toxic substances, solvents, etc.	27
Radiation hazards (X-ray, radioactivity, etc.)	23
Difficult working position	21

TABLE 18.20

Nervous disorders and mental strain in work

	Nervous disorders (per cent)		
	high	average	low frequency
Often mental strain in work (N = 241)	15	37	48
Seldom or never mental strain in work (N = 126)	2	15	83

Table 18.21 shows that almost ¾ of the hospital and public health workers are exposed to contagious substances in their work and that about one-half lift heavy loads which can cause serious injuries. About ¼ run the risk of accidents and about as many work with toxic substances and solvents, while almost ¼ are exposed to radiation hazards by means of X-ray, radioactivity, etc. and as many have to work in difficult positions.

The environmental hazards in work are therefore considerable in the case of large groups of hospital and public health workers. Anxiety about health hazards and occupational injuries is also considerable. About one-third (36 per cent) of hospital and public health workers often feel anxious about health hazards and occupational injuries.

Apart from direct health hazards there are also troublesome failings in the working environment. As indicated by Table 18.22, these refer primarily to availability and size of work and personnel premises and to various temperature conditions.

SHST's demands regarding the physical working environment In the light of their own experience and the survey results, *SHSTF demands the following:*

That employers pay more attention to obvious health hazards which occur in hospital and public health work

such as radiation hazards, chemical substances, contagious substances, heavy loads, lone work, and poor ventilation;

That employers take the steps required to protect employees;

That employees at places of work where health hazards are obvious be given the opportunity to carry out varied tasks;

That the employees involved be consulted prior to the purchase of new equipment, introduction of new substances, etc.;

That hospital and public health workers be given regular medical check-ups.

TABLE 18.22

Failings in the working environment (N = 610)

	Per cent
Working premises too small	20
No or too few personnel rooms	33
No or too few rest rooms	33
Dry air	33
Poor ventilation	28

REFERENCE

WAHLUND, I. and NERELL, G. (1976). *The salaried employee's working environment: health wellbeing.* TCO, Stockholm.

19. STRESSORS AND STRAIN IN WHITE COLLAR WORKERS

GUNNAR NERELL and INGRID WAHLUND

TOTAL ENVIRONMENT

Research in recent years has improved our knowledge of the importance of stress factors in the working environment and their influence on workers' well-being and health. In the modern view, the concept of the working environment, which was formerly above all concerned with physical aspects, has come to comprise the total environment of the employee. Therefore a discussion of hazards in the working environment can no longer be confined to the traditional occupational hazards, which may be caused by physical, chemical, biological, or ergonomic factors, or accident risks. As the new concept of the working environment gains ground in practice, efforts will also have to be made to evaluate the psychological and social potentialities of the work place and to chart the risks arising out of the shortcomings of the psychosocial environment.

Physical factors in the environment have long been known to be capable of injuring the health and well-being of employees, and preventive measures have therefore focused above all on traditional occupational hazards. Today a discussion of the importance of the psychosocial functions in the working environment can be based on a fairly comprehensive body of research. It is perfectly clear that psychosocial factors can affect satisfaction and well-being in the work situation and connections with mental and physical functional disturbances have also been established. So far, however, the role of the psychosocial factors in the origin of direct organic injuries, analogous to the role of physical factors, has not been fully proved. But the modern view of the working environment as a total environment embracing physical and psychosocial factors—a view founded on the knowledge we possess today—should occasion preventive measures, not only for the prevention of injury and disease but also to achieve a positive work experience and job satisfaction. This view implies that both physical and psychosocial factors in the working environment should be explored and analysed in connection with evaluation measures and preventive programmes.

Promotion of health

In its definition of health, adopted in 1946, the World Health Organization (WHO) speaks of health as a state of physical, mental, and social well-being. With this in mind, the principal aim of measures for the improvement of the working environment should be the promotion of health in the broad sense. Although working life is aimed at the production of goods and services and at giving workers an income, these matters should not be ends in themselves but rather means whereby as many people as possible can achieve health, well-being, and a quality of life; these latter conditions are to be regarded as the overriding objectives of working life.

The importance of the above thoughts concerning the psychosocial environment has been brought out in recent years in a large number of national and international contexts. Both the International Labour Organization (ILO) and the WHO have initiated action programmes in the sphere of psychosocial factors and health.

Recent trends in Scandinavia

At national level, these new tendencies in the working environment sector have had various manifestations. In the Scandinavian countries, working environment legislation is being drafted which includes physical, psychological, and social factors in its definition of the working environment. The greatest progress in this sector has been made by Norway, but the same approach can be seen in the new Swedish *Work Environment Bill*. The report of the Swedish Commission on the Working Environment, which contains the draft text of the new legislation, also includes an appendix in which a number of prominent experts on psychosocial conditions in the working environment have described relevant factors and their practical significance in the legislative context.

An *Industrial Injuries Insurance Act* recently passed in Sweden opens up possibilities of compensation for completely new types of injury, besides those previously incorporated in the concept of industrial injuries. Among other things, compensation is now payable for mental or psychosomatic injuries incurred at work. The rules of evidence concerning mental and psychosomatic diseases, however, are stricter than those applying to the harmful effects due to physical factors in the environment and occasioning compensation.

Further manifestations of the broader concept of the working environment can be found in the collective agreements recently concluded in the Swedish labour market. *Working environment agreements* were concluded both in the private and in the public sector in 1976. These agreements govern working environment activities at individual work places, the tasks of the safety committee and the safety delegates, and the organization of industrial health services. The agreements emphasize that both physical and psychosocial factors in the environment are to be included in the scope of safety organization and industrial health services. In the public sector a decision has been taken to include in the organization of employee health services a social function of personnel welfare which, parallel to medical and technical activities, will above all be concerned with charting and evaluating psychosocial factors in the environment.

SALARIED EMPLOYEES

It is understandable that the widening concept of the working environment and the consequences thereof should have increased the commitment of salaried employees and their associations in matters concerning the working environment. It is of course important to emphasize that the psychosocial factors do not exclusively concern salaried employees but can affect all employee categories. Relatively speaking, though, the psychosocial factors in the environment weigh heavier in the salaried sector, and this is probably the reason why salaried employees have taken such a vigorous line on the subject. Recent years have witnessed a transformation of the working conditions and working environment of large groups of salaried employees, often quite a drastic transformation. Organizational changes, administrative rationalization, the introduction of computer systems and automatic routines have brought changes in work content, in relations at work, and in the allocation of roles between different groups of employees.

In spite of this, researchers who have investigated the effects of technical development on job satisfaction have mainly studied manual workers. The salaried sector has no clear counterpart to mechanization, although organizationally speaking one can identify a corresponding pattern of development in this sector too. At the lowest level of mechanization, the craftsmanship stage, salaried employees were relatively few in number and had such duties as bookkeeping, supervision, and sales. At a medium level of mechanization, line/staff organizations emerge, bringing with them specialist functions employing salaried staff, e.g. personnel department, finance department, production department, and sales department. During this period there is a steep rise in the number of salaried employees. The number declines at the third and highest level of mechanization, at the same time as the demand for specialist qualifications increases. New routines, perhaps those based on computerization, can render traditional knowledge worthless, and create widespread redundancy among elderly salaried employees.

New demands; risk of unemployment
There is an increase both in the need for adaptibility and the risk of unemployment. Where other groups of salaried employees are concerned, the new organization may mean a fragmentation and thinning out of duties in a process reminiscent of a medium-high level of mechanization in manufacturing industry. Thus, somewhat paradoxically, modern organizations can both generate a need for growing numbers of specialists and increase the number of humdrum, machine-controlled routine tasks. These tendencies may be presumed to create various kinds of psychosocial problems in the working environment of the salaried employee. Structural changes and rationalization processes are a threat to job security. Organizational changes and technical rationalization lead to frequent changes in working conditions, style of management, and work organization. These changes can cause the skill acquired within a narrow subject sector to become completely obsolete.

Promotion prospects
Promotion prospects are often regarded as a benefit in the salaried sector. On the other hand these prospects demand, by definition, efforts to achieve promotion, and failure in this respect can be disastrous to the self-esteem of the individual. Our society is dominated by the competitive ethos. Social pressure compels young salaried employees to work overtime as a matter of routine in order to become eligible for promotion, it forces good teachers to look for headships, and it forces able engineers to try to become managers. As a rule there is no chance of stopping or of climbing down one step. Instead one is forced to go the whole way.

Career systems can lead to social isolation, because one does not readily discuss personal problems with competitors one's own age, with managers who are to choose new managers, or even with subordinates, in relation to whom one has a position of authority to maintain. This underlines the fact that relations at a work place are for the most part a reflection of the scheme of work organization applying there. A problematic psychosocial environment causes problems in human relations.

Role conflicts in foremen, nurses, police, and teachers
The salaried sector provides many examples of role conflicts or buffer roles, an intermediate position at work between groups which are liable to have contradictory interests.

The work situation of the *foreman* is a classic instance of role conflict. Most foremen are recruited from the shop floor and appointed to direct their former mates. The foreman has to match up to the employer's demand for efficient production and the workers' expectation of fair and humane supervision. Many surveys have identified the role of the *foreman* as a situation of psychosocial risk.

In the medical sector, the work situation of the *nurse* often implies competition between conflicting interests. The employer organizes the ward, work schedules, and personnel pool; the patient expects continuity of care and human contact. The actual business of medical work is fragmented by a host of paperwork routines, as a result of which the nurse barely recognizes the profession she has been trained for. At the same time her situation as a foreman involves problems because she is often forced to delegate responsibilities to personnel who are not trained for such tasks.

Policemen too occupy an awkward intermediate position in modern society. They carry out the decisions of a democratic community but are often accused of going by undemocratic principles of their own. They are exposed to menaces, danger, and insults, all of which are often directed at their families as well as themselves. Both the nursing profession and the police are characterized by a high standard of loyalty to their employers and to third parties, and this results in frequently recurring overtime, inconvenient shift work, etc. Sweden is seriously discussing the introduction of three shifts in the nursing sector.

The work situation of *teachers* is similarly characterized to a great extent by a conflict of roles. Teachers have to strike a balance between the demands of their pupils, the expectations of parents, and the varying curricula introduced by school authorities. In addition to this balancing trick, the teacher is expected to cope with a classroom situation which can often be very pressing.

A SURVEY OF OCCUPATIONAL ENVIRONMENT AND HEALTH

Against this background, the Swedish Association of Salaried Employees (TCO) conducted a survey of the work environment conditions of salaried employees. The survey was conducted by us in 1975 and 1976 and was partly financed by research grants from the Swedish Workers' Protection Fund (Wahlund and Nerell 1976). The survey was planned in close collaboration with a steering group comprising trade union representatives and scientists, the latter including Professors Bertil Gardell and Lennart Levi and Dr. Ricardo Edström.

The main points of enquiry were as follows:

To what extent do different salaried groups experience satisfaction and involvement in their work? Which factors contribute to this?
To what extent is work experienced as physically strenuous? Which factors contribute towards this?
What connections are there between working conditions, work experience, and various medical complaints and absenteeism?

The theoretical structure of the survey (cf. Fig. 19.1) is

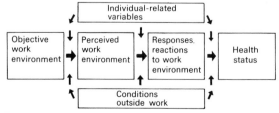

FIG. 19.1. The theoretical structure of the survey.

closely related to hypotheses formulated by the French–Kahn group (cf. Chapter 7).

The survey further comprised the employees' self-reported reactions to the objective and subjective working environments. These reactions may be psychological, behavioural, or medical, e.g. an experience of physical strain at work, absenteeism, psychosomatic symptoms, and the like. The final stage of the project involved an analysis of connections between reactions to the work environment and more long-term changes in the employee's state of health. Both individual-based factors and social background conditions were used as interacting variables.

Material and methods

The survey was carried out in the form of a postal questionnaire, comprising about 100 questions, which was sent to a random sample of every seventieth registered member of the various TCO member unions. The size of the sample, about 12 000 persons, was justified by the wide range of occupations and working conditions covered by the survey. The response frequency turned out to be 87 per cent, which is very satisfactory for a survey of this kind. The respondents were subdivided with regard to pay, age, and association membership as well as according to 17 occupational groups.

Roughly one-third experienced work as very often or quite often mentally strenuous, while a quarter replied that they seldom or never found their work a strain. Experienced mental strain is particularly common among teachers, policemen, and journalists (60, 49, and 48 per cent of respondents respectively) (Fig. 19.2). To arrive at a picture of the distinctive features of work involving mental strain, the two groups with high and low mental stress respectively (Table 19.1) have been compared in different respects.

TABLE 19.1

Respondents feeling *very often or quite often* that their work is mentally strenuous	32 per cent of all respondents
Respondents *seldom or never* feeling that their work is mentally strenuous	24 per cent of all respondents

Confinement to work

Confinement to work, as reflected in difficulties in getting away from one's job for a short while or in taking half a day or a whole day off at short notice, proved to be statistically related to experienced mental strain (Fig. 19.3). Almost three times as many people in the 'frequent stress' group as in the control group reported being unable to leave their duties for 5–10 min. Twice as many of those experiencing their work as mentally strenuous felt that they were unable to leave their place of work for half an hour to an hour or to take a day or so off at short notice.

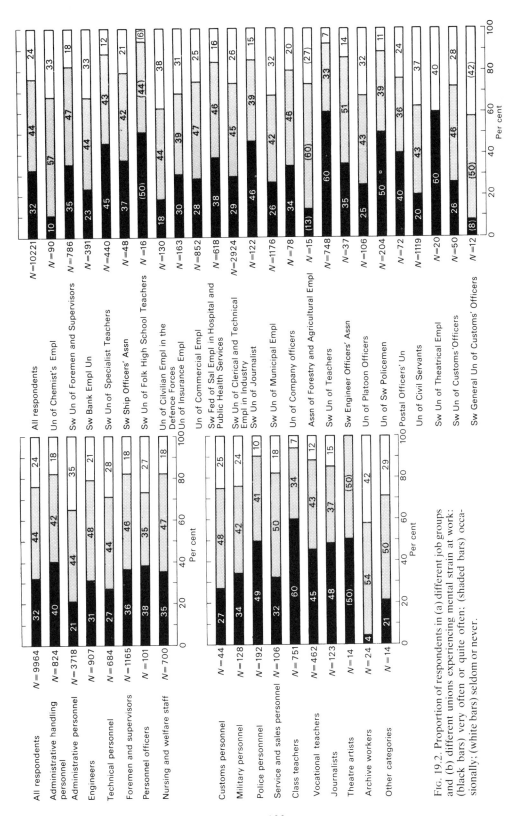

Fig. 19.2. Proportion of respondents in (a) different job groups and (b) different unions experiencing mental strain at work: (black bars) very often or quite often; (shaded bars) occasionally; (white bars) seldom or never.

123

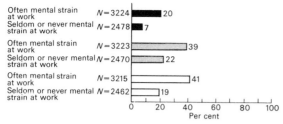

Fig. 19.3. Confinement to work of respondents experiencing different degrees of mental strain in their work: (black bars) cannot leave the job for 5–10 min; (shaded bars) cannot leave the place of employment for 0·5–1 hour; (white bars) cannot take 0·5–1 day off at short notice.

Influence at work

The possibilities of making one's own decisions about the planning and conduct of work play a very important part in work experience. The proportion of persons feeling that they were too closely controlled in their everyday work was twice as large in the 'mentally strenuous' group as in the other group (Fig. 19.4). The differences between these two groups are still more pronounced concerning questions as to whether work is excessively controlled by customers, patients, pupils, superiors, or authorities. Thus six times as many among those who often feel mental strain at work consider their work to be overly controlled by these conditions. Respondents finding these conditions particularly troublesome are to be found among members of the armed forces, policemen, teachers, and nursing staff.

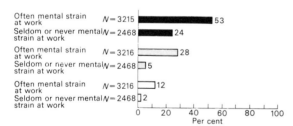

Fig. 19.4. Influence exerted on their work by respondents experiencing different degrees of mental strain at work: (black bars) work too closely controlled; (shaded bars) work too closely controlled by expectations and demands of persons not employed at the work place, e.g. by customers, patients, students, the general public; (white bars) work too closely controlled by superiors outside the work place, authorities, curricula, etc.

There are also salaried groups who find their work excessively controlled by conditions other than those mentioned above—for example, by instructions from superiors, demands for adjustment to co-workers, and excessive control of work by computerized routines. These types of control, unlike the factors mentioned earlier, are closely connected with the experience of work as monotonous and as affording little scope for individual initiatives and decisions.

Responsibility, influence

Great responsibility at work, opportunities of exerting influence and decision-making are often considered to be prerequisites of good job satisfaction. But these intrinsically positive factors can also contribute towards mental strain at work (Fig. 19.5). Presumably this happens when demands for decision-making and responsibility exceed the optimum level for the individual (overstimulation, overutilization). This is above all experienced by handling officers, administrative personnel ('decision-makers'), foremen, nursing staff, members of the armed forces, policemen, teachers, and journalists. Large groups of salaried employees are responsible for ensuring that certain duties are performed, regardless of time input, indisposition, or illness. When the employee is absent from work, there is no one else who can do his job, so that eventually he returns to a pile of work on his desk. Even if it comes as a positive experience to many people to feel that they are indispensable, this too can constitute a stress factor, and it may be the reason why many employees are 'delusively healthy' in the sense that their absenteeism is very low and possibly suboptimal.

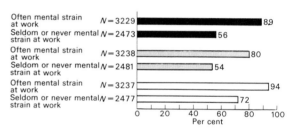

Fig. 19.5. Job content reported by respondents experiencing different degrees of mental strain at work: (black bars) often great responsibility; (shaded bars) frequent opportunities of independent initiatives and decision-making; (white bars) great concentration and alertness often required.

Work overload

The classical archetype of stress is the company president tearing from one meeting to another, puffing at big cigars, and answering several phones at once. We have learned that stress diseases are by no means the prerogative of senior management, and that they are not even commonest at this level. On the other hand factors such as shortage of time for the completion of duties and a large volume of tasks at work are universal stress factors. Often, too, people state that the department is understaffed in relation to its duties and that this is a cause of mental strain at work. Comparing the above-mentioned high and low mental stress groups, one finds that the proportion answering that they are often short of time in which to complete their duties is seven times as high in the former group (Fig. 19.6); administrative handling staff, teachers, engineers, and policemen bulk large in this group.

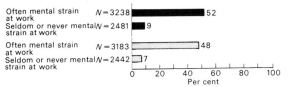

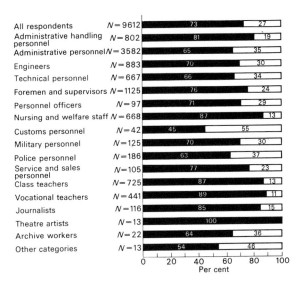

Fig. 19.6. Work loads of respondents experiencing different degrees of mental strain at work: (black bars) often too much to do at work; (shaded bars) often pressed for time at work.

Responsibility, concentration

If an attempt is made to arrange in rank order the factors the respondents feel are the main causes of mental strain at work, the most frequent include heavy responsibility and the need for close concentration. These are followed by shortage of time, excessive work load, and the demands and expectations of outsiders, e.g. customers, patients, pupils, and the general public.

Alienation, instrumental attitudes

Many scientists would say that opportunities of experiencing work as meaningful and conducive to development are important prerequisites of job satisfaction. Above all, industrial psychologists have warned of the effects which industrial work has proved capable of producing in the form of sensations of monotony, futility, and alienation or an instrumental attitude, implying that the worker abandons his hopes of deriving satisfaction from his work and, instead, sees in it nothing more than a means of satisfying his needs as a consumer, as a way of making a living. Researchers such as Blauner, Kornhauser, and Gardell have shown that this attitude towards work leads to a devaluation of work as a source of satisfaction and also to such reactions as resignation, absenteeism, loss of self-esteem, and social spin-off effects, i.e. less rewarding leisure, and a lower level of political and cultural activity. Previous views to the effect that people with tedious jobs are compensated by the use they made of their leisure have proved to be mistaken.

Experience in this sector mainly refers to industrial workers. It is therefore interesting to note that the present survey of salaried employees shows that 27 per cent declared that earnings were the main objective while 73 per cent worked primarily for the satisfaction they derived (Fig. 19.7) The instrumental attitude is commonest among junior salaried employees, administrative and technical personnel, and customs and police officers, while a larger proportion of people among administrative handling personnel, nursing staff, teachers, and journalists feel that their work affords them personal satisfaction. Those stating that they derive personal satisfaction from their work also feel that work content has an essential bearing on job satisfaction. In this group, the factors felt to contribute most towards job satisfaction are the ability to decide for oneself how work is to be done, the opportunity for a variety of work and for responsibility at work, and work which involves

Fig. 19.7. Evaluation by different job groups of the rewards of their work; (black bars) personal satisfaction from the job (white bars) earnings the main thing.

contact with people. These regarding work primarily as a means of making a living feel that the important factors influencing satisfaction are helpful colleagues, the possibility of deciding for oneself how work is to be done, good working hours, job security, and a fair-minded boss—in other words, factors which are connected with their surroundings, rather than with their duties as such. Three types of patterns of reaction to mental strain at work have been mentioned; namely psychological, behavioural, and medical.

Psychological and behavioural reactions

Psychological reactions are clearly connected with perceived mental strain. Twelve per cent of respondents in the high strain groups state that they often feel uneasy or reluctant about going to work, as against 1 per cent in the low strain group (Fig. 19.8). Forty-eight per cent of respondents in the high strain group state that they are too tired after work to engage in anything active, such as

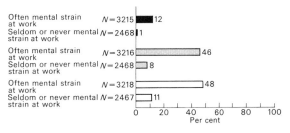

Fig. 19.8. Reactions to mental strain as reported by respondents experiencing different degrees of mental strain at work: (black bars) often worried or reluctant about going to work; (shaded bars) often difficult to get one's mind off the job during leisure hours; (white bars) often too tired after work to indulge in any activity.

hobbies or meeting friends and acquaintances, against 11 per cent in the low strain group. Forty-six per cent of respondents in the high strain group find it hard to get their minds off their work during their leisure hours, as against 8 per cent in the low strain group.

Behavioural reaction patterns are also found to be connected with mental strain. Of the people who often experience mental strain, 43 per cent have seriously considered changing jobs as against 24 per cent in the group of respondents seldom or never experiencing mental strain at work (Fig. 19.9). The group often experiencing mental strain at work, moreover, takes more drugs—above all more sedatives and tranquillizers—and smokes more than the group experiencing little mental strain. There is no great difference between the two groups where sickness absence is concerned. The main difference concerns absenteeism said to be due to weariness or tiredness in connection with work; the high strain group report three times as much absenteeism on this score as the low strain group. Thus, although mental strain as such does not appear to produce greater absenteeism, one finds that there is a close connection between psychological reactions and absenteeism. For example, those who very often feel uneasy or reluctant about going to work are absent far more than those who do not display this attitude.

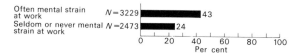

Fig. 19.9 Plans for changing jobs as reported by respondents experiencing different degrees of mental strain at work: (black bars) have seriously considered changing jobs.

A far greater difference emerges if one compares those experiencing their work as satisfying with those who display an instrumental attitude. Those experiencing satisfaction in their work have a lower rate of absenteeism in terms both of the number of spells of absence and total duration of absence than those who are absent because of distaste or reluctance.

Medical reactions

Concerning medical reactions to the working environment, one finds that those who often experience mental strain at work tend far more often than those who do not experience such strain to suffer from nervous and gastric complaints (Fig. 19.10). The differences are greatest with regard to nervous complaints, roughly four times as many people in the high strain group having definite complaints (15 and 4 per cent for the two groups, respectively). Those displaying an instrumental attitude to their work suffer from medical complaints to a greater extent than those who derive personal satisfaction from their work; they have twice the amount of gastric trouble, back trouble, and nervous complaints.

We have already mentioned distaste or reluctance and uneasiness about work, as well as difficulties in getting

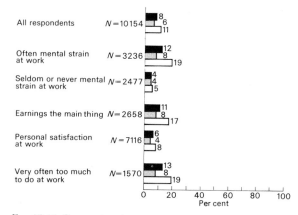

Fig. 19.10. Connections between mental strain, valuation of the rewards of work, heavy work load, and medical complaints: (black bars) percentage with high frequency of gastric complaints; (shaded bars) percentage with high frequency of back trouble; (white bars) percentage with high frequency of nervous trouble.

one's mind off the job during leisure hours as being psychological reactions to mental strain at work. Persons reporting these psychological reactions, compared with those not reporting them, have a much higher frequency of medical complaints, above all in the form of gastric and nervous troubles. This suggests that psychological and psychosomatic reactions occur to a great extent simultaneously. One is bound to wonder whether persistent troubles of this kind give rise to manifest states of illness, such as mental illness, high blood pressure, cardiac infarctions, or peptic ulcer.

A high frequency of nervous complaints occurs in 11 per cent of respondents. The corresponding figure among those experiencing their work as mentally strenuous is 19 per cent, while among those not experiencing their work in these terms it is 5 per cent. In the 'perceived mental strain' group one finds an even higher frequency of nervous complaints among those feeling that their work is excessively controlled (24 per cent), excessively tied to computer routines (29 per cent), or excessively dominated by adjustment to a colleague's style and pace of work (30 per cent). The same goes for respondents who find their work excessively monotonous (43 per cent) or insufficiently qualified (44 per cent) and those who feel that they have little opportunity of deciding for themselves how their work is to be done (39 per cent). About 35 per cent of respondents experiencing mental strain and uncertainty concerning the way in which work is to be done, unclear working instructions, and a conflict of roles suffer from nervous complaints.

Type of job and nervous complaint

The results suggest that monotonous and rigidly controlled jobs and jobs involving uncertainty and conflict lead to nervous complaints. The frequency of nervous complaints among these groups is greater than in the group with a general experience of mental strain and greater than for respondents as a whole. Perhaps these findings can be taken to imply that mental strain gives rise to medical reactions and sickness absence if the duties experienced as mentally strenuous do not afford scope for personal initiatives, the regulation of one's own style and pace of work, and the personal assumption of responsibility.

Other results pointing in the same direction are those obtained from a comparison of the absenteeism of respondents who feel that they are definitely able to influence decisions concerning their work, and respondents who definitely have no such opportunity. Those who are unable to influence decisions heavily predominate, as regards both the number of spells of absence and total absence, and also as regards absence due to weariness or tiredness connected with their work. Similar differences exist between those who never experience responsibility at work. Underlying these results there is probably a combination of mental strain and intellectual understimulation.

Confirmation of hypotheses

The survey findings suggest that the hypotheses formulated in the survey model are essentially correct. Conditions in the objective work environment, in the organization of work, and in job content are related to the individual's experience of his work and to his psychological and behavioural reactions as well as his medical complaints. The psychosocial working environment has repercussions on the employees' well-being and health. It is, though, important to remember that a cross-sectional survey, however well conducted, yields primarily statistical relationships. A single survey does not justify the inference that the statistical relationships are also causal connections. Previous research, however, has furnished evidence to suggest that the type of connection described here is actually a causal relationship.

Studies of this kind have been carried out by the research groups led by Lennart Levi and Bertil Gardell and have entailed longitudinal investigations of risk groups with comparable reference groups. There is good reason, therefore, to suppose that the connections found in this survey are causal. This should be verified, however, and a follow-up survey is therefore planned.

FOLLOW-UP STUDY

The follow-up will be based primarily on available statistics, and the following sources are conceivable:

(1) Statistics from the National Social Insurance Board concerning sickness absence, diagnoses, and hospitalizations;
(2) Medical statistics based on data from the National Social Insurance Board;
(3) The register of causes of death maintained by the Central Bureau of Statistics.

Thus, the purpose of the follow-up survey will be to try to establish whether the connections found in the cross-sectional survey can stand up to a longitudinal investigation.

Discussion of following up the survey should not prevent the survey findings from being used here and now. The survey verifies the views which TCO has put forth concerning the importance of the psychosocial working environment as a field for preventive measures. Collective agreements and legislation are slowly changing in this direction, and it is therefore important for the survey findings to be transmitted to local level, to individual work places. Interest in these measures has also been stimulated by the survey. For example, discussion groups have been organized and information material compiled. Study material has been prepared with the aim of providing safety delegates with properly composed training, and this, finally, must be the principle aim of the survey— namely, to transmit knowledge concerning the effects of the psychosocial environment to management as well as the local safety organizations with a solid foundation for concrete improvements to the working environment.

REFERENCE

WAHLUND, I. and NERELL, G., (1976). *Work environment of white collar workers, work, health, well-being.* Central Organization of Salaried Employees in Sweden (TCO), Stockholm.

SESSION 3

Mental, physical, and social disability possibly associated with psychosocial stressors at work

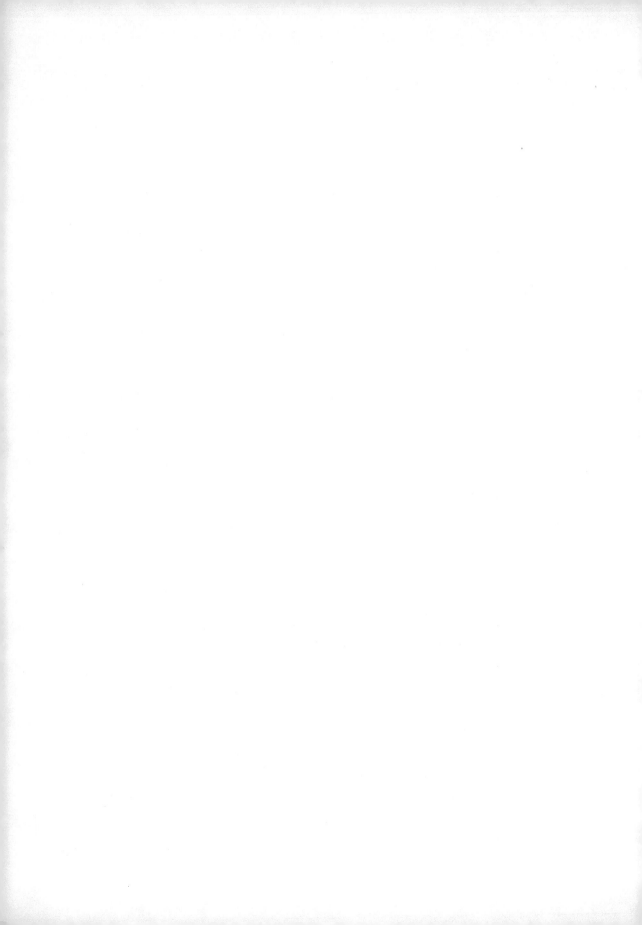

20. OCCUPATIONAL STRESS, ENDOCRINE CHANGES, AND COPING BEHAVIOUR IN THE MIDDLE YEARS OF ADULT LIFE

DAVID A. HAMBURG and BEATRIX A. HAMBURG

The middle years of adulthood constitute a neglected phase of the life cycle from the standpoint of biobehavioural research. There are fragments of evidence indicating characteristic stress—occupational, interpersonal, medical—during the age period 40–60. Even less is known of the individual and institutional strategies for coping with these stressful experiences. The present chapter sketches several lines of evidence and calls attention to promising directions of inquiry.

INTRODUCTION

Although biological and behavioural scientists recognize that the organism changes significantly in the course of the life cycle, most research is unsystematic in dealing with these changes. Many studies give minimal information about age of the subjects or phase of the life cycle. Nevertheless, the study of behaviour has gradually come to acquire a developmental perspective, albeit implicit in most research. With respect to explicit development research, much attention has been focused on the early years of life, reflecting the assumption that the long-range effects of early experience are probably profound. Next, considerable attention has been given to adolescence by workers in several fields, including the present authors. This work has mainly reflected concern with the special problems of this era, but has also paid some attention to the plasticity of the adolescent years and the possibilities for personal development. Recently, the life sciences have been stimulated by the concern of the public and policy-makers to examine the problems of ageing. The human studies have mainly dealt with retirement and beyond. So, several phases of the life cycle have received substantial attention. But major gaps remain. Most striking among these is the middle years of adulthood, variously specified but always including the decade of the 40s.

Taking account of this neglect of the middle years, the Social Science Research Council of the United States undertook an assessment of significant needs and promising approaches to problems of mid-life. The present paper is a direct outgrowth of the SSRC stimulus. An introductory statement of the SSRC Committee on Work and Personality in the Middle Years, prepared under the leadershop of O. Brim (1973), stated:

The major life events that characterize the middle part of the life span—reaching the peak of one's occupational career, the launching of children from the home, the death of parents, climacterium, grandparenthood, illness, retirement, widowhood—while they tend to proceed in a roughly predictable sequence, occur at varying intervals of time. Most behavioral scientists therefore concur that chronological age is not a meaningful index by which to order social and psychological data of adulthood; and the individual's own awareness of entry and exit from middle age seem to emerge from a combination of biological and social cues rather than from a fixed number of birthdays.

The SSRC committee has designated the middle years as the chronological age period between 40 and 60, and we shall follow this designation in the present paper.

The SSRC committee views mid-life as a developmental period of the life cycle in which the person faces new dilemmas and new possibilities for change. These years bring broadly predictable changes in work, family, and health. These changes involve complex mixtures of stressful experience, valued opportunity, and challenge to coping resources. In general, events that are highly unexpected tend to be most stressful in these years.

The SSRC committee emphasizes the place of work in personal identity.

Work still takes the largest single percentage of one's waking hours and constitutes for most a fundamental influence on the development of and change in the sense of self through the life cycle. The search for self-esteem—to be valued by others who matter, and to be valued by oneself; to feel in control of the world, one's life course, time, and self in its values and behaviour; to believe one is distinctive, unique even, that one counts for something special in the common pilgrimage of man; to sense personal growth and development so that one is something more than as of a week ago—the pursuit of these and other elements in the summary sense of self-esteem pervades the work of most people.

STRESSFUL EXPERIENCE IN THE MIDDLE YEARS

Economic stress

Some of the stresses of this era are economic. These have been recently studied by Jaffe (1971) in the population of the United States. He chose the age period 35–54. A major task of the period is providing adequate income while raising the children. By and large, the family's children have been born by the beginning of this period and have left the parental home by the end of it. Jaffe points out that occupational mobility, even after early success, tends to end early in the middle years. Earnings show little progress thereafter. In a culture emphasizing occupational and financial achievement, many men interpret this slowing of progress as something akin to failure.

Education is a factor in the duration of upward occupational mobility. More highly educated persons tend to advance in their forties and sometimes in their fifties. Those with less education tend to slip during the middle years. Earnings reflect the level of occupational advancement. Relatively high increases in earnings, five to seven per cent per year, occur prior to or during the early middle years concomitant with maximum upward occupational mobility. Later in this period, earnings tend to increase only as fast as the general economy grows, perhaps two to three per cent per year. This situation may elicit concerns about family, health care, unfulfilled ambitions, and regrets about prior education and/or occupational choices.

Sofer (1974) has recently completed a major review of occupational stresses in different social groups. Much of this review touches on mid-life problems, and some of it has implications for coping behaviour. In the next section of this paper, we rely heavily on Sofer's excellent review. Sofer states:

Large, complex organizations appear to have certain typical forms of psychological stress associated with their functioning. . . .

Two major stress-producing conditions appear to be the pressure of role conflict and role ambiguity and these appear largely as an outcome of employees being required to cross organizational boundaries, to produce innovative solutions to non-routine problems and to take responsibility for the work of others. . . .

The endemic nature of these 'stressor conditions' is incontrovertible. In a national survey in the United States of 725 persons representing that part of the labor force employed during the Spring of 1961, about half the respondents reported that they were caught in the middle between two conflicting persons or factions: in 88% of these cases at least one of the persons involved was an organizational superior of the respondent. Almost half of all respondents reported work overload, that is, conflict among tasks or problems in setting priorities. Four forms of ambiguity were particularly reported as troublesome: uncertainty about the way one's superior evaluates one's work, about opportunities for advancement, about scope of responsibility and about the expectations of others regarding one's performance. The difficulties people had with their organizational roles increased as conflict and ambiguity increased (Kahn *et al.* 1964).

Sofer points out that:

blue collar jobs have their own typical sources of anxiety and stress: such jobs are less secure than others, the posts held by an individual are typically not related to each other in an orderly sequence, and earnings do not rise concurrently with increasing family needs, being related more to strength, skill and speed than to the improvements in judgment, experience or to the capacity for looking after others that is generally accepted to come with age. The industrial worker is more subject to occupational vicissitudes than persons in more skilled or senior posts,

is likely to experience or perceive randomness in occupational success, is likely to fear machines and technological improvements for their possible effects on him, is not likely to see a close connection between ability, effort and success, is prone to develop a philosophy of life that attributes such success to luck, pull, discrimination or the power of others in a better position to manipulate society. There is a distinct ideology of the underdog or underprivileged worker which expresses hopelessness, resignation and unwillingness to believe that one matters as much as other people and that one's needs and wishes will be taken into account (Knupper 1947; Stouffer *et al.* 1949).

Stresses affecting white collar workers and middle executives

White collar workers and executives are usually able to take for granted the job security and adequacy of income that are uncertain for blue collar workers. At higher occupational levels, concerns tend to focus on different questions: the extent of personal autonomy, the use of distinctive individual capacities, and recognition for one's own contribution. This latter point is especially interesting since large organizations involve complex networks of persons who contribute to a particular task or project. Often it is difficult for anyone to know what the distinctive contribution of any individual has been. This ambiguity impacts on the high aspirations in upper occupational groups—work is often the major basis for self-esteem. This orientation puts a premium on identification with the employing organization and makes personal satisfaction vulnerable to vicissitudes in work situation and career trajectory. This vulnerability is often enhanced by high dependence on one employer. At higher occupational levels, effectiveness may rest substantially on knowledge of the administrative and political nuances of a particular organization. Typically, the executive becomes strongly identified with his employing organization and privately doubtful of his capacity to do as well elsewhere.

A national survey in the United States has found links between rank, conflict, and tension in occupational settings. The peak of conflict occurs at the upper middle levels of management. This finding partly reflected the unfulfilled mobility aspirations of middle management. Such persons are subject to formidable pressures from their own internal standards, and also from certain key relations in the organization: those who are in the same unit and are in higher positions, who are sufficiently dependent on the individual's performance to care about his adequacy without being so completely dependent on him as to be inhibited in making their demands known (Kahn *et al.* 1964).

The middle manager's work often involves a struggle for power, autonomy, and influence in relation either to other individuals in his own unit or in relation to other units or occupational groups. The emotional investment in these struggles may be intense because:

(a) The individual has formulated his self-esteem heavily on his work;

(b) He is identified with his unit, organization, or profession;

(c) He cannot readily make drastic occupational shifts.

Not all middle managers can become top-level executives; not all promising young faculty members can become professors. Career disappointment in the middle years is a poignant form of stress. These are typically people whose sense of personal worth rests heavily on long-range career trajectories of distinction. When they sense a downward turn in the trajectory—especially one that had not been anticipated—much depression is likely to ensue. The person who has expected much is faced with the unwelcome prospect of settling for less; the lifelong optimist may become disillusioned. Sofer notes:

A career disappointment can then come to constitute a disturbance in self-conception, involving the necessity to re-assess or re-classify oneself, and an embarrassing withdrawal of the image of the prospective self that one may have held out to intimates. Seniors may be felt to have betrayed one. Personal and familial sacrifices may have been made in the vain pursuit of illusory occupational goals.

Stresses affecting high-level executives

High-level executives have their own distinctive occupational stresses. Though they have much auto-nomy and financial security, their decisions are relatively visible and mistakes have far-reaching consequences. The organizational stakes are very high. Moreover, they often are constrained by organizational practices that have evolved over the years and have considerable force of tradition. These may involve roles in the organization, ways in which these must be filled or vacated, and the conditions under which staff may be employed or dismissed (Crozier 1964).

The senior administrator often faces the requirement for a major occupational transition in mid-career. Such transitions are typically stressful. Earlier, he usually has specialized competence based on technical skill. In due course, he adds to this the ability to manage a group of technically-oriented subordinates. But as he moves upward administratively, he usually must become a generalist, managing a wide range of specialized groups in the organization. While this entails greater recognition and higher earnings, it may undermine a long-established basis for self-esteem, i.e. technical competence and demand qualities of judgement and wisdom in which the persons feels privately unsure of himself. The administrator must show that he respects the skills of diverse groups in the organization, can take their views into account, yet make crisp decisions that often favour the interests of some at the expense of others. He may find it necessary to increase distance from previously close associates in an effort to maintain objectivity and fairness in decision-making. But the emotional cost of this for the executive and his wife may be significant.

In the middle years, poignant events may, in un-anticipated ways, highlight disappointments and elicit deep personal regrets. In the hectic pace of occupational events in the early part of a career, long-term con-siderations may be pushed aside and remain vaguely formulated. Then a vivid, unusual occasion may sharply bring into focus some long-term concerns or regrets. The college reunion is one such occasion (Menninger 1974). At such a time, concerns about ageing, health, and mortality may be elicited by noting the changes in some old friends who have not been seen for years, or learning of the death of peers from an earlier day. Concerns about marital status may be stimulated by learning of divorces among those previously thought to be happily married. Occupational concerns may be elicited by making un-favourable comparisons of one's own progress with that of peers. Experiences of this kind may elicit anxiety and lead to self-assessment. In due course, the assessment process may bring about mid-course corrections in occupation, marriage, or other activities. Such modifications in life course may offer refreshing opportunities but also involve major transitions that tend to be stressful.

ENDOCRINE AND PSYCHOLOGICAL CHANGES IN MID-LIFE

The menopausal era

We turn now to stressful events of the menopausal era. The term menopause refers to cessation of menses; climacterium refers to involution of the ovaries and associated processes; involutional period refers primarily to advancing age. These terms overlap and are often used interchangeably. We focus here on the meno-pause and the era in a woman's life surrounding the menopause. Cessation of the menses takes place gradually in most women over a two- to five-year period. Symptoms of the normal menopause, such as hot flushes and increased irritability, probably have some relation to changes in ovarian hormones and gonadotrophins, but the relationship between endocrine changes and the severe involution psychiatric disorders remains obscure. (Koran and Hamburg 1975).

The menopause usually takes place between ages 45 and 49. With advancing age, the decline of ovarian secretory activity occurs gradually over several years. Ovulation and menstruation become irregular. Menses cease when the amount of oestrogen secreted is too little to stimulate uterine endometrial growth. In due course, oestrogen levels become so low that they fail to inhibit the pituitary and large quantities of pituitary gonado-trophins, mainly FSH are secreted. These high, sus-tained levels of gonadotrophins may have adverse effects in some women. But it is not clear that they cause hot flushes. Indeed, one of the leading neuroendocrinolo-gists interprets the evidence as indicating that hot flushes and associated mental symptoms probably reflect an oestrogen-withdrawal condition analogous to drug withdrawal syndromes (Reichlin 1968).

133

There is a tendency towards decline in sexual activity around the age of 60. This decline is often related to the male spouse's diminishing sexual interest which tends to begin at about the same age. However, many menopausal women experience a loss of sexual interest which can be reversed by oestrogen replacement therapy. The decrease in sexual interest may be due to regressive changes in the female genitalia induced by oestrogen deficiency, predisposing to discomfort in sexual intercourse. Oestrogens in small doses may also be helpful in the treatment of hot flushes and associated anxiety, irritability, and depression.

At the end of a woman's reproductive period, other events frequently occur in her life that may have threatening implications. We can only summarize them very briefly here.

(1) The likelihood of serious illness is greater at this time of life than it had been before;
(2) This is an era where is a rather high probability of having chronically ill parents;
(3) Concerns about the loss of youthfulness may be personally threatening, especially in cultures which place great value on youth and manifest strong ambivalence toward the elderly;
(4) This is a time when children are likely to be 'lost' in the sense that they have more or less disappeared from the home and intimate contact has diminished;
(5) When faced with the 'empty nest', a woman must decide what to do with the time made available by the departure of her children;
(6) The woman's husband may well be undergoing concurrent transitions in his own life, making him less available in time and emotional commitment than he had been in some earlier phases of their marriage.

The menopausal era may thus pose difficult and distressing tasks for the individual living through it. Indeed, several of these psychosocial tasks may occur at about the same time. Those women who are concomitantly undergoing the most drastic or distorted endocrine changes have additional burdens. Nevertheless, most women cope effectively.

The menopausal-equivalent era for men
Although the male endocrine changes of the middle years are less striking than those of women, the psychological ramifications of a menopausal-equivalent era in men are no less difficult. The concomitant occurrence of major transitions in several spheres— occupational, family, and health—often make this a stressful time. To what extent the endocrine changes *per se* may contribute to individual vulnerability remains largely a matter for future investigation. These changes have recently been well reviewed by Timiras (1972).

From about age 30 onward through the remainder of the life span, there is a gradual decline in the secretion of the male sex hormones, androgens. This decline in hormone output reflects the diminishing number of secretory cells in the testis (Hamburger 1948; Pincus *et al.* 1954; Gherondache *et al.* 1967). The accessory sex glands, such as the prostate, depend for their physiological activity on androgens secreted by the testis. Therefore, the gradual decrease in androgens leads to atrophic changes in structure and function throughout the male reproductive system.

In general, the termination of the adult reproductive period is more gradual than that of females. Indeed, this difference has embryologic roots. In women, the formation of gametes is an embryonic process that results in a fixed number of egg cells, discharged one per month over the adult reproductive span, completed at menopause. In contrast, spermatogenesis begins at puberty in males and continues throughout life. Similarly, the decline in secretion of oestrogens and progesterone by the ovary of the mid-life woman is relatively abrupt in comparison with the decline in androgen secretion by the male testis. Nevertheless, physicians do observe men experiencing hypofunction of the testes associated with loss of sexual potency and motivation, cardiovascular symptoms, especially flushes and tachycardia, chills, sudden perspiration, numbness, vertigo, and emotional instability. This syndrome has been considered a male 'climacteric'. When it occurs, it usually is in the late fifties or early sixties—i.e. later than the menopause in women. Little is known of individual differences in androgen secretion and metabolism that might be partly responsible for this syndrome. With the recent advent of precise, reliable techniques for measuring gonadal and pituitary hormones, as well as the discovery and characterization of hypothalamic hormones that regulate the reproductive system, it becomes possible to identify such individual differences that may have considerable bearing on vulnerability to stressful events of the 40–60 age period (James *et al.* 1973).

The earlier work of Kinsey and associates (1948, 1953), as well as the more recent work of Masters and Johnson (1966, 1970) has enlarged the knowledge of sexual behaviour and physiology in mid-life. In both sexes, coital frequency decreases with age, gradually in most people though abruptly in some. Effective sexual responses can be maintained into advanced years, and sexual activity in the middle years remains vigorous in most people. Most men age 40–60 maintain the patterns of erection, mounting, and ejaculation without difficulty, though individual differences are striking. These responses become slower after 60; the vasocongestive response of the scrotum and testes is reduced and more stimulation is required to elicit penile erection. But once erection occurs, it is maintained for a longer time than is characteristic of young men. The intensity of orgasmic experience tends to be reduced in both sexes, but under favourable circumstances may still be highly satisfying. Much depends on the quality of interpersonal relationship between the participants.

PROMISING DIRECTIONS FOR RESEARCH ON HORMONE–BEHAVIOUR RELATIONS IN MID-LIFE

Recent reviews on hormonal changes with ageing provide useful information on present knowledge and its limitations (Gregerman and Bierman 1974; Eisdorfer and Raskind 1975). Examining the frontiers suggests some needs and opportunities for future investigations.

The tendency toward decline in male sexuality cannot be related to declining levels of plasma or urinary testosterone before age 50, if then. On the average, such relations seem plausible only after the mid-life period.

Relation between behaviour and testosterone levels

It is important to note that, at the time of this writing, there are no published studies relating sexual behaviour, age, and testosterone levels in specific individuals. This is a kind of study that needs doing. From early adolescence to young adulthood, there is a marked increase in the circulating concentration of testosterone. For the American population as a whole, there is no evidence of a declining level before age 50, and even then the decline is very gradual. In the 80–90 age group, testosterone has declined to 40 per cent of the level found in adult men below age 50. But there is remarkable variation among individuals. Some men past age 80 have higher testosterone levels than young adult men. Other elderly men have such low levels that they are in the adult female range. It is precisely this fact of large individual difference which invites study in relation to behaviour —not only sexual activity, but other variables such as mood, vigour, alertness, and persistence.

There are other parameters of individual difference as well. With advanced age, the concentration of testosterone-binding globulin increases. Hence, more testosterone is bound and so the concentration of *free* (physiologically-active) testosterone decreases considerably more than the *total* testosterone. Kinetic studies indicate testosterone *production* is diminished in later life. There are also changes in metabolism; e.g. changes in the pattern of testosterone metabolites (androstanediols). The individual differences in these parameters, and especially their *rates of change* over time, have drawn little attention; and the relation of such differences to changes in behaviour has scarcely been examined.

Relation between behaviour and oestrogen levels

In women, testosterone does not change with age. It remains at a low (though not necessarily functionally insignificant) level throughout adult life. The oestrogen decline described above is much more predictable than the decline in male testosterone. Nevertheless, there are important limitations in available data. Most of the information is cross-sectional. Hardly any data are available on the exact time sequence or rate of decline in oestrogen levels in specific individuals. Here again, this approach is worth while for examining hormone–behaviour relations. Are precipitous changes associated with psychological vulnerability?

After the menopause, there is a further decline in oestrogen levels in the 50–60 age range. Oestrogen production generally falls with advancing age. Women at age 70 have, on the average, about one-half the production of young adult women. This production reflects the secretory activity of adrenal cortex and testis in oestrogen production in later life. Some investigators suspect from clinical observations that individual variations in post-menopausal oestrogens may influence vulnerability to depression.

Relation between age and endocrine stress responses

Do endocrine stress responses change with age? Although there is no evidence of general decline in excretion of the adreno-medullary catecholamines, adrenalin and noradrenalin, there may well be a change in the *dynamics* of adrenal response to stress, as well as the response of the sympathetic nervous system. Some clinical investigators believe that there is a reduction in hypothalamic reactivity in the elderly. Although resting levels of corticosteroids do not change remarkably with age, their response to ACTH diminishes (Eleftherion and Sproutt 1975). In rodents, there are major strain differences in this response. Thus, it is plausible that genetic factors might determine significant human individual differences in such responses. Similarly, there are fragments of evidence suggesting a decline in brain noradrenalin and an increase in the enzyme monoamine oxidase (MAO) in the elderly. If true, these developments could predispose to depression. Such possibilities are only on the threshold of systematic investigation. The advent of new technology for measuring brain and adrenal amines, such as mass fragmentography, can provide much more information than could previously have been obtained.

Overall, ageing probably affects various endocrine subsystems—but at different rates and to different extents. The available information is scattered—regrettably non-specific with respect to age categories, rates of change, and hormone–behaviour linkages.

For the future, important opportunities exist in lines of enquiry that focus on:

(1) Long-term rates of change (i.e. individuals studied repeatedly over several years);
(2) Responsiveness to stimulation (i.e. effects of experimentally administered hormones and of environmentally-induced stressful experience upon endocrine and autonomic responses);
(3) Patterns of hormone metabolism over extended time;
(4) Binding protein in hormone transport;
(5) Excretion via kidneys;
(6) Target-tissue sensitivity.

All of these are subject to change over time and marked individual differences. By studying these parameters, it may become possible to sort out different kinds of vulnerability to mid-life crisis and other disorders.

New developments in biology and behavioural science should greatly facilitate such investigations. These include mass fragmentography and radio-immunoassay. These techniques utilized together (and with closely related techniques) permit the measurement of a much wider array of hormones and their metabolites with greater precision and sensitivity than ever before—including peptides, steroids, and amines.

The availability of hypothalamic hormones and their synthetic analogues for experimental and clinical purposes is an important additional tool for research on these problems. The feedback effects of these hormones on the brain, both indirectly via stimulation of steroid secretion and directly in their own right, deserve special attention. Since hypothalamic hormones serve as neurotransmitters or at least neuroregulators in brain circuits far beyond the hypothalamus, and since steroids affect biogenic amines that are so important as neurotransmitters and neuroregulators, a whole new vista is opening up for relating hormones and neurotransmitters to behaviour. To seek such relations in the context of age-linked biological transitions, such as menopause and puberty, is of great clinical interest.

It is worth bearing in mind that individual differences in endocrine function affecting brain and behaviour might arise from several sources:

(1) Genetic factors influencing endocrine variation (which we have written about in other contexts, especially differential susceptibility to psychological stress);
(2) Concurrent stress (e.g. powerful effects on hypothalamus, adrenal cortex, and adrenal medulla, triggered in mid-life by the unexpected loss of an important person);
(3) Early experience (based chiefly on experimental data in rodents indicating that early environmental conditions may have an enduring effect on the adrenal response to stress, and perhaps on other endocrine parameters as well).

Several recent experimental and clinical investigations augment knowledge of pituitary and gonadal hormone changes with age (Judd *et al.* 1974); Isurugi *et al.* 1974; Rubens *et al.* 1974; Vermeulen *et al.* 1972). While informative, these reports are typical in lacking certain information highly pertinent to the problems under consideration here:

(1) They contain no behavioural data;
(2) They lack longitudinal data on individual subjects;
(3) They focus little attention on individual differences, though the attention they do give suggests wide individual differences.

A recent comprehensive review and analysis of genetic variations in endocrine systems is valuable as a framework for future investigations of the sort being suggested here (Shire 1976). But it gives only modest explication of the potential significance of these genetically determined endocrine variations for behaviour.

Clinically, there are several known circumstances of sharply diminished testicular function:

(1) Mumps orchitis;
(2) Surgical interference with blood supply;
(3) Klinefelter's syndrome.

Clinical endocrinologists observe behavioural changes under these conditions:

(1) Hyperirritability;
(2) Depression;
(3) Diminished sexuality;
(4) Difficulty in concentration;
(5) Cardiovascular symptoms: intense sweating episodes, 'hot flushes', tachycardia.

Can this sort of response occur—probably to a less extreme degree—on a genetic basis in a larger percentage of men, thus making them vulnerable to stress? These are questions for future research.

Systematic longitudinal studies of mid-life individuals, linking endocrine and behavioural measures, offer significant promise of clarifying differential susceptibility to the vicissitudes of stressful experience. Experimental interventions may usefully be superimposed on such longitudinal observations. Research of this sort might usefully include:

(1) The interplay of various hormones;
(2) The interplay of hormones and neurotransmitters;
(3) The interplay of these biological processes with learned coping strategies.

The general significance of these biological variations is not likely to be in grotesque distortions of behaviour but in subtle and complex processes of vulnerability to stressful experience, especially when it is of long duration. At any rate, the current situation offers unprecedented opportunity for research—albeit difficult research—to clarify hormone behaviour relations in mid-life, and in other phases of the lifespan as well.

COPING BEHAVIOUR IN THE MIDDLE YEARS

Educational factors have a bearing on status and income—and hence on personal coping resources—throughout the career trajectory (Jaffe 1971). Extensive education permits entry into the labour force at relatively high levels and provides better opportunities.

on the average, throughout the course of life. As we shall see, coping responses tend to differ at different occupational levels. Nevertheless, workers at all levels have a remarkable capacity for adapting to the levels of satisfaction actually available in their jobs (Blauner 1964). Moreover, most individuals even adapt effectively to circumstances in which few satisfactions are available on the job and must be found elsewhere (Sofer 1974). In surveys, few workers describe themselves as highly dissatisfied. In a given job, individuals vary widely in the extent to which their self-esteem is based on work; put differently, persons differ greatly in their distribution of self-esteem commitments. Where job satisfactions are meagre, formulation of self-esteem on other bases is personally valuable. Sofer (1974) points out

Meaning can be introduced into jobs and job contexts found boring or unsatisfactory by those performing them. This is done, for example, by elaborating the movements required, by unofficial exchanges of duties between workers, by working to targets defined by the worker himself or by groups of workers, by introducing social rituals or games, or by thwarting supervisors and managerial groups (Roy, 1953, 1959–1960; Walker and Guest (1952). . . . Once they have become established in their occupations, the job aspirations of blue collar workers are typically not high and their definitions of what constitutes success have to be judged by job needs as they perceive them, that is, largely in terms of security of employment and reasonableness of hours, colleagueship and supervision.

Coping behaviour of industrial workers

The mental health of industrial workers varies with situational factors such as opportunity to use their abilities in the work, feeling of interest, sense of accomplishment, and personal growth (Kornhauser 1965). The exercise of skills, their continuing development, and recognition for competence all loom large in the maintenance of self-esteem in industrial workers as well as at higher occupational levels.

In most industrial societies, a large proportion of industrial workers belong to trade unions. Among blue collar workers, the union tends to have considerable psychological significance, especially as the middle-aged worker reduces his aspirations, hoping for a steady job and depending on the union to protect his interests. Increasingly, such workers look to the union to improve not only their financial position but their working conditions. Higher occupational aspirations tend to be shifted to their children who, with more educational opportunity, will hopefully reach attainments not possible for their parents.

Coping behaviour of white collar workers and executives

In contrast to blue collar workers, white collar workers and executives enter relatively clear-cut channels and follow visible steps over the years (Glaser and Strauss 1971). Institutional support and facilitation for career development of executives goes beyond that available to other workers. Individual alertness to these oppor-

tunities has a bearing on long-term occupational effectiveness. These higher occupational groups share with lower groups certain basic values: economic security, occupational continuity, interaction with others at work, and formulation of the job in ways that support self-esteem. In general, executives and white collar workers have more occupational scope and institutional resources for implementing these values than do blue collar workers.

Middle-level managers and professionals in organizations must integrate two general tasks: fostering personal advancement and co-operating in joint activities. Contrary to a common stereotype, excessive competitiveness may well hinder long-range advancement. Sofer (1974) points out:

Most organizational tasks are carried out by groups which develop solidarity, shared definitions of their mission and status and shared conceptions of how they should relate to other task groups, to subordinates and superiors: the individual must be an acceptable colleague on easy terms with equals, prepared to give credit to their contributions and to refrain from pressing his own claims to special consideration and merit. But if he is to advance it is also necessary that he differentiates himself from his peers and convey that he is potentially able to distance himself enough to view their organizational contribution objectively or, if required, to control it from a position of greater authority. Both task performance and career building make high demands on interpersonal competence.

The development of such skills is typically a task of earlier years; the rewards of such efforts may be fully appreciated in the middle years.

Since it is hard to assess an individual's specific contribution in large organizations, evaluation of performance of executives and professionals tends to rest heavily on personal characteristics such as enthusiasm, confidence, initiative, and readiness to co-operate. Technical competence, scope of information, and capacity for problem solving are also valued. Thus, long-term recognition rests heavily on interpersonal as well as substantive criteria.

Coping behaviour of high-level executives and professionals

In empirical studies, persons at higher occupational levels report greater satisfaction with their work than those at lower levels. This partly reflects satisfaction with status *per se*. Executives and professionals have a relatively high degree of control over their use of time and organization of effort. In the middle years, they value these assets and often sense a rewarding competence in making use of them. Moreover, they are less subject to direct scrutiny and day-to-day criticism than they had been in earlier years. They have considerable scope for defining occupational roles in idiosyncratic ways and for making their own priorities. For such individuals, work is a major source of self-esteem—often the single most important component of self-esteem. Under these conditions, work shapes the entire life style (Sofer 1970; Blauner 1960). A considerable body of systematic studies indicates that satisfaction with jobs is higher for managerial than non-managerial persons; satisfaction is higher at successive levels within management (Porter and Lawler 1965). A study of managerial attitudes in fourteen countries shows that higher levels of management report greater job satisfaction than lower levels. So, despite distinctive high-level problems, achievement has potent rewards around the world. Moreover, studies in the United States reveal that, within management, the needs for esteem, autonomy, and self-actualization are better met at each higher level (Porter and Lawler 1965).

Large organizations often inform their executives of personal assets and limitations as perceived by senior executives. The ability to make use of such feedback is an important factor in coping with the stresses of higher occupational positions. An expectation of lifelong learning, an openness to new possibilities, a premium on what one can become—all this has significance for the growth of self-esteem and for occupational effectiveness. These periodic self-assessments, continuing into the middle years, may be particularly acute and poignant then because of the growing sense of limited time remaining for mid-course corrections and because of concomitant stressful events in health or family spheres. Yet they offer great potential in the sense of personal renewal and effective use of one's capacities.

Occupational disappointments of the middle years may be profound. Ways of coping with such disappointments have been inadequately studied. A deeper understanding of effective coping in this context would be helpful not only in fostering occupational effectiveness but also in relieving family strains and, medically, in treating depression.

The disappointed individual may bolster self-esteem by mobilizing supportive beliefs—e.g. that he would not resort to unethical modes of behaviour used by others in obtaining advancement. He may draw upon shared group-beliefs by centring on the concept that personal merit is not the main factor in success (Sofer 1970). For many, a crucial process lies in finding alternate satisfactions, such as the reawakening of familial, recreational, political, or community commitments. Relationships with spouse, children, grandchildren, and old friends may be enormously helpful in these stressful circumstances.

George's (1974) studies of stress in high-level decision-makers

In recent years, some behavioural scientists have studied stress and coping in high-level decision-makers, typically in the middle years of life. A good example is the work of George (1974) who focuses on major political leaders under stress. He examines coping behaviour in individual, group, and organizational contexts. Although he centres on high-level political decision-making, it is likely that his analysis applies to other similar situations. In studying presidential decisions,

George uses an extreme case to highlight a set of processes that are important over a much wider range of situations involving executives or others in leadership positions. His analysis illuminates the importance of social support, guidance, and facilitation for individual coping efforts.

The decision-making model utilized by George is one that links the individual to his small group and organizational settings. When multiple, conflicting stakes are aroused in a difficult situation, the individual decision-maker undertakes a sort of 'balance-sheet' assessment, comparing his current policy with proposed new ones. In doing so, he examines the anticipated utility of these alternative policies, both for himself and for other people who are particularly significant to him. He similarly examines the various policies in relation to anticipated approval and disapproval, again both in the way he views himself and the way he will be viewed by others. The political decision-maker, and the individual decision-maker in many difficult situations, often has to operate under the following limitations:

(1) Incomplete information about the situation;
(2) Inadequate knowledge of the relation between ends and means, so that he cannot predict with high confidence the consequences of choosing a given course of action;
(3) Difficulty in formulating a single criterion for use in choosing the best available option.

In such a setting, strategies for dealing with cognitive complexity become essential. George describes a set of such strategies that have been illustrated in research on political decision-making. They have much overlap with strategies employed in other situations of cognitive complexity.

These difficult situations typically pose multiple stakes for the decision-maker that cannot readily be reconciled. He must, therefore, have ways of dealing with such decisional conflicts. George describes three broad strategies:

(1) Avoiding the conflict;
(2) Resolving the conflict;
(3) Accepting the conflict.

For each of these strategies, he delineates several tactics through which they can be implemented. In the small group context, effective coping with decisional stress is facilitated by certain kinds of relationships with other persons and communications with them. The nature of such facilitating relationships in face-to-face groups have a good deal in common with the recent research literature on group psychotherapy (Yalom 1970).

The administrative decision-maker typically copes with the difficult problems he faces within the framework of a large organization. All large organizations have structural characteristics of hierarchy, specialization, and centralization that have herent risks and constraints. But George points out that organizations also provide opportunities for facilitating the individual's constructive problem-solving capacities. Organizations can assist a political leader in a stressful situation in seeking and utilizing relevant information and advice. Organizations can also compensate for some of the disruptive influences of small groups.

A major theme running through George's analysis both of small groups and of the organizational context has to do with the strong advantages of explicitly considering a wide range of alternatives, including unpleasant ones, before making a major decision. This issue appears to be of great importance over a wide range of coping issues and by no means limited to stressful political decisions. There are many processes in the small group and the large organization that may inhibit or facilitate a consideration of multiple alternatives. For instance, George says:

since advocacy is inevitable, the solution lies in the direction of ensuring that there will be multiple advocates within the bureaucratic politics systems who, among themselves, will cover the range of interesting policy options on any given issue.

There are advantages of planning procedures that encourage critical, broad-gauged consideration of many overlapping and competing factors that are embedded in a particular problem. In so doing, alternative courses of action can be formulated with increasing clarity; the advantages and limitations of each can then be assessed in a way that draws upon the best available evidence, involving not only protection of the decision-maker himself, but also giving serious consideration to the welfare of others.

Improving decision-making processes

There are ways in which organizations can improve the quality of decision-making processes. For example, there is practical utility in organizational early warning systems. Since it is so difficult under most stressful circumstances to make anything like an optimal decision, there is an urgent need for monitoring the course of the transaction with the environment in such a way as to detect early warning signals, when untoward consequences are beginning to appear but before irreversible damage has occurred. This has great relevance both for individuals making personally important decisions in stressful situations, e.g. regarding organizational or family transitions, and for social problems in a rapidly changing society.

Recent studies of historical cases suggest several factors that increase the risk of malfunction in decision-making processes. These malfunctions tend to occur under the following conditions:

(1) When the decision-maker and his advisers agree too readily on the nature of the problem and on a single response to it;

(2) When advisers take up alternatives with the decision-maker, but only cover a narrow range of options;
(3) When there is no advocate for an unpopular option;
(4) When advisers work out their own disagreements over alternative possibilities without the decision-maker's knowledge and then present him with a single recommendation;
(5) When advisers agree privately among themselves that the decision-maker should face up to a distressing situation, but no one is willing to alert him to it;
(6) When the decision-maker is largely dependent upon a single channel of information;
(7) When the underlying assumptions of a plan have been evaluated only by the advocates of that option;
(8) When the decision-maker does not arrange for a well-qualified group to examine carefully the negative judgement offered by one or more advisers on a preferred course of action;
(9) When the decision-maker is impressed by a consensus among his advisers but does not thoroughly examine the adequacy of its basis.

Making explicit these sources of interference with effective problem-solving enhances future opportunities for coping with stressful decision-making situations. The heavy responsibilities of such decision-making typically occur in the middle years. While certainly stressful at times, they can also be deeply gratifying, culminating in a sense of profound competence and social worth.

Coping behaviour for women in the menopausal era

While women in most societies have not had such grand responsibilities—vividly moving and shaking the levers of power—they nevertheless have always in the long course of human evolution had major commitments and vital responsibilities. By our criteria, these qualify as occupational commitments even when not technically a part of the labour force. In the more-then-three-million years in which humans lived in hunting-and-gathering societies, women not only had the principal parental responsibilities but also the task of obtaining a major part of the food supply by gathering edibles (Lee and DeVore 1968). In the past few thousand years, as agriculture became established, women still had a role in subsistence as well as in care-of-young. The present chapter is not the place for an extended discussion of the very recent changes in occupational commitments of women. These deserve serious attention in the framework of stress and coping. Biologically, the menopause constitutes a major transition; it is embedded in a different social context than ever before in history. While this social change is stressful, it also provides new and potentially gratifying opportunities for women in the middle years.

Research is badly needed to clarify coping behaviour

in the menopausal era (Koran and Hamburg 1975). A few coping strategies may be summarized here:

(1) Avoidance tendencies, involving psychological processes through which people minimize awareness of threatening implications of their life-circumstances;
(2) Patterns of behaviour that have the functional effect of reassuring oneself about the persistence of youthfulness;
(3) Seeking of information about the menopause itself, about new bases for self-esteem, and about changes in interpersonal relationships;
(4) The making of new friendships or the deepening of existing ones;
(5) The initiation or deepening of occupational and recreational activities;
(6) A search for 'substitute children', both within and beyond the family;
(7) Exploring new ways of relating to one's children;
(8) Seeking out new satisfactions in the role of grandparent;
(9) Intensifying religious commitment;
(10) Self-appraisal, especially in placing greater value on personal qualities of experience, judgement, and maturity.

LONGITUDINAL STUDIES: A LIFE COURSE PERSPECTIVE ON STRESS AND COPING IN THE MIDDLE YEARS

Long-term studies of human development into the adult years have been undertaken at several universities, including the Terman study at Stanford, the Growth and Guidance studies at the University of California, Berkeley, and the Grant study at Harvard. A recent report from the latter study provides some new evidence on the life course extending into the middle years (Vaillant and McArthur 1972). Despite the difficult methodological problems of very long-term studies, they provide important clues to factors influencing the development of behaviour through the life cycle.

The Grant study
The Grant study is one of the longest prospective studies of adult development in the world. Begun in 1938 when the average subject was 18, it has continued to the present time. The average subject is now past 50 years of age. Like Terman's group, the subjects were selected in ways that maximized valued characteristics. Thus, the Grant study shows how the male adult life cycle proceeds under favourable circumstances.

Broadly speaking, these men, after obtaining their college education at Harvard, concentrated on marriage when they were in their twenties, on job accomplishment in their thirties, and on their children in their forties. This is of course an oversimplification, meant to convey differing emphases in different phases of the life cycle.

The authors believe that the data generally support an Eriksonian sequence: (1) intimacy, followed by (2) career consolidation, followed by (3) generativity.

Images of adolescent and mid-life behaviour are examined. A stormy adolescence in itself does not seem to be predictive of mid-life difficulty. But the relatively rare severe identity crises of adolescence tended to remain largely unresolved through the adult years.

In college each adolescent was rated for psychological soundness. Retrospectively, he also was rated for childhood adjustment by a researcher kept blind to this rating and to adult outcome. For each adolescent a check list of 25 traits was also completed. . . . The adolescent traits that were significantly associated with subsequently healthy rating in mid-life were 'well integrated', and 'practical organizing'. Conversely, the traits 'asocial' and 'incompletely integrated' and 'cultural interests' were associated with a poor mid-life outcome.
. . . The 30 men who at 47 received the highest scores in overall adult adjustment were compared to the 30 men whose middle-aged lives seemed most maladapted. In this way, the value of mastering intimacy during the decade from 20 to 30 could be documented. For example, of the best adapted men, 93% had achieved a stable marriage before 30 and had stayed married until 50. Of the worst adapted men, only 23% had married before 30 and had continued to live with their wives.

These observations may be related to the substantial body of health statistics indicating the vulnerability to many diseases of relatively isolated men (Kramer and Redick 1974).

One of the most striking observations in the most recent Grant study follow-up is the change that occurred in many lives at about 40 years of age. Most of these men actually viewed their 40s as more tumultuous than their adolescence. The intensity of these reactions involved not only emotional distress but also challenge and opportunity, satisfaction and growth. Indeed, the men considered best adapted by the staff tended to appraise the age period 35–49 as the happiest in their lives. On the whole, their health was good; they were vigorous; they had acquired substantial experience, competence, and recognition; were open to new possibilities, and had hopes for further growth. The 40–50 decade involved much reordering of past experience and reassessment of personal priorities. These processes heavily involved occupational commitments, social contribution, and relations with wife and children. Much of this worked out well by the end of the decade, and some of it yielded new satisfactions. But in mid-passage, periods of depression were evident. Indeed, overt depression was much more common in this decade than in the prior one.

As they mature, delinquents and addicts are more apt to acknowledge formerly latent depression. The same pattern occurred in the Grant study. But if these Grant study subjects were conscious of more depression, they also in mid-life appeared far more able to accept their own tragedy and that of others. If the subjects were dissatisfied with their careers, it was because they longed to be of greater service to those around them, not because they saw themselves as failures. . . . Perhaps

140

the most important conclusion of the Grant study has been that the agonizing self-reappraisal and instinctual reawakening at age 40—the so-called mid-life crisis—does not appear to portend decay. However marred by depression and turmoil middle-life may be, it often heralds a new stage of man. (Vaillant and McArthur 1972).

The studies of Levinson *et al.*

In ongoing research involving intensive personality study over four years, Levinson, Darrow, Klein, Levinson, and McKee are obtaining interview and Thematic Apperception Test data on a sample of 40 men, all of whom are currently in the age 35–45 decade (Levinson *et al.* 1974). Their sample includes 10 men in each of four occupational groups: blue and white collar workers in industry; business executives; academic biologists; and novelists. These authors distinguish several chronological periods in the adult life course: early adulthood, ages 20–40; middle adulthood, ages 40–60; and late adulthood, age 60+. They are studying early adulthood and the 'mid-life transition'—i.e. the several years on either side of age 40 that they consider a transitional period between early and middle adulthood.

Their view of the adult life course involves several psychological phases, each of which influences subsequent ones:

(1) *Leaving the family* is seen as a transition between adolescent life, centred in the family of origin, and entry into the adult world;

(2) *Getting into the adult world* occurs when the centre of gravity of one's life shifts from the family of origin to a new home base and an effort to form an adult life of one's own—This phase usually starts in the early 20s and extends until age 27–29;

(3) *Settling down*—this phase usually begins in the early thirties, and the person 'now makes deeper commitments, invests more of himself in his work, family, and valued interests and, within the framework of this life structure, makes and pursues more long-range plans and goals';

(4) *Becoming one's own man*, which tends to occur in the middle to late thirties. During this phase, there is a tendency to become independent of mentors who had earlier been highly significant. During this phase, 'a man wants desperately to be affirmed by society in the roles that he values most. He is trying for that crucial promotion or other recognition. At about age 40—we would now say within the range of about 39 to 42—most of our subjects fix on some key event in their careers as carrying the ultimate message of their affirmation or devaluation by society' (Levinson *et al.* 1974);

(5) The *mid-life transition*. They formulate this phase as centring on an intimate, personal assessment of the goodness-of-fit between a guiding life structure and an appraisal of self. To what extent has he become the kind of person he would ultimately like to be? 'He is having a crisis to the extent that he questions his life structure and feels the stirrings of powerful forces within himself that lead him to modify or drastically change the structure (Levinson *et al.* 1974). In this view, one of the main issues underlying the mid-life transition is

the sense of bodily decline and the more vivid recognition of one's mortality. The necessity to confront one's mortality and to deal in a new way with wounds to one's omnipotence fantasies, to overcome illusions and self-deceptions which relate to one's sense of omnipotence. Greater freedom in experiencing and thinking about one's own and other's death, and greater compassion in responding to another's distress about decline, deformity, death, loss, bereavement.

In the mid-forties Levinson *et al.* find a tendency towards restabilization. Over several years, the mid-life transition comes to an end. Some reorganization of behaviour occurs, the life structure is modified, and stable patterns for living the middle years usually emerge.

Men such as Freud, Jung, Eugene O'Neill, Frank Lloyd Wright, Goya and Gandhi went through a profound crisis at around 40 and made tremendous creative gains through it. There are also men like Dylan Thomas, Scott Fitzgerald and Sinclair Lewis, who could not manage this crisis and who destroyed themselves in it.

These dramatic instances highlight the divergent paths opened up by a mid-life crisis, and raise fundamental questions about underlying processes of stress and coping. It should be noted, however, that we have little idea of the incidence of mid-life crisis in general populations of different countries.

CLINICAL OBSERVATIONS ON MID-LIFE CRISIS: OCCUPATIONAL AND INTER-PERSONAL COMMITMENTS

Over two decades, we have been consulted often by persons experiencing a mid-life crisis. Indeed, it constitutes a significant portion of psychiatric practice in the United States. Clinically, these problems seem to be increasingly frequent, but there is no way of knowing at present what the true incidence and prevalence might be. Although psychiatric practice undoubtedly overstates the scope of the problem in the general population it nevertheless provides some understanding of underlying processes in mid-life adaptation and clues for future systematic investigation. Our own experience, like that of most psychiatrists, is mainly with relatively highly educated persons characterized by high occupational aspirations—mostly men, but some women as well. By mid-life crisis, we refer to episodes of intense and persistent emotional distress concomitant with drastic changes in occupational and interpersonal commitments

141

occurring in the age period 40–60. We certainly do not suggest that crisis is an inevitable event in the middle years of adulthood; rather, we attempt to sort out factors that tend to exacerbate or relieve distress in this age period, events that are stressful and strategies that tend to be effective in coping with these stresses. We are impressed, here as elsewhere, with the immense variety of human responses to a particular situation and the multiplicity of factors influencing human adaptation (Hamburg *et al.* 1975). We wish here only to sketch briefly a few mid-life events that have been stressful for one or another of our patients, and a few strategies that have been useful for one or another of our patients in coping with such stressful experiences. Overall, we are encouraged by the favourable long-term outcome in most of these patients.

Occupational dissatisfaction

Commonly, occupational dissatisfaction looms large in precipitation of mid-life crisis. Some people feel they have attempted too much, have over-reached, have scattered their energies, have not been fully effective; others feel they have attempted too little, have not stretched themselves, have not responded vigorously to opportunities. In either case, there is a discrepancy between aspiration and attainment in such persons. This is usually accompanied by a deep concern that there is no longer enough time for correction, for reducing the discrepancy.

Many responses to such a personally-threatening appraisal of one's life situation are possible. We mention here only a few. One possibility is to scale down one's aspirations—usually in small steps over several years, gradually accommodating to a new image of self. Another response is renewed effort, a fervent commitment to make full use of time remaining. Both these responses centre on the occupational sphere in persons for whom occupational achievement has been an important source of self-esteem. But sometimes the arena of principal concern shifts from occupational to interpersonal commitments.

Interpersonal commitments during the mid-life crisis

A special new relationship may be formed under the stimulus of mid-life doubts and concerns. This relationship may be a deep friendship, a love affair, or a new marriage. It may be formulated as an alternate source of satisfaction, replacing the prior emphasis on occupational satisfaction, and providing a vital new basis for self-esteem. However, it may be viewed as facilitating renewed occupational efforts, providing a new stimulus, encouragement, assistance, even inspiration.

Such a relationship may have many other connotations. It may relieve old burdens. It may add new satisfactions. It may provide a sense of recapturing youth. It may open new vistas—information, ideas, shared experiences. The person in mid-life may find he has fewer inhibitions than he had in his youth, less

uncertainty, more confidence in taking advantage of new opportunities. His self-esteem may be renewed by the fact that he has been able to earn the respect of someone to whom he attaches a special value; moreover, his old assets now elicit new responses—a storehouse of past experiences, skills, and knowledge to be shared with the new person. This relationship may be felt as a kind of special accomplishment. It may elicit favourable reactions from others. It may be experienced as invigorating—sexually, occupationally, and in other ways.

For all that, it is a high-risk strategy. For one thing, it is typically based on a selective view of the other person— seen in the best circumstances, with fewest burdens, and refreshing novelty. The relationship may happily extend beyond this period—but all too often the exciting phase of novelty is followed in due course by a bitter phase of disillusion. But even if the relationship endures, there are very difficult problems to be faced: guilt over violating long-internalized standards of acceptable behaviour; concern over possible damage to significant others; distraction from deep and enduring commitments to family, friends, and occupation. Divorce and remarriage appear to be increasingly common in this age group, but these problems go beyond the scope of the present paper.

In the middle years, some persons seek new gratifications in the interpersonal sphere while holding occupational commitment essentially constant. Others seek new gratification in the occupational sphere while holding interpersonal commitments essentially constant. Some make major changes in both concomitantly. This latter is a particularly high-risk strategy though it may on occasion yield high gains.

Resolution of the crisis

More commonly, there is—after a period of doubt, perplexity, even anguish—a renewal or confirmation of existing commitments—occupational and interpersonal. Often, this is accompanied by a modest, personally significant reformulation of these long-established commitments—new points of emphasis, heightened appreciation of aspects previously taken for granted, additional dimensions of experience. Such reformulations, strengthening existing occupational and interpersonal commitments, tend to centre on several themes:

(1) On being useful—to younger people in the same occupation, to children, to grandchildren, to the sick, or to the disadvantaged;
(2) On tradition, kinship, a sense of belonging in a valued group—occupational, family, recreational, ideological;
(3) On competence and skill, now extended or embellished or renewed;
(4) On recognition, especially by significant others, though sometimes in a wider arena;
(5) On experience, judgement, even wisdom.

It is a poignant dilemma of contemporary circumstances that social change of unprecedented rapidity casts doubt on the relevance of the mid-life adult's knowledge for the tasks of a person half his age or younger (D. Hamburg 1975). Still, experience has its uses (B. Hamburg 1975).

As the years pass, physical vigour counts for less, knowledge and judgement more; grand exploits less, integrity more; technical skill less, compassion more. And always, even in the drastically changed context of the modern world, satisfaction depends on the network of enduring and dependable human relationships that has been at the heart of human evolution for millions of years.

REFERENCES

BLAUNER, R. (1960). Work satisfaction and industrial trends in modern society. In *Labour and trade unionism: an inter-disciplinary reader* (ed. W. Galenson and S. M. Lipset). Wiley, New York.

—— (1964). *Alienation and freedom: the factory worker and his industry*. University of Chicago Press, Chicago.

BRIM, O., Jr. (chairman) (1973). Description of proposed activities, report of the Committee on Work and Personality in the Middle Years, Social Science Research Council, May meeting, New York.

CROZIER, M. (1964). *The bureaucratic phenomenon.* (An examination of bureaucracy in modern organizations and its cultural setting in France.) University of Chicago Press, Chicago.

EISDORFER, C. and RASKIND, M. (1975). Aging, hormones and human behaviour. In *Hormonal correlates of behavior, Vol. I: A lifespan view* (ed. B. Eleftherious, and R. Sproutt). Plenum Press, New York.

E LEFTHERIOU, B. and SPROUTT, R. (eds.)(1975). *Hormonal correlates of behaviour, Vol. I: A lifespan view*. Plenum Press, New York.

GEORGE, A. L. (1974). Adaptation to stress in political decision making: The individual, small group, and organizational contexts. In *Coping and adaptation* (ed. G. Coelho, D. Hamburg, and J. Adams). Basic Books, Inc., New York.

GHERONDACHE, C. N., ROMANOFF, L. P., and PINCUS, G. (1967). Steroid hormones in aging men. In *Endocrines and aging* (ed. L. Gitman). Charles C. Thomas, Springfield, Ill.

GLASER, B. G. and STRAUSS, A. (1971). *Status passage. A formal theory*. Aldine Atherton, Chicago.

GREGERMAN, R. and BIERMAN, E. (1974). Aging and hormones. In *Textbook of endocrinology* (fifth edn.) (ed. R. H. Williams). W. B. Saunders, Philadelphia.

HAMBURG, B. (1975). Social change and the problems of youth. In *American handbook of psychiatry, Vol. 6* (ed. D. A. Hamburg and H. K. H. Brodie). Basic Books, Inc., New York.

HAMBURG, D. (1975). Ancient man in the twentieth century. In *The quest for man* (ed. V. Goodall). Phaidon Press Limited, London.

——, HAMBURG, B., and BARCHAS, J. (1975). Anger and depression in perspective of behavioral biology. In *Parameters of emotion* (ed. L. Levi). Raven Press, New York.

HAMBURGER, C. (1948). Normal urinary excretion of neutral 17-ketosteroids with special reference to age and sex variations. *Acta Endocrinol.*, **1**, 19–37.

ISURUGI, K., FUKUTANI, K., TAKAYASU, H., WAKABAYASHI, K., and TAMAOKI, B. I. (1974). Age-related changes in serum luteinizing hormone (LH) and Follicle-stimulating hormone (FSH) levels in normal men. *J. clin. Endocrinol. Metab.*, **39**, 955.

JAFFE, A. J. (1971). The middle years. Neither too young nor too old, special issue *Industrial Gerontology*.

JAMES, V. H. T., SERIO, M., and MARTINI, L. (1973). *The endocrine function of the human testis, Vol. I.* Academic Press, New York.

JUDD, H. L., JUDD, G. E., LUCAS, W. E., and YEN, S. S. C. (1974). Endocrine function of the postmenopausal ovary: concentration of androgens and estrogens in ovarian and peripheral vein blood. *J. clin. Endocrinol. Metab.* **39**, 1020.

KAHN, R. L., WOLFE, D. M., QUINN, R. P., and SNOEK, J. D. (1964). *Organizational stress. Studies in role conflict and ambiguity*. Wiley, New York.

KINSEY, A. C., POMEROY, W. B., and MARTIN, C. E. (1948). *Sexual behavior in the human male*. W. B. Saunders Co., Philadelphia.

KINSEY, A. C., POMEROY, W. B., MARTIN, C. E., and GEBHARD, P. H. (1953). *Sexual behavior in the human female*. W. B. Saunders Co., Philadelphia.

KNUPPER, G. (1974). Portrait of the Underdog. *Public Opinion Quart.* **11**, (1).

KORAN, L. M. and HAMBURG, D. A. (1975). Psychophysiologic endocrine disorders. In *Comprehensive textbook of psychiatry* (2nd edn) (ed. A. M. Freedman, H. I. Kaplan, and B. J. Sadock). The Williams and Wilkins Co., Baltimore.

KORNHAUSER, A. (1965). *Mental health of the industrial worker, a Detroit study*. Wiley, New York.

KRAMER, M. and REDICK, R. W. (1974). Epidemiological indices in the middle years. Presented at the February meeting of the Committee on Work and Personality in the Middle Years, Social Science Research Council, New York.

LEE, R. B. and DEVORE, I. (1968). *Man the hunter*. Aldine Publishing Co., Chicago.

LEVINSON, D. J., DARROW, C. M., KLEIN, E. B., LEVINSON, M. H., and MCKEE, B. (1974). The psychosocial development of men in early adulthood and the mid-life transition. In *Life history research in psychopathology, Vol. 3* (ed. D. R. Ricks, A. Thomas, and M. Roff). University of Minnesota Press.

MASTERS, W. H. and JOHNSON, V. E. (1968). *Human sexual response*. Little, Brown and Co., Boston.

—— and —— (1970). *Human sexual inadequacy*. Little, Brown and Co., Boston.

MENNINGER, W. (1974). Class reunions and mid-life crisis. Personal communication.

PINCUS, G., ROMANOFF, L. P., and CARLO, J. (1954). The excretion of urinary steroids by men and women of various ages. *J. Gerontol*, **9**, 113–32.

PORTER, L. W. and LAWLER, E. E. (1965). Properties of organization structure in relation to job attitudes and job behaviour. *Psychol. Bull.*, **64**, (1).

REICHLIN, S. (1968). Neuroendocrinology. In *Textbook of endocrinology* (4th ed.) (ed. R. H. Williams). W. B. Saunders Company, Philadelphia.

ROY, D. F. (1953). Work satisfaction and social rewards in quota achievement: An analysis of piecework. *Amer. sociol. Rev.*, **18**, (5).

—— (1959–60). 'Banana Time'. Job satisfaction and informal interaction. *Human Org.,* **18,** (4).

RUBENS, R., DHONT, M., and VERMEULEN, A. (1974). Further studies in leydig cell function in old age. *J. clin. Endocrinol. Metab.,* **39,** 40.

SHIRE, J. G. M. (1976). The forms, uses and significance of genetic variation in endocrine systems. *Biol. Rev.,* **51,** 105.

SOFER, C. (1970). *Men in mid-career.* Cambridge University Press.

—— (1974). Occupational difficulties. In *American handbook of psychiatry* (ed. S. Arieti). Basic Books, Inc., New York.

STOUFFER, S. A., SUCHMAN, E. A., DE VINNEY, L. C., STAR, S. A., and WILLIAMS, R. M. (1949). *The American soldier, Vol. 1, Adjustment during army life.* Princeton University Press, Princeton.

——, LUMSDAINE, A. A., LUMSDAINE, M. H., WILLIAMS, R. M., BREWSTER SMITH, M., JANIS, I. L., STAR, S. A., and COTTRELL, L. S. (1949). *The American soldier, Vol. 2, Combat and its aftermath.* Princeton University Press, Princeton.

TIMIRAS, P. S. (1972). *Developmental physiology and aging.* The Macmillan Company, New York.

VAILLANT, G. E. and McARTHUR, C. C. (1972). Natural history of male psychologic health. I. The adult life cycle from 18–50. *Seminars Psychiat.,* **4,** (4).

VERMEULEN, A., RUBENS, R., and VERDONCK, L. (1972). Testosterone secretion and metabolism in male senescence. *J. clin. Endocrinol. Metab.,* **34,** 730.

WALKER, C. R. and GUEST, R. H. (1952). *The man on the assembly line.* Harvard University Press, Cambridge, Mass.

YALOM, I. D. (1970). *The theory and practice of group psychotherapy.* Basic Books, Inc., New York.

21. THE MEASUREMENT, EVALUATION, AND IMPORTANCE OF ELECTROENCEPHALOGRAPHY AND ELECTROMYOGRAPHY IN ARDUOUS INDUSTRIAL WORK

INGEMAR PETERSÉN, PETER HERBERTS, ROLAND KADEFORS, JAN PERSSON, KERSTIN RAGNARSON, and BJÖRN TENGROTH

INTRODUCTION

In recent years, a growing tendency has been observed for research workers in a number of medical and other disciplines to leave the shelter of their laboratories in order to carry out studies in industrial medicine in the work place itself. There are examples of many different types of workplaces like this, not least in heavy industry.

Heavy industrial work exhibits a number of characteristic profiles of difficulties for the workman. It is here that one finds the monotony of the assembly line, the heavy loads, the fumes from welding, the dust, the din, the taxing working positions, heat and cold; here are the precarious positions high up on the scaffolding, on the ship's hull.

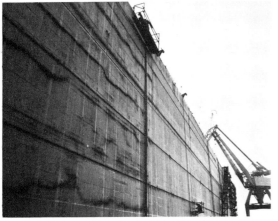

FIG. 21.1. Risky working sites in shipyard environment.

Some types of irksome working environment may be seen in Fig. 21.1, 21.2 and 21.3. The pictures are taken in one of Götaverken Ltd.'s ship-building yards in Göteborg, Sweden. Fig. 21.1 shows working positions high above the ground. Fig. 21.2 shows an extremely trying working position for a welder. Fig. 21.3 represents a general view of a workshop, with its huge dimensions, its multiplicity of factors demanding attention, its smoke-filled atmosphere. We do not hear the banging of the sledge-hammers, but this amounts to almost 140 dB. These pictures demonstrate the importance of increasing our knowledge of the functioning of the nervous system during work that makes great demands on alertness and attention, on muscular strength, on precision, and so on. It is evident that industrial labour challenges us in many ways to make the most of neurophysiological methods, for instance electromyography (EMG) for studying muscular exertion in exacting working positions, and electroencephalography (EEG) for studying the individual variations of alertness during work. Neurophysiological studies can lay bare the risk factors involved in work, thus contributing to measures for improving the working environment. The knowledge obtained, for example about working positions, may cause demands to be made for a change in the technique of working or for an alteration in the construction of the product or in the planning of the work.

There are many reasons why such working studies have been carried out to date on far too small a scale. Recording EEG and EMG signals without the use of cables which obstruct the work has posed considerable dificulties. The variability of the EEG signal and the

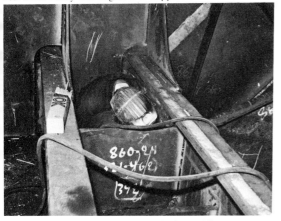

FIG. 21.2. Trying working position during welding.

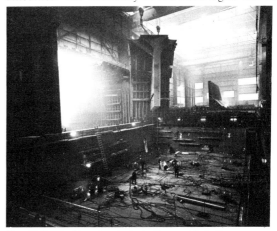

FIG. 21.3. Working sites in the hull assembly hall.

abundance of data involved have made it necessary to develop successful methods for objective automatic signal analysis. Clinical electroencephalography has also been considerably encumbered by a number of factors. Information about normal variations, even in less complex situations, has been extremely insufficient, while knowledge of the electroencephalogram's mean values and dispersion in different forms of strenuous and exacting professional work is non-existent.

As regards EEG in the laboratory, where the individual sits relaxed, with closed eyes, we in Göteborg have been systematically collecting information for more than a decade, from persons who fulfil strict criteria of health, exposure to injury, etc., and from others who deviate more or less from these criteria. The material is arranged for statistical analysis of problems concerning the effect of drowsiness and sleep and of certain provocative measures such as hyperventilation and inter-mittent photic stimulation. Special attention has been paid to age and sex. These EEG data, recorded on tape, provide valuable comparative material for use in the evaluation of EEG working recordings (see Selldén 1964; Petersén and Eeg-Olofsson 1971; Eeg-Olofsson 1971; Matousek and Petersén 1973; Persson 1972).

On the technical side, development in recent years has made it possible to record biosignals of quality, even in very demanding environments, where it is a question of disturbances of various kinds. Thereby new possibilities have been created for electrophysiological studies in industrial environments (Stalberg and Kaiser 1972; Petersén et al. 1976). The means of using electro-physiological methods in heavy industrial work have also been greatly improved through the development of methods for objective analysis of biosignals (Larsen et al. 1973; Viglione and Martin 1973).

What, then, can we expect from EMG and EEG in arduous industrial work? The question is easier to answer in the case of EMG. This method has been used particularly in kinesiological studies of bodily move-ments and movements of the extremities (Lundervold 1951; Carlsöö 1961). With the development of objective methods for analysing the myoelectric signal with its modifications in sustained muscular contraction (Kaiser and Petersén 1963; Kadeforts et al. 1968; Lindström 1970), new paths have been opened for the description and evaluation of muscular exertions in industrial work (Petersén and Magnusson 1971; Magnusson and Petersén 1971; Broman et al. 1973; Petersén et al. 1976).

The question of using EEG as a method for describing and evaluating arduous industrial work is much more complicated. Preparatory investigations are required to ascertain the appearance of the electroencephalogram when the subject has his eyes open, and how it varies with alertness, breathing, sound and light stimulation, and so on. It is also necessary to acquire further knowledge about variations in the electroencephalo-gram according to daily rhythm, before we can esti-mate its value as an instrument for recommendations as to working hours, shift work, breaks, etc. When, for

good enough reasons, arduous industrial work is to be studied with modern medico-technical electrophysio-logical methods such as EMG and EEG, apart from the difficulties of method mentioned above, several other factors have to be taken into consideration. One must get a clear idea from the beginning of what is unique about any particular workplace and what is more or less of general application. Before investigating a number of different workplaces it is important to think over the possibility of preparatory model experiments for study-ing fundamental phases of the work. It is important to fit the results of one's investigations, for instance of the working position during a spell of work, into the general picture. Even if, by various methods, one discovers signs of difficulties in the working position itself, it may be that the underlying cause is to be found in the smoke from the welding, in the tempo of the work, in the noise, and so on. It is evident that a research representative using special methods can easily go astray among the multi-factorial array of causes of accident, injury, and dis-comfort in an environment of arduous industrial work.

The present project chiefly concerns the welder in ship-building work. From the beginning of the project at Götaverken a project team was set up, consisting of engineers Kadefors and Persson, a medical man, Petersén, a safety supervisor, Andreasson, and welders, Fagerbrant, Köhler, and Pettersson at Götaverken. These persons are in continuous collaboration over questions such as the planning of the research pro-gramme, choice of work places to be investigated, etc. The members of the team also draw up joint reports on the investigations carried out as well as joint proposals for improvements to the working environment. The team also makes decisions as to the co-option of new members as the project develops further, for example with new subjects of study and new workplaces.

By bringing together, in these ways, a number of areas of competence for work, planning, and decision, our team aims to acquire experience that may have validity and value, not only for its own yard but also for other ship-building yards and, preferably, for other types of industry as well.

ELECTROMYOGRAPHY—EMG

EMG: basics
The nerve connecting the spinal cord to the muscle contains a great number of motor nerve fibres. Each nerve fibre, on entering the muscle, branches into a number of fine nerve endings, each one connected through an end-plate to an individual muscle fibre. These muscle fibres, the nerve fibre, and its cell body in the spinal cord constitute a functional unit, the motor-unit (Sherrington 1925). When a depolarization wave propagates along the nerve fibre and reaches the muscle fibres belonging to the motor-unit, contractile muscle filaments associated to the muscle fibres are excited, causing the muscle fibres to twitch almost synchro-

nously. After a short period of relaxation and recovery, a new impulse arrives and a new twitch is initiated. A skeletal muscle motor-unit may fire at a maximal rate of 20–30 discharges per second.

The firing of a motor-unit can be detected by means of electrophysiological methods. The depolarization wave propagates along the muscle fibre membranes with a velocity of approximately 5 m/s. An electrode located in the vicinity of the fibre detects a portion of the voltage evoked by the transmembrane currents at depolarization. The passage of a depolarization wave is registered by the electrical measuring instrument as a pulse. The event is called an action potential. In intramuscular EMG, the terms *muscle fibre potential* and *motor-unit potential* are frequently employed. Due to the high electrical conductivity of muscle tissue, the potentials can be picked up at some distance from the fibre or even on the surface of the skin above the muscle under study. The greater the distance between the source and the electrode, the lower the signal amplitude. Only rarely are single motor-unit potentials recognizable on the skin surface.

Relations to force and fatigue
The normal muscle is electrically silent at rest. At a low level of activation, only a few pulses are seen in the EMG (see Fig. 21.4(a)). As the contraction level rises, the number of events per unit time in the EMG increases (Fig. 21.4(b)) until the whole baseline is filled and the signal assumes the character of random noise (Fig. 21.4(c)). The rectified average of the EMG—a convenient measure of signal level—has a relationship to muscle force which is sometimes almost linear (Bigland and Lippold 1954; see, however, Lindström *et al.* 1974). The rectified average (also called the 'integrated' value) of the EMG signal thus bears information on muscle contraction level.

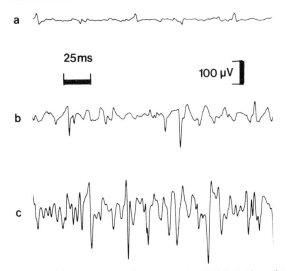

FIG. 21.4. Electromyogram from m. capri radialis in (a) low, (b) medium, and (c) strong contraction.

At sustained muscle contractions with a high voluntary effort, the EMG pattern modifies. Fig. 21.5 shows the EMG from m. brachioradialis in maximal voluntary contraction. It is seen that there is a change in the general shape of the signal as the muscle comes into a state of fatigue. After 30 s, the wave forms have slowed down (Cobb and Forbes 1923) and tend to group into bursts with a repetition rate of 8–12 Hz (Lippold *et al.* 1957).

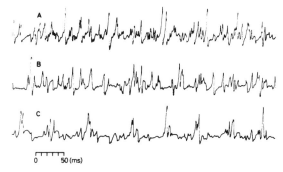

FIG. 21.5. EMG derived from m. brachioradialis in maximal contraction, (A) at the beginning of the contraction, (B) after 15 seconds, and (C) after 30 seconds. Note the variations in the pattern as the muscle is fatigued. (From Kadefors, Kaiser, and Petersén 1968).

Application of EMG in vocational studies
Monitoring of myo-electric signals provides a sensitive index of muscle tension and has been widely applied in psychological stress research, particularly in psychiatric patients (e.g., Malmo *et al.* 1951; Noble and Lader 1971). The technique has proved very sensitive in studies of muscle relaxation (de Vries and Adams 1972). Person and Kudina (1967) studied workers in manual tasks calling for high motor capability, concluding that acquisiton of skill involves relaxation of antagonist muscles.

The potential use of EMG as a quantifier of localized muscle fatigue has been observed by several authors. The augmentation in the rectified average seen has been used as a fatigue index (e.g., de Vries 1968). It was noted that this augmentation was limited to the low-frequency band (Kogi and Hakamada 1963) and that the high-frequency band showed a simultaneous decrease (Kaiser and Petersén 1963; Sato 1965). The spectral changes were given a detailed treatment (Kadefors *et al.* 1968) revealing that the phenomenon is more pronounced for intramuscular than for surface-derived signals, that it occurs in virtually all skeletal muscles and that it is succeeded by a recovery phase which for a 30-s exhaustion extends over several min.

The effect on the myo-electric signal of strenuous work has been investigated by few authors. Lundervold (1951) studied the changes in EMG patterns provoked by intense typewriting. The spectral modifications occurring in assembly-line work were studied at Volvo

(Broman *et al.* 1973), and effects of static load on muscles active in routine soldering work were investigated by Chaffin (1973), employing the power increase in the low-frequency band as a measure of 'localized muscle fatigue'.

In basic investigations on 'inexperienced' and 'experienced' welders (Petersén *et al.* 1976; Herberts *et al.* 1974) responses to standardized tasks in certain postures were recorded. It was found that welding of four consecutive electrodes caused significant shifts in the EMG spectrum from certain muscles, particularly in 'inexperienced' welders in overhead work.

What, then, is the physiological significance of the spectral EMG changes? It has been shown (Lindström 1970; Lindström *et al.* 1970) that the form of the spectrum is inherently determined by the depolarization wave source function and the geometrical lay-out of the pick-up electrodes. The action potential propagation velocity of the muscle fibres is a major parameter in the spectral modifications. A certain decrease in high-frequency content is associated with a decrease in conduction velocity which might be as high as 50 per cent. It was shown (Kadefors *et al.* 1969) that muscle ischemia plays an important role in the mechanism and in the cat that accumulation of muscle metabolites causes the propagation velocity of muscle fibres to decrease (Mortimer *et al.* 1970). The EMG changes quantified in spectrum analysis are therefore indicative of conduction velocity changes caused by insufficient clearance of muscle metabolites.

Notes on methodology

In spectrum analysis, various frequency components can be separated and displayed independently. Fig. 21.6 shows how the spectral components of the signal displayed in Fig. 21.5 are modified. The shaded area can be computed and studied as a function of time in an automatic way by means of filters, signal rectifiers, and graphic recorders.

The octave filter-bank analyser developed by Örtengren (1970) is a convenient instrument for spectrum analysis of myo-electric signals. Here, the rectified averages of the signal components within various frequency bands are displayed as a function of time. The fraction of the total signal contained within a certain band can be monitored if desired.

Fig. 21.7 shows an example of a record covering an overhead welding. For clarity, several frequency components are included. It is seen that during the course of completion of the task there is a tendency towards a decline in the high-frequency domain which is matched by a simultaneous augmentation for low fre-

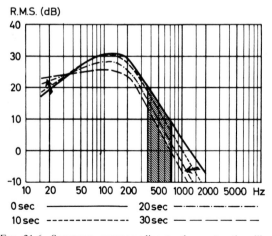

FIG. 21.6. Spectrum corresponding to the contraction illustrated in Fig. 5. The high frequencies vanish in the fatiguing state. The signal power within the 500-Hz octave band (shaded area) is computed and studied as a function of time.

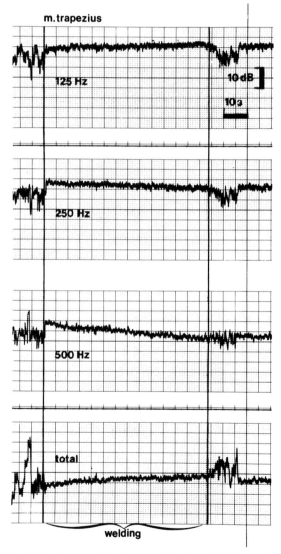

FIG. 21.7. An example of an analysis of an EMG recording obtained during work in the flat-section workshop.

148

quencies. It should be noted that the amplitude is in dB, i.e., in a logarithmic scale: a change of $+3$ dB corresponds to an amplitude factor modification of $\sqrt{2}$.

The amount of myo-electric signal activity might interfere with the spectral characteristics, causing the spectral development to be contraction-dependent. For interference pattern EMG (which is present at about 10 per cent of maximal voluntary contraction and onwards) it has been shown that the changes are small to moderate (Walton 1952); Kaiser et al. 1968). Lindström et al. (1974) have shown that the dependence for various muscles and electrodes ranges between -3.2 (biceps brachii; surface electrodes) and $+2.0$ (trapezius; needle electrode) dB/log(load) for the 500-Hz component. This means that the fraction of the total signal power contained within the 500-Hz octave band may vary 2–3 dB as the contraction level is changed by a factor 10. It is therefore unsuitable to make measurements during the course of a welding task: the melting away of the electrode and the slowly changing postures make such comparisons doubtful. A more suitable method is to compare the situation before and after completion of the task by means of standardized test loads.

An electromyographic investigation of welders in overhead work

As an example of and a model for EMG analysis applied to vocational studies, a project concerning shoulder muscle response to overhead welding work during production was carried out.

The workplace is briefly characterized as a station in the flat-section workshop between two automatic welding machines along an assembly line. The one-side welding performed in the first machine is imperfect at the back side, which is downward. Repairs in the welds are performed manually. The work pace depends on the current assembly line situation and is at times very high. Each time a new plate comes up for attachment, 10–20 min of continuous welding takes place, virtually all of it overhead; the interval between successive plates may be as short as 2–3 min. Fig. 21.8 illustrates the situation.

Method and material. Myo-electric signals were collected from m. trapezius (upper portion), m. deltoideus (ventral portion), and m. supraspinatus. The signals from the trapezius and deltoid muscles are readily detected on the skin surface by means of bipolar surface electrodes (Medelec, Ltd.) affixed with adhesive tape. The supraspinatus muscle was reached by applying fine-wire intramuscular electrodes (Basmajian and Stecko 1962). A reference electrode was placed on the skin above the spine on level Th 5. Fig. 21.9 shows the applied electrodes with wires for connection to the external equipment. Amplification and display of the signals were handled by means of an electromyograph (Medelec M6). The amplified signals were stored on magnetic tape (Honeywell 3600B; 1 7/8 in/s) for further analysis.

The subjects, six healthy welders aged 25–40, were trained and experienced on the particular workplace studied.

In order to establish an adequate basis for judging the effect of exposure to overhead work, the workmen were asked to assume a standardized posture with the upper arm in a forward horizontal and the forearm in a vertical position, for 10 s before and after a sequence of weldings. The recordings made during the standardized postures were compared in the analysis. In order to establish a standard for the reproducibility of the myo-electric signal levels obtained in different runs with standardized postures, a sequence of about 20 postures

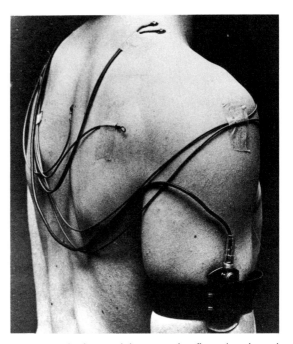

FIG. 21.9. Surface and intramuscular fine wire electrodes applied.

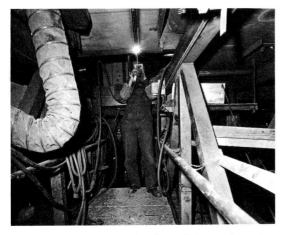

FIG. 21.8. Photograph showing the workplace under study.

was studied. Fig. 21.10 shows part of the graphic recording obtained in the analysis. The study concentrated on the 500-Hz component (S_{500}). It is seen that the reproducibility is good; a statistical analysis showed that readings obtained in different runs had a standard deviation of 0·50 dB.

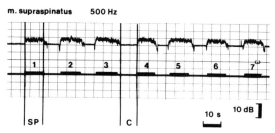

m. supraspinatus   500 Hz

10 s   10 dB

SP   C

FIG. 21.10. Recording of the 500-Hz component during a sequence of standardized postures (SP) as defined in the text (elevated arm, no load applied). C: calibration.

Results. In the present investigation, recordings were made in actual production work. This means that the number of welds in a sequence was subject to large variations. It is therefore inadequate (and certainly it was never the intention) to use the data in a comparison of the characteristics of the individual workers. The set-up and the number of measurement channels varied somewhat during the course of the experiments, partly due to occasional disturbances from neighbouring equipment and interference with adjacent production activities.

The results of comparative measurements taken in the standardized posture situations are summarized in Table 21.1. Here, a small number of readings have been omitted following application of the EMG level constancy criterion. The numbers in Table 21.1 indicate the modifications encountered in the S_{500} recording. Negative values pertain to a decrease in activity concomitant with lowered muscle fibre propagation velocity. As indicated above, standard deviations in the single S_{500} readings amounted to $\sigma = 0·50$ dB. The figures in Table 21.2 represent differences between two such readings; two standard deviations will consequently correspond to $2\sigma\sqrt{2} \approx 1·4$ dB. It will be seen from the table that for the deltoid muscle this level was exceeded in only one case, whereas the corresponding numbers for m. supraspinatus and m. trapezius are two and four, respectively.

The occasional variability of neighbouring readings is a striking feature of Table 21.2. This is by no means surprising in view of the large variations encountered in the actual production situations; sometimes the recorded sequence is preceded, for example, by intense overhead work with pneumatic hammers or blasting equipment, or at times by a few minutes of rest and relaxation. Table 21.1 therefore only indicates whether or not spectral modifications do occur, their order of magnitude and muscle preference. In order to cover the important aspect of the cumulative effect of exposure to overhead work, a separate analysis was carried out. Here, the first and last standardized posture runs were compared for each subject. Table 21.2 shows the results.

TABLE 21.1

Spectral modification in the 500-Hz filter band (dB).
Overhead welding, flat-section workshop.

Subject	Number of welds in a sequence	Muscle		
		Deltoideus	Trapezius	Supraspinatus
1	6			−0·3
	4	−0·8	−2·7	−2·3
	7	−0·8		−0·7
2	9	−1·2		
3	9	+1·0	−1·5	−2·2
4	7	−0·5	−2·8	−0·2
	5	−2·5	−3·0	
5	4	−0·8	−0·5	0·0
6	3	−0·5	−0·8	
	7	−0·5	−0·2	−1·0

It is obvious that for the deltoid muscle, no systematic cumulative effect is present irrespective of the exposure to overhead work. In the trapezius and supraspinatus cases, however, virtually all numbers are negative. There is a trend showing a more pronounced effect at higher levels of exposure. Fig. 21.11 visualizes this property of the data in the two muscles concerned.

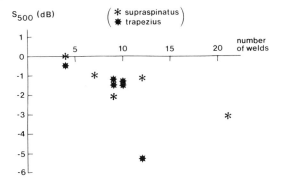

FIG. 21.11. Total spectral modification in the 500-Hz band as a function of the number of completed welds. Six subjects were studied.

Conclusions. The present investigation has shown that spectral variations indicative of localized muscle fatigue (Chaffin 1973) are indeed found in experienced welders in overhead production work. The effect is present and significant in m. supraspinatus and m. trapezius but generally not in m. deltoideus. There is a strong tendency in the data towards accumulation of the effect over prolonged sequences of overhead work. The breaks of a few seconds between successive welds must certainly be deemed insufficient for recovery, and not even the minute or two allotted between plates can be deemed satisfactory in this respect.

The results are in agreement with previous investigations in a model set-up for the study of myo-electric

TABLE 21.2

Accumulated effect in $S_{500}(dB)$ over the time of observation for the various subjects. Number of welds in brackets ( ).

Subject	Muscle		
	Deltoideus	Trapezius	Supraspinatus
1	0·0 (15)	−1·3 (10)	−3·2 (21)
2	+0·2 (13)	−1·2 (9)	—
3	+1·0 (9)	−1·5 (9)	−2·2 (9)
4	−1·2 (12)	−5·3 (12)	−1·2 (12)
5	+1·2 (4)	−0·5 (4)	± 0·0 (4)
6	−1·2 (10)	−1·4 (10)	−1·0 (7)

signals in welding work (Petersén *et al.* 1974; Herberts *et al.* 1974). Here, overhead studies were carried out on a number of muscles, including m. biceps brachii, m. trapezius (middle portion), m. rhomboideus, and the muscles investigated here. It was found for inexperienced welders that only the latter muscles displayed significant changes in the EMG. In a group of experienced welders (such as those employed in the present study), only m. trapezius (upper portion) and m. supraspinatus showed a significant effect.

It is of note that elderly welders frequently complained to us about chronic shoulder pains. A special investigation, focused on the diagnosis and aetiology of such pains in welders aged 50–65, is being carried out.

It can be concluded that the rationale for applying EMG in studies of welders is as follows:

(a) Welding work is essentially static, with a slow, superimposed movement due to the gradual melting away of the welding electrode. It is reasonable that this type of working activity causes localized muscle fatigue, as evidenced in the spectral changes.

(b) Many welders have complaints about shoulder muscle fatigue. It is observed that chronic shoulder pains are common in elderly welders.

(c) Welding is a vocational activity which calls for high physical fitness, strength, skill, and a high degree of motor co-ordination. Muscle fatigue interferes with the ability to pursue a weld all the way (which takes approximately 2 min) and there is no doubt that fatigue sensations constitute an important stressor in this type of welding. EMG spectrum analysis provides an objective measure of the local physiological response to sustained muscular work, clearly of interest in evaluation of work places in terms of stress.

ELECTROENCEPHALOGRAPHY

Introduction

When one considers many of the risk factors to be found in arduous industrial work, it is easy to realize how important is the degree of alertness and attention in the workman for the avoidance of accident and injury. In this connection, it should be of interest as a matter of principle to be able to characterize individual variations in alertness. We all know, among our acquaintances, of individuals to whom it would never occur to take a little rest, even if the opportunity arose, while others we know take a nap now and then even when there is no real opportunity. There seems to be a pattern of alertness reactions that is not necessarily coupled to efficiency. In arduous industrial work, the same individual variations in alertness must reasonably occur within there necessarily being a work plan which allows for them. The possibility of elucidating the very high frequency of accidents—in certain sections more than 140 accidents, with consequent absence from work, per million working-hours—is naturally of the greatest interest. Problems to attack that seem particularly apparent are shift work, breaks, and the length of the working day.

It is well known that the electroencephalogram varies with the degree of alertness. It is thus reasonable to adopt this method when studying variations in alertness during work. Studies of EEG in industrial work, however, involve a number of problems. Our knowledge of EEG recorded in individuals with open eyes is inadequate. This is already true of recordings made in the laboratory, but the individual variations of the electroencephalogram with closed and open eyes in different types of work, for instance in arduous industrial work, are completely unknown to us.

Arduous industrial work of various kinds obviously involves a number of stress factors—noise, light stimuli, etc. It is thus of great interest to see what the literature has to offer on the subject of the effects of stress on the electroencephalogram. Unfortunately it does not include much about the EEG reactions of individuals in industrial work.

Reports on EEG responses to stress are fairly few. In spite of this, the range with regard to aim, study situations, and results is considerable. Electroencephalographic studies of pilot stresses in flight showed substantial, partly paroxysmal EEG changes (Sem-Jakobsen 1959, 1971). Of particular interest is the statement that certain effects related to the G-force during flight could not be reproduced in simulators on the ground; the feeling that a situation involves a real or a simulated risk is thus a matter of importance for the effect on the EEG and other things.

Adey et al. (1963) and Schoenbrun and Adey (1967) reported on EEG in simulated stresses of space flight with special reference to problems of vibration. In subcortical and in cortical structures of macaques they found driving of brain rhythm due to shaking, the driving being maximal in the frequence range 9–15 Hz. This rhythmic driving was abolished by phenobarbital anaesthesia.

These studies provide examples of important EEG responses to considerable strains on the individual. Other studies give accounts of discrete EEG changes with less dramatic strains on the individual. With such physical and mental loads on experimental persons Kamp et al. (1970) found only slight shifts of the peak in the alpha frequency band. Storm van Leeuwen et al. (1967) described how the connection between certain so-called specific subcortical and cortical activities in dogs were changed with stress, and how different types of stress could affect these connections in different ways. General stress, active or passive, was accompanied by a decrease in the amplitude of all specific activities. Partial stress was accompanied by coincidence of activities that usually alternated. EEG changes of an entirely different type from those described above have been associated with 'severe metabolic and other stress' (Roth et al. 1967). The authors refer to high-voltage, bilaterally

synchronous, slow activity during hyperventilation, hypoglycaemia, in acute anoxia, in association with liver disease, increased intracranial pressure, centrencephalic epilepsy, and during the course of electroconvulsive treatment.

A connection between a slow posterior rhythm (Pitot and Gastaut 1956; Nayrac and Beaussart 1956; Aird and Gastaut 1959; Petersén and Sörbye 1962) and stress factors has been discussed. Selldén et al. (1965) found this activity after heart surgery in children who had not shown it pre-operatively, whereas it did not appear following minor surgery. Petersén et al. (1965) found an increased occurrence of such rhythms in patients with severe burns. The rhythm was found in all of seven patients demonstrating syndromes of myoclonic epilepsy (Petersén and Hambert 1966; Hambert and Petersén 1970). The possibility of a connection between the appearance of the slow posterior rhythm in these materials and a common stress factor was pointed out by the authors mentioned.

As far as can be judged from the literature, knowledge of electroencephalographic changes on account of stress is not of any great value for the application of the electroencephalographic method in arduous industrial work, though this does tend to have an abundance of stresses. Consequently, in our EEG studies in industrial environments we have had to start from scratch in several respects not least as regards the development of methods.

This part of the chapter reports a pilot investigation, aiming at a description of dissimilarities in neurophysiological signals during different circumstances such as rest in laboratory environment and rest and work situations in the shipyard during exposure to mild and trying environment respectively. It is hoped that it will be possible to discriminate among mental states corresponding to different environmental loads by means of a study of a number of neurophysiological signals.

Glare recovery or readaptation time (RAT) has been found to depend upon factors such as the subject's age and the oxygen concentration in the breathing air as well as physical fatigue. Preliminary investigations have indicated a relation between RAT and welding. RAT was adopted in our study to further investigate changes in the subject's mental condition. The evaluation will proceed as the relations mentioned are further elucidated.

Material and measurements
Each of five welders were studied for two days. The measurements from the first day were taken as a habituation procedure and were not used in the subsequent analysis. However, the measurements were distributed over the day and carried out in exactly the same way during the two days. The investigation was accomplished during three situations, viz., rest with eyes closed, rest with eyes open, and welding. Three different environmental conditions were covered, viz., quiet

laboratory (QL), quiet shipyard (QS), and shipyard during full work (FS). The QL recording was made in the morning before the start of work, the QS recording during a lunch pause (after the meal), and the FS recording at about 1.15 p.m., when the subject had worked hard for about one hour and a half. The number of individuals with records of sufficient quality for more than 36 s is shown for each occasion in Table 21.3. The reduced number of satisfactory recordings during welding is due to one subject using alternating current welding, which caused too much electrical interference, and two subjects with a large amount of muscle artefacts.

TABLE 21.3

Number of individuals with recordings of sufficient quality for analysis for different situations during different environmental conditions

| Situation | Environmental condition (Class in the pattern recognition procedure) | | |
	Quiet laboratory QL	Quiet shipyard QS	Full work shipyard FS
Rest, eyes closed	5	5	5
Rest, eyes open	5	5	5
Welding	—	3	2

After the morning and afternoon recordings, RAT was measured.

Methods

Recording of electroencephalogram, eye movements, electrocardiogram, and respiration was carried out by means of a portable, light-weight radio-telemetry system (Persson *et al.* 1973). The receiver and a display system, making the signals move over a TV screen, is shown in Fig. 21.12. The system, which has a range of about 100 m and transmits up to 8 channels, does not restrain the worker in his task (Fig. 21.13). The stress imposed by the measurement procedure is minimal. Four bipolar EEG derivations, placed according to the international ten–twenty system (Jasper 1958), were used, viz., Fp1-F7, F7-T3, P3-01, and T5-01. Horizontal and vertical eye movements were recorded. The respiration was picked up by a probe, using a number of thermocouples in series, exposed to the air flow in the nose. This component may cause the worker only slight discomfort. The recordings were stored on magnetic tape for subsequent analysis.

In order to investigate whether the welding gave rise to any electrical activity which might interfere with the bioelectric activity in the frequency range of interest (0–30 Hz), one pair of electrodes was replaced by a resis-

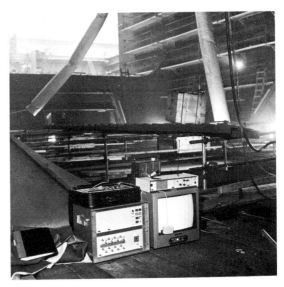

FIG. 21.12. Telemetry receiver, tape recorder, display unit, and TV monitor (Kaiser Laboratories, Copenhagen).

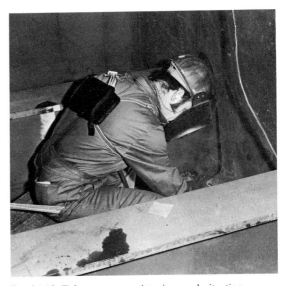

FIG. 21.13. Telemetry transmitter in a work situation.

tor of a magnitude approximating twice the electrode resistance (4·7 kΩ). The resistor was attached to the forehead, about 0·2 m from the welding place. The electrical interference was found to be negligible except during starting up and interruption of the welding, when spike-like artefacts appeared.

The signal analyses were performed on a PDP-15 computer. Before digitization, each channel was bandpass-filtered to the range 0·1–40 Hz by means of filters of a high-frequency roll-off of 12 dB/octave. The signals were digitized at a rate of 256 Hz/channel in an analog-to-digital converter of 12 bits resolution.

153

Although changes in a number of signal properties, e.g., spectral measures, were to be studied in relation to a change in environmental conditions, the main objective was to investigate whether the complete picture of a large number of signal parameters could be used to discriminate between registrations obtained during the different environmental conditions. This was accomplished by means of a pattern recognition technique, using linear discriminant analysis (Larsen *et al.* 1973; Nilsson 1965).

The pattern recognition process comprises two stages (Fig. 21.14): (1) feature extraction, i.e., estimations of a number of signal properties, constituting a *pattern*, by means of digital signal analyses; (2) pattern classification, i.e., the pattern is determined to belong to one of a number of classes (here: QL, QS, and FS).

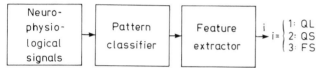

FIG. 21.14. The pattern recognition process. QL: Quiet laboratory environment; QS: quiet shipyard environment; FS: full-work shipyard environment.

The pattern recognition procedure comprises two main phases. The first is a *training phase*, aiming at the determination of discriminant functions on the basis of a number of patterns of known class belonging. The second is a *test phase*, where unknown patterns are classified by means of the discriminant functions, found in the training phase.

Here, the main objective is a discussion of the feature extraction of neurophysiological signals and the training of a pattern classifier, intended to discriminate the classes QL, QS, and FS. This classifier has been used to test patterns collected from three subjects.

Since muscle artefacts were often present in the frontal EEG derivations, the feature extraction comprised the EEG derivations P3-01 and T5-01, the EGG, and the respiration. Epochs of length 12 s of the EEG signals were investigated concerning power spectrum and amplitude probability density function. A total of 22 parameters, including pulse and respiration rate, were obtained. These parameters constituted patterns for the subsequent pattern classification.

From the power spectra of the EEG signals, a number of spectral parameters were derived as described in Appendix I. Parameters, related to the amplitude distribution function of the EEG, were estimated according to Appendix II. The parameters used in the pattern recognition are shown in Table 21.4.

The parameters, derived in the feature extraction stage (Table 21.4), were used to determine discriminant functions as described above. One pattern recognition was performed in each of the three situations: rest with eyes closed, rest with eyes open, and welding. A stepwise multiple discriminant analysis was applied (Dixon 1971,

TABLE 21.4

Parameters used in the pattern classification

No.			No.				No.	
1	P3-01	δ	11		T5-01,	δ	21	pulse rate
2		θ	12			θ	22	resp. rate
3		α_1	13			α_1		
4		α_2	14			α_2		
5		β_1	15			β_1		
6		β_2	16			β_2		
7		Z_{med}	17			Z_{med}		
8		N_{rej}	18			N_{rej}		
9		G_1	19			G_1		
10		G_2	20			G_2		

programme BMD07M). Under the assumption that the parameters have normal joint distribution functions, the programme selects in each step that parameter which gives the greatest improvement in the classification. The procedure is interrupted either after a specified number of steps or when the improvement in the classification, due to the inclusion of a new parameter, is below a specified level. When the procedure is interrupted after d steps, each pattern (i.e., the set of parameters for a certain case) corresponds to a point in a d-dimensional pattern space. Each class (see also Table 21.3) is represented by a decision region in the pattern space. The position of a test pattern determines its class membership. In order to illustrate the separation between classes, the first two canonical variables are plotted, thus giving an optimal two-dimensional representation of the dispersion.

The measurements of RAT were performed by means of a study of opto-kinetic nystagmus. The dark-adapted eye was exposed to moving vertical strips of black and white colour with a subdued background light. Immediately after the exposure to a flash, the direction of the fence was changed. From the blocking of the opto-kinetic nystagmus, seen in a recording of horizontal eye movements, the recovery time was obtained (method described by Blomberg 1959, modified by Högman *et al.* 1972).

Results

Acceptable recordings, including at least three 12-s epochs afflicted with a negligible amount of artefacts, were derived according to Table 21.3. Only the parieto-occipital and temporal-occipital leads were used in the analyses, because of the abundance of muscle artefacts in the frontal leads, especially during work. An example of a telemetric recording during welding is shown in Fig. 21.15. Here, the horizontal eye movement channel is afflicted with muscle artefacts. Otherwise, the signals are of satisfactory quality.

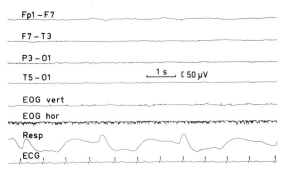

Fp1 – F7
F7 – T3
P3 – O1
T5 – O1   1 s   [50 µV
EOG vert
EOG hor
Resp
ECG

FIG. 21.15. Registration during welding.

Spectral dissimilarities between the situations rest with eyes closed, rest with eyes open, and welding in the EEG lead P3-01 are illustrated by Fig. 21.16. With eyes closed, an accentuated spectral peak, corresponding to the 'alpha rhythm', appears at about 9 Hz. With eyes open and during welding the alpha peak has decreased or vanished. Instead, a large amount of activity appears in the β, δ, and θ bands. The differences of the individual parameters studied (Table 21.4) between the environmental conditions OL, QS, and FS were very small for all of the situations investigated (Table 21.3). Discriminant analyses were performed for each of the situations rest with eyes closed, rest with eyes open, and welding. The ten parameters, yielding the maximum separation between the classes QL, QS, and FS, are shown in Table 21.5.

The performance of the classification was examined for five and ten parameters. Based on normality assumptions, equality between the classes was tested at the 5 per cent level of significance (F-statistic). The result is shown in Table 21.6. With five parameters, significant differences between the classes QL and FS were not obtained for rest with eyes closed and rest with eyes

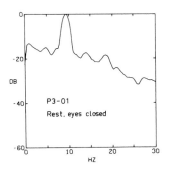

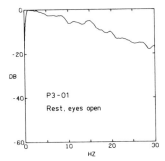

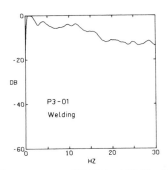

FIG. 21.16. Power spectra of EEG lead P3-01, all recorded in quiet shipyard environment. (Subject RQ).

TABLE 21.5

The ten 'best' parameters, in order giving the greatest improvement to the separation between classes in a pattern classification

	Rest, eyes closed	Rest, eyes open	Welding
1	P3-01, β_2	P3-01, β_2	T5-01, G_1
2	Resp. rate	Pulse rate	P3-01, δ
3	T5-01, α_1	T5-01, θ	P3-01, β_2
4	P3-01, N_{rej}	Resp. rate	Resp. rate
5	T5-01, G_1	T5-01, δ	Pulse rate
6	P3-01, θ	P3-01, G_1	T5-01, α_2
7	T5-01, β_2	P3-01, G_2	T5-01, α_1
8	T5-01, G_2^2	P3-01, β_1	T5-01, Z_{med}
9	P3-01, α_2	P3-01, Z_{med}	T5-01, G_2
10	T5-01, α_2	T5-01, G_1	P3-01, α_1

TABLE 21.6

Pairs of classes, showing a significant difference at the 5 per cent
level of significance. QL: quiet laboratory; QS: quiet shipyard;
PS: full-work shipyard

No. of parameters	Rest, eyes closed	Rest, eyes open	Welding
5	QL–QS QS–FS	QL–QS QS–FS	QS–FS
10	QL–QS QL–FS QS–FS	QL–QS QL–FS QS–FS	QS–FS

open. Otherwise, significant differences between pairs of groups were obtained in all cases.

Transformations from the five- and ten-dimensional pattern spaces to two-dimensional ones with a preservation of optimal dispersion between classes (Dixon 1971) were accomplished by means of the first and second canonical variables. The transformed patterns are shown in Figs. 21.17–21.19. The improvement in classification by increasing the number of parameters is evident.

The classifier derived on the basis of ten parameters was used to test records from three subjects. The registrations in quiet and in full-work shipyard were followed by recordings in the laboratory. Laboratory recordings in the morning and afternoon were mainly classified as QL recordings, whereas recordings at noon were grouped into QS. This might indicate a circadian factor in the patterns studied. The results also indicate that possible circadian effects are overshadowed by environmental effects in FS recordings. Registrations in quiet shipyard were mainly grouped in the class QS as regards the states rest with closed and open eyes respectively as well as welding. Registrations in full-work shipyard were mainly classified to QS, a result which seems incorrect. This may be due to inefficiency of the classifier. However, it might be caused by registrations of less environmental exposure than the reference

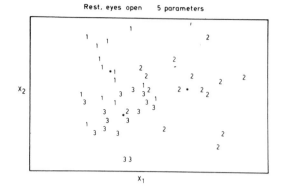

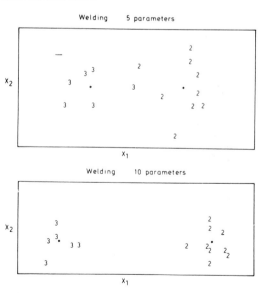

FIG. 21.18. Optimal representation in two dimensions of the dispersion between classes. Rest, eyes open. X^1: first canonical variable. X^2: second canonical variable. 1:QL, 2:QS, 3:FS. * indicates class mean.

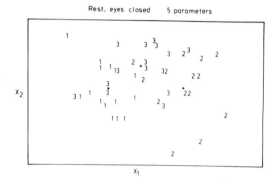

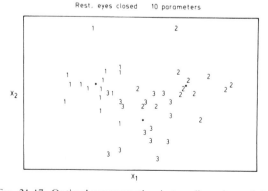

FIG. 21.17. Optimal representation in two dimensions of the dispersion between classes. Rest, eyes closed. X^1: first canonical variable. X^2: second canonical variable. 1:QL, 2:QS, 3:FS. * indicates class mean.

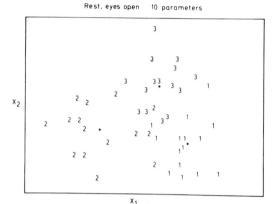

FIG. 21.19. Optimal representation in two dimensions of the dispersion between classes. Welding. X^1: first canonical variable. X^2: second canonical variable. 2:QS, 3:FS. * indicates class mean.

group FS. The test phase reported was applied to a small sample. However, the results are promising and further investigations will be carried out.

RAT is subject to an increase from the morning to the afternoon measurements for all subjects (Table 21.17). Each figure for recovery time is the result of three measurements.

Discussion

The pilot investigation described, which comprises five subjects, has shown that it is possible to derive high quality recordings of EEG, ECG, eye movements, and respiration even during such work situations as welding, where electromagnetic fields could be expected to give severe interference with the bioelectric phenomena studied. The main problem turned out to be artefacts in the EEG from other bioelectric signals, such as muscle and eye movement artefacts. Even if some of the subjects showed artefact-free recordings from all over the scalp, the investigation had to be restricted to the EEG derivations P3-01 and T5-01 in order to permit a pattern classification comprising the whole sample.

A comparison of a number of signal parameters between the environmental conditions QL (quiet laboratory), QS (quiet shipyard), and FS (full-work shipyard) yielded very small differences. By using ten parameters in a pattern classification by means of discriminant analysis, it was possible to represent the classes QL, QS, and FS by decision regions, which were significantly discriminated. It should, however, be noted that the conclusion of significant separation is based upon normal assumptions, which might be violated. Accordingly, the picture of the possibility of classifying unknown patterns may be over-optimistic. The ultimate determination of the efficiency of the classifier is provided by an investigation of the error rate during classifications of further patterns. This testing will use the discriminant functions, which are based on the material presented here. Such a test phase was tried successfully on a sample of registrations from three subjects.

RAT has been shown to increase from the morning to the afternoon recording. It is not yet clear which component in the environment causes this increase.

However, preliminary investigations indicate an influence of welding as well as physical fatigue. Where this influence is a reaction to the eventual toxicity of the fumes or an anoxia is not clear. This point will be further examined.

Discussion

When pursuing an investigation in industrial medicine, or industrial psychology, or some other type of study of men at work, it is relevant to define or characterize both the men and the work. Age, sex, personality, experience, development, health, previous illness, social conditions, type of work, special strains and stresses involved in the work—these are only a few of the many factors that are important. Not least where the strains and stresses of work are concerned, of course, the workman's own appreciation is of fundamental importance. For this purpose we have, as mentioned earlier, a consultative group consisting of workmen, safety supervisor, technicians, and medical men. Members of this group had a conversation with the six welders whom we studied by means of electromyography with regard to the working position at a particular work station.

During this conversation, the following opinions about the work place were put forward, some of them being more, and others less, characteristic of this particular workplace.

Too short meal breaks. You have to gulp down your food and go back to work immediately. No time to give your stomach a rest. The worst time of the day is two hours after a meal.
Uneven distribution of work. Sometimes there is no work. Then all of a sudden you're up to the neck in it. Slow working pace for a couple of days. Then everything has to be ready very quickly. You are more done up than usual after these changes of tempo.
Welding fumes. You feel more tired after a day's work with a lot of fumes than after a day with not much fumes from the welding.
Working clothes. It is important to have clothes that protect you against the welding sparks. The pain from the burns takes it out of you.
Noise is troublesome, wherever you find it.
Psychological factors. The whole job becomes worse if things get into a jam in some way, for instance if your tackle disappears, if you cut yourself on something, if you get angry, if

TABLE 21.7

Recovery time after glare (s)

		1	2	Subject no. 3	4	5	Grand mean
Morning	m	3·40	6·03	5·53	6·66	4·06	5·13
	s	0·34	0·11	0·20	0·80	0·51	
Afternoon	m	4·56	7·40	10·40	9·83	6·75	7·78
	s	0·63	0·36	1·90	1·10	0·07	
Difference		1·16	1·37	4·87	3·17	2·69	2·65

there's a row with the foreman. You feel bad-tempered and dog-tired when you get home in the evening those days when everything goes wrong.

Working position. It is particularly risky to stand at the edge of the position, where you have to lean backwards all the time. It's hard work keeping your arms up in the air all the time you're working. The design of the workplace makes no allowances for workmen of different heights.

It is clear that the results of the electromyographic study of working positions have to be fitted into a complicated picture of the whole to make any effective contribution to the improvement of the work place. The same reasoning, of course, applies to the results of the electroencephalographic studies. The electromyographic investigations of experienced and inexperienced welders showed that the former's technique of working involved another type of less tiring muscular strain than the latter's. This possibility had been foreseen when planning the investigation. We therefore filmed a number of phases in the various working sequences— low vertical welding, high vertical welding, and overhead welding. It is our hope that, by combining electromyographic and filmed studies, we may bring about an improvement in the learning of welding techniques.

Our object is to study a number of workplaces in the ship-building industry by our methods, in the first instance with reference to the welders. These studies will conclude with reports containing recommendations for measures aimed at the improvement of the working environment. The results of any measures towards such improvement will thereafter be judged by the workmen concerned. If necessary, check measurements will be undertaken at the same time. A report has been given above of the results obtained by a model study in the flat-plate workshop at the first of the workplaces in question.

After that we propose to enlarge out experience of workplaces in other industries. It is, of course, important to pay particular attention to and form a judgement of the transition from research work to routine investigation in our project. It is necessary for the firm's doctor to take part in forming this judgement. If a practicable routine for judging working positions in different work stations and measures regarding them can be worked out in accordance with what has been said here, the authorities concerned must make up their minds on the question whether, if necessary, an ergonomic service organization for workplace classification should be set up, for example, within the framework of industrial medicine.

In accordance with the earlier results of our group's work, quoted above, we have taken particular note of changes in the spectrum of effects in different frequency areas at certain phases of the work and in certain workplaces. Naturally, there are other approaches possible for EMG studies in arduous industrial work, for instance, those which aim at acquiring knowledge of muscle tension due to stress factors of various kinds or to an accumulation of these in the working environment.

In the electroencephalographic investigation presented, no attempts have been made to differentiate between the effects of the many strains. The working situation has been regarded as a totality to which the individual reacts. Nor are the individual patterns of perception and reaction, due to e.g., personality, motivation, aspiration, and experience, included in the report. The interaction of one strain with others, be they sequential or simultaneous, is another aspect which has not yet been surveyed. The effects may in some cases be additive, in others counteracting, and they may depend on the context of the strain, or of the individual.

A successive adaptation to the environment and to the working group may cause a successive diminution in the physiological and psychological response patterns (Frankenhaeuser *et al.* 1962; Frankenhaeuser *et al.* 1967; Monat *et al.* 1972). Relatively small changes can be expected in the reaction patterns between temporally close registrations of the type obtained in the present study.

Adaptation means an adjustment to the environment, resulting in a diminution of the immediate level of strain. In fact, an experienced welder in the experiment stated that he could even occasionally fall asleep during long, monotonous welding work in spite of the complex and offensive environment. Nevertheless, changes in the EEG-pattern have been found to persist after predominantly mental activity (Sickel 1962; Rogge 1972) but also subsequent to predominantly physical activity (Sickel 1962). These findings indicate that complex sustained strains, to which experienced welders are exposed, may evoke changes in the EEG which remain or accumulate even during short rests, in spite of subjective adaptation to the environment.

The capacity to adapt also has implications for security and precision aspects of the work. An increased degree of stress elicits higher amounts of rigidity in behaviour in, e.g., problem-solving (Cowen 1952). A situation perceived as risky tends to cause a 'narrowing of attention' (Baddeley 1972). Other factors may influence the behaviour in the same negative direction.

Since only experienced workers are included in the present investigation, some effects in the physiological response-patterns may be concealed. A comparison between experienced and inexperienced workers and a longitudinal investigation of new welders are planned to shed light on these effects. A completion of the investigation with regard to personality ratings, an examination of the influence of motivation, aspiration, experience, and other psychosocial variables, and a mapping of the mutual strain level of different environmental variables on the individual have been started.

APPENDIX I. SPECTRAL ESTIMATION

The power spectra were calculated from epochs of 4 s by means of the fast Fourier transform. Before Fourier transformation, the signal sequence was modified by a parabolic data window, thus reducing interference between disparate frequency bands (Persson 1972). The average spectrum from three non-overlapping segments of length 4 s was smoothed by means of a weighting sequence of triangular shape with nine weights. The resulting spectral window had a half-power bandwidth of about 1·25 Hz. In the case of a Gaussian signal, the normalized standard error s.d.$[\hat{P}]/E[\hat{P}]$ for the spectral estimator $\hat{P}$ is about 0·196 (see Persson 1974a). The corresponding equivalent number of degrees of freedom (Blackman and Tukey 1958) is 52.

From the power spectrum, the power in six frequency bands of conventional notations were calculated (Table 21.8). The power parameters yield the power in the different frequency bands related to the total power in these bands.

TABLE 21.8

Frequency ranges for EEG power parameters

δ	1·0– 3·5 Hz
θ	3·5– 7·5 Hz
α_1	7·5– 9·5 Hz
α_2	9·5–12·5 Hz
β_1	12·5–17·5 Hz
β_2	17·5–25·0 Hz

APPENDIX II. ESTIMATION OF PROPERTIES OF THE AMPLITUDE PROBABILITY DENSITY

Tests of normality of the EEG sequences were accomplished by means of the Kolmogorov–Smirnov test for samples of unknown mean and variance (Lillie fors 1967). For the validity of the test, it is important that it is applied to a sequence of independent sample points, obtained from a stationary signal. In order to achieve a sufficiently low dependence between adjacent samples (Persson 1974b), the sampling frequency was set to 8 Hz. The 12-s epoch was divided in 2-s segments and a test carried out on the sample of size $N = 16$, constituting one segment. It should be noted that the low sample size yields tests of very low power.

In the Kolmogorov–Smirnov test one investigates the variable

$$Z = \sqrt{N} \max_{-\infty < x < \infty} |F_N(x) - F(x)|,$$

where $F_N(x)$ is the sample distribution function and $F(x)$ is the normal distribution function of mean and variance equal to the sample mean and sample variance. If the value of Z exceeds a critical value, the hypothesis that the sample has a normal distribution function is rejected. In the present analyses, the tests were performed at the 10 per cent level of significance. The average Z_{med} of the

test variables and the number of rejections N_{rej} of the hypothesis of normal distribution were calculated for each epoch of length 12 s. In addition to the test of normality, two measures of the shape of the amplitude distribution function were estimated, viz., the skewness and the excess (Cramér 1961).

Let μ_v denote the central moment of order v of the variable ξ of mean m and variance σ^2, i.e.

$$\mu_v = E((\xi - m)^v).$$

Then the coefficient of skewness is defined as

$$\gamma_1 = \frac{\mu_3}{\sigma^3}$$

and the coefficient of excess as

$$\gamma_2 = \frac{\mu_4}{\sigma^4} - 3.$$

Now consider a sample $(x_1, x_2 \ldots, x_N)$, i.e. a sequence of mutually independent variables x_i of mean $\bar{x}$. Then, the central moment of order v of the sample is

$$m_v = \frac{1}{N} \sum_{i=1}^{N} (x_i - \bar{x})^v.$$

From the sample the coefficients of skewness and excess may be estimated by

$$g_1 = \frac{m_3}{m_2^{3/2}}$$

and

$$g_2 = \frac{m_4}{m_2^2} - 3.$$

Since these estimators are biased, analogous quantities were used in the present analysis. Thus, the skewness was estimated by means of the variable

$$G_1 = \frac{\{N(N - 1)\}^{\frac{1}{2}}}{N - 2} g_1$$

and the excess by means of

$$G_2 = \frac{(N - 1)}{(N - 2)(N - 3)} ((N + 1)g_2 + 6).$$

For a sample from a normal distribution it holds that (Cramér 1961, p. 386)

$$E[G_1] = 0,$$
$$E[G_2] = 0,$$

$$\text{Var}[G_1] = \frac{6N(N - 1)}{(N - 2)(N + 1)(N + 3)},$$

and

$$\text{Var}[G_2] = \frac{24N(N - 1)^2}{(N - 3)(N - 2)(N + 3)(N + 5)},$$

With a sequence of length 12 s, a sample size of $N = 96$ was obtained and accordingly s.d.$[G_1] \approx 0.25$ and s.d.$[G_2] \approx 0.49$.

159

SUMMARY

In recent years, electroencephalography (EEG) and electromyography (EMG) have received growing interest in non-clinical applications such as the evaluation of the impact of industrial environment on the physiology of the working man. In the present project, part of a large-scale undertaking to improve environmental conditions at Götaverken shipyard, EEG analysis was applied to achieve discrimination between patterns of neurophysiological parameters recorded under different environmental conditions. Analysis of EMG likewise proved useful in a model investigation to objectify muscle fatigue in arduous overhead welding work.

REFERENCES

ADEY, W. R., WINTERS, W. D., KADO, R. T., and DELUCCHI, M. R. (1963). EEG in simulated stresses of space flight with special reference to problems of vibration. *Electroenceph. clin. Neurophysiol.*, **15**, 305–20.

AIRD, R. B. and GASTAUT, Y. (1959). Occipital and posterior electroencephalographic rhythms. *Electroenceph. clin. Neurophysiol.*, **11**, 637–56.

BADDELEY, A. D. (1972). Selective attention and performance in dangerous environments. *Brit. J. Psychol.*, **63**, 537–46.

BASMAJIAN, J. V. and STECKO, G. A. (1962). A new bipolar indwelling electrode for electromyography. *J. appl. Physiol.*, **17**, 849.

BIGLAND, B. and LIPPOLD, O. C. J. (1954). The relation between force, velocity and integrated electrical activity in human muscles. *J. Physiol.*, **123**, 214–24.

BLACKMAN, R. B., and TUKEY, J. W. (1958). *The measurement of power spectra.* Dover Publications, New York.

BLOMBERG, L.-H. (1959). A simple objective method for determination of the glare effect. *Experentia*, **15**, 358.

BROMAN, H., MAGNUSSON, R., PETERSÉN, I., and ÖRTENGREN, R. (1973). Vocational electromyography: methodology of muscle fatigue studies. In *Developments in electromyography and clinical neurophysiology* (ed. J. E. Desmedt), pp. 656–64. Karger, Basel.

CARLSÖÖ, S. (1961). The static muscle load in different work positions: an electromyographic study. *Ergonomics*, **4**, 193–211.

CHAFFIN, D. B. (1973). Localized muscle fatigue—definition and measurement. *J. occup. Med.*, **15**, 346–54.

COBB, H. and FORBES, A. (1923). Electromyographic studies of muscular fatigue in man. *Amer. J. Physiol.*, **65**, 234–51.

COWEN, E. L. (1952). The influence of varying degrees of psychological stress on problem-solving rigidity. *J. abnorm. soc. Psychol.*, **47**, 512–19.

CRAMER, H. (1961). *Mathematical methods of statistics.* Princeton University Press, Princeton.

DE VRIES, H. A. (1968). 'Efficiency of electrical activity' as a physiological measure of the functional state of muscle tissue. *Amer. J. phys. Med.*, **47**, 10–22.

—— and ADAMS, G. M. (1972). Electromyographic comparison of single doses of exercise and meprobamate as to effects on muscular relaxation. *Amer. J. phys. Med.*, **51**, 130–41.

DIXON, W. J. (1971). *Biomedical computer programs*, pp. 214a–214t. University of California Press, Los Angeles.

EEG–OLOFSSON, O. (1971). The development of the electroencephalogram in normal adolescents from the age of 16 through 21 years. *Neuropädiatrie*, **3**, 11–45.

FRANKENHAEUSER, M., STERKEY, K., and JAERPE, G. (1962). Psycho-physiological reactions in habituation to gravitational stress. *Percept. Motor Skills*, **15**, 63–72.

——, FRÖBERG, J., HAGDAL, R., RISSLER, A., BJÖRKVALL, C., and WOLFF, B. (1967). Physiological, behavioral and subjective indices of habituation to psychological stress. *Physiol. Behav.*, **2**, 229–37.

HAMBERT, O. and PETERSÉN, I. (1970). Clinical, electroencephalographical and neuropharmacological studies in syndromes of progressive myoclonus epilepsy. *Acta Neurol. Scand.*, **46**, 149–86.

HERBERTS, P., KADEFORS, R., and PETERSÉN, I. (1974). Electromyographic study of shoulder muscles in welding. *Acta Orthop. Scand.*

HÖGMAN, B., TENGROTH, B., and ÖRNBERG, G. (1972). Metod och teknik för studier av bländning med hjälp av optokinetisk nystagmus (OKN). *FOA 2 rapport C2517—E1 E3 E4 H5.* Stockholm.

JASPER, H. H. (1958). The ten twenty electrode system of the International Federation. *Electroenceph. clin. Neurophysiol.*, **10**, 371–5.

KADEFORS, R., KAISER, E., and PETERSÉN, I. (1968). Dynamic spectrum analysis of myo-potentials with special reference to muscle fatigue. *Electromyography*, **8**, 39–74.

——, MAGNUSSON, R., NILSSON, N. J., and PETERSÉN, I. (1969). Effects of ischemia on the myoelectric signal spectrum. *Acta Physiol. Scand.*, *Suppl.* **330**, 110.

KAISER, E. and PETERSÉN, O. (1963). Frequency analysis of muscle action potentials during tetanic contraction. *Electromyography*, **3**, 5–17.

——, KADEFORS, R., MAGNUSSON, R., and PETERSÉN, I. (1968). Myoelectric signals for prosthesis control. *Myo-electric control of prostheses*, pp. 14–44. Medicinsk Teknik-Medico Teknik, Stockholm.

KAMP, A., TROOST, J., and VAN RIJN, A. J. (1970). Influence of mental and physical stress on the alpha rhythm in normal subjects and patients. *TNO-niews* Medisch–Fysisch Instituut TNO, Utrecht, the Netherlands, **25**, 368–70.

KOGI, K. and HAKAMADA, T. (1963). Slowing of surface electromyogram and muscle strength in muscle fatigue. *Rep. Inst. Sci. Lab.*, **60**, 27–41.

LARSEN, L. E., RUSPINI, E. H., McNEW, J. J., WALTER, D. O., and ADEY, W. R. (1973). Classification and discrimination of the EEG during sleep. In *Automation of clinical electroencephalography* (ed. P. Kellaway and I. Petersén), pp. 243–68. Raven Press, New York.

LILLIEFORS, H. W. (1967). On the Kolmogorov–Smirnov test for normality with mean and variance unknown. *J.A.S.A.*, **62**, 699–402.

LINDSTRÖM, L. (1970). On the frequency spectrum of EMG signals. *Report 7:70*, Research Laboratory of Medical Electronics. Chalmers, University of Technology, Göteborg.

——, MAGNUSSON, R., and PETERSÉN, I. (1970). Muscular fatigue and action potential conduction velocity changes studied with frequency analysis of EMG signals. *Electromyography*, **10**, 341–56.

—, —, and —— (1974). Muscle load influence on myoelectric signal characteristics. *Scand. J. rehab. Med.*, **3**, 127–48.

LIPPOLD, O. C. J., REDFEARN, J. W. T., and VUĈO, J. (1957). The rhythmical activity of groups of motor units in the voluntary contraction of muscle. *J. Physiol. (Lond.)*, **137**, 473–87.

LUNDERVOLD, A. J. S. (1951). *Electromyographic investigations of position and manner of working in typewriting*. A. W. Broggers Bogtrykkeri A/S, Oslo.

MAGNUSSON, R. and PETERSÉN, I. (1971). Vocational electromyography. In *Proc. 2nd Nordic Meeting on Medical and Biological Engineering* (ed. O. Lorentsen), pp. 174–6. Norwegian Society for Medical and Biological Engineering, Oslo.

MALMO, R. B., SHAGASS, C., and DAVIS, J. F. (1951). Electromyographic studies of muscular tension in psychiatric patients under stress. *J. clin. exp. Psychopath.*, **12**, 45–66.

MATOUSEK, M., and PETERSÉN, I. (1973). Frequency analysis of the EEG in normal children and adolescents. In *Automation of clinical electroencephalography* (ed. P. Kellaway, and I. Petersén). Raven Press, New York.

MONAT, A., AVERILL, J. R., and LAZARUS, R. S. (1972). Anticipatory stress and coping reactions under various conditions of uncertainty. *J. Personality soc. Psychol.*, **24**, 237–53.

MORTIMER, J. T., MAGNUSSON, R., and PETERSÉN, I. (1970). Conduction velocity in ischemic muscle: effect on EMG frequency spectrum. *Amer. J. Physiol.*, **219**, 1324–9.

NAYRAC, P. and BEAUSSART, M. (1956). A propos des rythmes à 4 c/s postérieurs chez les anciens traumatisés craniens. *Rev. Neurol.*, **94**, 849.

NILSSON, N. J. (1965). *Learning machines*. McGraw-Hill, New York.

NOBLE, P. J. and LADER, M. H. (1971). An electromyographic study of depressed patients. *J. psychosom. Res.*, **15**, 233–9.

ORTENGREN, R. (1970). A measurement system with simultaneous read-out for spectrum analysis of myoelectric signals. *Proc. 1st Nord. Meeting on Med. and Biol. Engineering*, pp. 139–41. Otaniemi, Finland.

PERSON, R. S. and KUDINA, L. P. (1967). Application of cross-correlation analysis of interferential EMG's for the study of time relations of motoneuron discharges in man. *Digest of International Meeting on Electromyography*, p. 37. University of Glasgow, Glasgow.

PERSSON, J. (1972). A computerized spectral analysis of electroencephalograms from normal children during the first year of life. *Technical report No. 20*. School of electrical engineering, Chalmers University of Technology, Göteborg.

—— (1974a). Variability and covariability of modified spectral estimators. *IEE Trans. Acoustics, Speech Signal Processing*, **ASSP-22**, 158–60.

—— (1974b). Comments on estimations and tests of EEG amplitude distributions. *Electroencep. clin. Neurophysiol.*, **37**, 309–13.

—, KADEFORS, R., and PETERSÉN, I. (1973). Telemetry of physiological signals during heavy industrial work. *Digest 10th ICMBE*, p. 235. Dresden.

PETERSÉN, I. and EEG–OLOFSSON, O. (1971). The development of the electroencephalogram in normal children from the age of 1 through 15 years. *Neuropädiatrie*, **3**, 247–304.

—— and HAMBERT, O. (1966). Clinical and electroencephalographic studies of responses to Lidocaine and Chlormethiabole in progressive myoclonus epilepsy. *Acta Psychiat. Scand.*, **42**, (Suppl. 192) 45–64.

—, KADEFORS, R., and PERSSON, J. (1976). Neurophysiologic studies of welders in shipbuilding work. *Environ. Res.*, **11**, 226–36.

—— and MAGNUSSON, R. (1971). Vocational electromyography. Methodology of muscle fatigue studies. In *Digest 9th ICMBE*, p. 163. Melbourne.

—— and MATOUSEK, M. (1972). EEG-Breitband-frequenzanalyse bei normalen Kindern und Jugendlichen. *EEG-EMG*, **3**, 134–8.

—— and SÖRBYE, R. (1962). Slow posterior rhythm in adults. *Electroenceph. clin. Neurophysiol.*, **14**, 161–70.

—, —, JOHANSSON, B., AVELLAN, E., and GELIN, L.-E. (1965). An electroencephalographic and psychiatric study of burn cases. *Acta Clin. Scand.*, **129**, 359–66.

PITOT, M. and GASTAUT, Y. (1965). Aspects E.E. Graphiques inhabituels des séquelles des traumatismes craniens: II. Les rythmes postérieurs à 4 cycles-second. *Rev. Neurol.*, **94**, 189–91.

ROGGE, K.-E. (1972). EEG-Veränderungen nach verzögerten akustischen Rückmeldung der Lautsprache. *Z. exp. Angew. Psychol.*, **19**, 641–70.

ROTH, M. OSSELTON, J. W., and GIVENS, J. G. (1967). Some common features of the EEG changes associated with severe metabolic and other stress and their bearing on the problem of homeostasis. In *Recent advances in clinical neurophysiology* (ed. L. Widén). *Electroenceph. clin. Neurophysiol., Suppl.* **25**, 276–81.

SATO, M. (1965). Some problems in the quantitative evaluation of muscle fatigue. *J. anthropol. Soc. Nippon*, **73**, 20–7.

SCHOENBRUN, R. L. and ADEY, W. R. (1967). Space-flight-related stresses on the central nervous system. *Radiat. Res. Suppl.*, **7**, 423–38.

SELLDÉN, U. (1964). Electroencephalographic activation with *Megimide* in normal subjects. *Acta Neurol. Scand.*, **40**, Suppl. 12.

—, OLANDERS, S., and CARLGREN, L.-E. (1965). EEG examination at heart operation on children with congenital heart disease. *Commun. 6th Internat. Congr. Electroenceph. Clin. Neurophysiol.*, pp. 149–58. Vienna.

SEM-JACOBSEN, C. W. (1959). Electroencephalographic study of pilot stresses in flight. *Aerospace Med.*, **30**, 797–801.

—— (1971). Physiological aspects of aircraft accident investigation. *Aerospace Med.*, **42**, 199–204.

SHERRINGTON, C. S. (1925). Remarks on some aspects of reflex inhibition. *Proc. roy. Soc. (Lond.) Ser. B*, **97**, 519.

SICKEL, W. (1962). Über das menschliche Electroenzephalogram nach mehrstündiger psychischer Aktivität. *Arch. gesamte Psychol.*, **114**, 1–54.

STORM VAN LEEUWEN, W., KAMP, A., KOK, M. L., DE QUARTEL, F., and TIELEN, A. (1967). EEG of unrestrained animals under stressful conditions. In 'Recent advances in clinical neurophysiology' (ed. L. Widén). *Electroenceph. clin. Neurophysiol., Suppl.* **25**, 212–25.

STALBERG, E. and KAISER, E. (1972). Long term EEG-telemetry. In *Biotelemetry* (ed. H. P. Kimmich and J. A. Vos). Meander, N.W., Leiden.

VIGLIONE, S. S. and MARTIN, W. B. (1973). Automatic analysis of the EEG for sleep staging. In *Automation of clinical electroencephalography* (ed. P. Kellaway and I. Petersén), pp. 269–85. Raven Press, New York.

WALTON, J. N. (1952). The electromyogram in myopathy: Analysis with the audio-frequency spectrometer. *J. Neurol. Neurosurg. Psychiat.*, **15**, 219–26.

22. PSYCHOLOGICAL STRESS AND COPING IN PSYCHOSOMATIC ILLNESS

R. S. LAZARUS

INTRODUCTION

To many, stress involves any strain on, or deformation of, psychological processes and tissue systems resulting from difficult-to-handle environmental demands. When viewed in psychological terms, stress also includes certain emotions that we can call 'stress emotions' such as anxiety, fear, anger, grief, guilt, shame, etc. We assume that these play an essential role in the production of psychosomatic illness. This is so because one of the hallmarks of stress emotion is the body's mobilization to cope with a situation of actual or potential psychological or physical harm. Although this mobilization can be seen as an adaptive evolutionary mechanism facilitating species survival, under conditions creating massive and continuous or frequent bodily disturbances, the adaptive mechanism also results in disease. There are those who consider all disease as having psychosomatic components in that the tissue systems are functioning less effectively or in a less integrated fashion because of stress than ought to be the case.

If the above reasoning is accepted, then anything we can learn about the psychological processes concerned with emotion will contribute to an understanding of psychosomatic illiness, and indeed, is a necessary prelude to such understanding. Although we know much about what happens to the tissues when a person or animal is aroused or undergoing a stress emotion, the details of the psychological determinants of emotion and its regulation, and hence their ultimate role in bodily disease, have remained somewhat elusive. Psychosomatic medicine as a research discipline must go beyond the physiological processes conducive to disease and try to understand:

(1) The psychological processes which make a person's encounters with the environment stressful;
(2) The self-regulation processes brought to bear in the management of stress;
(3) Each step in the subsequent sequences leading to those bodily states that Levi and Kagan (1971) have called 'precursors to disease';
(4) Ultimately disease itself.

COGNITIVE APPRAISAL

How is a stress emotion brought about? From my theoretical perspective (Lazarus *et al.* 1970; Lazarus 1966; Lazarus 1975) emotion arises from certain kinds of adaptive *commerce* a person has with his environment. This implies that emotions represent a two-way interaction involving on the one hand needs and motives and other psychological properties of persons, and environmental settings that provide opportunities for gratification as well as potentials for frustration and harm on the other. Furthermore, the presence, intensity, and quality of the emotional reaction and the nature of coping activities reflect the way this adaptive commerce is evaluated by the person. The main categories of evaluation producing emotions are as follows:

(1) Threat;
(2) Challenge;
(3) Positive well-being.

In addition, negatively-toned emotions also depend on judgements by the person about whether and how the commerce can be coped with and mastered.

Thus, the psychological processes of perception and judgement are crucial for emotion, and therefore ultimately play a role in psychosomatic disorders. The concept of *cognitive appraisal*, expresses such judgement or evaluation of one's ongoing adaptive commerce. Emotions flow from the appraisal which, in turn, is determined by the continuous and constantly changing interplay between person and environment.

A definition of emotion

From this cognitive–phenomenological perspective I define emotion as a complex disturbance resulting from adaptive commerce between the person and the environment, a disturbance which includes three loosely interrelated components, namely, subjective affect, physiological changes related to species-specific forms of mobilization for action, and the action impulses (having both instrumental and expressive qualities) generated by the appraisal. This action impulse varies from one emotion to another and helps define the specific emotional process. For example, in anger, the action impulse is attack while in fear it is escape or avoidance. We must speak of impulse here because the action may be inhibited by internal and social or physical constraints. The somatic disturbance arises from this action impulse which, in part, reflects the mobilization for action. In short, the quality and intensity of the emotion and its action impulse all depend on the cognitive appraisal of the person or animal's well-being. In lower animals, for example those studied by Tinbergen (1951), the evaluative feature of the perception that elicits the emotion is evidently built into the species nervous system; in higher mammals such as man, symbolic thought processes and learning play a predominant role.

Notice that this way of looking at things is an attempt to specify the psychological processes at work when a person somehow perceives or senses danger, or harm to himself, or whatever. In his monograph, *The problem of anxiety*, when Freud (1936) spoke of anxiety as arising from the perception of danger, he was pointing toward such cognitive processes in emotion, though he never really addressed the principles by which such perception, or I would prefer to say appraisal to emphasize the evaluation, operates. To determine such principles requires that ultimately we can say what it is about a given sort of person, having a particular pattern of commerce with a specific environment, that leads to a specific emotional reaction pattern. If we are truly to understand psychosomatic diseases, each facet and stage of the emotional process from its initiation to its self-regulation (e.g., coping) and its somatic effects must be understood.

GENERALITY AND SPECIFICITY IN PSYCHOSOMATIC DISORDER

Probably no man in recent decades has more influenced theory and research on psychosomatic or stress disorders than Hans Selye (1956). Selye based his research on the once revolutionary theme that physiological stress reactions to noxious agents or stressors were not tied to the type of noxious agent or stressor, but rather occurred as a universal, organized defence against any type of assault on the tissues. He called this syndrome of defence the *general adaptation syndrome* (GAS), and attempted to demonstrate that it proceeded in a series of stages: If the noxious condition and the bodily defences mobilized against it persisted beyong the initial stage of *alarm* into the second stage of *resistance*, various forms of tissue damage would occur. Selye referred to this damage as the 'diseases of adaptation'. The continuing process of resistance would lead to depletion of bodily defences and ultimately to the stage of *exhaustion* and death. When the GAS functions efficiently, the defensive reaction is commensurate with the seriousness of the environmental assault. Occasionally, however, the reaction is out of proportion to the potential harm of the noxious agent, as in the case of allergy, and the defence itself is then more of a danger than the very assault it was designed to overcome. And in what I consider a somewhat fanciful notion, Selye also argued that ageing represents the gradual wearing out of the adaptational resources of the system from use over its lifetime.

Selye brought a sense of integration into the arena of physiological stress and disease, and he connected psychology with the problem of stress disorders by maintaining the generalist position that any noxious agent could mobilize the GAS, even purely psycho-

logical demands and threats. His emphasis was thus on the universality of the defensive reaction in the animal world and on its generality across all noxious stimuli; in other words, it did not matter what noxious stimulus started the process since it would run off in essentially the same way, involve essentially the same hormones, and produce the same tissue reactions regardless of the type of assault. A similar generality theme is found in Levi's (1965) research using catecholamine excretions (adrenal medullary hormones). Levi showed that subjects would secrete adrenalin and noradrenalin not only in response to threatening movies (such as *The devil's mask*, *An occurrence at Owl Creek bridge*, and *Paths of glory*) but also a comical film (*Charley's aunt*). In commenting on this Levi states, 'There seems to be a positive correlation between the intensity of emotional arousal, whatever its quality, and the urinary excretion of adrenalin and possibly of noradrenalin. Such a statement highlights the influence of Selye, although in Levi's research the focus is on secretions of the adrenal medulla, while Selye's focus was on pituitary-adrenal cortical hormones. Still, the general outlook is the same, that the hormonal reaction does not depend on the particular nature of the stressful or arousing stimulus.

There is an opposing position which centres on the other end of the polarity between generality and specificity and which argues that different stressors, or the adaptive processes that are generated, produce divergent patterns of response. The specificity of stress reactions has been emphasized by this writer (1966) and by Mason (1971). This position contains two interrelated themes. First, it is argued that the bodily response is frequently different depending on the type of assault. Mason (1963; p. 328) puts it as follows:

Along with psychological stimuli such as conditioned avoidance and adaptation to the restraining chair, physical stimuli such as cold and hemorrhage also do indeed appear to elicit an elevation in 17-OHCS levels. On the other hand, exercise appears to produce little or at least questionable changes, fasting even less change, and heat actually elicits suppression of 17-OHCS levels.

The findings cited by Mason (which Mason regards as somewhat tentative) suggest that Selye may have over-stated the generality of the stress response in asserting that all noxious environmental conditions will produce the same general adaptation syndrome.

The second theme is that the GAS may depend on psychological rather than physiologically noxious stimuli. Since it is extremely difficult in the laboratory to isolate noxious stimuli, such as exercise, fasting, heat, and cold, from the psychological states that might go along with them (e.g., cognitive appraisals), virtually all of the research on the GAS has managed to confound the physiologically noxious with psychological variables. Selye has paid attention only to the bodily defensive process *after* they have been aroused neuro-humorally, and not to the physiological and psychological signalling system that 'recognizes' the noxious effects or potential and distinguishes it from benign events. In an earlier work (Lazarus 1966; p. 398), for example, I made the comment that:

It is altogether possible that the extensive findings of stress biochemists that physiologically noxious agents produce changes in the homonal secretion of the adrenal cortex are the result of their psychological impact.

And Mason (1971; pp. 328–9) has put the matter thus:

. . . While much more new research is needed before we know the full extent to which psychological factors have entered into 'physical stress' research, even those findings on fasting, heat, and perhaps exercise are sufficient to cast serious doubt at present upon the concept of physiological 'non-specificity', which is the very foundation upon which much of stress theory rests. . . .
    What I am suggesting, in the other words, is that the 'primary mediator' underlying the pituitary-adrenal cortical response to the diverse 'stressors' of earlier 'stress' research may simply be the psychological apparatus involved in emotional or arousal reactions to threatening or unpleasant factors in the life situation as a whole. The 'primary mediator' may simply be a common body mechanism brought into operation by an experimental variable which was essentially overlooked or underestimated in 'stress research,' namely, the great sensitivity of the endocrine systems to psychological influences which have contaminated many experiments of 'physical stressors'. Perhaps one of the principal points of historical importance concerning 'stress' theory will eventually prove to be in the early calling attention to the sensitivity and ubiquity of psychoendocrine mechanisms.

There is some limited but provocative empirical evidence consistent with the above assertion that the essential mediator of the GAS could be psychological, and not merely *any* assault on the tissues of the body. Symington *et al.* (1955) suggest, for example, that an animal that is unconscious can sustain bodily harm without the endocrine mechanisms of the GAS becoming active. They observed that patients who were dying from injury or disease, and who remained unconscious (comatose) during this terminal condition, showed a normal adrenal cortical condition as assessed by autopsy. However, patients who were conscious during the fatal disease process did show adrenal cortical changes. And as a partial control, Gray *et al.* (1956) provide evidence that anaesthesia by itself does not produce a significant adrenal reaction. Such studies support the possibility that it is the *psychological significance of the injury* rather than the tissue injury itself that produces the adrenal cortical changes associated with the GAS.
    Another version of the specificity position, centred however on autonomic nervous system reactions, is the research by Lacey (1967) on beat-to-beat heart rate changes under divergent stimulating conditions. The basic point is simple. The heart rate response is bidirectional, rising when a person is oriented to shut out or ignore environmental input, but dropping when one is expecting or looking for a stimulus whose time of appearance can be anticipated. Such a decrease in heart rate occurs even when the anticipated stimulus is threatening, as in the case of an electric shock (e.g. Folkins 1970). This psychologically-based bi-directionality is not seen in other autonomic nervous system and organ reactions such as the electrodermal response which rises and falls solely in relation to level of activation. The implications are clear. Autonomic nervous system activity does not operate solely as a unified expression of general activation or arousal under conditions of stress or relaxation, but rather, the end organ reactions of autonomic activity pattern themselves in accordance with the nature of the demands or the psychological process taking place. Although there may be some degree of generality as expressed in the concept of activation or arousal, there is also considerable specificity, with the bodily response also differing sharply depending on the type of psychological activity generated under different kinds of environmental load.
    Recent research on biofeedback in the regulation of somatic states further reinforces the view that there can be a surprising degree of specificity even among autonomic nervous system effects that are normally somewhat interdependent. Shapiro *et al.* (1970) have shown in operant conditioning biofeedback experiments, for example, that subjects rewarded only for increases or decreases in systolic blood pressure were able to raise or lower their blood pressure while their actual heart rates (a related cardio-vascular function) remained unchanged. Moreover, when the procedure was reversed so that only changes in heart rate were reinforced, heart rates were raised or lowered while systolic blood pressure remained essentially unchanged. On the other hand, Schwartz (1974) reports that it is easier for subjects to learn to make their systolic blood pressure and heart rate go up together than to make them go in different directions, a finding which supports a somewhat weak generality position. In any event, these and other studies suggest that there is a considerable degree of specificity in the self-regulation of these response systems, though the limits and consequences of such specificity have not yet been determined.
    In one sense, the debate about generality or specificity is unproductive, since it is reasonable to expect both principles to have some validity. Somewhat different adaptive processes must be called into play to manage diverse demands, and yet at the same time, the person also operates as an integrated psychobiological system. Separate organ systems are somehow pulled together in the service of the major adaptive requirements of living rather than separately going their own way. Classically too, many writers have emphasized health as integration of systems and pathology as lack of integration. Yet the debate is instructive in another sense because it has important implications for the way the psychobiological mechanisms underlying adaptation and psychosomatic illness can be viewed and studied. These implications can be made clear by asking two questions:

(1) 'Given something like a general adaptation syndrome, how might the various psychosomatic or stress disorders come about in different individuals or under different conditions?'
(2) 'How might various psychosomatic or stress disorders be understood given a degree of specificity in the stress reaction pattern?'

Stress disorder from the standpoint of generality

Since, the source of stress is given little or no importance, and the reaction pattern is always a uniform sequence of bodily defences, that is, a syndrome which unfolds epigenetically depending mainly on the severity and duration of the environmental demands, differences in the type of disorder (e.g. migraine, gastro-intestinal ulceration of mucous colitis, hypertension, etc.) are presumed to depend on particular vulnerabilities of the organ system of the individual rather than on the kind of stressful commerce with the environment. Genetic-constitutional factors evidently create variations among individuals in the vulnerability of organ-systems. When the individual is exposed to any severe or chronic stress, ailments will develop which reflect the impact of the GAS on such vulnerable organ systems. The resulting disorder should have little to do with the psychodynamics of stress itself, though certain factors such as individual differences in the severity of stress, its chronicity, and the stage of the GAS, could lead to different somatic outcomes.

Of the current research on stress disorders that appears to adopt the generality position, the work by Holmes and Rahe and studies growing out of it seem to be the most influential example. These researchers developed a measure of life changes and scaled it so that changes, both positive and negative, having the greatest impact (such as death of a spouse) were given high value while those involving small impact were given low value. Although there are many methodological problems connected with this research (Sarason 1978), somatic and psychological illness were found to be associated with a high life-change score for the period previous to the illness. This tends to support the idea that stress of any kind leads to an increased risk of illness in general. Little effort has been made as yet to link the type of stress, the type of emotional response, or the form or effectiveness of coping with the stress, to the type of illness. Dohrenwend (1973) has recently obtained some evidence that it doesn't matter whether the stresses are viewed as desirable or undesirable (distressing) by the persons involved, the magnitude of life changes being the critical determinant. Nevertheless, the possible role of the type of life change and of the effectiveness of coping remains at issue. In any event, the life-change approach implicity adopts a generalist position to stress and disease.

Stress disorders from the standpoint of specificity

Here the options are considerably more varied, as I see it, since the nature and severity of the stress disorder could depend on at least three factors:

(1) The formal characteristics of the environmental demands;
(2) The quality of stress—emotional response generated by the demands, or in particular individuals, facing these demands;
(3) On the processes of coping mobilized by the stressful commerce.

With respect to the first option, some time ago Mahl (1949, 1952, 1953) demonstrated that hydrochloric acid secretion in the stomach was minimal or absent in acute stress but marked in chronic stress. This is evidence that formal characteristics of stress are relevant to the physiological reaction and presumably, therefore to the type of stress disorder produced.

The second option deals with the fact that stress emotions vary in quality depending on the situation as well as on personality characteristics. Thus, given some heavy environmental demand or set of demands, some individuals will experience mainly a sense of helplessness, anxiety, and depression, while others might react with anger or some other emotional state. Although there is at best only weak evidence that the adrenal medullary and autonomic patterns vary with the quality of the emotion experienced, it is highly improbable that the overall pattern of somatic reaction would fail to reflect such very different emotional states as anger, fear, depression, and so on, especially when one takes the position, as I have, that diverse emotions are associated with different action impulses. From the perspective of specificity, we must concern ourselves with the various types of environmental social demands generating the stress emotion in the first place, as well as the personality characteristics of the person which lead to divergent appraisals of stressful encounters that are conducive to different emotions.

With respect to the third option, coping processes are integrally linked to the emotional and somatic outcome of a stressful transaction. Thus if a person successfully denies that he is in some kind of danger, or engages in other ways of neutralizing the stressful demands, he shows a lessening or absence of the expected stress emotion and the somatic disturbances related to it. I shall have more to say about coping in the subsequent section.

It seems unnecessary to adopt an either/or position with respect to the generality–specificity question at this stage of our knowledge. They are not mutually exclusive, and it seems wise to entertain the idea of some degree of generality and specificity in the sequence starting with disturbed commerce with the environment and eventuating in somatic illness. However, given the psychological approach to stress emotions with which I began this paper, I find the specificity arguments richer in the range of potential factors that might account for variations in the degree and type of somatic illness in different individuals and under different environmental conditions. Personality factors can enter into the equation at a number of places as the person addresses the demands and opportunities afforded by his environment, for example, in the appraisal of threat and challenge, and in the choice of coping processes whereby any stressful commerce is managed.

It must be said also that there has been little interest on the part of psychophysiologists in studying the activities of the various systems of neural and humoral regulation simultaneously in stress situations and in attempting to integrate them. Thus, autonomic reactions are almost never studied in association with even the adrenal medulla secretions which are closely linked with them physiologically, nor are adrenal medulla and autonomic reactions studied in association with the pituitary-adrenocortical axis. An exception is some research by Frankenhaeuser (1971). Mason (1970) especially appears to be deeply impressed with the complexity of hormonal mechanisms in stress and the interdependence of various levels of response, including the physiological and psychological. Limited understanding of the complex pattern of hormonal responses seem to encourage oversimplication of psychobiological mechanisms.

SELF-REGULATION IN THE STRESS EMOTIONS

As I have already noted, a key theme in my approach to the stress emotions is self-regulation (Lazarus 1975). The stress emotions, and emotion in general, are short-lived, ebbing, flowing, and changing over time as the commerce between the person and the environment changes. Such changes, especially the lowering or raising of intensity, as well as the quality of the emotional reaction, depend on changes in cognitive appraisal as the person obtains feedback from his own reactions and from cues in the environment, or as that person engages in intrapsychic forms of coping (usually called defences). In coping the person often redefines (reappraises) his relationship with the environment, constantly striving to master the situation by overcoming the damage, postponing or preventing the danger, or by tolerating it.

In the psychosomatic arena one of the most frequently cited examples is research studying the reactions of parents who experienced the tragedy of a child dying of leukaemia (cf. Wolff et al. 1964) in an NIMH research hospital in Bethesda, Maryland. Parents who were 'well-defended', that is, who coped by seeming successfully to deny the seriousness of their child's illness, showed far less 17-hydroxicorticosteroid secretion than those who faced the fatality of their child's illness without the protection of such defences. Related observations have also been made by Grinker and Spiegel (1945) with combat air crews, by Hamburg et al. (1953) and more recently Adreason et al. (1972) with patients with severe burns, by Visotsky et al. (1961) with paralytic polio victims, by Price et al. (1957) with surgical patients, and

by Weisman (1972) with terminally ill cancer victims. My own laboratory research (see Lazarus et al. 1970 for a review) has made it clear that encouraging denial or detachment coping strategies in subjects who watch disturbing motion picture films is capable of substantially lowering stress levels, presumably by leading to alterations in cognitive appraisals of the stressful events which 'short-circuited' the film-induced threats.

Much coping activity is also anticipatory—the person anticipates a future harmful confrontation, such as failing in an examination, performing in public, or whatever—and this leads to preparations, often successful, against the future possibility of harm. Such anticipatory coping is a form of regulation of the stress emotion that would otherwise be experienced. Although anticipatory coping itself may involve considerable mobilization and hence stress, it need not (cf. Monat et al. 1972), and one must weigh the cost of such preparation against the lowered stress level sustained in the actual confrontation when it occurs. Recently (Lazarus 1974) I have distinguished between two types of such self-regulation, one which might properly be called direct actions, the other involving cognitive or intrapsychic attempts to *control the emotion* itself or its somatic correlates. In direct action, the person tries to alter or master the troubled commerce with the environment, as, for example, when the person attempts to demolish, avoid, or flee the harmful agency, to prepare somehow to meet the danger. Thus, if a student faced with an important and potentially threatening examination spends the anticipatory interval reading relevant books and articles, rehearses understanding of the subject with others, tries to find out or guess what questions will be asked, etc., that student is engaged in direct action forms of coping, whether these are effective or ineffective. To the extent these are successful, the potential stress has been mastered before it is faced. To the extent to which such activity leads to a more benign appraisal of the potential outcome, say by giving him a sense of mastery and preparedness, and regardless of whether this benign appraisal is realistic or defensive, the stress reaction involved in the troubled or threatened commerce with the environment is mitigated by the preparatory action prior to the ultimate confrontation. On the other hand, *cognitive coping* takes place when action is either too costly or when the person is helpless to do anything about the troubled commerce. Such modes of self-regulation include taking tranquillizers, antispasmodics, alcohol, sleeping pills, or engaging in a variety of other techniques, such as muscle relaxation, transcendental meditation, biofeedback therapy, yoga, and hypnosis. These are palliative because they are focused on reducing the visceral or motor disturbances which are distressing the person rather than changing the environmental transaction itself. In helping the person regulate the emotional accompaniments of stress which interfere with adaptive functioning or are embarrassing, the prospects for effective coping with the basic problem can also sometimes be improved. For example, by owering the level of anxiety, the person may be able to think better, rest better, and to confront situations he would ordinarily avoid.

Self-regulatory processes, both anticipatory and during a stressful transaction itself, are normal features of stressful commerce, a continuous part of life itself: As such they are key intervening processes in the causation and prevention of psychosomatic disorders. In all likelihood, some of these will be effective under certain conditions, while others are not. The problem is to understand the ways the diverse forms of self-regulation work, and to be able to specify the antecedent conditions determining their use.

Unfortunately, the psychology of self-regulation and coping in general is not very far advanced. We are limited mainly to description rather than prediction. A wide variety of self-regulatory devices are employed by all of us throughout our lives, depending on personal characteristics, environmental demands and contingencies, and the way our commerce with the environment is appraised. However, we know little about the conditions under which any given mode of self-regulation will be successful in lowering stress levels or preventing somatic illness, or the relative costs of such processes, despite increasing research on the problem. Some recent research has employed dispositional measures of coping exclusively (e.g. Andrew 1970), that is, coping styles or traits as measured for personality tests, in trying to predict their impact on the outcome, say, of minor surgery, while other studies (e.g. Cohen and Lazarus 1973) have examined the active coping processes employed by the surgical patient the evening before the operation. Although both types of research have demonstrated a relationship between such variables and indexes of recovery from surgery, their findings are often contradictory in respect to the relationship between actual coping and coping dispositions and recovery. Moreover, there is evidence that a coping strategy which works in one context, or for one type of person, might have damaging consequences for another (cf. Speisman *et al.* 1964; Gal, unpublished study, discussed in Lazarus 1974).

SUMMARY

It is quite clear that self-regulation is an integral part of the problem of stress, disease precursors, and psychosomatic disorder, and we cannot hope to develop practical understanding without taking into account their function in stress-relevant environmental transactions. Moreover, each psychobiological step in linking an external stressor with a somatic response process needs to be spelled out and examined in the attempt to understand the psychodynamics of somatic precursors of illness and illness itself. The process begins from the moment a person appraises some given commerce with the environment as harmful, challenging, threatening, benign, or positive, and includes how such appraisals persist or change as events proceed, the manner in which the person chooses one or another form of self-regulation, and finally, the costs and effectiveness of given self-regulatory strategies in particular types of persons and environmental contexts. We need to see psychosomatic illness as an expression of repeated or persistent forms of commerce or transactions a person is having with an environment. Such commerce and the ways it is appraised depend both on the characteristics of environmental situations and personality characteristics, not on one or the other alone.

REFERENCES

ADREASON, N. J. C., NOYES, R., and HARTFORD, C. E. (1972). Factors influencing adjustment of burn patients during hospitalization.

ANDREW, J. M. (1970). Recovery from surgery with and without preparatory instruction for three coping styles. *J. Personal. soc. Psychol.*, **151**, 223–6.

COHEN, F. and LAZARUS, R. S. (1973). Active coping processes, coping dispositions, and recovery from surgery. *Psychosom. Med.*, **35**, 375–89.

DOHRENWEND, B. S. (1973). Life events as stressors: A methodological inquiry. *J. Hlth soc. Behav.*, **14**, 167–75.

FOLKINS, C. H. (1970). Temporal factors and the cognitive mediators of stress reaction. *J. Personal. soc. Psychol.*, **14**, 173–84.

FRANKENHAEUSER, M. (1971). Behavior and circulating catecholamines. *Brain Res.*, **31**, 241–62.

FREUD, S. (1936). *The problem of anxiety*. Norton, New York. (Also published as *Inhibitions, symptoms, and anxiety*.)

GRAY, S. J., RAMSEY, C. S., VILLARREAL, R., and KRAKANER, L. J. (1956). Adrenal influences upon the stomach and the gastric response to stress. In *Fifth annual report on stress, 1955–1956* (ed. H. Selye and G. Hensen), p. 138. MD Publications, Inc., New York.

GRINKER, R. R. and SPIEGEL, J. P. (1954). *Men under stress*. McGraw-Hill, New York.

HAMBURG, D. A., HAMBURG, B., and DeGOZA, S. (1953). Adaptive problems and mechanisms in severely burned patients. *Psychiat.*, **16**, 1–20.

LACEY, J. I. (1967). Somatic response patterning and stress: some revisions of activation theory. In *Psychological stress* (eds. M. H. Appley and R. Trumbull), pp. 14–37. Appleton-Century-Croft, New York.

LAZARUS, R. S. (1966). *Psychological stress and the coping process*. McGraw-Hill, New York.

—— (1974). A cognitively-oriented psychologist looks at biofeedback. Address given to the Biofeedback Research Society, Colorado Springs, Colorado, 15 February 1974.

—— (1975). The self-regulation of emotion. In *Parameters of emotion* (ed. L. Levi). Oxford University Press, London.

——, AVERILL, J. R., and OPTON, E. M. Jr. (1970). Towards a cognitive theory of emotion. In *Feelings and emotions* (ed. M. Arnold), pp. 207–32. Academic Press, New York.

LEVI, L. (1965). The urinary output of adrenalin and noradrenalin during pleasant and unpleasant emotional states: A preliminary report. *Psychosom. Med.*, **27**, 80–5.

—— and KAGAN, A. (1971). Adaptation of the psychosocial

environment to man's abilities and needs. In *Society, stress and disease* (ed. L. Levi), pp. 399–404. Oxford University Press, London.

MAHL, G. F. (1949). Anxiety, HCL secretion, and peptic ulcer etiology. *Psychosom. Med.*, **11**, 30–44.

—— (1952). Relationship between acute and chronic fear and the gastric acidity and blood sugar levels in macaca mulatta monkeys. *Psychosom. Med.*, **14**, 182–210.

—— (1953). Physiological changes during chronic fear. *Ann. N.Y. Acad, Sci.*, **56**, 240–9.

MASON, J. W. (1970). Strategy in psychosomatic research. *Psychosom. Med.*, **23**, 427–39.

—— (1971). A re-evaluation of the concept of 'non-specificity' in stress theory. *J. Psychiat. Res.*, **8**, 323–33.

MONAT, A., AVERILL. J. R., and LAZARUS, R. S. (1972). Anticipatory stress and coping reactions under various conditions of uncertainty. *J. Personal. soc. Psychol.*, **24**, 237–53.

PRICE, D. B., THALER, M. and MASON, J. W. (1975). Preoperative emotional states and adrenal cortical activity. *AMA Arch. Neurol. Psychiat.*, **77**, 646–56.

SARASON, I. G. (1978). Methodological issues in the assessment of life stress. In *Parameters of emotion* (ed. L. Levi). Oxford University Press, London. (In press.)

SCHWARTZ, G. E. (1974). Self-regulation of patterns of responses: applications to basic physiology, the study of consciousness and human performance, and clinical treatment. Presidential address read at the Biofeedback Research Society Meetings in Colorado Springs, Colorado, 18 February 1974.

SELYE, H. (1956). *The stress of life*. McGraw-Hill, New York.

SHAPIRO, D., TURSKY, B., and SCHWARTZ, G. E. (1970). Differentiation of heart rate and blood pressure in man by operant conditioning. *Psychosom. Med.*, **32**, 417–23.

SPEISMAN, J. C., LAZARUS, R. S., MORDKOFF, A. M., and DAVIDSON, L. A. (1964). The experimental reduction of stress based on ego-defense theory. *J. Abnorm. soc. Psychol.*, **68**, 367–80.

SYMINGTON, T., CURRIE, A. R., CURRAN, R. S., and DAVIDSON, J. N. (1955). The reaction of the adrenal cortex in conditions of stress. In *Ciba Foundation colloquia on endocrinology, Vol. VIII The human adrenal cortex*, pp. 70–91. Little, Brown, and Co., Boston.

TINBERGEN, N. (1951). *The study of instinct*. Clarendon Press, Oxford.

VISOTSKY, H. M., HAMBURG, D. A., GOSS, M. E., and LEBOVITZ, B. Z. (1961). Coping behavior under extreme stress. *Arch. gen. Psychiat.*, **5**, 423–48.

WEISMAN, A. D. (1972). *On dying and denying*. Behavioral Publications, Inc., New York.

WOLFF, C. T., FRIEDMAN, S. B., HOFER, M. A., and MASON, J. W. (1964). Relationship between psychological defenses and mean urinary 17-hydroxycorticosteroid excretion rates: Part I and II. *Psychosom. Med.*, **26**, 576–609.

23. MEDICAL ETHOLOGY IN RELATION TO OCCUPATIONAL HEALTH

J. P. HENRY, D. L. ELY, and P. M. STEPHENS

By employing complex, functionally-differentiated population cages and monitoring the occupants with a computer-operated magnetic tagging system, quantitative behavioural observations can be made of the effects of social ethological influences. In addition, measurements can be made of various neuroendocrine control mechanisms, in particular of the Cannon fight–flight response and of the depressive alarm reaction of Selye. The ensuing pathological changes can be relatively rapidly determined and contrasted with the control situation. A valid analogy can be made between the work situation in man and the dominant mouse that is busy patrolling a cage system once every eight min. Both are responding to the subtle patterns of arousal of an instinctual mechanism; both are engaged in an activity that is species-preservative, not a direct sequel of the basic self-preservative instincts for eating and drinking. The factors controlling the socialized, patrolling dominant may include his perception of the requirements of the group and do not appear to differ in kind from those motivating the man. Hence, we would view a population cage stocked with mice as a potential tool for the social–ethological study of the occupational as well as the reproductive activity of an ongoing mammalian colony.

SOCIAL DEPRIVATION AND CONFRONTATION

Social ethology is involved in the interactions that occur between the various members of a social grouping of mammals as they seek *desiderata*, such as food, nesting areas, and mates (Crook 1970). Studies along these lines can be carried out in the laboratory by using complex population cages in which there are separate nesting, feeding, water, and activity areas. For some time, we have been engaged in such work, using a CBA strain of mice which does not differ greatly in appearance from the wild domestic mouse *Mus musculus* (Henry *et al.* 1967: Henry *et al.* 1972; Henry and Stephens 1977).

By special arrangement of the cage design (Fig. 23.1) and by using 32 animals, half males and half females, that have been socially deprived from early weaning until fully mature at four months, we have been able to induce repeated social confrontations which resulted not only in agonistic behaviour, but also in physiological disturbances. Such animals do not develop a stable hierarchy, but stimulate each other a great deal. Not only is there an increase in catecholamine-synthesizing

enzymes in the adrenal medulla of such animals (Henry *et al.* 1971b), but they develop sustained high blood pressure, arteriosclerosis, and myocardial fibrosis (Henry *et al.* 1971a; Henry and Stephens 1977).

NORMALLY SOCIALIZED ANIMALS

We have also been much interested in the behaviour of normally socialized animals and in the social hierarchy that develops in a healthy colony composed of only 5 male siblings and 10 females. There is a clear-cut differentiation of role in such systems that is especially apparent in the males (Ely *et al.* 1972). Their behaviour characteristically falls into three distinct categories: a dominant; occasional presence of rivals; and there are subordinates. As these different types respond to the social pressures peculiar to their situation, they develop strikingly different physiological patterns. The combination of differences in behaviour and in physiology suggest that the emotions they are typically experiencing also differ (Ely and Henry 1978; Henry and Stephens 1977).

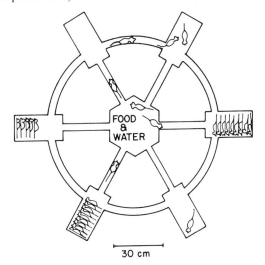

FIG. 23.1. Intercommunicating box system used to induce social interaction holds 16 male and 16 female mice. Lucite boxes are of standard size (23 × 11 × 11 cm) and are connected into a circle by flexible plastic tubes (internal diam. 3·8 cm). The central hexagon holds food and water and is connected to each box by radial tubes (internal diam. 3·2 cm). Thirty-two schematized mice are distributed in a typical pattern of aggregated groups.

First, consider the normal interaction between the members of a group of siblings in a colony started with mature adult siblings four months old. In the results to be reported a total of 16 colonies where box arrangement differs from the disorder-promotion design of Fig. 23.1 by providing only one entrance for each cage (Fig. 23.2) were used. These colonies were studied by terminating various groups on the 14th, 42nd, and the 104th day of normal social interaction. In all these colonies there was a certain amount of confrontation between the males. The females engaged in nesting and some became pregnant. The animals were evaluated for scarring on the hind quarters, which is a measure of the intensity of social interaction, and for the frequency of patrol activity of the different members. The emerging dominant is recognizable in terms of his far greater frequency of movement between boxes as well as the greater time spent in the female nesting areas (Fig. 23.2) and the feeding area (Ely *et al.* 1972).

MALE TERRITORIES

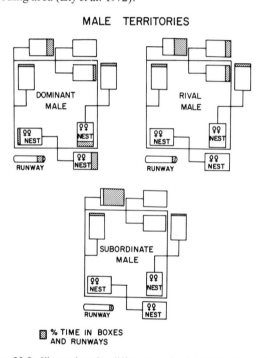

FIG. 23.2. Illustrating the different territorial distribution of dominants, rivals, and subordinate male mice in a population cage. In contrast to that shown in Fig. 23.1, this cage is designed to encourage territory formation.

DOMINANCE, SUBORDINATION, AND BLOOD PRESSURE

These behavioural distinctions between dominants and subordinates can be seen when a behavioural profile is made, using data provided by a computer that has followed the box-to-box movements of the magnetically tagged animals. The width of the pathways represents the number of passages in a sample 6-h period and the size of the circles is proportionate to the total time spent in that box. The frequent visits by a dominant to a sequence of boxes, i.e. 4 boxes in less than 8 min, is termed a patrol and is a good measure of the extent to which his position is established (Fig. 23.3) (Henry and Stephens 1977).

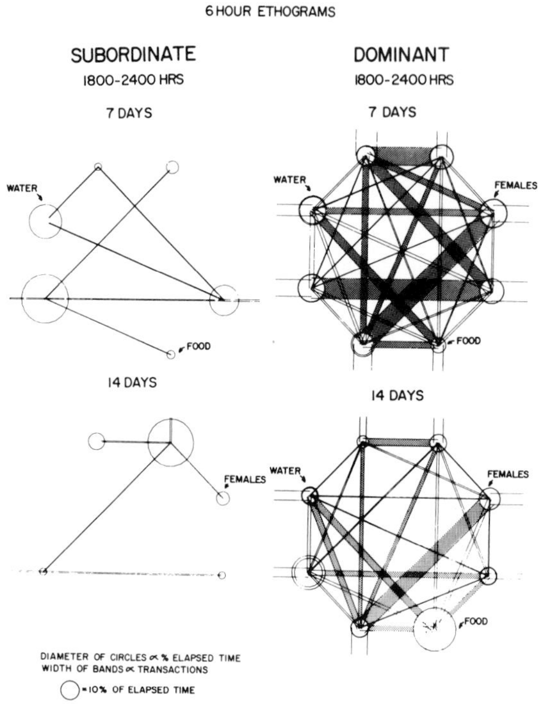

6 HOUR ETHOGRAMS

FIG. 23.3. Contrasting behaviour patterns in a population cage as plotted over a 6-h period by computer. The diameter of the circles is proportional to the time spent in the box and the width of the bands connecting boxes is proportional to the number of trips taken. The dominant animal has greater activity and visits more boxes.

The blood pressure of the dominant can be compared with that of the other four animals. The pressures are about the same until after 14 days of interaction. At this point, the hierarchy is well on the way toward being established, and patrol activity by the dominant diminishes, while the cumulative scarring of his subordinates increases slowly (Fig. 23.4). Despite the commencing stabilization of the social structure, the blood pressure of the dominant begins to rise (Fig. 23.5). It appears that the leading animals in these groups are making increasing efforts to drive off the other males. However, in closed population cages they cannot completely eliminate the subordinate males.

There is some evidence of mounting social tension, for there are increased rates of catecholamine synthesis. Thus the adrenal medullary response of Cannon (Mason 1968b), i.e., the content of the enzyme tyrosine hydroxylase (TH) responsible for the synthesis of

170

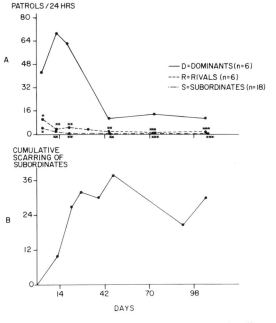

PATROLS / 24 HRS

A

— D=DOMINANTS(n=6)
--- R=RIVALS (n=6)
·—· S=SUBORDINATES (n=18)

CUMULATIVE
SCARRING OF
SUBORDINATES

B

DAYS

FIG. 23.4. Behaviour of the dominants, rivals, and subordinates from eight different colonies during normal socialization: (A) Contrasting the patrol activities (4 boxes in less than 8 min) of the three groups; (B) The cumulative scarring of the subordinates with passage of time in the colonies.

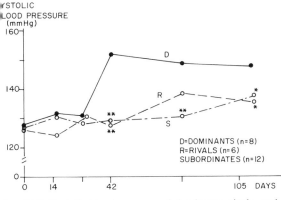

SYSTOLIC
BLOOD PRESSURE
(mmHg)

D=DOMINANTS (n=8)
R=RIVALS (n=6)
SUBORDINATES (n=12)

DAYS

FIG. 23.5. Systolic blood pressure of dominants, rivals, and subordinates from eight different colonies during normal socialization. Measurements were followed on the same animals at specific intervals throughout the 105-day period (* = $p < 0.05$; ** = $p < 0.01$). (D = dominants ($N = 8$); R = rivals ($N = 6$); S = subordinates ($N = 12$.)

noradrenalin, increases (Fig. 23.6). In all three subgroups, the dominant, the rival, and the subordinates, the first 14 days of social interaction of these formerly normally socialized animals saw a good deal of confrontation. With the rise in the TH there is also an increase of the phenylethanolamine N-methyltransferase (PNMT), the adrenal enzyme which converts

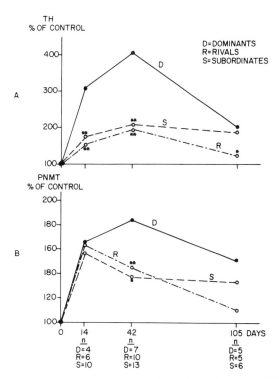

TH
% OF CONTROL

A

D=DOMINANTS
R=RIVALS
S=SUBORDINATES

PNMT
% OF CONTROL

B

DAYS
D=4   D=7   D=5
R=6   R=10   R=5
S=10   S=13   S=6

FIG. 23.6. (A) Adrenal content of tyrosine hydroxylase (TH) and (B) adrenal content of phenylethanolamine N-methyltransferase (PNMT) in dominants, rivals, and subordinates after 14, 42, and 105 days of normal socialization in a population cage. (D = dominants; R = rivals; S = subordinates.)

noradrenalin to adrenalin. The increase in PNMT continues in the dominant, despite a return in the subordinated animals toward control values. Then at 42 days, when the behavioural data shows that the social structure is stabilized, the TH and the PNMT in the dominant finally attain a maximum and by 105 days the values have returned toward base line. By this time, i.e. after three months of social interaction, there is stability in the colony and fighting is at a minimum.

As Christian (1971) has shown, we confirm from our studies of other mouse colonies fighting with significant intensity that their adrenals will greatly increase (Henry and Stephens 1977; Henry et al. 1971b). Since the adrenal weights of our various groups of normally socialized animals do not increase, even after three months of interaction, this indicates that conflict during socialization has not involved sufficiently intense fighting to stimulate cortical hypertrophy, despite some increase in the level of the adrenocorticotropic hormone (ACTH). Furthermore, the rise seen in the adrenal catecholamine-synthesizing enzymes does not indicate an equivalent stimulation of the adrenal cortex. The level of corticosterone in these animals, however, does show an important differentiation in the early days of socialization. For this hormone, which reflects the

171

ACTH activity, is significantly elevated in the subordinates as compared with the dominants (Fig. 23.7).

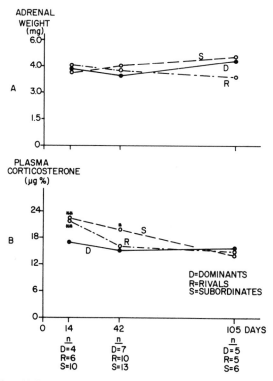

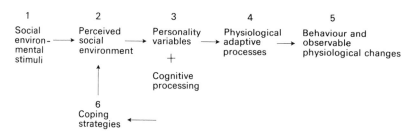

FIG. 23.7. Adrenocortical responses of dominant, rival, and subordinate males after different periods of normal socialization in a population cage. (A) Absolute adrenal weight measured at autopsy. (B) Plasma corticosterone fluorometrically measured. The N's are not identical for each social rank at 14, 42, and 105 days because different colonies were terminated at each period ($* = p < 0.05$; $** = p < 0.01$). (D = dominants; R = rivals; S = subordinates.)

A THEORY OF SOCIAL STIMULI AND PHYSIOLOGICAL CHANGES

Such findings combined with the growing evidence in the literature have led us to the following theoretical formulaton which originates from Christian (1971) Frankenhaeuser (1975), Mason (1968a,b), and other contemporary neuroendocrinologists (Sassenrath, 1970 Rose et al. 1972; for a review see Henry and Stephens 1977). First we subscribe to the hypothesis that a probable course of the complex sequence of events that intervene between the social environmental stimuli and the observable physiological changes is as shown in Fig. 23.8.

Diagrams with these principles have been independently formulated by Harris and Singer (1968), by Levi (1972), and most recently by Kiritz and Moos (1974). In area 4 of Fig. 25.8, that of the physiological adaptive processes, we would propose that two responses are at work—the defence response of Cannon (1929), Hess and Brügger (1943), and Folkow and Neil (1971), and on the other hand, the alarm response of Selye (1971).

REALITIES NOT MEETING EXPECTATIONS

These two separate neuroendocrine mechanisms have been comprehensively defined by Mason in his review studies; they are the sympathetic adrenal-medullary of Cannon (Mason 1968b) and the pituitary adrenal-cortical alarm reaction of Selye (Mason 1968a). It is becoming increasingly apparent that the mechanisms which activate them within the hypothalamus can be differentiated. We suggest that the two responses reflect different reactions to social environmental stimulation. Here we would introduce one other symbolic system to help explain the complex processes at work—the old saying that:

$$\text{Satisfaction is proportional to} \quad \frac{\text{Reality}}{\text{Expectations}}$$

would appear relevant for mice as well as men. Recently Levine et al. (1972) and Weiss (1972) have both shown in their studies of operant conditioning with rats that the corticosterone level of the animal rises when the realities of the situation fail to meet the animal's expectations based on prior experience. This broad concept would include the general theme that when the organism, be it a rodent or a higher primate, perceives that his expecta-

FIG. 23.8. Diagram of a probable sequence of events that intervene between the social environmental stimuli and the observable physiological changes.

tions are not being met, his behaviour will be one of engagement of the fight–flight mechanism with the consequent possibility that he may improve his situation. If the behaviour that follows involvement of the sympathetic adrenal-medullary response mechanism results in a successful re-establishment of the security of the organism's expectations, then the responses settle down. If the Cannon response is not effective and the expectations are simply not being met, then the organism must accept defeat. In this case, the physiological changes will tend to follow the classical Selyean alarm–response pattern. Behaviourally there will be withdrawal, decreased motor activity, and the stage is set for the behaviour characteristic of endogenous behavioural depression (Sassenrath 1970; Sachar 1970).

This withdrawal is accompanied by increased corticosterone output and by the classical depressive emotional response. Price (1969) perceived this depressive or yielding reaction as being of evolutionary value because it decreased social conflict and tended to stabilize the control of the hierarchy.

DOMINANCE, CORTICOSTERONE, AND GONADOTROPHINS

The animal model with which we are working provides us with the opportunity to test these theoretical ideas. Not only does the dominant male have a lower level of corticosterone than the subordinate, but evidence from other sources suggests that his gonadotrophic activity is enhanced. The work of Rose and his associates shows that the testosterone levels of a low status 'depressed' monkey will sharply increase when he is placed in a colony of receptive females where he can assume a dominant role (Rose et al. 1972). On the other hand, Bronson (1973) showed that the gonadotrophins decrease during agonistic social interaction among male mice. Thus a successful challenge to a dominant, which leaves him with a lowered social status, should be associated with the adoption of subordinate, depressed–withdrawn behaviour and we could expect an increase in corticosterone levels. These predictions were tested in a recent series of observations.

LOSS OF DOMINANT STATUS

Former dominants were placed in colonies where there already was a dominant in residence. In the six 'intruder' dominants there was a sharp decrease in the relative level of PNMT, i.e. the adrenaline-synthesizing enzyme, and TH remained at a very high unchanged level. However, corticosterone increased very significantly, i.e., from 15 to 23 μg per cent, and the already elevated blood pressure increased from nearly 150 mm Hg to some 200 mm Hg (Fig. 23.9).

The behaviour of these animals was very similar to that of another set of dominants which were given the active

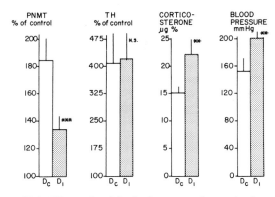

FIG. 23.9. Effects of social rejection upon a former dominant. Open column: the levels of PNMT, the adrenl enzyme controlling adrenalin synthesis; TH, the rate-limiting enzyme for noradrenalin, plasma corticosterone, and blood pressure in a group of normal dominants. Hatched column: represents the same parameters in former dominants that have been placed in a strange social group as solitary intruders. (D_c = dominant controls ($N = 7$); D_i = dominant intruders ($N = 6$.)

ingredient of marijuana Δ-9 tetrahydrocannabinol. If there was a rival present in the colony, the hours spent by the dominant under the influence of the drug permanently cost him his status in the colony and he was reduced to a low subordinate rank (Fig. 23.10). The behaviour records demonstrated this with a dramatic reversal and permanent loss of his patrol activity, while the rival took over. The record of his other activities showed that he had not rendered even temporarily ataxic by the drug and his feeding time was only temporarily and slightly impaired (Ely et al. 1975).

The accompanying physiological changes have not been followed in detail, but in a few cases these deposed former dominants showed extremely high levels of corticosterone. In an accompanying study of colonies in which there was no rival, the dip in patrol activity and temporary neglect of his normal activity pattern cost him nothing. In these thoroughly stable colonies, he reassumed his usual high levels of patrol activity within a few hours (Fig. 23.11) (Ely et al. 1975).

Finally if a strange animal is introduced during the period that the dominant is lightly intoxicated, i.e., with 0·5 mg/kg, he will nevertheless fail to do his job (Fig. 23.12). Unlike the subordinate, a part of the role behaviour or work assignment of the dominant is to drive off intruders. It is striking that this social role behaviour is neglected when under the influence of the drug. Certainly there is full recovery when the effect has worn off (Fig. 23.11) (Ely et al. 1975).

EFFECTS OF SOCIAL ISOLATION

In two recent papers, our group has contrasted the behaviour of animals that have been raised in isolation until they were adult instead of commingling in a

173

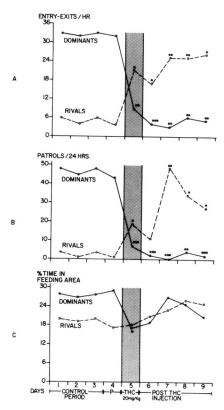

Fig. 23.10. Dominant ($N = 3$) and rival ($N = 3$) males' behavioural responses to a single injection (IV) of 2 mg/kg Δ9-THC given to the dominant ($* = p < 0.05$; $** = p < 0.02$; $*** = p < 0.001$).

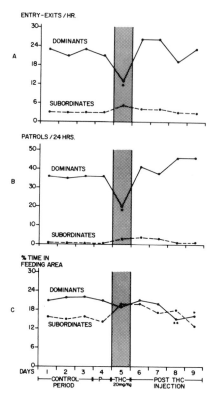

Fig. 23.11. Dominant ($N = 6$) and subordinate ($N = 6$) males' behavioural responses to a single injection (IV) of 20 mg/kg Δ9-THC given to the dominant. In these colonies there were no rival males present ($* = p < 0.05$; $** = p < 0.01$, as compared to placebo values).

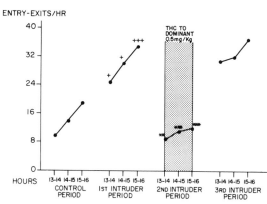

Fig. 23.12. Dominant male's ($N = 6$) aggressive response (entry–exits/h) to an intruder before, during, and after a single injection (IV) of 0.5 mg/kg Δ9-THC. The increase in activity during the control period from 1300 to 1600 h is due to the normal circadian activity rhythm ($+ = p < 0.05$; $+++ = p < 0.001$, as compared to control values and $** = p < 0.01$; $*** = p < 0.001$, as compared to first intruder values).

common box as siblings (Ely and Henry 1974; Watson *et al.* 1974). Both groups were followed by magnetic tagging and this monitoring device incorporated with the Reimer–Petras design (Ely *et al.* 1972) was used to follow the development of social differentiation (Fig. 23.2). Isolated males consistently failed to develop normal social behaviour and were hyperaggressive. The normal social hierarchy was missing and it was not possible to identify a clear-cut dominant with unobtrusive subordinates. The constant struggle between the members of the colony led to the necessity to rank them in terms of aggressivity rather than specify their roles as dominant, rival, and subordinate. A concomitant of the ensuing social disorder was fewer pregnancies and an increased litter mortality.

The foregoing observation of murine colony social patterns can be summarized as follows:

1. Healthy socialized colonies differentiate into a dominant, sometimes a rival, and a number of subordinates;
2. While the hierarchy is being established, the dominants show an increased sympathetic adrenal-medullary activity. At the same time, the future

subordinates' plasma corticosterone level is increased;

3. Disordered colonies result if they are stocked with animals that have been socially deprived by raising them in isolation from weaning until fully adult at four months. Such animals are hyperaggressive and will not accept a subordinate role assignment;

4. If social status is radically lowered by putting a dominant into a strange colony which already has a dominant, the intruder-dominant will show a large increase in plasma corticosterone and in blood pressure. He will exhibit the withdrawal behaviour of a depressed animal and may die within a few days, despite adequate access to food and water.

HUMAN APPLICATIONS

We would regard the endless series of patrols that the active dominant carries out, visiting four or more boxes in the course of every eight min, as an example of role behaviour that is an occupational task. The failure of the drugged or downward-socially displaced animal to perform the expected social organizational tasks is compatible with endogenous depression (Sachar 1970) and the raised 17-OHCS levels would confirm this (Ely and Henry 1978; Ely et al. 1975).

There appear to be close parallels between the human and the animal social behavioural patterns which also show up when appropriate living space arrangements are considered. The precise design both of human working areas and of complex animal population cages is critical for the successful development of a smoothly working hierarchy with successful differentiation of roles and a minimum of confrontation and fighting. Some designs foment social tension by forcing the various members of the group to infringe on territory in order to gain access to some critical function. If food and water are only available in one central region, there is more fighting and the blood pressure is higher, than if it is placed in every box (Henry et al. 1967). If the young are to be successfully reared, it is helpful to provide easily defended, single-entry, dark nesting boxes (Henry et al. 1967). In addition to social disorder due to failure of socialization during youth, there is then the factor of appropriate architectural design. These rules apply to the field of human occupational health, and well designed working areas provide appropriate facilities for food, for elimination, and for the various role players without forcing any one group or member to encroach unduly upon the territory of others.

BIOLOGICAL COMPONENTS IN CONFRONTATION BEHAVIOUR

Certain recent studies have drawn attention to various aspects of these behavioural patterns and needs which man shares with the other animals. In the work of Maclay and Knipe (1972) on the pecking order in human society, which they have called the dominant man, they make the cogent point that, even in man, there are very clear-cut inherited patterns of behaviour that play a critical part in confrontation behaviour. They discuss the role of body size and eye contact. The deference behaviour of the subordinate and the subtle signalling of the dominant by facial display, eye contact, and body posture are reviewed in detail. The role of dominance and subordination in the post-industrial society is extensively discussed in the context of an ethological viewpoint.

The imperial animal by Tiger and Fox (1971) is an ethologically-oriented discussion of the social system of modern technology. It contrasts male and female behaviour patterns and bonding behaviour. They review social roles and discuss the methods by which the child is integrated into society and learns how to play the assigned social roles. They discuss the repertoire of signals, postures, and gestures, and other non-verbal behaviour that bonds the group: much of this, man shares with the higher primates. Despite its unbelievably elaborate proliferation, culture, they argue, is based upon the basic biology of man. That is, it rests upon his primate and hunter–gatherer patterns of behaviour. Because they are built-in, post-industrial man must still use the remarkably simple and uniform pattern of social relationships designed to permit him to survive under the hunter–gatherer conditions in which his social brain evolved—and to whose precise nature, the life of the few remaining Bushmen of the Kalahari and the nomads of the great Australian desert still bear vivid living witness.

Other important ethological texts include Lorenz (1966), On aggression, in which he discusses the aggression and territoriality of man and the two-volume work of Bowlby (1970, 1973) on Attachment and loss. In this he discusses attachment behaviour in primates and man and the mother–child attachment mechanism is reviewed. He shows how with maturation these same bonds come to extend to the other members of the basic group. Finally the society in which the individual is raised receives the benefit of the attachment behaviour. These bonds hold the aggressive drives in check and are responsible for the successful development of a social hierarchy. Eibl-Eibesfeldt's (1972) recent study of the natural history of behaviour patterns which he entitles Love and hate points to the positive affiliative mechanism by which stable working groups of both mice and men are welded together. If the attachment behaviour is disrupted during the development period, the individual develops disturbed emotional patterns ranging from excessive fear and anxiety to an aggressive 'psychopathic' lack of attachment that leads to the chronic disorder of any murine or human community that is unfortunate enough to include in its make-up a sufficient proportion of persons who are socially deprived.

SOCIAL SETTING AND PHYSIOLOGICAL RESPONSE

Kiritz and Moos (1974) have discussed the various factors determining the influence of a social setting upon the physiological responses of an individual. Their diagram outlining the probable sequence of events was described earlier. They discuss factors from those which determine the perceived social climate referring to a relationship dimension involving support, cohesion, and involvement, to those of a personality development dimension in which responsibility for group activity was important, and, finally, to a factor concerned with maintenance or change of the system. This evaluates the pressure under which the individual is working as well as the predictability and consistency of the environment.

The above dimensions would also apply to a colony of mice. The influence of the relationship of the animals to each other and their support and cohesion can be seen in terms of the blood pressure of a group the members of which are socially adapted to each other by virtue of being raised together from infancy in the same population cage. The indirectly measured systolic arterial pressures are far less elevated than those of a group of formerly isolated animals that consistently fight each other. The levels of the catecholamine-synthesizing enzymes and of arteriosclerosis in the two groups also differ radically. Thus the discussion of support, cohesion, and involvement, which characterizes the socialized group, refers to the very basic mammalian instinct of attachment when given its extension from immediate parents and siblings to the social group.

LEADERSHIP AND RESPONSIBILITY

Kiritz and Moos's (1974) personality development dimension in which leadership and responsibility for group activity is involved can be applied to the role of the dominant who not only controls the movement of the subordinates, but is also the representative of the group attacking and driving off those intruding on the confines of the population cage.

Parallels can be drawn between other human and social–ethological situations. For example, the above authors comment on the increased level of urinary 17-hydroxycorticosteroids in field officers who were having difficulty handling confusing and interfering orders from their staff superiors during a crisis. A similar situation could be the increased corticosterone level of a former dominant mouse trying to cope in a colony in which it is unfamiliar (Ely and Henry 1978) or the increased corticosterone of a dominant that received Δ9-THC and is attempting to regain control (Ely and Henry, unpublished data).

Kiritz and Moos (1974) cited the high heart rates of space agency executives who had just been put in charge of a critical project. The increased blood pressure of a dominant that is trying to shape up a group of subordinates is due to activation of the same sympathetic adrenal-medullary system (Ely and Henry 1978).

WORK STRESS AND PREDICTABILITY OF THE ENVIRONMENT

Finally, the pressure under which the individual is working and the predictability of the environment are both factors that affect the mouse as well as the man. The presence of a rival ready to move in, in the case of a failure to perform, determines whether the loss of role of a dominant mouse will be permanent if he even temporarily abandons the contest (Figs. 23.10 and 23.11). Levine and Weiss have both emphasized the importance of predictability if the organism is to control the environment and not develop the physiological disturbances which we have shown will lead, for example, to hypertension and coronary artery disease (Levine *et al.* 1972; Weiss, 1972).

THE ROLE OF THE HOME

An important area of concern to the human physician is the role of the home as opposed to the work environment. One can argue that if both are disturbed then the chances that man will be able to function effectively are greatly decreased. We have not yet investigated the role of the female in determining the stability of a social situation in any detail. However, we have been struck by the interesting fluctuations in TH and PNMT in colonies of socially deprived male CBA that were mixed with normally socialized sibling females. Colonies that were exposed to social interaction in a six-box population cage for 21 days show an increase in TH and PNMT. Colonies that have only been together for 21 days will still be fighting vigorously and the raised adrenal-medullary enzyme levels are no surprise. However, it is intriguing that there is no increase in the 2-month-group (Figs. 23.13 and 23.14). An explanation might be in the fact that females in these colonies would be 6 months old and just about at the peak of their breeding activity. They would be highly receptive and would readily become pregnant at this stage. Perhaps the aggression of the socially disordered males was temporarily inhibited. However, the 6-month-group would be 10 months old and the females would by then be past the breeding period. It is possible the presence of the older females may not have inhibited the aggressive activity of the ageing, socially depressed males, and it may be for these reasons that the TH is raised in the 2- and the 10-month-groups.

PHYSIOLOGICAL CONCOMITANTS OF SOCIAL INTERACTION

The medical ethologic approach involves study of the physiological concomitants of behaviour elicited by the social interaction that occurs as members of a group seek things that they need, such as food, nesting areas, and mates. It has been shown that the physiological arousal

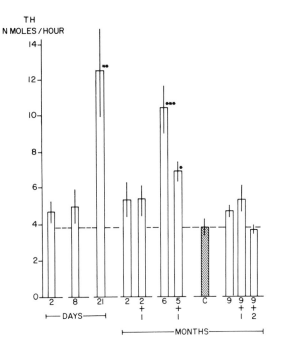

FIG. 23.13. The tyrosine hydroxylase (TH) activity of an $N = 8$ random sampling of the male members of each of the 10 colonies. The asterisks denote significant differences from the C_4 ($N = 15$) control value. ($* = p < 0.05$; $** = p < 0.01$; $*** = p < 0.001$.)

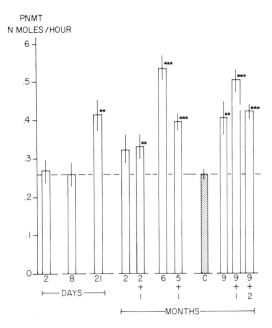

FIG. 23.14. The phenylethanolamine N-methyltransferase (PNMT) activities of the male members of each of the 10 colonies. The asterisks denote significant differences from control values.

that ensues involves activation of the neuroendocrine system. The subsequent biochemical patterning is determined by the social role of the individual. A dominant in a large closed-system population cage will show increased sympathetic adrenal activity and a raised systolic blood pressure. If he loses status and his expectations are not met, as when the dominant is moved into a system to which he does not belong, then there is a further elevation of blood pressure. Plasma corticosterone will also be significantly elevated. The animal loses weight and may die within a few days. Similar observations have been made by Barnett (1964) and Von Holst's (1972) observations of the death from uraemia of tree shrews that are confined to intense subordinate status indicate that in this species at least the intense renal vaso-constriction may have irretrievably damaged the kidney.

SUMMARY

Using the same principles that apply to man, we have outlined the factors controlling various types of sustained emotional arousal in social groups of animals. We have referred to the Cannon fight–flight and to the depressive-alarm response of Selye. Useful observations can be made of the effect of social ethological influences upon these physiological control mechanisms and the ensuing pathological changes can be relatively rapidly determined and contrasted with the control situation. A valid analogy can be made between the work situation in man and the dominant mouse that is busy patrolling a cage system once every eight min. Both are responding to the subtle patterns of arousal of an instinctual mechanism; both are engaged in an activity that is species-preservative, not a direct sequel of the basic self-preservative instincts for eating and drinking. The factors controlling the socialized patrolling dominant may include his perception of the requirements of the group and do not appear to differ in kind from those motivating the man. Hence, we would view a population cage stocked with mice as a potential tool for the social ethological study of the occupational as well as the reproductive activity of an ongoing mammalian colony.

REFERENCES

BARNETT, S. A. (1964). Social stress: The concept of stress. In *Viewpoints in biology* (ed. J. D. Carthy, and C. L. Duddington), Vol. 3, pp. 170–218. Butterworths, London.

BOWLBY, J. (1970). *Attachment and loss, Vol. 1: Attachment.* Hogarth Press, London.

—— (1973). *Attachment and loss, Vol. 2: Separation, anxiety and anger*. Hogarth Press, London.

BRONSON, F. H. (1973). Establishment of social rank among grouped male mice: relative effects on circulating FSH, LH, and corticosterone. *Physiol. Behav.*, **10**, 947–51.

CANNON, W. B. (1929). *Bodily changes in pain, hunger, fear and rage: an account of recent researches into the function of emotional excitement* (2nd edn.). Appleton, New York.

CHRISTIAN, J. J. (1971). Population density and reproductive efficiency. *Biol. Reprod.*, **4**, 248–94.

CROOK, J. H. (1970). Social organization and the environment: Aspects of contemporary social ethology. *Anim. Behav.*, **18**, 197–209.

EIBL-EIBESFELDT, I. (1972). *Love and hate: the natural history of behavior patterns* (trans. by G. Strachan). Holt, Rinehart, and Winston, New York.

ELY, D. L., HENRY, J. A., HENRY, J. P., and RADER, R. D. (1972). A monitoring technique providing quantitative rodent behavior analysis. *Physiol. Behav.*, **9**, 675–9.

—— and HENRY, J. P. (1974). Effects of prolonged social deprivation on murine behavior patterns, blood pressure, and adrenal weight, *J. comp. Physiol. Psychol.*, **87**, 733–40.

—— and —— (1978). Neuroendocrine response patterns in dominant and subordinate mice. *Horm. Behav.*, **10**, 156–69.

——, ——, and CIARANELLO, R. D. (1974). Long term behavioral and biochemical differentiation of dominant and subordinate mice in population cages. *Psychosom. Med.*, **36**, 463.

——, ——, and JAROSZ, C. J. (1975). Effects of marihuana (9-THC) on behaviour patterns and social roles in colonies of CBA mice. *Behav. Biol.*, **13**, 263–76.

FRANKENHAEUSER, M. (1975). Experimental approaches to the study of catecholamines and emotion. In *Emotions: their parameters and measurement* (ed. L. Levi), pp. 209–34. Raven Press, New York.

FOLKOW, B. and NEIL, E. (1971). *Circulation*, pp. 344–9. Oxford University Press, London.

HARRIS, R. E., and SINGER, M. T. (1968). Interaction of personality and stress in the pathogenesis of essential hypertension. In *Hypertension: neural control of arterial pressure*, Vol. 16, Proceedings of the Council for High Blood Pressure Research, pp. 104–14. American Heart Association, New York.

HENRY, J. P., MEEHAN, J. P., and STEPHENS, P. M. (1967). The use of psychosocial stimuli to induce prolonged systolic hypertension in mice, *Psychosom. Med.*, **29**, 408–32.

——, ELY, D. L., STEPHENS, P. M., RATCLIFFE, H. L., SANTISTEBAN, G. A., and SHAPIRO, A. P. (1971a). The role of psychosocial factors in the development of arteriosclerosis in CBA mice: observations on the heart, kidney, and aorta. *Atherosclerosis*, **14**, 203–18.

——, STEPHENS, P. M., AXELROD, J., and MUELLER, R. A. (1971b). Effect of psychosocial stimulation on the enzymes involved in the biosynthesis and metabolism of noradrenaline and adrenaline, *Psychosom. Med.*, **33**, 227–37.

—— and —— (1977). *Stress, health, and the social environment. A sociobiologic approach to medicine*. Springer-Verlag, New York.

——, ELY, D. L., and STEPHENS, P. M. (1972). Changes in catecholamine-controlling enzymes in response to psychosocial activation of the defence and alarm reactions.

In *Physiology, emotion and psychosomatic illness*, Ciba Foundation Symposium 8 (new series), pp. 225–46. Associated Scientific Publishers, Amsterdam.

——, ——, WATSON, F. M. C., and STEPHENS, P. M. (1975). Ethological methods as applied to the measurement of emotion. In *Emotions: their parameters and measurement* (ed. L. Levi), pp. 209–34. Raven Press, New York.

HESS, W. R. and BRÜGGER, M. (1943). Das subkortikale Zentrum der affektiven Abwehrreaktion, *Helv. Physiol. Acta*, **1**, 33–52.

KIRITZ, S. and MOOS, R. H. (1974). Physiological effects of social environments, *Psychosom. Med.*, **36**, 96–114.

LEVI, L. (ed.) (1972). Stress and distress in response to psychosocial stimuli. *Acta Med. Scand. (Suppl. 528)*, **191**.

LEVINE, S., GOLDMAN, L., and COOVER, G. D. (1972). Expectancy and the pituitary-adrenal system. In *Physiology, emotion and psychosomatic illness*, Ciba Foundation Symposium 8 (new series), pp. 281–96. Associated Scientific Publishers, Amsterdam.

LORENZ, K. (1966). *On aggression* (trans. by M. K. Wilson). Harcourt, Brace and World Inc., New York.

MACLAY, G. and KNIPE, H. (1972). *The dominant man: the pecking order in human society*. Delacorte Press, New York.

MASON, J. W. (1968a). A review of psychoendocrine research on the pituitary-adrenal cortical system, *Psychosom. Med.*, **30**, 576–607.

—— (1968b). A review of psychoendocrine research on the sympathetic-adrenal medullary system, *Psychosom. Med.*, **30**, 631–53.

PRICE, J. S. (1969). The ritualization of agonistic behaviour as a determinant of variation along the neuroticism/stability dimension of personality, *Proc. roy. Soc. Med.*, **62**, 37–40.

ROSE, R. M., GORDON, T. P., and BERNSTEIN, I. S. (1972). Plasma testosterone levels in the male rhesus: influences of sexual and social stimuli, *Science*, **178**, 643–5.

SACHAR, E. J. (1970). Psychological factors relating to activation and inhibition of the adrenocortical stress response in man: a review. In *Progress in brain research, Vol. 32: pituitary, adrenal and the brain* (ed. D. de Wied and J. A. W. M. Weijnen), pp. 316–24. Elsevier, Amsterdam.

SASSENRATH, E. N. (1970). Increased adrenal responsiveness related to social stress in rhesus monkeys. *Hormone Bahav.*, **1**, 283–98.

SELYE, H. (1971). The evolution of the stress concept—stress and cardiovascular disease. In *Society, stress and disease, Vol. 1: the psychosocial environment and psychosomatic diseases* (ed. L. Levi), pp. 299–311. Oxford University Press, London.

TIGER, L. and FOX, R. (1971). *The imperial animal*. Secker and Warburg, London.

VON HOLST, D. (1972). Renal failure as the cause of death in *Tupaia belangeri* (tree shrews) exposed to persistent social disease. *J. comp. Physiol.*, **78**, 236–73.

WATSON, F. M. C., HENRY, J. P., and HALTMEYER, G. C. (1974). Effects of early experience on emotional and social reactivity in CBA mice, *Physiol. Behav.*, **13**, 9–14.

WEISS, J. M. (1972). Influence of psychological variables on stress-induced pathology. In *Physiology, emotion and psychosomatic illness*, Ciba Foundation Symposium 8 (new series), pp. 253–80, Associated Scientific Publishers, Amsterdam.

24. HEALTH, WELL-BEING, AND DISEASE IN RELATION TO THE WORKING SITUATION. A REVIEW OF FINDINGS IN DANISH SOCIO-MEDICAL STUDIES

OLE SVANE

Until recently research in Denmark on the effects of the working situation has been split into a medical and a behavioural-science tradition. In the following I shall outline some findings and methodological considerations in the last 15 years' research.

MEDICAL RESEARCH

In contrast to activity in neighbouring countries the output of occupational medical research in Denmark has been very sparse in the last fifteen years. Occupational medicine is a field of application of diverse medical disciplines. Yet it is astonishing that a specification of the total Danish medical research leads to the conclusion that maximally two out of every thousand scientific publications by Danish medical authors concern occupational medicine (Svane 1973). The manpower in and financial support for the field have been very scarce, possibly because the well-established family doctor system has not catered for the development of a network of industrial physicians.

One can distinguish three kinds of research in occupational medicine during the last fifteen years: studies stemming from the biological tradition, socio-medical studies, and pamphlet-like 'critical' studies.

The best representatives of the biological tradition are the toxicological pieces of research. In a study of respiratory symptoms and pulmonary functions in welders, it is concluded that it is not possible to demonstrate differences in the symptomatology of welders and non-welders. One of the explanations might be the use of classical definitions of bronchitis and of measuring the functional capacity of the lungs with highly specific but low-sensitivity methods.

The socio-medical studies have been published by the Danish National Institute of Social Research. The series *The physically handicapped in Denmark* (Andersen *et al.* 1964, 1966, 1967) was aimed at throwing light on the process of rehabilitation. The main conclusion of the study was that medically defined disability has little significant for people who are not totally crippled. The two factors that lead to a high probability of rehabilitation are the level of education (leaving school with some sort of passed exam) and confidence in one's own ability to cope with difficulties. In a study of three shift workers (Andersen 1970) conclusions are close to those of the contemporary pieces of research concerning the medical and psychosocial effects of working in continual three-shift work. The most interesting part is the comparison between shift workers who are recruited

only if they pass a medical test and other shift workers, i.e. between policemen and industrial workers. The job contents are so different that this admittedly impairs the conclusions. The difference was primarily a lower frequency of ulcer-like complaints, while the psycho-social picture of the two groups was nearly the same, only the features of the industrial worker's group being drawn more distinctly.

A survey of Danish workers' health, working conditions, and job satisfaction has been concluded (Redder *et al.* 1972) in which the aim was to get an overall impression of the working situation and its consequences as seen by the workers themselves. A sample of 10 000 names was drawn from the registers of the Danish Trades Union Council. 75 per cent of the questionnaires were returned. A follow-up on the non-respondent group indicated that the figures referred to in this paragraph would be representative for the whole population of the Danish TUC with small modifications. The TUC covers one million persons out of the two and a half million employed in trade and industry. The physical and chemical working conditions were described as shown in Table 24.1.

The most significant complaints concerned noise, physical burdens, draught, and dust. In a comparable Swedish survey (Bolinder *et al.* 1970) the same conditions were most frequent. On average 3·4 physical/chemical complaints were mentioned. The health situation of the respondents was measured in two ways: answers to general questions and to 38 questions concerning specific symptoms. The general health results are: 84 per cent of the total described their health situation during the last year as good or comparatively good; 8 per cent had to take care of their health difficulties. The second general measure was a question about taking medicine several times a week. The main types of medicine were pain-relieving and pills for nervous troubles. 18 per cent took medicine several times per week—women 22 per cent, men 16 per cent. The answers to questions on symptoms showed another picture: 80 per cent of all indicated some symptom or other. The average per person was 4·9 symptoms.

30 per cent had five symptoms or more. Table 24.2 lists the symptoms. The frequencies in three age groups are shown separately for men and women. The symptoms concerning the motor apparatus constituted nearly one-quarter of all mentioned symptoms, as did the nervous symptoms, including 'feeling stressed'.

42 per cent had one or more of the four dorsal symptoms. These symptoms are characterized by often

Table 24.1 Frequencies of physical/chemical complaints. Total population

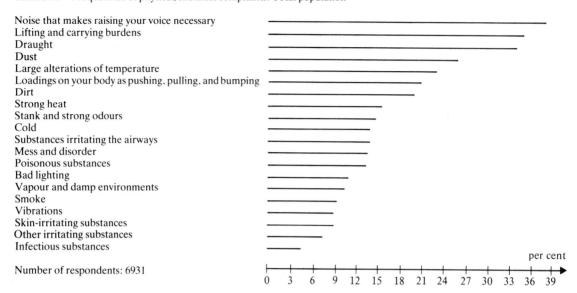

Noise that makes raising your voice necessary
Lifting and carrying burdens
Draught
Dust
Large alterations of temperature
Loadings on your body as pushing, pulling, and bumping
Dirt
Strong heat
Stank and strong odours
Cold
Substances irritating the airways
Mess and disorder
Poisonous substances
Bad lighting
Vapour and damp environments
Smoke
Vibrations
Skin-irritating substances
Other irritating substances
Infectious substances

per cent

Number of respondents: 6931

0 3 6 9 12 15 18 21 24 27 30 33 36 39

being related to the working situation. For all symptoms mentioned, the distribution of answers to the sub-question on the cause of the symptoms was as shown in Table 24.3.

The symptoms from the motor apparatus, in particular, were often indicated as being caused by the working situation. The nervous symptoms were characterized by being related to the category 'both–and' in between 40 and 50 per cent of the cases. The symptom 'feeling stressed' was related to work in 39 per cent of the cases, not to work in 6 per cent, 38 per cent answered 'both–and', and 17 per cent had no answer or could not indicate the cause.

The third facet of the description of the working situation in the survey was a measurement of job satisfaction. The index of job satisfaction consisted of six items with three categories each. The lowest job satisfaction, i.e. indicating the worst alternative to all six questions, had the index value 6, the highest job satisfaction had the index value 18. The questions concerned (1) monotony of work, (2) pace of work, (3) autonomy at work, (4) opinion of supervisors, (5) opinion of work mates, and (6) possibility of contact with work mates during work. Table 24.4 shows the distribution of the index values: 89 per cent of the total had an index score higher than the arithmetic mean value of the index, i.e. they had a high job satisfaction by definition. In the section on socio-psychological studies I will return to these results.

A description of a fourth facet of working conditions was attempted by constructing a 'stress-index' consisting of the answers to seven items: (1) feeling stressed, (2) difficulties with sleep, (3) constantly tired, everything overwhelming, (4) fits of fear, (5) nervous and unbalanced, (6) headache without visual pheomena, and (7) ulcer-like pains in upper stomach. The highest index

value was 7, being maximally 'stressed', the lowest 0, indicating none of the seven symptoms. Table 24.5 gives the distribution of index values. 50 per cent of the total indicated one item or more. 91 per cent had an index score lower than the arithmetical mean value of the index.

Comparing the four facets: physical/chemical complaints, the number and distribution of symptoms, job satisfaction, and 'stress index' values, gives rise to the question of how to describe the working conditions in numerical terms. A provisional answer is that the measure of job satisfaction gives a different result from normative measures such as the number of symptoms and of physical/chemical complaints. There is a significant covariance between the four measures, as expected.

The population can be divided into fifty groups according to the union membership. The differences between groups in respect to each facet are considerable. The industrial workers in the footwear, ceramic, clothing, and sweets industries had 6 symptoms or more, their job satisfaction index values were less than 14·5, and they indicated 1·4 stress items or more. But the same workers were not in the high score group when asked about physical/chemical complaints. The high scoring unions on physical/chemical complaints were the plumbers' and tinsmiths', shipwrights', painters', leather-dressers', and dental mechanics' unions. The unions mentioned in connection with the three other facets scored mean frequencies on chemical/physical complaints. A definite explanation for these findings cannot be given. A possible way to explain the process of accumulating symptoms and producing a high 'stress index'—score might be to assume that all or some of the items constituting the job satisfaction index determine

TABLE 24.2

Frequencies of symptoms distributed by sex and age

Symptoms	Males			Females		
	–24 years	25–49 years	50 years–	–24 years	25–49 years	50 years–
Lumbar pains during lifting	19	25	30	16	22	31
Dorsal pains extending to the legs	8	16	23	9	15	24
Muscular pains in upper back	18	22	25	32	41	39
Other dorsal pains	21	23	26	16	21	27
Pains in knee or hip	11	14	23	4	11	24
Pains in wrist or arm	15	14	16	18	23	30
Bent fingers	1	3	6	1	1	4
Swollen joints of hands or fingers	2	2	4	1	4	12
Numb white fingers	2	3	7	2	5	11
Hand or arm eczma	8	6	5	12	8	4
Foot or leg eczma	4	5	6	3	2	2
Impaired hearing (conversation)	7	10	21	3	4	13
Impaired hearing (telephone or door bell)	3	5	15	1	1	8
Smarting eyes	11	15	15	21	19	21
Tired and painful eyes	8	10	11	16	14	15
Nausea	5	4	4	8	6	8
Pains in upper stomach	15	15	15	14	16	16
Pains in lower stomach	9	10	10	8	8	10
Constipation or diarrhoea	5	9	9	8	14	15
Pains or itching at the anus	8	13	13	2	7	5
Fits of coughing several times per day	7	7	14	4	5	10
Fits of asthma	1	1	3	1	1	2
Shortness of breath by effort	8	12	22	8	9	13
Chest pains by effort	3	5	9	3	3	7
Difficulties of sleep	10	15	19	10	14	29
Constantly tired— everything overwhelming	8	11	17	15	21	26
Fits of fear	3	4	4	6	6	7
Nervous and unbalanced	12	14	13	19	22	20
Dizzy or fainting	3	3	4	7	6	6
Sexual problems	7	8	9	6	8	7
Feeling stressed	16	27	23	23	30	33
Varicose veins	2	10	18	3	18	33
Cold feet	11	10	13	37	31	21
Headache without visual phenomena or nausea	8	9	8	16	19	18
Headache with visual phenomena or nausea	15	18	13	28	28	20
Frequent common colds	23	16	16	19	12	13
Itching or painful urination	2	1	3	2	3	3
Difficulties in self-control	4	2	5	2	4	7
Number of respondents	600	2700	1500	440	1300	450

TABLE 24.3

The respondents' indication of the causes of symptoms

Causes are to be found:	per cent
especially at work	26
especially not at work	5
both at work and not at work	37
no answer or cause can be indicated	33
Total	100

Number of indicated symptoms: 34 501

TABLE 24.4

Job satisfaction. Distribution of index values
Total investigated population

Index value	Per cent	Number of respondents
6 (lowest)	0	1
7	0	8
8	0	14
9	1	59
10	2	99
11	2	152
12 (mean)	6	349
13	8	490
14	12	709
15	16	964
16	23	1387
17	21	1272
18 (highest)	9	551
Total	100	6055
Number of respondents	6055	

TABLE 24.5

'Stress index'. Distribution of index values
Total investigated population

Index value	Per cent	Number of respondents
0 (not stressed)	50	3296
1	22	1423
2	12	817
3	7	470
4	5	320
5	2	156
6	1	74
7 (stressed)	1	24
Total	100	6580
Number of respondents	6580	

the influence of the physical/chemical factors or are determining factors themselves. It is reasonable to exclude genetic and non-work factors until we have explained differences between unions as we do not think that selection for different jobs and union membership gives more than a small part of the explanation.

The third kind of medical research which has to be mentioned consists of pamphlet-like 'critical' studies. These studies have had an immense political effect as they alerted public opinion to the medical, psychological, and social problems connected with the work situation. The reports on bacon factories, breweries, and the working conditions of painters (e.g. Bryggeri-rapporten 1972) have not made any contributions to knowledge seen from a positivistic point of view. But their findings have focused attention on the experiences of the workers themselves, with the effect of introducing behavioural science methods into occupational medicine.

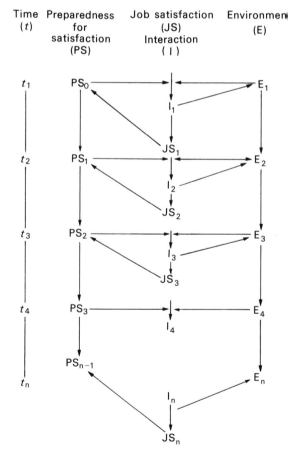

FIG. 24.1 A concept of job satisfaction (Petersen *et al.* 1968).

182

RESEARCH ON JOB SATISFACTION

During the last ten years a special analytical tradition has dominated Danish research in the fields of job satisfaction. The analytical tool has been constructed in collaboration between a psychologist and a statistician. As an outsider of medical origin I have not the ability to evaluate the tool. My object is simply to account for the most essential features of the research.* For further information the reader is referred to Petersen et al. (1968). Eggert Petersen defines his concept of job satisfaction as 'the current, dynamic preparedness for satisfaction than in interaction between a given individual and a given, current environment has left in the individual'. Schematically he describes the process leading to a current preparedness as follows (Fig. 24.1).

The essential content of Petersen's theory of job satisfaction is that job satisfaction is not a stable trait, but a dynamic state of mind. The theory explains how it is possible to have high job satisfaction even if the environment is not good as seen from a normative point of view, namely by emphasizing experience as the determining factor.

The analytical tool devised to work up the data has been called a 'model for measurement'. The actual data are answers to a certain number of questions (items). The questions are put in a rigid way: How contented are you with . . . .? The alternatives to the questions are: (1) excellently; (2) well; (3) quite; (4) not especially. The purpose of the model for measurement is to assume a functional relationship between the variables investigated and to control whether the actual data are able to fit into the model. The special strength of Rasch's model is that both the questions and the persons answering them can be characterized by the parameters of the statistical model. As the questions deal with the different qualities of the job, you will get a parameter concerning the single quality. The mode of estimating the parameters allows a comparison between the items by comparing the numerical value of the parameters. In the same way one can describe each individual's general tendency to answer the questions in the affirmative or the negative, i.e. you get an overall measure of the individual's job satisfaction.

In their basic research on job satisfaction Petersen et al. (1968), using the concept of job satisfaction and the

TABLE 24.6

Factors contributing to job satisfaction

Empirical factors	Interpreted factors:
(1) The factory's internal managerial function	The measure of individual-oriented 'modern' managerial initiative, existing in the social system of the factory as concerns physical environmental conditions, organization, establishing of roles, recruitment, adjustment, intercommunication, and sanctioning.
(2) The factory's policies regarding co-operation and welfare	The factory management's individual-oriented attitude toward welfare and co-operation.
(3) The number of positive variants for the supervisor†	The supervisor's current tendency to create job satisfaction among his co-workers.
(4) Supervisor's place of recruitment	To what degree the supervisor's position is marginal.
(5) Percentage of supervisors in work group	Supervisional intensity in group per group member.
(6) Size of work group	Intensity of contact in work group (including supervisor)
(7) Solidarity parameter for workers	Group dynamics as expressed by solidarity within the group.
(8) Physical space available	The group members' requirements as regards freedom of movement.
(9) Wages	Only job satisfaction factor with negative effect in the sense that the factor can primarily cause lack of job satisfaction (when the wages are considerably lower than expected) and only has a job satisfaction producing effect during short periods (e.g. immediately after a raise in wages).
(10) Predisposition for job satisfaction††	Expression of worker's current set of general expectations of his work.

†Established on the basis of nine biological personal factors proved to correlate with the work's experienced job satisfacton.

††Established on the basis of nineteen biological personal factors proved to correlate with the workers experienced job satisfaction.

*A list of reports and publications from the Research Institute of Mental Hygiene is available from: Professor Eggert Petersen, Arhus Universitet, DK 8000, Arhus C, Denmark.

analysis outlined above, arrive at the relevant job satisfaction factors tabulated in Table 24.6.

The 19 biographical personal factors mentioned in the second footnote to Table 24.6 are described as follows:

It is, incidentally, surprising from an everyday point of view to see what in a factor may be a positive variant, and what may constitute a negative variant. Thus, in the sex factor 'female' is a positive variant and 'male' a negative one—in other words, women in general thrive better than men. Correspondingly, unskilled, for instance, thrive better than skilled, younger workers better than older ones, persons from homes that have been broken up by divorce better than persons from normal homes, persons with only elementary schooling better than more highly educated ones, workers who have undergone some kind of post-school training thrive less well than persons without such additional training; workers who have not participated in study groups thrive better than those who have; workers who have worked at several different places thrive

better than workers, who have only worked at one and the same place; workers with low seniority thrive better than those with a greater length of service; unmarried persons thrive better than the married; childless persons better than those with children; persons, who hold no position as shop stewards or other positions of trust, better than those who have positions of this kind.

These 'surprising' correlations—the development of which is 'contrary' to what might seem plausible from an everyday point of view—are explained in the investigation on the basis of the conceptual model for job satisfaction. . . .

A considerable number of public and private enterprises have been investigated by the method described. The astonishing result has been that the job satisfaction measured has been quite high in nearly every place. As a consequence of these findings the group is now undertaking a study including a set of medical symptoms. It seems as if medical and behavioural science research will be unified in the future.

REFERENCES

ANDERSEN, R. *et al.* (1964–7). *The physically handicapped in Denmark. Vol. I-VI*, Publications from the Danish National Institute of Social Research, Copenhagen.

ANDERSEN, E. (1970). *Three-shift work.* Publications from the Danish National Institute of Social Research, Copenhagen.

BOLINDER, E., MAGNUSSON, E., and NYRÉN, L. (1970). *Risker i jobbet*: LO-enkäten, Lund.

BRYGGERIRAPPORTEN (1972), Copenhagen.

PETERSEN, E. *et al.* (1968). *Trivsel pa arbejdspladsen.* Publ. from the Research Institute of Mental Hygiene, Copenhagen.

REDDER, K. W., SVANE, O., and WESTERGAARD, P. W. (1970). *Report on the survey of working conditions.* Published as part of Rapport nr. 2 Arbejdsmiljogruppen af 1972, Copenhagen.

SVANE, O. (1973). A paper presented to a symposium arranged by The Danish Medical Research Council and the Danish Social Science Research Council on community medicine.

25. RELATIONSHIP BETWEEN ORGANIZATIONAL STRUCTURE AND OCCUPATIONAL MENTAL HEALTH. A REVIEW

ERLAND MINDUS

INTRODUCTION

Multiple causation

Occupational health services are rapidly changing their conceptions and goals with the increasing awareness of the multitude of factors operating and the intricate relation between them. This means that attention is not only directed at the classical objectives, such as the relation between specific occupational hazards and specific disorders, e.g., between quartz dust and silicosis, but also, increasingly, on the still more complex relationship between non-specific factors in the job situation and the accentuation of a number of non-specific disorders, such as musculoskeletal, cardio-vascular, and nervous disorders. These ailments are the main incapacitating disturbances on the labour market and the results of the impact of a number of psychosocial factors which accentuate the basic pathogenic causes.

As a consequence, occupational health services have to observe and try to identify those groups of employees who are at high risk: those who lack adequate occupational fitness and training, the elderly, mental high-risk groups, especially in the lower socio-economic field, and all those whose aspirations and mental make-up need a specific work setting to keep healthy.

Three facets

Besides this individually directed approach, attention has to be paid to the various facets or stages which constitute the work environment. Three sets of factors have to be integrated and manipulated: the set of technical hygiene factors with their biological impact; the social system which constitutes the work place, with a number of psychological factors and social roles directing the attitudes and behaviour in groups of employees; and, lastly, the impact of society with its norms and values, which not only set limits within which the organizations have to operate but also constitute an essential element in the individual's needs to find identity, security, and means to control anxiety. All these three sets of factors are constantly changing at an increasing rate, which means that the capacity to adjust to permanently changing situations is a major problem.

Occupational mental health

As a result of this trend, occupational health activities are splitting up into a number of subspecialities, of which occupational mental health is one that is rapidly growing. A second consequence is the organization of health services in order to be able to cope with the psychosocial problems involved in the work setting.

Occupational mental health has to integrate medical with psychological and sociological aspects. The expertise involved must be adequate to handle emotional problems and mental disturbances in their social setting. The main activity is, however, directed at training and the main groups of trainees are not emotionally sick. The goal is to train those responsible for the organization of work and for management in order to avoid factors in the job which produce conflicts and block co-operation. The long-range target is to help as many as possible to an optimal emotional development. This type of work calls for specialists on sub-conscious motivation and reaction-forming, on personality-developing factors, and on the relationship between environment and personality. A great deal of attention has to be paid to the effect of the actual organization in which the job is set, since the organization in itself has a tendency to affect the attitudes and behaviour of man and thus to influence mental and physical health.

Integrated services

The second consequence of the need for increased attention to psychosocial factors is the change in the organization of the occupational health services. One major implication is that these services have to be integrated in the business organization. Unless this is done the relationship between those who try to give service and those who are supposed to receive it will be negligible. If you are not a permanent member of the organization you will always stay in a consultant position and the effects of the services will be much less marked. (It is hardly necessary to mention that very small work places with a few employees need other types of services and that the goals have to be lowered.) The consequence of these principles, which are quite broadly accepted in Sweden, is that outside organizations such as various types of community health services, even if they are sophisticated and expertly directed, will have consider-able difficulty in achieving results in the life of the working organizations. This does not obviate the great need for some kind of co-operation between these occupational health activities and the health services organized at national level.

Occupational health services: three aspects

Up till now the main parts of the occupational health services have rested on two pillars, one technical and the

185

other medical. The first takes care of classical safety problems, technical hygiene, and ergonomic activities and has to control the factors which have direct biological consequences. The medical part is concerned with prevention, treatment, and rehabilitation as well as with various counselling health information programmes. As a result of the development described earlier, these two parts have to be combined with a third group of activities, mainly directed at observing and handling psychosocial problems. These specialists are supposed to study attitudes and values which are operating in the various groups of employees, and the degree and different types of adjustment to work and life which can be observed in the organization, to help to minimize conflicts and disturbances in adjustment, to analyse and give advice when relationships between individuals or groups are upset, and to observe effects of changes in the organization of work.

This trend to develop occupational health services into a more refined tool is now very much accepted in Sweden. These principles are characteristic of the services which are organized in the public administration. In the organization of the National Road Board with 15 000 employees, seven regional teams of doctors, technicians, and psychosocial experts try to handle the problems of health in relation to work in an organization. The background for being able to get resources like these is the general public awareness of the importance of occupational mental health activities. One factor which improved the general interest was a national campaign on occupational mental health, which was run in Sweden in the years 1968–70. In this campaign almost twenty thousand persons took part in study groups on their jobs, discussing various aspects of their job situation in relation to health and satisfaction. Another background factor is the general and very intense public interest in various facets of the work environment, which interest is condensed in a steady and very rapid refinement of the laws regarding safety and health. A third aspect of considerable importance has been the results achieved at the Laboratory for Clinical Stress Research in Stockholm, as well as those of the Swedish Council for Social Science Research.

On the international level, much interest has been focused in the International Committee on Occupational Mental Health, which has been active since 1964. In this group experiences have been pooled from the European countries as well as from the United States. The emphasis on the psychosocial parameters of occupational health has constantly been stressed.

ORGANIZATIONAL STRUCTURE AND OCCUPATIONAL MENTAL HEALTH

The relationship between organizational structure and ocupational mental health can be described in three parts: the relationship between personality and type of job, the type of organization and the interplay of expectations, and dependence between the enterprise and those working in it, the so-called 'psychological contract'.

Personality

When the labour market is functioning reasonably well, which means that there is a sufficient diversification for people to choose between professions and jobs, people try to find types of job which are in accordance with their prerequisites and their personality's needs. If the selection process is effective the choice of vocation will satisfy these needs and fit into the specific ways in which each personality reacts. The result is that, to some extent, in different occupations we will find different persons with different personality types. In department stores, in steelmills with the shift-workers around the furnaces, in the consulting business, and the other free enterprises the difference between people may be extreme. There is nothing very special in this observation. But the practical consequences are largely overlooked, and this creates problems for occupational mental health.

When discussing the need for changes in the structure of business and administration, both private and public, there is a lot of discussion about the necessity for everybody from time to time being forced to change profession. But very little is said about the difficulties which may arise if the relationship between personality and type of job is broken. People are looked upon as plugs which can fit any type of hole without losing effectiveness or incurring personal losses. In reality, the breaking up of this relationship between personality and type of job is in many cases intensely traumatic and the personal losses are never compensated. The end results are easily studied in the work of occupational health officers and in the rapid increase of disablement pensions.

The prevention of these mishaps involves training for change, training in accepting new roles, in giving long-range support during the change, and explaining to those involved the types of reactions noted. In these respects occupational mental health experts may be able to give advice and help management to make their decisions more in accordance with the personal needs of those involved.

Just as individuals choose types of job in order to satisfy specific needs, so if possible they choose the type of organization which fits their individual personality. The drives that make people look for 'their' special type of organization have much to do with dependence, security, and obsessive–compulsive traits. Institutions with a high degree of stability and a lot of red tape attract a different kind of personality from those with a minimum of organization and a lot of variation in the structure. Inside all organizations a gradual selection process concentrates a number of personalities who are similar in character and who act more or less uniformly. This tendency is accentuated by the common social background of the participants, their training and acceptance of common policies, and a certain amount of inbreeding'. The end result will be that those employed in an organization often perceive the enterprise as unique and having a 'personality'. Thus it is possible to note a kind of similarity between the personalities of those employed and the style of the organization.

Subconscious interplay

From the occupational mental health view this more or less subconscious interplay between the needs of people and the type of organization has a profound influence. The rapid change of the industrialized and urbanized society tends to break up old relations, disintegrate the family structure, bring loss of identity, and make people anonymous. The result is that they rely more on their work and the organization to retain identity and keep down anxiety. The relation between the organization and those employed in it consequently will have an emotional tone and does not only imply employment and maintenance. This emotionally charged interplay colours the perception of almost everything that happens inside the organization. Praise, promotion, and increased salary, as well as criticism, transfer, or dismissal are all heavily charged with emotions of the same type that coloured our relations to our parents and others during our childhood. We are all projecting feelings and experiences from early days on our relations on the job.

In every type of organization a number of people are seen who were hired under quite different conditions, who run into trouble and were transferred to other and very often lower positions, and who cannot accept what happened to them. Bitter, unhappy, and more or less paranoid, they are never able to turn their backs on what happened and try to make a new career. At the centre in all these cases is a feeling of a breach in the relation between employee and employer. They do not even accept that they are not fired out of consideration for their bad position on the labour market and for their families. All these cases are clear illustrations of the relationship between organization and occupational mental health activities.

Reciprocity in expectations and dependence

The third part of the relationship being described is that the enterprise also has expectations and is dependent on its relationship with its employees. The result is a reciprocity in expectations and dependence. If this proceeds in a healthy way, this interdependence will foster identification with job and organization and at the same time a feeling of freedom and mastery, which in itself is a condition to develop. It is easy to understand how such a relationship will promote job satisfaction, increase self-esteem, and thus promote mental health.

Conflicts

The interrelations between personality, job, and organization may frequently be subject to conflicts of various origin. Very often there is a combination of conflicts, which intermingle and add to the strain that is perceived. Those conflicts which are subconscious and chronic are more deleterious. Some conflicts are only formal, others are real, and some are pseudo-conflicts related to insufficient or distorted information.

Common and most difficult are the conflicts which are generated inside the personality. Problems with identity, difficulty in handling aggressions, free-floating or focused anxiety, distortion of reality, and projections will all start disturbances in the relationship. A very marked trend is the expression of neurotic anxiety by way of phobic reactions. In all these cases, distortions of relations to others are the central factor and consequently these types of problems are not seldom found at the roots of conflicts at the work place. The phobic panic effectively blocks co-operation. Thus in the very real conflicts centred around the constant fight for a larger part of the invariably insufficient resources, bitterness is not seldom added because one or perhaps several of those involved put extra heat in their arguments from unsolved internal conflicts of the type described. To these two causes of conflicts may not seldom be added a third: the classical types of conflicts generated by supervisory behaviour. By this is meant not only the ordinary problems of insufficient information or delegation, etc., but also the general attitude that the logical and rational aspects of a job can be discussed but only seldom the feelings and psychological relations between people. To discuss feelings is not rational and thus the conflicts stay unsolved. This attitude has not changed very much in spite of all the sensitivity training and other types of learning experiences which have been given in recent years.

To these three types of individual-centred conflicts may be added such which are inherent in the type of job, the type of organization, and the structural changes of both. One of the most discussed problems has been how modern industrialized society will be able to produce jobs that can satisfy psychological needs and keep people motivated. As long as this is not done, people experience the job situation as a conflict, expressed in low job satisfaction and various types and degrees of alienation. The relationship between the psychological job-structure and various mental health factors has been stresssed over and over again.

Reconstruction of jobs

In the last ten years in the Scandinavian countries a remarkable development has started to restructure jobs and their organization in order to break the almost automatic correspondence between job fragmentation and various indicators of low morale and decreasing mental health. It is a very hopeful sign that production engineering has added a new dimension to its thinking by integrating medical, sociological, and psychological aspects with the technological aspects. Production is now planned along socio-technical lines in order to satisfy the following needs:

The job must require something more than endurance and give variation in relation to the perceived subjective demands.

The job has to give the worker a possibility to learn something and go on learning.

The job must give possibilities to make decisions among alternatives.

The job and how it is done must give chances for gaining respect, recognition, and confidence.

The layout of the job has to allow the worker to see the connection between his job and the finished product which motivates the job.

The job must be part of personal growth and be in accordance with the values expressed in the personnel policies.

Comprehensive cost-benefit analysis
It is hard to exaggerate the importance of this improvement and to find how obsolete all those excuses are regarding the impossibility of changing production lines and techniques. It is clear that a high productivity can be maintained and perhaps increased if the design of the particular job makes the job-holder motivated. It is also quite clear that if the calculation of production costs includes the costs involved in labour turnover, absenteeism, conflicts, and dissatisfaction, including strikes, these ambitions to improve the job will be seen as a necessity. It is also quite clear that a modern developed society will not stay passive and just watch how people on the job lose their ambitions and potential for growth, become resigned, and develop various signs of decreasing physical and mental health.

Adapting to rapid changes
At the same time as the design of jobs is changing, it is noticeable how rapidly the structure and organization is changing. Both in private companies and in public utilities the trend is towards greater and greater flexibility, with continual restructuring as the only constant element. This means that conflicts produced by defects in the organization will frequently be noted but the time required to deal with them will not be available since this particular part of the organization will soon be reshaped. Consequently, besides the dominant demand to live with and adjust to a constant change, all the classical and very frequent problems arising from role conflicts, role ambiguity, working in marginal positions, and so on will act as stressors. To work in an everchanging organization means being able to establish and break relations and at the same time be strained by role conflicts or other shortcomings of the organizational structure.

Conflicting trends
Decentralizing and dispersing responsibility to regional parts of an organization are the ambitions of everyone and consequently there are great expectations of sharing increasing parts of authority. In reality the trend is very

much in the opposite direction. Computerized data collecting always gives the important information first to the central administration and, having this information nobody will be able to dispute authority or the right of this administration to make the necessary decisions on behalf of those in regional departments. This clash between ongoing centralization of power and the expectations of sharing responsibility is a constant source of conflicts.

One important respect of redesigning the job and the organizational structure is that those working in enterprises, private or public, more and more frequently demand to express their opinions on how it should be done. In reality they are fighting for a contributory influence. The more this influence is felt, the less strained by conflicts will the participants be. They share the responsibility, and this is excellent psychotherapy.

As noted earlier, one or more of the above-mentioned conflicts may be present at the same time, adding to the pressure that is experienced. The resulting reactions will be determined by a number of factors.

Interaction within the group
One of these is the interplay between the strained person and the group around him. In time there is a kind of feedback between the person with his conflicts and those around him, who suffer from the symptoms of his personal stress. For instance the aggressiveness of the strained individual might produce hostility from those around him and thus increase temperature. The same situation is very often found around the paranoic personality.

Another set of factors which determine the type of reaction is the stability of the way in which the individual adjusts to his situation. This is often expressed by the term frustration tolerance. This kind of tolerance has much to do with training to meet and handle conflicts. It is clear that far too many people do not get the necessary amount of this training.

Ego strength
Besides conflict training, ego strength is a most important element. One aspect of ego strength is to be able to use the same rational and low-risk way of handling conflict situations. There is a kind of hierarchy of adjustment mechanisms for solving conflicts according to which, if the strain is low, the adaptive mechanisms are mild, not very radical, and involve no risks. If the conflict is not solved and the strain increases, the attempts to adjust become more radical but at the same time involve some risk. At the far end of this hierarchy of adaptive mechanisms is the destructive one with maladjustment, fixation in a sick role, or flight into a psychosis. Ego strength means that even if the strain is considerable or intense, the adaptive mechanisms used are not destructive.

Types of reactions
The types of reactions might be divided into social and

clinical symptoms. The first are observed by the fellow workers, the supervisors, the personnel department, and to an increasing extent by the unions and outside organizations such the national boards for the labour market, health, safety, and others. The clinical symptoms are registered by the occupational health departments in collaboration with the supervisors and the personnel departments.

The social signs are, besides high labour turnover, all kinds of absenteeism and different types of flight mechanisms, passing over into sick roles, grumbling, expression of aggressions, including strikes, and lastly and most dangerous of all, the loss of potential for personal growth. The last is in the long term a mortal threat to the survival of any enterprise.

The clinical symptoms are weariness, emotional reactions, depressions with their apathy, the release of other types of mental disturbances, and psychosomatic diseases and the accentuation of other ailments.

Complex interconnections

In the introductory part of this paper I stressed the multifactorial genesis of occupational diseases. At this point it is necessary to discuss the connections between work and mental health. The number of factors operating in this relation are many and it is difficult to get a clear picture of the relative importance of each one. Numerous studies have been done concerning these problems, but many of them have not avoided the pitfall of confusing statistical correlation with causal connection. Parts of this relationship appear to be reasonably clear, other are only assumptions but fit into a frame of reference.

First of all there is the nature of the job, estimated from the psychological view as described earlier. The content of factors motivating the worker's contribution to the enterprise bears a relationship to job satisfaction. Job satisfaction is influenced by the amount of aspirations and expectations that are centred on the job. This means that some kind of job satisfaction may be noted for a particular worker simply because the worker has no aspirations or has become resigned to having none and is therefore not actively dissatisfied. Assuming that real job satisfaction is observed, its quality will affect the attitude to the job and to the job-holder. If the attitude to the job is good, it is reflected in an equally good attitude to the ego. Here, too, mediating factors intervene, such as those related to status. The quality of the attitudes derived from the job act as a reinforcement or the reverse for self-esteem. To the medical profession it is clear that maintaining good health in a person with low self-esteem is impossible. The degree of self-esteem or its total absence influence the perception of pains or other symptoms and determine where on the continuity from health to sickness and sick role the person in question will stay.

Stamping out

This is easily demonstrated by what is happening to large groups of employees who lose their jobs or are transferred to jobs which are worse or are perceived as worse. Most of them have been working happily and with reasonable capacity in spite of some kind of disorder, for instance musculoskeletal or cardiovascular. They have had their low-back pain or chest pain without the interpretation that they are sick or passing into a sick role. As soon as their job situation is changed in the above manner, the same ailment will no longer be accepted. From this moment they are not merely complaining but suffering and consequently accept the sick role. Shorter and shorter work spells will be interfoliated with longer and longer sick-leaves and after two or three years whole segments of this part of the population will have taken their disability pensions and left the labour market. In thinly populated areas with little work available, this process will start as soon as notice is given of dismissal.

There are thus reasons to believe that how the job is shaped and in which structure the job is placed have a profound bearing on mental health. Consequently one of the essential goals of occupational health is to promote mental health.

Finally two examples will be cited to illustrate these discussions. They are both from the occupational health services in the National Road Board in Sweden.

Job organization and health

In these services regular health checks are made of all employees. The results from one region with 1300 persons have been compared with those from 80 000 health checks in the private construction business, all examined with the same technique. Corrections were made for age and smoking habits. The examinations were based on extensive health interviews and interviews concerning the job situation, including the work environment. All the individuals have been medically examined. From the physical findings the employees of the Road Board have more obesity, higher blood pressure, more chronic bronchitis and more diabetes than the controls. There are furthermore a number of disorders related to their type of work. Compared with the controls the group has a lower incidence of nervous complaints, fewer cases of depressions, has less often seen doctors, for these complaints, and fewer times been in hospital. The social background of both groups and the type of job they are doing are identical. There is a difference in the terms of employment. The primary group of 1300 are employed by the state, which mostly means lifelong employment. The second difference is that this same group has a different job organization in that they all work in very small groups dispersed around the country. These groups, of mostly around twenty persons, have a high degree of autonomy in how they arrange their work, who does what, and how this is done. This is reflected in a high degree of job satisfaction and in an exceedingly high stability of this population. There are strong reasons for believing that the low incidence of mental disorders in the examined group is related in some way to the organizational structure of the job.

Overtime, conflicts, and health

The second example is taken from examinations of supervisors and a corresponding control group of shop foremen, both groups being matched for social background age, and so on. The first study was done ten years earlier and the result showed that the supervisors had a higher incidence of cardiovascular and nervous disorders than the controls. The two groups differed in one respect: the supervisors had more overtime and more conflicts with the public. The analyses showed that these stressors reasonably well explained the increased incidence of nervous and cardiovascular disorders.

Ten years later the same examination was done with another sample of supervisors and their controls and with very much the same technique. In the meantime overtime had been considerably reduced and the earlier conflicts with the public had lost their character of stressors. Everything else was identical with the first study. The higher incidences of nervous and cardiovascular disorders had now disappeared. There are reasons for believing that the improved job situation had improved both mental and physical health in the observed group.

SUMMARY

Aims, policies, and organization of occupational mental health are discussed as well as the stressor roles of problems in the structure of the job and the organizations. Types of reactions are described and relationships between job factors and health are outlined.

26. THE INDIVIDUAL AND HIS WORK IN RELATION TO A MYOCARDIAL INFARCTION

TÖRES THEORELL, EVY LIND, ULF LUNDBERG, TONY CHRISTENSSON, and OLOF EDHAG

WORK ADDICTION AND CHD

'Hard work never killed anybody' has been a common notion in work-oriented, urbanized societies. This statement, however, has been challenged recently by several authors. Hinkle (1974) and co-workers showed the men who combined 'night college' and full-time work in the Bell company had a significant excess cardiac mortality.

Since the onset of a myocardial infarction implies a risk of cardiac death, studies on cardiac morbidity in relation to the work situation are also relevant to this question. Buell and Breslow (1960), Biörck et al. (1968), Weiss et al. (1957) and Russek and Zohman (1958) have found in retrospective studies that men who developed myocardial infarctions before regular retirement age had been working excessively long hours for long periods more often than control subjects.

The above-mentioned studies dealt with objective criteria such as number of hours of work in relation to coronary heart disease. However, a number of studies also indicate that potential candidates of coronary heart disease at a young age seem to have had different attitudes to work than comparable non-candidates. Bonami and Rimé (1972) made projective personality tests (thematic apperception tests) in 11 000 industrial workers and followed them up seven years later. Among the findings they reported was the observation that men who developed myocardial infarctions had been much more preoccupied with thoughts about work than had comparable men who did not develop the disease. This preoccupation with work took place at the expense of thoughts about family and recreation.

Rosenman and co-workers have reported a 'behaviour pattern', which they call type A, to be associated with excess morbidity in coronary heart disease below the age of 60. It is characterized by 'drive', 'ambition', and 'impatience'. This behaviour pattern also has a dimension of seriousness and competitiveness in the work situation, and this was associated per se with the probability of developing coronary heart disease—the greater the competitiveness, the greater the risk (Jenkins 1974).

Liljefors and Rahe (1970) have studied retrospectively a group of monozygotic twin pairs discordant for coronary heart disease— one twin had manifest clinical coronary heart disease, and the other did not. They found that the twin who had developed the disease tended to be the one who reported himself to have shown the greater devotion to work. Wolf (1969) and co-

workers have pointed out that the combination of working hard and being dissatisfied with work (Sisyphus pattern) may be crucial.

Medalie et al. (1973) were able to show, in a large prospective study, that a feeling of lack of appreciation from superiors is indeed a 'CHD risk factor'. A related finding may be that of Hinkle (1974), who demonstrated that a low level of education may be associated with an elevated risk of developing premature coronary heart disease.

To summarize the literature on a person's work situation and his risk of developing 'premature' manifestations of coronary heart disease: 'Work addiction' seems to elevate the risk of developing the disease. It is not known whether 'work addiction' in a person mainly reflects a genetic trait or whether environmental work conditions form this 'behaviour'. Ongoing research on monozygotic twin pairs may provide information about this question (Rahe et al. 1974; Flodérus 1974).

So far the problem has been described only from the point of view of the individual in his work. The next question is: How is the work situation related to other factors relevant to the development of an acute myocardial infarction?

PREDISPOSING AND PRECIPITATING FACTORS

In order to probe this question we have to distinguish between predisposing and precipitating factors. Among circumstances known or supposed to increase the risk of developing 'premature' myocardial infarction are the following predisposing factors:

(a) Ageing
(b) High serum cholesterol — genetic traits diet, environment
(c) High blood pressure — genetic traits, environmental influences
(d) Cigarette smoking — genetic traits, link with personality, environmental influences
(e) Behaviour pattern A — genetic traits, environmental influences

Precipitating factors may be defined as factors which may increase a susceptible person's risk of developing a myocardial infarction within a short period of time, e.g.

within a year. Such factors may be divided into the following groups:

(a) Diseases which increase the demands on the organism, e.g. anaemia, infectious diseases, abnormal hormonal production (e.g. pheochromocytoma and adrenocortical tumours);
(b) Physical overload, e.g. heavy manual work (Elmfeldt 1974);
(c) Psychosocial stressors, e.g. accumulation of important life events within a short period of time.

The precipitating factors may act by increasing the demands on the myocardium (e.g. catecholamines increase the pulse rate and the blood pressure; these hormones have an increased output during periods of distress and/or adaptation) or by facilitating the formation of clots in the coronary arteries (Ardlie *et al.* 1966). The effects of the behaviour pattern may be mediated by several mechanisms, one of which may have to do with the propensity to *react* physiologically to psychosocial or physical stimuli (see below). All the factors may be influenced by both the genetics and the environment of the individual. Pertinent to the work environment are the following findings. An increased work load as well as dietary factors have been associated with an elevated serum cholesterol (Friedman *et al.* 1958). The feeling of a lack of appreciation at work has been related to an elevated blood pressure (Groen *et al.* 1968). Finally, it is well known that the amount a person smokes is influenced to a large extent by pressures and strains at work as well as by the habits of workmates (Frith 1971). Thus, in predisposing factors we have indirect evidence for the assumption that the interplay of the actual work environment and the individual's acting in it may profoundly influence his probability of developing a 'premature' myocardial infarction through effects on known risk factors.

Psychosocial factors may also be *precipitating* in the sense mentioned above. Being widowed was associated with an increased risk of dying a cardiac death within half a year after the spouse died in an English study (Parkers *et al.* 1969). In a similar way, retirement (Jores and Puchta 1959) and marriage (Lew 1957) have been associated with an increased mortality in cardiac death. Thus, it may be that significant life events may act as precipitators. This hypothesis has been supported in retrospective studies using the life change measurement technique proposed by Holmes and Rahe. These studies demonstrated a build-up of reported life changes during the last half-year prior to disease onset (Theorell and Rahe 1971; Rahe and Paasikivi 1971; Rahe and Lind 1971; Rahe *et al.* 1974a).

With regard to changes in the work environment as a *precipitating* factor, Hinkle (1974) and co-workers have studied transitions, promotions, and demotions in the Bell company in relation to mortality and morbidity in coronary heart disease. They were not able to demonstrate any excess mortality or morbidity in these work change situations. They did conclude, however, that periods of unusually hard work often preceded the acute attacks. Russek and Zohman (1958) also concluded, from a retrospective study, that a period of work overload often preceded the onset of a myocardial infarction.

Our own studies

The studies presented below focus on the following problems:

(1) If there are unexpectedly many changes in the life situation of people who develop a myocardial infarction, during the year before disease onset, do these changes tend to occur at work, in the family, or in some other area of life?
(2) What are the areas of life which the myocardial infarction patient claims that he has had a problem with? Is it work, family life, or some other area?

In a nation-wide defined population with one employer (the co-operative chain) the persons who had developed a myocardial infarction during 1970 or 1971 were selected for study. They were matched individually for age, sex, and kind of employment with subjects in the same population who had *not* developed a myocardial infarction. Both groups were asked to fill out a modified version of the schedule of recent experiences (Lind and Theorell 1973a)—a list of questions concerning life changes during the last 12 months preceding the disease onset or the enquiry, respectively. All the questionnaires were checked in a telephone interview. Table 26.1 shows how the reported changes for the last year were distributed in the two groups. The rates of participation for both steps were 56/69 (patients; 5 deaths since the original selection) and 65/69 (controls). The proportion with work change prior to illness onset was much greater in the patient group than in the control group (41 vs. 17 per cent $p < 0.01$). Most of the changes at work during the year prior to the onset of a myocardial infarction implied more *responsibility* or *more conflicts*. For non-work-related areas only marginal differences were observed.

The patients and controls in this study were also asked to rate how *upsetting* they considered that the listed changes would be if they happen to them and also how much adjustment the respective changes would require. The ratings were made graphically on a horizontal line. Table 26.2 shows ratings of upsettingness of the changes in the two groups. Some areas, particularly those related to work, were considered much more upsetting by the patients Examples of this were the start of an extra job (20 versus 2, $p < 0.01$) and decreased responsibility at work (49 versus 29, $p < 0.05$). The amount of *adjustment* required by the changes at work was also claimed to be larger by the patients than by the control subjects, e.g. increased responsibility (48 versus 25, $p < 0.01$).

Out of five significant differences (at least $p < 0.05$), three concerned working life. The expected ratio would be 12/46, which represents the listed number of items concerned with work divided by the total number of listed items. Thus, in these subjective retrospective self-reports, working life stands out as a crucial area (Lind and Theorell 1973a).

In general, several of the retrospectively reported differences between patients and control groups may be due to the patient's own knowledge of his diagnosis. Therefore, a prospective study was undertaken. This study (Theorell and Flodérus–Myrhed 1977) started in September 1972. The study group consisted of all male members aged between 41 and 61 of the union of build-ing construction workers in greater Stockholm ($N = 8973$). They were asked by post to fill out a psychosocial questionnaire. All those who did not respond to the initial request were reminded once and then again, if necessary, but after this 25 per cent had still failed to respond. However, the non-responders were demon-strated not to differ significantly from the responders with regard to occupational group, age, number of sick-leave days during the past year, marital status, and income. Furthermore, in a follow-up of their health records, both groups were observed to have com-parable incidences of myocardial infarction. 219

TABLE 26.1

Frequency of reported life change items during the year prior to a myocardial infarction

	Patients ($N = 56$)	Controls ($N = 65$)
Change of profession	2	1
Retirement	0	0
Change in work schedule	7	1
Increased responsibility	6	2
Decreased responsibility	2	2
Conflict with superiors	7	2
Conflict with colleagues	8	4
Out of work > 1 month	0	3
Other changes at work	10	7
Start or end of extra job	5	4
Courses for the job	6	15
Change of income	15	26
Other changes in financial state	9	8
Marriage	0	0
Separation or start of divorce	0	1
End of divorce	1	1
Conflict with spouse	3	3
Conflict within family	5	3
Conflict with relatives	3	1
Temporary separation from spouse > 1 month (no conflict)	0	2
Spouse start or stop working	9	3
Addition of family member	0	0
Change in sexual habits	13	13
Spouse seriously ill	5	5
Spouse deceased	0	0
Child seriously ill	1	2
Child deceased	0	0
Close relative seriously ill	14	14
Close relative deceased	4	4
Close friend seriously ill	6	7
Close friend deceased	3	3
Change of residence	2	2
Addition of member of household (not family)	0	0
Exit of member of family or household	9	11
Change in living conditions	15	17
Change in social habits	12	7
Accidents leading to more than 3 weeks sick leave	5	0

retired subjects and 1317 subjects who had had a long-lasting illness episode during the last year were excluded from the study which thus comprised 5187 subjects.

The questionnaire comprised about 60 items regarding

TABLE 26.2

*Ratings of the 'upsettingness' of individual
'life change items'*

	Patients	Controls
Change of profession	41	36
Retirement	41	27
Start of extra job	35	22
End of extra job	20	2
Attending a course for the job	18	7
Change in work schedule	59	48
Increased responsibility	34	20
Decreased responsibility	49	29
Conflict with superiors	59	47
Conflict with colleagues	47	53
Out of work > 1 month	62	75
Other changes at work	55	48
Increased income	11	3
Decreased income	62	64
Decreased expenses	9	5
Increased expenses	58	47
Marriage	51	58
Start of divorce	81	88
End of divorce	77	77
Conflict with spouse	75	72
Conflict within family	81	75
Conflict with relatives	53	44
Temporary separation from spouse > 1 month (no conflict)	43	37
Spouse start work	20	30
Spouse end work	22	11
Addition of family member	44	31
Change in sexual habits	53	23
Spouse seriously ill	90	86
Spouse deceased	98	98
Child seriously ill	88	90
Child deceased	97	98
Close relative seriously ill	58	62
Close relative deceased	66	70
Close friend seriously ill	48	57
Close friend deceased	61	64
Change of residence	32	17
Addition of member of household (not family)	39	37
Exit of member of family or household	39	25
Change in living conditions	10	7
Change in social habits	17	9
Change in personal habits	25	20

life events during the last year, psychological attitudes, and social background. Factor analysis revealed three clusters of variables. One of these comprised only work variables and was designated 'workload'. Table 26.4 shows the variables included in it, as well as the frequencies in the total study group, in the group of men who developed a myocardial infarction (deaths and survivals) during the initial two-year follow-up and among men who survived a myocardial infarction during the same period. For the majority of variables, higher frequencies were observed in the prospectively ill groups. This was particularly true for the survivors of a myocardial infarction. Table 26.5 shows the observed and age-adjusted expected frequencies of 'workload' (i.e. reporting at least one of the items included in the cluster shown in Table 26.4 in subjects who developed a myocardial infarction during the follow-up. The most marked differences between observed and expected frequencies were found for the survivors (53 vs. 25 per cent, $p < 0.001$) and among those for whom statements regarding previous history of coronary heart disease were *available and negative* ($N = 31$, 48 vs. 25 per cent, $p < 0.01$). No difference was found for the group of subjects who *died* from the infarction ($N = 19$, 11 vs. 23 per cent, n.s.).

The prospective study of middle-aged building construction workers thus demonstrated an association between factors such as extra work, changes in extra work, changes in responsibility, 'wrong' amount of responsibility, conflicts at the work place, and threat of unemployment during one year, on the one hand, and elevated risk of myocardial infarction during a subsequent two-year period on the other. As in Hinkle's (1974) study of the Bell telephone company, *objective promotion* (i.e. becoming the boss of a team of workers) was not associated *per se* with increased risk. Thus, it could be concluded that an interplay of environmental and individual factors is important in the pathogenesis.

It should be pointed out that the recording of myocardial infarctions comprised only cases with definite evidence of this illness and also that the incidence of myocardial infarction in this group was the same as that of the age-comparable male population of greater Stockholm. Two other 'clusters' of psychosocial variables, 'unsatisfactory family conditions' and 'changes in family structure last year', were not associated with risk of myocardial infarction. Nor was psychosocial 'work load' associated with risk of subsequent 'serious accident', 'ulcer or long-lasting gastritis', or 'degenerative joint disease' during the follow-up.

The workers with the physically heaviest work, the concrete workers, were demonstrated to have about twice the myocardial infarction incidence of the other building construction workers. This was particularly evident in the older half of the studied population. A closer examination of the job situation of the concrete workers (Theorell *et al.* 1977a; Theorell and Olsson 1955) indicated that they had been forced to start this unskilled work during early childhood due to poor financial circumstances, that they thus had less education at the start than other workers, that their work had been and was still markedly more strenuous than other construction work, and that their present work had lower status than other building work (even though concrete work today requires as much technical skill). Thus, a number of psychosocial and physical factors may be involved.

One way of illuminating the relative importance of the work environment from a pathophysiological standpoint is to monitor physiological changes during discussions about work, family, finances, and other possible problem areas with the patient. 22 interviews were performed with the same number of male patients below 55 years of age who had all survived a myocardial infarction at least 3 months but not more than 6 months before the study. Electrocardiograms were recorded

TABLE 26.4

Prevalence (per cent) of the single items included in the 'workload' index for the total study group and the MI subjects

		MI-group	
	Total study group $N = 5187$	Deaths and survivals $N = 51$	Survivals only $N = 32$
Change of profession	1·3	0	0
Extra job	4·6	8·2	13·3
Start of extra job	4·1	2·0	3·1
End of extra job	4·3	6·0	9·7
Change of work hours	3·4	2·0	0
Increased responsibility	10·2	15·6	21·9
Decreased responsibility	1·9	2·0	3·1
Too little or somewhat too little job responsibility	3·3	7·9	12·5
Too much or somewhat too much job responsibility	12·5	9·8	15·6
Problems with superiors	5·2	7·8	9·4
Problems with work mates	3·7	3·9	6·3
Unemployed for more than 30 consecutive days	14·3	17·6	21·9

All questions concern the last 12 months before the study.

TABLE 26.5

Age-adjusted comparisons — 'workload' and MI

	Total MI group	Deaths	Survivals	No prior history
N	51	19	32	31
Median age	55	55	52·5	53
Observed frequency (per cent) of workload (O)	37·3	10·5	53·1	48·4
Age-adjusted expected frequency (per cent) of workload (E)	22·7	22·7	24·9	24·5
Ratio O/E	1·64	0·46	2·13	1·98
Z-value	2·49	1·27	3·69	3·09
$p <$	$<0·01$	N.S	$<0·001$	$<0·01$

during a rest period of at least 10 continuous min. None of the subjects was receiving antiarrhythmic drugs at the time when the interview was made. Topics being discussed were noted on the electrocardiogram.

The interviews all followed the same structure and covered the following topics:

(1) Work;
(2) Family and sexual life;
(3) Disease problems; and
(4) Financial state.

Statistically significant variations in the number of premature ventricular contractions in specific relation to the topics discussed were noted in two subjects. Their interviews are presented in Figs. 26.1 and 26.2. In each of these cases discussion about work was associated with ventricular arrhythmias. In patient A a description of all the responsibilities at work even elicited multifocal ventricular premature contractions, once three in a row.

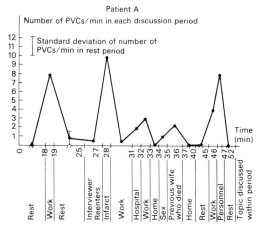

FIG. 26.1. Arrythmias recorded during stress interview with patient A.

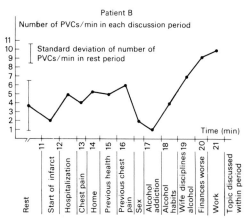

FIG. 26.2. Arrythmias recorded during stress interview with patient B.

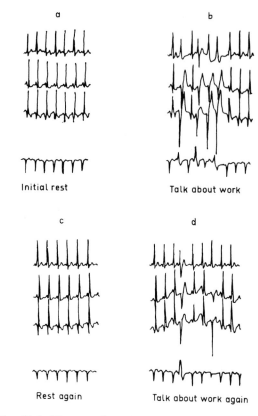

FIG. 26.3. Electrocardiographic recordings during interview with patient A.

Fig. 26.3 shows

(a) Initial rest period;
(b) First work discussion (18th to 19th min);
(c) Rest period around the 40th min;
(d) Work discussion (46th to 47th min).

The sequences a–b and c–d have in common that work discussions followed a period of rest. Furthermore, during both of these work discussions the patient, who is a manager at a department store, was emotionally upset when he talked about problems related to his personnel at the department. This aspect of his work was not touched upon around the 30th and 33rd min, respectively, when the work situation was also discussed. In patient B, a discussion about the work situation was associated with multiple premature ventricular contractions. Thus, although this applied to only a limited number of patients (2/22) in this sample of relatively young survivors of a myocardial infarction, the mere discussion or thought of important work matters could elicit potentially life-threatening arrhythmias. Both increased sympathetic and parasympathetic nerve stimulation to the heart may play a role in the production of such arrhythmias.

In a study of 30 subjects of working age who had had a myocardial infarction ($N = 25$) or some other acute manifestation of coronary heart disease one to two weeks previously, an interview was performed covering three areas: illness, work, and family. Non-invasive recordings of heart rate, arrhythmias, blood pressure, and a ballistocardiographic index of stroke volume (IJ amplitude) were made after each segment of the interview. In three cases, arrhythmias of benign nature started during the work segment of the interview, whereas no arrhythmias started during the illness segment and only one additional arrhythmia started during the family segment. Furthermore, an index of increased heart performance—increase in heart rate (HR) multiplied by increase in IJ amplitude (IJ)—showed a striking association with an index of myocardial infarction size, maximal GOT level, during the work discussion. The change in HR × IJ from resting levels showed a product–moment correlation with maximal GOT level of 0.58 ($p < 0.01$) during the 'work' discussions. The corresponding correlations for 'illness' and 'family' were 0.44 and 0.41 ($p < 0.05$), respectively (Theorell *et al.* 1977b). Thus, particularly during talk about work, those with large infarcts exhibited striking elevations in heart performance. The numbers in the last two studies are small, but they point to the rather specific important *work* for this group of patients.

In a longitudinal study, the output of urinary catecholamines was studied from week to week in relation to reported life changes during the past week. Information about life changes was obtained in a standardized interview utilizing the schedule of recent experiences. The measurement of the catecholamine output was made in a standardized way, taking diet, smoking, alcohol habits, and diurnal variations into account. Despite this, considerable variations were observed in the amount of catecholamines excreted, and these variations were mostly correlated with the total life change score (Theorell *et al.* 1972) during the previous week. Strains resulting from changes in the work situation formed a large part of this score.

Thus, from an electrocardiographic and physiological standpoint, psychological problems related to the work situation may be potentially as important (dangerous) as problems related to other areas in the individual's life. We have performed three studies relevant to 'problem areas' on survivors of premature myocardial infarction below 60 years of age in comparison to age-matched subjects.

The first study was performed on 106 male patients below the age of 60 years admitted to our hospital for a myocardial infarction. They were compared with 96 age-matched randomly selected subjects living in the greater Stockholm area. A structured interview was performed with each patient and subject about the life situation prior to the time of onset of myocardial infarction. The sociological variables that significantly differentiated the patients from the control subjects were the following:

(1) Being born as a late child in a large family (at least number five);
(2) Having been unable to do military service;
(3) Conflicts with teachers at school during childhood and adolescence;
(4) Excessive overtime work (of a long-standing nature);
(5) Conflicts with superiors at work (of a long-standing nature) (Lind and Theorell 1973b).

The other study was performed on 67 subjects actively employed in a nation-wide system (the co-operative chain) who had survived a myocardial infarction during the years 1970 and 1971. The group for comparison was a sample of subjects individually matched with regard to age, sex, and kind of employment. All patients and subjects received questionnaires with items regarding life changes (see above) and 'problem areas'. These questions were validated in a telephone interview with all subjects and patients available half a year after the initial questionnaire had been sent out. High agreement was found (Theorell *et al.* 1973). The results from the patients' self-reports in the questionnaires are presented in Table 26.3.

In this study, family life was the area in which the patients claimed the most dissatisfaction, but work was also claimed to have been 'too responsible' and to give 'little satisfaction' more often by the patients than by the controls.

In a third study, 62 consecutive patients admitted to our hospital were given a questionnaire with questions about problem areas prior to the onset of a myocardial infarction. They were compared with healthy subjects living in Stockholm and all employed in a large Stockholm city agency, comparable as to age and professional status. In this study, again, work dissatisfaction and overtime work were claimed to be experienced more often (prior to the onset of myocardial infarction) by the patients than by the control subjects. Questions about responsibility (subjective estimation) and amount of time spent in supervising others at work indicated that the patients in this study saw their work as entailing relatively little responsibility (Theorell and Rahe 1972).

In discussing the conflicting evidence regarding work responsibility in the second and third studies, respectively, it should be pointed out that the second study primarily concerned unskilled workers outside urban areas, whereas the third mainly covered professionals and skilled workers. It is possible that the 'wrong' amount of responsibility may be the crucial factor involved and that the *direction* (too much or too little) is different in different socio-economic groups but makes no difference to the risk of myocardial infarction. A similar result has been obtained in the study of work responsibility in relation to serum cholesterol (Cobb 1973).

Thus, the individual's *way of acting* in his work as well as his *actual work environment* seem to be important factors for the likelihood of developing a myocardial infarction before retirement age. Long working hours, feelings of overload, lack of appreciation from superiors, competitiveness, long-standing conflicts at work, and a relatively low level of education seem to be key factors in this process in the urbanized countries.

Support for this statement is derived from a number of retrospective small-scale studies as well as from a couple of large-scale prospective studies. These factors operate partly through established 'risk mechanisms' and partly through other mechanisms.

It should be pointed out that work conditions *per se* have a small likelihood of 'causing' a myocardial infarction if no other risk factors are present. On the other hand, a person who is dissatisfied and has 'too much' responsibility in his work will have a greater likelihood of dying from a heart attack or surviving it at a young age than most other persons of the same age, sex, serum cholesterol, blood pressure, and cigarette consumption. Therefore, an implication of the findings mentioned above may be that the physician should be particularly thorough in his 'preventive' evaluation and treatment of risk factors in persons with known 'Sisyphus syndromes'. Another implication may be that persons with many known risk factors ought to be taught to avoid excessive overtime work, etc. A third possible implication: We may start efforts to *change* a 'Sisyphus pattern' or a 'type A behaviour' in a person. We do not know how large a role genetics play in this behaviour pattern, although preliminary results from on-going research on monozygotic twins indicate both a genetic and an environmental component in behaviour pattern are associated with the development of a premature myocardial infarction (Rahe *et al.* 1974; Flodérus 1974). If the genetic part is large, efforts to modify behaviour would be of marginal success. Otherwise, they should be more successful.

The last implication of the findings discussed above concerns changes at work. A crisis or a major change in the work situation may be considered a 'risk situation'. This does not, of course, mean that we have to avoid all changes at work but implies that a person who is susceptible to or has coronary heart disease should be

TABLE 26.3

Psychosocial background variables in patients who have survived a myocardial infarction and in controls (co-operative chain study)

	Patients ($N = 65$) (56 re-interviewed)	Controls ($N = 65$) (64 re-interviewed)
Hostility when slowed down		
Hostile	41 (38)	32 (31)
Not hostile	24 (17)	32 (31)
Not significant, initial study		
($\chi^2 = 4\cdot39, p < 0\cdot05$, re-interviewed data)		
	Patients	Controls
Number of changes of residence since age 15		
5 times or more	31	17
Less than 5 times	32	43
$\chi^2 = 5\cdot63, p < 0\cdot05$		
Subjective feeling of responsibility at work		
Too much	23	12
Just right or too little	41	52
$\chi^2 = 4\cdot76, p < 0\cdot05$		
Ability to relax after a normal work day		
Sometimes or less frequently	27	16
Nearly always or always	38	49
$\chi^2 = 4\cdot20, p < 0\cdot05$		
Satisfaction at work		
Sometimes or less frequently	13 (10)	6 (4)
Nearly always or always	51 (46)	59 (60)
Not significant, initial study		
($\chi^2 = 3\cdot90, p < 0\cdot05$, re-interview data)		
Satisfaction with family life		
Always	29 (27)	50 (49)
Less than always	36 (28)	15 (15)
$\chi^2 = 14\cdot23, p < 0\cdot001$, initial study		
($\chi^2 = 9\cdot67, p < 0\cdot01$, re-interview data)		

handled with greater care than others when he has a major change at work. For instance, his manager should pay more attention to his work problems, and his physician more attention to his physical condition and also be informed about the problems at work. The reasons for giving special attention to coronary heart disease are many. Risk of death and serious disability are the most obvious. The general strategy could be applied to other diseases as well.

The person who has developed a myocardial infarction not only encounters an entirely novel *personal* situation when he gets out of the hospital—he is afraid of dying suddenly, his physical, social, and sexual capacity is severely limited, and his life gets encircled by many rigid pieces of advice—but also, when he is supposed to start working again, he encounters several social problems. The percentage of subjects who return to work after a myocardial infarction varies in different samples but is usually around 50–80 per cent. A large proportion of those who are unable to return to work do not have clear-cut somatic reasons for this—but appear to stay away from work for other reasons. Some have physically demanding work that they cannot perform despite only moderately extensive damage to the myocardium; others stay away out of anxiety (Cay *et al.* 1973).

However, even in the patients who do start some kind of job after the myocardial infarction, serious problems arise. Colleagues and employers are often badly informed about the patient's disease. They may suspect that the patient is trying to 'get out of' uncomfortable jobs by complaining about disease symptoms. Even though this may not frequently be the case, the patient's *suspicion* that he is being looked upon in this way creates a problem. This is just one example of problems which the patient may encounter when he returns. In addition to the work problems which existed before the disease onset—such as lack of appreciation, demanding strains, etc.—the patient also has to struggle with his somatic symptoms. A depressive reaction is common in this situation, and it takes an average of three years to overcome (Bruhn *et al.* 1971).

In a larger perspective, it could also be asked whether *reducing reasons* for feelings of overload, lack of appreciation, long hours, and conflicts at work may influence the coronary heart disease morbidity and mortality. Thus, 'hard work' *per se* probably does not kill very often, but those who work hard *and* get little satisfaction from it may die from coronary heart disease earlier than others!

REFERENCES

ARDLIE, N. G., GLEW, G., and SCHWARTZ, C. J. (1966). Influence of catecholamines on nucleotide-induced platelet aggregation. *Nature (London)*, **212**, 415.

BIÖRCK, G., BLOMQVIST, G. L., and SIEVERS, J. (1968). Studies in myocardial infarction in Malmö 1935–1954. Infarction rate by occupational group. *Acta med. scand.*, **21**.

BONAMI, M. and RIMÉ, B. (1972). Approche exploratoire de la personnalité precoronarienne par analyse standardisée de donnée projective thematique. *J. psychosom. Res.*, **16**, 103.

BRUHN, J. G., WOLF, S., and PHILIPS, B. U. (1971). A psychosocial study of surviving male coronary patients and controls followed over nine years. *J. psychosom. Res.*, **15**, 305–13.

BUELL, P. and BRESLOW, L. (1960). Mortality from coronary heart disease in California men who work long hours. *J. chron. Dis.*, **11**, 615–26.

CAY, E. L., VETTER, N., PHILIP, A., and DUGARD, P. (1973). Return to work after a heart attack. *J. psychosom. Res.*, **17**, 231–43.

COBBS, S. (1973). Role responsibility: A differentiation of a concept. *Occ. Mental Health Notes*, **3**, 10–14.

ELMFELDT, D. (1974). Hjärtinfarkt i Göteborg 1968–1970. Chapter 13. Doctoral thesis, Göteborg.

FLODÉRUS, B. (1974). Psychosocial factors in relation to coronary heart disease and associated risk factors. *Nord. Hyg. Tidstr.*, Suppl. 6.

FRIEDMAN, M., ROSENMAN, R. H., and CARROL, V. (1958). Changes in the serum cholesterol and blood clotting time in men subjected to cyclic variation of occupational stress. *Circulation*, **17**, 852.

FRITH, C. D. (1971). Smoking behavior and its relation to the smoker's immediate experience. *Brit. J. soc. clin. Psychol.*, **10**, 73–8.

GROEN, J. J., MEDALIE, J. H., NEUFELD, H. N., GOLDBOURT, U., RISS, E., and SNYDER, M. (1968). An epidemiological investigation of hypertension and ischemic heart disease within a defined segment of the adult male population in Israel. *Israel J. med. Sci.*, **4**, 477.

HINKLE, L. E., Jr. (1974). The effect of exposure to culture change, social change, and changes in interpersonal relationships on health. In *Stressful life events — their nature and effects* (eds. B. S. Dohrenwend and B. P. Dohrenwend), Chapter 2. Wiley and Sons, New York.

JENKINS, D. (1974). Toward a redefinition of the coronary-prone behavior pattern: Inferences from test items which predict future coronary disease. Lecture at the Annual Meeting of the American Psychosomatic Society, Philadelphia.

JORES, A. and PUCHTA, H. G. (1959). Der Pensionierungstod. Untersuchungen an Hamburger Beamten. *Med. Klin.*, **54**, 1158–64.

LEW, E. A. (1957). Some implications of mortality statistics relation to coronary artery disease. *J. chron. Dis.*, **6**, 192–209.

LILJEFORS, I. and RAHE, R. H. (1970). An identical twin study of psychosocial factors in coronary heart disease in Sweden. *Psychosom. Med.*, **32**, 523.

LIND, E., and THEORELL, T. (1973a). Levnadsförändringar ('life changes') året före infarkt. *Soc. Med. Tidskr.*, **4**, 233.

—— and —— (1973b). Sociological characteristics and myocardial infarctions. *J. psychosom. Res.*, **17**, 59–73.

MEDALIE, H. J., KAHN, H. A., NEUFELD, H. N., RISS, E., and GOLDBOURT, U. (1973). Five-year myocardial infarction incidence – II. Association of single variables to age and birthplace. *J. chron. Dis.*, **26**, 329.

PARKERS, C. M., BENJAMIN, B., and FITZGERALD, R. G. (1969).

Broken heart. A statistical study of increased mortality among widowers. *Brit. med. J.*, **1**, 740.

RAHE, R. H. and PAASIKIVI, J. (1971). Psychosocial factors and myocardial infarction — II. An outpatient study in Sweden. *J. psychosom. Res.*, **15**, 33–9.

—— and LIND, E. (1971). Psychosocial factors and sudden cardiac death: a pilot study. *J. psychosom. Res.*, **15**, 19–24.

——, ROMO, M., BENNETT, L., and SILTANEN, P. (1974a). Recent life changes, myocardial infarction and abrupt coronary death. *Arch. int. Med.*, **133**, 221–8.

——, ROSENMAN, R. H., and BORHANI, N. (1974b). Heritability and psychological correlates of behavior pattern types A and B. *CVD Epidemiology Newsletter*, **16**.

RUSSEK, H. J. and ZOHMAN, B. L. (1958). Relative significance of heredity, diet and occupational stress in coronary heart disease of young adults. *Amer. J. med. Sci.*, **235**, 166–77.

THEORELL, T. and RAHE, R. H. (1971). Psychosocial factors and myocardial infarction — I. An inpatient study in Sweden. *J. psychosom. res.*, **15**, 25–31.

—— and —— (1972). Behavior and life satisfactions characteristics of Swedish subjects with myocardial infarction. *J. chron. Dis.*, **25**, 139–47.

——, LIND, E., FRÖBERG, J. L., KARLSSON, C-G., and LEVI, L.
(1972). A longitudinal study of 21 subjects with coronary heart disease: Life change, catecholamine excretion and related biochemical reactions. *Psychocom. Med.*, **34**, 505–16.

——, ——, and LUNDBERG, U. (1973). Hjärtinfarkt inom den svenska kooperationen. *Soc. Med. Tidskr.*, **10**, 568.

—— and FLODÉRUS-MYRHED, B. (1977). 'Work load' and risk of myocardial infarction — a prospective psychosocial analysis. *Int. J. Epidem.*, **6**, 17–21.

—— and OSSON, A. (1977). Concrete work and myocardial infarction. *Scand. J. Work Environ. Hlth.*, **3**, 144–53.

——, ——, and ENGHOLM, G. (1977a). Concrete work and myocardial farction. *Scand. J. Work, Environ., Hlth*, **3**, 144–53.

——, SCHALLING, D., and AKERSTEDT, T. (1977b). Circulatory reactions in coronary patients during interview — a non-invasive study. *J. Biol. Psychol.*, **5**, 233–40.

WEISS, E., DLIN, B., ROLLIN, H. R., FISCHER, H. K., and BEPLER, C. R. (1957). Emotional factors in coronary occlusion I. Introduction and general summary. *Arch. int. Med.* **99**, 628–41.

WOLF, S. (1969). Psychosocial forces in myocardial infarction and sudden death. *Circulation*, **4** (Suppl. 4), 74.

27. WORK AND PEPTIC ULCER

J. J. GROEN

INTRODUCTION: THE PSYCHOSOMATIC ULCER THEORY

The progress in our knowledge and concepts of the etiology of peptic ulcer is an illustration of the development in thinking and research in medicine during the past two centuries. The disease was first described by the pathologists Morgagni (1789) and Cruveilhier (1829) and it was apparently a rare condition at that time, although we are not quite sure whether this rarity was only apparent, due to the fact that the clinicians did not recognize the condition, as e.g. in the case of Napoleon (Groen 1971a).

At the time of these first descriptions the aetiology was unknown, as it still is. It is understandable that the first theories were based on those mechanisms which were known to the contemporary pathologists. Virchow (1853) believed that the disease was caused by an embolus or thrombosis in one of the nutrient arteries of the stomach. Faber (1953) and Konjetzny (1930, 1931) advocated the role of gastritis but all attempts to isolate a causative micro-organism have failed. Gradually the concept developed that peptic ulcer could be the result of circumscribed digestion of the mucosa by its own secretion products: hydrochloric acid and pepsin. The question why such an autodigestion occurred only in some people took a long time to answer. With the introduction of methods to determine the amount of acid and pepsin in the gastric juice came the hypothesis (still valid (Mirsky 1952, 1958) that some people who for some reason on other secrete more pepsin and acid in their gastric juice than others, might be more prone to develop an ulcer. However, it again took time before anybody dared to offer a hypothesis for the cause of this hypersecretion in some people. The most commonly accepted theory, widely held up to this day, is that this is a genetic characteristic of the individual. However, how such a genetic factor works remained unclear.

Almost a century ago Talma, (1889, 1890, 1895), Professor of Medicine at the University of Utrecht in the Netherlands and, in many respects, a pioneer of psychosomatic medicine, formulated the so-called neurogenic ulcer theory. He and his co-workers Lichtenbelt 1912; van Ijzeren 1901) had performed experiments on rabbits and had observed that electrical stimulation of the vagus nerve produced an increased secretion and tonic contractions of the stomach musculature with closure of the pylorus and, in a few experiments, even shallow ulcerations of the mucosa. This work, together with the clinical observation of 'nervous tensions' in his patients, led Talma to suppose that during life, intense 'vagal activity', as a result of these nervous tensions, could be the cause of gastric ulcer in man. I have been told by one of Talma's former students that he used to carry on conversations with the patients while holding his hand on their abdomen. He maintained that if he discussed certain topic with them (e.g. their relation to their wife) he could feel a sudden contraction of the antrum of the stomach. This was long before the introduction of X-ray examinations revealed that such contractions do occur under emotional circumstances (Westphal 1914; Westphal and Ketsch 1913).

The neurogenic ulcer theory was extended and became widely known in Germany through the work and writings of von Bergmann (1913, 1936; see also Bober and Schröder 1956). In the United States the great authority of Cushing (1932) brought the neurogenic theory under general attention when, in a paper on gastric ulcer in patients with brain tumours and after neurosurgery, he postulated that similar processes may play a role in the pathogenesis of peptic ulcer. In doing so he broke through the mind–body barrier, when he wrote:

Those favourably disposed toward the neurogenic conception of ulcer, have, in process of time, gradually shifted the burden of responsibility from the peripheral vagus to its centre in the medulla, then to the midbrain, and now to the interbrain, newly recognized as a highly important, long-overlooked station for vegetative impulses, easily affected by psychic influences. So it may easily be that highly-strung persons, who incline to the form of nervous instability classified as parasympathetic (vagotonic), through emotion or repressed emotion, incidental to continued worry and anxiety and heavy responsibility, combined with other factors, such as irregular meals and excessive use of tobacco, are particularly prone to chronic digestive disturbances with hyperacidity, often leading to ulcers.

Only those who have lived through the time when the dichotomy between spirit and matter, between soul and body, and between psychiatry and medicine was absolute and adhered to as an almost religious dogma by all 'scientific authorities', can understand what these lines meant in those days. Only very few realized their fundamental importance or were inspired by them to put this, by now psychosomatic, theory to the test. The hypothesis became even more daring when Alexander (1934, 1950; Alexander *et al.* 1968) added a new aspect by postulating that ulcers were not caused merely by 'nervous instability' but by a *specific* psychogenic constellation. He supposed, in other words, that the relationship between 'psychic tension' and peptic ulcer was just as specific as that of a certain species of bacteria to one specific type of bodily disease. Not nervous tension in general, but a specific type of nervous tension was supposed to be the cause of ulcer and other kinds of tension were considered to be the cause of other 'psycho-somatic' or non-psychosomatic disorders. In formulating this theory, Alexander not only gave a new aspect to the aetiological hypothesis of peptic ulcer, he also intro-duced a new fundamental concept in psychosomatic thinking. Thus the specificity ulcer theory became historically linked with the development of theory formation in psychosomatic medicine in general.

Alexander based his hypothesis on the psycho-analytical study of a number of patients who suffered from ulcers; he thought that he could detect in their personalities a certain 'core' consisting of a number of 'traits' which he considered as specific for these patients, that is to say, by which they differed from other patients and healthy individuals. In addition, he proposed that this specific personality structure had developed in these patients as a result of their youth experiences. The main features of this ulcer-predisposing personality were a combination of strong passive 'oral' strivings for love reception (largely subconscious) and (as a substitution) a manifest conscious, active, competitive urge to achieve gratification by work, and by exemplary, independent, dutiful, social behaviour. Goldberg (1958) in a classical study of the family relations in young ulcer patients, illustrated the role of a demanding, 'detached' mother in producing in her son this tendency to substitute active achievements by dutiful behaviour for the original unfulfilled passive attempts to obtain from her love and attention (van der Heide 1940; van Nieuwenhuyzen 1961; Ruesch 1948; Wretmark 1953).

Before Alexander, George Draper and co-workers (Draper and McGraw 1927; Draper and Touraine 1932) had already formulated a similar hypothesis about personality as a predisposing factor in the production of disease.

Groen (1947, 1971a) extended Alexander's specificity concept. He formulated the theory that an ulcer was the result of a constellation of *three* specific factors:

(a) a certain predisposing personality structure, more or less of the same type that Draper and Alexander had described;
(b) an interhuman conflict situation by which the individual was frustrated on both levels of his strivings, i.e., in which both the passive wishes for love reception were not satisfied and the inde-pendent dutiful strivings did not yield success in either work or social activities;
(c) an exaggerated self-control, also a result of their upbringing, by which these individuals in such a situation did not act out their frustrations by violence, depression, weeping, or complaining behaviour and often did not even tell their parents, marriage partners, or friends about their troubles.

The three factors are mutually dependent. The predisposing personality structure makes these individuals more vulnerable and thereby more sensitive to a conflict because they need gratification, either by love reception or success in work, more than others, and because, by their not complaining or acting out, the conflict is not solved.

By introducing into the aetiological hypotheses both the specific constellation of a predisposing personality and a precipitating interhuman conflict situation, the psychosomatic hypothesis became analogous to the common concept of how a disease is produced in general. There is always a 'host' ('*le terrain*', as Pasteur called it) and an external noxious 'agent' ('*le grain*' in Pasteur's terminology, which was obviously derived from the well known biblical parable of the Sower). A disease is the result of a physico-chemical, biological, or human pathogen (a stressor as it was later designated) which acts on a sensitive organism. Disease is always produced by at least two causes; the specific response of any organism, i.e. the type of the disease, is determined both by the nature of the sensitive organism (the 'personality') and of the stressor. These two causal factors are interdependent because it depends on the nature (the sensitivity) of the organism whether a noxious factor is a stressor or only a neutral unimportant stimulus.

In the case of ulcerogenesis a certain type of personality, as determined by both genetic and acquired factors, is supposed to be sensitive to certain interhuman stressors. The result is a certain behaviour, which, like all behaviour of the organism, is both outwardly and inwardly directed. In most patients with a psychosomatic disorder, ulcer patients among them, the patient inhibits the motor, mimic, and vocal (verbal) components of his behaviour and this inhibition is supposed to reinforce, as an inwardly directed substitution, the discharges into the visceral organs.

In this chapter we will not deal further with the pre-disposing personality but concentrate on the precipi-tating external circumstances and conflict situations.

These external factors are supposed to be the *social circumstances*, which determine the interhuman com-munications of the individual in the social subgroups to which he belongs, especially in his family and work situation. In this concept peptic ulcer is the result of a 'soluble level' interhuman conflict. If an individual is frustrated either in his family, or in his work situation, no ulcer will develop because the social gratification in one field of communication may compensate the frustration in the other. Ulcers arise only in individuals who are frustrated *both* in their strivings for attention and love reception in their family *and* in their efforts to obtain social success and gratification by their work. *Thus, work, or rather the emotional frustration caused by failure the work-associated strivings and anticipations of the individual*, is postulated as a factor in the multicausal etiology of peptic ulcer.

This means that the assiduous study of patients with peptic ulcer has introduced into the field of vision of medicine an aetiological factor which is not simply biological but connected with the function of work in the social and economic structure of the cultural group and its influence on the psychobiological behaviour of the individual. This makes it necessary to examine this aspect of work for our society and the individual in a volume on *Society, stress, and disease*. Work is not only of interest for economists. Work is also an important factor in health or disease, and peptic ulcer may serve as a paradigm of the psychobiological aspects of this importance.

BIOLOGICAL AND SOCIAL ASPECTS OF WORK

One of the most striking differences between the behaviour of man and almost all other social animals is the important role of work in the daily activities of the individual and the group. Certain animals perform work, like spiders building a web. The work performed by ants and bees has been an object of both admiration and study since earliest times, and we marvel at the 'ingenious' way in which birds build nests or certain mammals dig holes. These work activities by animals are performed in some species individually and in others in co-operation by social groups. In general, however, the work behaviour of animals is immediately related to one of the fundamental biological processes of nutrition or reproduction.

In the human we find this immediate relationship between work and the gratification of the primordial needs only in so-called primitive societies where hunters or shepherds provide food for the family or tribe. In simple agricultural communities food is also produced for immediate consumption by the group. Production of clothing also serves an immediate purpose and the same is true for building one's own home, providing fuel, etc.

With the evolution of human societies into more complicated organizations, however, this direct relationship between work and immediate biological needs was replaced by production for customers or market or, as in the case of work in modern Western industry, for purposes which the worker does not even know: modern Western man is alienated from the aim of his work. In modern Western society work is an activity which the group requires the individual to perform as a duty within the framework of certain technical and economic production systems and organizations. In addition to the manual work in industrial production, more and more people work in offices, where they perform administrative functions but otherwise under largely similar interhuman conditions. In this type of work, the ultimate purpose is also often far away from the actual performance. Only a minority of people: small farmers, craftsmen, shopkeepers, and the so-called free and serving professions have an opportunity to find in their work direct communication with the clients for whom they work, but the number engaged in these middle-class 'free' occupations is rapidly diminishing in Western society. However, even for them the work is, next to a source of gratification, a socially enforced duty.

Another difference between human society and other animals living in social groups concerns the importance and scope which work behaviour has acquired as a required or enforced activity. In Western societies children are educated by their parents to work and this part of their education becomes more important as they grow up. They are conditioned at a very early age to go to school regularly, and to work there at tasks specially designed to train them for their future work as adults. They are given homework, tests, and obtain rewards or punishment both in school and at home depending on how they work. At a later age they are sent to more and more difficult schools, all the time as a preparation for their later work behaviour in the society. Thus the parents and teachers fulfil the function of social educators who produce the workers which our society needs. Work is in Western society a universal activity, a duty from which even royalty and rich people from the so-called leisure class cannot escape and which they have to perform in order to keep their social status, the respect of their parents and later on of their marriage partners, their fellow men and, perhaps most important of all, their self-respect. The biblical commandment to work for six days and rest on the seventh, which in the old days put most emphasis on the necessity of leisure on the seventh day, is now more and more interpreted with the accent on the duty to work on all the other days!

The pressure and social compulsion to work vary widely in different human societies; although more or less present in all human groups, this culturally enforced labour became most marked in Western society in the second half of the nineteenth and first half of the twentieth century. However, even in Western society itself there is a large difference in the motivation or devotion (in Pavlovian terms 'in the reinforced conditioning') of different people to their work, both by their external life situation and by an 'inner' urge. Just as is the case in other forms of human behaviour, work behaviour is determined by endogenous predisposition or 'drive' and by exogenous 'signals', 'inducers' or 'releasers'. Both these endogenous and exogenous factors are partly derived from man's inborn biological structure and potentialities, partly shaped and modified by the cultural and psychological processes of imprinting, conditioning, and learning. Especially the process which has been named 'instrumental conditioning' in the experimental studies of behaviour seems to be the mechanism along which Western modern man has learned to devote so much of his time and energy to a form of behaviour which, even though it ultimately serves his nutrition, sexual activities, and aggression, has become far detached from the immediate gratification of these fundamental biological drives. For many individuals in modern Western society work has superseded all other activities; many people strive more for gratification in their work than in their 'natural' biological activities. In the nineteenth century and first half of the twentieth century work had become one of the most highly valued activities in the social morale and religious ethics of Western society: work was proclaimed one of the highest virtues in life, compared to which the biological gratifications of eating and copulation were at best tolerated for pleasure during off hours.

Another manifestation of how important the drive to work has become in Western society is the fact that a lot of our play behaviour, whether in children or as hobbies in adults, is performed with the same intensity, in the framework of similar social organizations and for similar rewards, either money (professional sportsmen) or fame and social status, as industrial work.

Only recently (after the Second World War) is a minority of people in the Western world beginning to reflect whether work will *eo ipso* lead to well-being and happiness and whether the performance of more and more work (like the accumulation of more and more wealth) is indeed the universal social value for which we should all strive. The clinical observation that certain diseases like peptic ulcer seem to occur especially in people who work very hard, has also induced us to reconsider the effects of work from the point of view of both bodily and mental health. Therefore it seems worthwhile to devote some considerations to the causes of why people work and why Western people work so hard.

GRATIFICATION FROM WORK

Money and what one can buy with it in a money-worshipping society is probably the most important gratification people try to obtain through work. Other gratifications should not be left out of consideration, however, for instance the joy of creating a product with one's own hands. This is an especially important gratification in the creation of works of art and in so-called do-it-yourself' hobbies. It also serves as a reward in small-scale agriculture and manufacture but as said before, this form of gratification is rapidly disappearing in modern industrial production and administration. A third source of gratification through work is the reward obtained in the form of praise from a key figure who serves as the leader of the production group or/and from one's co-workers in the group. All these rewards may be understood in the psychological concept of assuring one's personal and social *security*. Next to this gratifying function, work in Western society offers possibilities to fulfil strivings for *self-fulfilment by development*, e.g. by ascent on the social scale thereby increasing both income, social status, power (sometimes leadership), and self-respect. If successful in his work, the Western individual, especially the male, achieves not only

promotion in the work situation; work also offers him way to improve his position in society at large, whic means that he becomes more dominant over his fello men and also (by being more respected as a provider) his own family. Here we encounter in our consideratio an analogy with animal societies where also, next t security, social rank and power are coveted gratific tions. But whereas animals obtain their higher soci status by age, display, or aggression, in the life of th modern human, work achievements have substituted fe these forms of competitive behaviour.

In summary, work has become, especially in Wester societies, a form of human behaviour which, part because it is socially required and partly because of th possibilities it offers for gratification, has become at lea as important as the 'original' biological drives nutrition, procreation, and aggression. *Work serves, lik these drives, both the fundamental strivings for securi (homeostasis) and development (self-fulfilment) of th individual* (Gardell 1971; de Wolff 1972). We have trie to express these multiple gratifications which can b obtained through work in Table 27.1 in diagrammat form and in terms and concepts which are used both biology, psychology, and sociology.

TABLE 27.1

Gratifications obtainable by work behaviour

_____

(1) Reward in the form of money and what it can buy (ind pendence, security).
(2) Creation of a product (preferably not monotonous) wi one's own hands or assembling a more complicate product.
(3) Communication with fellow workers, mutual confidenc support and security derived from 'belonging' to homogeneous group.
(4) Reward from appreciation of one's clients and/or th leader and/or co-workers in the working group.
(5) Self-respect, social respect, and status in the community large and in the family (as provider) by being a goc worker.
(6) Opportunity to act out one's strivings for furthe development, self-fulfilment, and expansion, often competitive aggression with others for higher status, mor responsibility, power, dominance, and leadersh ('actuation of self-concept'), both inside and outside th group, and the increase in social and self-respect that g with it.

_____

The manifold forms of gratification in Table 27. which can be obtained by successful work explain wh some people are so highly motivated by or even obsesse by their work and why they devote more time to it tha for instance, to their wife and the education of the children. This is the case especially when, as ofte happens in Western society, the wife is 'cool 'detached', 'independent' and does not play a submissive, obedient, loving role. In this type of marriage the husband often tries to substitute gratification in his work for his frustrations in the family. On the other hand, for those men who do not succeed in finding one of the above gratifications, the work in our society may be an equal source of frustration (Gardell 1971; Groen 1971b; Levi 1971).

FRUSTRATION BY WORK

Frustration in the work situation may come about through several factors. One is that most people are not conditioned during their childhood and adolescence for the 'cold' environment, the impersonal human relations in industry and offices, and the alienation from the product of their work. Many are frustrated when they find out that their co-workers are actually more competitors than comrades and that these rivalries are quite different from what they had expected. The relationship between the managers (whom many workers do not even know or see) and the workers is often impersonal and sometimes inhuman, and their mutual distrust is encouraged by the stereotyped generalizations which employers believe in about the workers and the workers believe in about the employers. A sign of appreciation from a boss or foreman, expected by a worker when he does his best, may never come; on the contrary he may be rebuked or unjustly passed over for promotion. These types of frustrations undermine the security of the worker and diminish his confidence in his bosses, fellow men, and/or himself. For ulcer patients it seems to be especially difficult to cope with the frustration that their tendency to work in an exemplary way, to do more than their duty, to improve production and working methods are not appreciated or rewarded. They may be hurt by dishonest tactics of their chiefs or rivals because they themselves, while also trying to actuate their self-concept, strive by 'honest' competition for promotion and leadership. Often ulcer patients have been, until their disease broke out, hard workers very devoted to their work and duties but expecting for their exemplary behaviour reward, promotion, and other signs of social appreciation. When these anticipations were not realized they felt hurt in their confidence in bosses or co-workers and frustrated both in their strivings to improve the work and to improve their own status with it. It is quite possible that the strong devotion of ulcer patients to their work and their compulsive urge to improve their own status through the high quality of their work is a result of their education by a stern, demanding, driving, but honest mother. Just as they wanted to please and induce this mother to give them love and appreciation by fulfilling her wishes by exemplary behaviour at school, they later try to obtain appreciation from the boss in their work.

Thus the ulcer patient as a worker distinguishes himself on the one hand by the high quality of his work,

but he is also difficult because he demands from bosses and co-workers that they appreciate him and follow his suggestions for improvement of the work, and he is soon disappointed when this is not the case. 'A good but difficult worker' was how an industrial physician characterized the typical ulcer patient in the factory. In contrast to the high devotion to work is also the high level of absenteeism of many of them when, therefore, after a frustration, the ulcer has manifested itself. This makes the worker with an ulcer often, in spite of his high motivation, both a medical and a managerial problem.

The question is often asked: Why do people with a personality structure as described, under the stress of a frustration in their work, react by the development of an ulcer? Why do they not develop one of the other reactions to frustration: aggressive violence, protest behaviour like strikes or sabotage, anxiety states, depressions, indifference and apathy, or alcoholism or other drug additions? Or why do they not develop another psychosomatic disease like functional pains, migraine, hyperthyroidism, hypertension, or ischemic heart disease? This brings us back to the problem of the specificity of the response of different individuals to a psychosocial stressor. The theoretical answer to this question has partly been given in the introduction of this chapter: in these patients the tendency to hard work developed as a substitute for their original craving for love and attention from their mother, which she only gave as a reward for dutiful, virtuous, well-mannered, exemplary behaviour. It is supposed that this educative behaviour of the mother suppressed in the son the tendencies to aggressive violence, dishonesty, sabotage or any show of bad temper, anxiety, or bouts of alcoholism. Later in his life the patient, even when frustrated, cannot behave otherwise than like the well-mannered boy his mother expected him to be. In biological terms: *both fight and flight behaviour were suppressed and punished rather than reinforced during their youth, whereas conflict avoidance (submissive) behaviour was encouraged and rewarded* (Alexander 1934; Goldberg 1958; Groen 1947; Hamilton 1950; van Nieuwenhuyzen 1961; Ruesch 1948; Weiner 1971, 1973).

Many physiologists have confirmed Cannon's (1909, 1929) original observations that fight and flight diminish gastric secretion and contractions (Beaumont 1833; Wolf and Wolff 1943; Wolf 1965; Weiner 1973). These behaviour patterns are associated with high arousal levels and sympathetic (nor-) adrenergic activation and are thereby associated with increased cardiac output and/or blood pressure. This might be the reason why individuals who inhibit aggression when frustrated do not develop ulcers, but are more at risk for e.g. hypertension and coronary heart disease. Avoidance or submissive behaviour is more associated with para-sympathetic cholinergic activation, which acts mostly on the gastro-intestinal system (Mittelman and Wolff 1942; Westphal and Ketsch 1913; Wolf and Wolff 1943) and this might be the reason why the more submissive and conflict-avoiding type of personality, when frustrated and inhibited in his acting out, is more predisposed to the development of peptic ulcer (Weiner 1973; Wolf and Wolff 1943; Wolf 1965; Yager and Weiner 1971). As most people (like animals) are utilizing, depending on their development and present situation, either aggressive or submissive behaviour patterns, the 'choice' or alternation of peptic ulcer rather than these cardiovascular disorders can be understood both in terms of excessive psychological and physiological 'coping mechanisms'.

FRUSTRATION IN WORK AND PREVALENCE OF PEPTIC ULCER: EPIDEMIOLOGICAL STUDIES

That frustration in the work situation plays a role in the aetiology of peptic ulcer is amply supported by biographical-anamnestic studies of individual patients and by clinical experience; other kinds of evidence are mostly indirect and relatively scarce. In general the influence of psychosocial factors in the production of disease is difficult to test e.g. by epidemiological methods. Many modern epidemiologists are insufficiently trained in the validation of the social-psychological questionnaire techniques and/or are *a priori* sceptical about the value of such techniques or of the basic psychosomatic concepts. As a result they often do not even try to test the psychosomatic hypotheses and limit their epidemiological studies to prevalence or incidence surveys, or they register the social circumstances, which are easier to measure, but not (as the theory postulates) the psychological impact of the social factors on the emotional life and the nervous system of the individuals. Recently Pflanz (1962, 1971) has written a practically complete review of all epidemiological studies carried out so far on the role of socio-cultural factors in the aetiology of duodenal ulcer. Because of the different methods used in the different surveys, he found it impossible to draw well-founded conclusions. However, in spite of this methodological difficulty, a few pertinent observations appear from at least the majority of the studies.

In the first place, the prevalence of the disease is very different in the different geographic areas of the world. This must mean that peptic ulcer cannot be the simple result of one universally present biological pathogenic factor. Pflanz also documents the peculiar fluctuations which have occurred in the prevalence and incidence of the disease since it became known in Western countries in the course of the past two centuries: It was rare in the first half of the nineteenth century, and it increased during the second half, mainly in the form of ventricular ulcer, both in males and females. In the first half of the twentieth century duodenal ulcer became a frequent disease, much more common than ventricular ulcer, especially among young males (Alsted 1939); recently since the Second World War a modest decrease in prevalence has been described in the English literature

(Morris and Titmus 1971; Susser 1961, 1967; Susser and Stein 1962). This recent decline coincides with the observation that duodenal ulcer in Western countries is no longer a disease of predominantly young people, but that it now occurs about equally among all adult age groups. This suggests that the rise in incidence of duodenal ulcer among young males in the first half of the nineteenth century might have been a 'cohort phenomenon' of their generation (which has now become older), possibly due to environmental factors, which shaped the personality of these young people during their formative years.

Similar fluctuations in prevalence, or at least in clinical manifestation, have been described during and after the Second World War. In most countries the incidence increased during the war, especially among the civilian non-combatant population (Kalk 1943; Melton 1940, Sallström 1945; Spicer *et al.* 1942, 1944). Groen (1971b) has drawn attention to the rarity of peptic ulcer among inmates of the German concentration camps and the population of Holland during the famine of 1944–5. Pflanz *et al.* (1956) described the same situation among German soldiers. All these observations are compatible with a role in the aetiology of a special type of emotion tension or social stressor, which seems to be somehow related to the structure of society (Halliday 1948; Aakster 1972). As far as the influence of the work situation is concerned, the following data have been established by epidemiological studies:

1. Duodenal ulcer is more prevalent in city dwellers than among the inhabitants of rural areas. This would fit in with the possible role of a frustration, which occurs more frequently in the impersonal, alienated work situations in the industry of the big cities, than in small rural agricultural units.

2. In the United States the coloured population has a lower prevalence of peptic ulcer than the whites, which may be due to the fact that, especially in the south, a larger number of the negro population has not yet been conditioned in the same proportion to work under industrial conditions as the whites. In India Hindus suffer more than Christians or Moslems. In South Africa, the Bantus have much less peptic ulcer than the whites and in Uganda the Indians have more than the Africans, possibly due to similar socio-economic differences between these groups. In 1930 Kouwenaar published a survey from Sumatra, which showed that ulcer of the stomach and duodenum was much more prevalent among the Chinese than among the Javanese workers both living on a large plantation. He pointed out that this could not be explained by the external circumstances as such, which were exactly the same, but by the emotional attitudes and ways of life, which are very different among these two ethnic groups. Several studies have demonstrated differences in prevalence of duodenal ulcer between higher and lower social

206

classes of society, but other workers have not been able to confirm this. This might be due to the fact that certain patterns of life which once were characteristic of the upper classes, have now been adopted by the so-called lower social groups, especially in Western affluent society. With the increase in prosperity and change in ways of life in Western countries, the so-called lower social classes have now acquired both the advantages and the social stressors which used to be the privilege of the better classes.

3. Several observations in different countries have shown a different prevalence in peptic ulcer in immigrants, compared to the native population. This may be due to the impact of the strange and difficult interhuman situations under which immigrants have to work in most countries. However, as explained in the introduction of this chapter, it need not be the work situation only, but also the changes in family life which occur in the new environment that are the main frustrations for new immigrants.

4. Marked differences in prevalence of peptic ulcer have been found between members of different occupations (Logan and Cushion 1958; Levy 1959; Levy and Fuente 1963). The findings of Avery Jones and Doll (Jones 1957; Doll and Jones 1951, 1958) in this field have been confirmed by many others. The prevalence has been found to be especially high in white-collar workers, civil servants, foremen in industry, employees of the transportation industry, and skilled workers. In the medical profession, surgeons have a higher prevalence than other specialists. These observations support the supposition that some factor, associated with the work situation, plays a role in the aetiology of ulcer, but they do not allow more pertinent conclusions about the nature of the factor. The available evidence, however, does not suggest that it is related to physically hard work or unhygienic conditions in the work shops, but rather to some stressor associated with responsible work. Pflanz (1971) expresses his impressions, after reviewing all these papers, as follows:

It is not the profession or occupation *per se* which seems to predispose to the development of peptic ulcer but rather the demands made upon the person by his occupation, and/or the responsibilities which a particular line of work entails. It should not be concluded *a priori* that manual work carries with it no responsibilities, the critical variable is how a particular worker perceives his work. Other intervening variables between the demands of and the responsibility (real or imagined), for a particular line of work, are competition with others, the various frustrations of being an unskilled rather than a skilled worker, or the social isolation which certain kinds of work produce.

Thus the epidemiologist arrives at a similar hypothesis to the psychosomatically-oriented clinician; unfortunately the two have not yet succeeded in supporting each other's hypotheses by independent statistically significant evidence!

EXPERIMENTAL WORK; STRESS AND DUODENAL ULCER IN MONKEYS

Interesting support for the hypothesis that mental stress in the work situation may lead to peptic ulceration was described by Brady in 1958 under the suggestive title of 'Ulcers in executive monkeys'. In the course of research on operant avoidance conditioning it was found that a number of the experimental animals (*Macaca iris*) died from duodenal ulcers with haemorrhage or perforation. That this was not due to the immobilization in the restraining chairs in which the animals were kept in or to the electric shocks which they received but indeed to the stress of the 'work' necessary to avoid punishment was made likely by the following experiment. Two monkeys were placed in 'yoked chairs'; both received shocks at irregular times but only one could prevent the shocks to himself and his partner by pressing a lever. Thus both animals were exposed to the same physical situation but only the 'executive' monkey was exposed to the psychological stressor of having to press a lever to avoid this unpleasant event. Only some of these 'executive monkeys' developed an ulcer. A further interesting finding was that when the animals were on a schedule of six hours-on, six hours-off for a period of 3–6 weeks, ulcers developed more often than when they were on a 30 minutes-on, 30 minutes-off schedule, or even when the experiments were continuous. The executive monkeys also had higher acid secretion. The personality of the animals seemed to play a role because only some of them developed ulcers (Porter 1958; McRioch 1971).

It is an interesting parallel that in a similar experiment on two human volunteers (Davis and Berry 1971), only the one who could prevent an electric shock by pressing a button after a warning signal (a noise) manifested an increase in gastric motility during these avoidance experiments. This work is not only interesting because of its results but also because it is one of the few researches in which the conditions under which people work in industry (and in which conflict avoidance is often required) are imitated in animal experiments.

PEPTIC ULCER AND ABSENTEEISM FROM WORK

Peptic ulcer does not play a great role as a cause of mortality but it is an important reason for admission to hospitals and above all for absenteeism from work. In most statistics peptic ulcer is responsible for about 10 per cent of all medical reasons for absenteeism (Bykov and Kurzin 1954; Morris and Titmuss 1971; Philipsen 1969; Susser 1961, 1967; Talma 1889; Weyel 1974a; Vertin 1954). Also in this respect peptic ulcer is a paradigm of the way in which, in modern Western society, psychosomatic diseases are becoming more and more important reasons for absenteeism from work and thereby have become a real problem in industrial medicine and social insurance.

Because of their great devotion to their work, most ulcer patients begin their industrial careers as excellent workers with a low absenteeism record and even a tendency to work extra hours or to take work home from the office. Usually when their pain begins they continue to work, out of their high sense of duty and motivation. In the early stages, however, they already fight against the frustration in their work and this brings them into an ambivalent position, partly still driven to work by their sense of duty and partly with the tendency to stay home as a flight from the conflict-loaded work environment.

The first absenteeism usually occurs when their doctor tells them to stay home or to go to a hospital for medical or surgical treatment. It is important to realize that it is the doctor's advice which introduces the absenteeism, because in many discussions about the alarmingly high rate of absenteeism from work through psychogenic conditions in modern industry, the role of the medical profession in keeping people absent instead of trying to solve their conflicts, while keeping them active, is insufficiently realized. The important question therefore is whether in the medical treatment of peptic ulcer a cure of bed-rest at home or in the hospital is indeed as essential as is now generally believed. Most clinical experience confirms the psychosomatic concept that bed-rest operates mainly because it removes the patient from his conflict situations in the home or in the work and instead provides him with attention and loving care from his wife, the nurse, the dietitian, and the doctor. Several series of ulcer patients have been treated with equally good results on an ambulatory basis when the doctor saw the patient frequently and, in addition to antacids and anticholinergics, helped the patient to find a solution for conflict situations. This appears not only more rational; it also does not open the gate to repeated bouts of absenteeism.

In today's practice of medicine most patients with peptic ulcer, however, are still prescribed by their doctors to stay away from work for the traditional, arbitrarily determined period of six weeks. In many cases the success of this symptomatic treatment is temporary and after one or two recurrences the desirability of an operation is brought up. This 'solution' is then accepted by doctor and patient because neither of them sees another way and often because both have the exaggerated confidence in surgery which characterizes our Western preference for technical ways of solving problems in general. Thus after the medical indication for absenteeism has proved inefficient, comes the surgical indication. In a fairly high percentage of cases gastric resection does away with the pain and restores the patient to 'health' and working capacity. These are the cases where just enough of the stomach is removed to abolish or greatly diminish acid secretion. An important factor is also that surgical patients, especially when the operation is dangerous, receive more attention (flowers!) from the hospital staff, their relatives, and co-workers than almost any other group in our society. Previous competitors and cool wives show attention and kindness which they were unprepared to give to healthy fellow men. From the point of view of health and further absenteeism the surgical treatment can, when the result is successful, be considered as having been worthwhile (Glen and Cox 1968; Smell and Cay 1973; Thoroughman et al. 1964, 1966, 1967).

In a not inconsiderable number of patients, however, the acid secretion remains high and, when the patient returns to his frustrations at home and in the work situation, the ulcer recurs or a new ulcer may form in the jejunum. This usually leads to new periods of absenteeism, first for 'rest' and, if that does not help, for another operation.

Not rare are other patients who because the mutilation of their stomach is too extensive, develop other symptoms and signs. The so-called dumping syndrome can be extremely cumbersome; the impaired possibility for an adequate nutritional intake causes emaciation and fatigue, and this, added to the disappointments of the patients in what their doctors have promised them but not fulfilled, produces a new syndrome of a peculiar combination of bodily discomfort and mental frustration. Many of these cases are both medical and social failures. They have now become chronically so ill that they are more or less continuously absent from work, and the result is often dismissal or a certification of chronic invalidity. This is a miserable end-result to which psychosocial factors, first working through family and work conflicts, later through the one-sided somatic and technical approach of modern medicine, have contributed (Bastiaans and Groen 1952; Ely and Johnson 1966; Glen and Cox 1968; Throughman et al. 1964, 1966, 1967).

The present situation in the treatment of peptic ulcer, which might seem favourable in view of the low mortality, is therefore far less satisfactory when one considers the figures for sickness and absenteeism rates. This fact in itself should already call for a serious reconsideration by the medical profession of its at present still predominantly negative attitude towards what the psychosomatic approach could offer. Fortunately, there are at present more doctors, surgeons, and industrial physicians who, aware of this unsatisfactory state, treat their patients not only by medical-technical measures but also by a psychosocial approach, which means the elucidation and amelioration of the situation in the family and at work. But this can be successful only when both the family physician (or the gastro-enterologist) and the industrial physician regard this as a part of the regular treatment and if both have acquired the experience necessary for such a psychosocial approach. It is not within the scope of this paper to outline the forms of psycho- and sociotherapy which are applicable here. It was our aim, however, to point to these curative possibilities for the industrial physicians in the treatment of workers with peptic ulcer and above all how such treatment could also be an important form of secondary prevention of further illness and absenteeism.

PEPTIC ULCER AND SOCIAL INSURANCE

A few words must be added about the importance which peptic ulcer, like many other psychosocially induced diseases, has now acquired in countries, like Holland, with a highly developed system of social insurance (Weyel 1974a,b). In the olden days (they are not all that far behind us, viz. before the Second World War) most European countries and the United States had no (or only limited) systems of reimbursing the workers for the loss of income when they were absent from work. In most of the countries of the Third World the situation is still as it used to be in Europe and the United States in the nineteenth century: no work, no pay. This meant that a recurring or chronic disease automatically brought with it poverty for the worker and his wife and children. Philanthropy and relief provided only small compensation for the social disaster which accompanied the disaster to health. Partly through the increasing influence of workers on legislation, partly due to a change in ethical concepts in Western society, this situation has now changed. An elaborate system of premiums and provisions assures the worker in many countries now of a continued income while he is ill. For this he needs only a medical certificate. The social insurance system works well on the whole but it has also given rise to repeated conflicts between industrial physicians and those workers in whom, from a discrepancy between their subjective feelings and the objective signs, the doctor may feel that there is no reason for absenteeism. This means that some doctors suffer more under the burden of these conflicts than from the advantages the social insurance offers to the worker.

The issue has even produced political consequences. The average total absenteeism rate in the Western European countries has now reached a figure of about 10 per cent. Large amounts of money are paid out regularly to a non-working section of the population. Actually social insurance is now one of the channels along which a considerable part of the total national income is redistributed to non-working people, partly for medical, partly for social indications. The costs of this social support are borne relatively more by those with the higher incomes. From the so-called conservative parties more and more voices are heard about what they consider to be the abuses of the social insurance system. It is claimed that the system offers to the workers an opportunity to stay away from work too easily without any risk of a loss in income. It is indeed very likely that workers who do not feel well may use this as an excuse not to go to work when the work itself offers no gratification to them. This may be one of the reasons why the absenteeism rate in the United States (where there is no such system of complete reimbursement of pay for absenteeism) is only half that of the European countries, and why the absenteeism rate in Europe has risen recently to such a high figure, more or less parallel with the introduction of complete social insurance. Several doctors, especially those who have to sign absenteeism certificates which they feel are not or are only partly justified, have also voiced their objections to the system. They claim that if the worker were to be punished for absenteeism by a decline in income, it would be a stimulus for him to stay at work, often in his own interest. Thus the problem of the pros and cons of total social insurance has both moral, political, and medical aspects.

The problem also plays a role in the certification of patients with peptic ulcer. It can be very difficult or indeed impossible to decide whether the pain is really so severe that the worker for this reason needs to interrupt his work. That the absenteeism is also caused by inter-human conflicts and frustrations in the work situation is often not realized by the doctor. The problem becomes alarming when, as we described, operated patients either do not improve or develop the post-gastrectomy syndrome, in which not pain but fatigue and feelings of weakness are the main subjective symptoms. It does not seem just to impose on patients whose symptoms and signs are at least partly due to a medical failure or inefficiency, a fine by also taking away from them and their family a part of their income. It is for this reason that among physicians who work in the social insurance system and industry, other ideas have originated about how to maintain the advantages and do away with the drawbacks of our social system.

It is realized and documented by several researches that conflicts in the work situation are important contributing causes of disease and absenteeism in general and of peptic ulcer in particular (Gadourek 1965; Philipsen 1969). If this is the case, a therapy by medical and surgical measures is at best symptomatic but not a rational or causal form of treatment. *In addition to the treatment of the disease in the individual patient it is to the human relations in the family and in industry that our treatment must be directed.* This makes the doctor side with those industrial psychologists and experts of management who demonstrated long ago that inter-human frustrations in the work situation diminish output. It now appears that, just as unsatisfactory human communication is responsible for unrest, strikes, insufficient motivation, and sabotage, it also contributes to sickness absenteeism. It means that industrial medicine, which in the early years saw its main purpose in the improvement of hygienic conditions in the workshop and the prevention of accidents and exposure to toxic substances, that is, in protection against the bodily health hazards, will now have to direct its efforts to the mental hazards that threaten the worker. Just as in the other fields of medicine, this can be achieved by a combination of general measures directed at the whole of the industrial population and special precautions for the so-called exposed or high-risk individuals. Ulcer patients and those predisposed to the development of an ulcer should therefore be recognized early as a special risk group and their personal circumstances and frustrations detected and adjusted. It would be an interesting task for a research project to carry out such a combined medical, psychological, and industrial approach to the ulcer problem in one factory and choose an otherwise comparable factory as a control, where the treatment would be continued in the traditional way. If our hypotheses about the role of psychosocial factors in the causation and course of peptic ulcer are correct, the prediction can be tested that such a combined medical and psychosocial approach would bring about a diminution in both sickness and absenteeism from the disease. (Gardell 1971; Groen 1974; Rexed 1971).

REFERENCES

AAKSTER, C. W. (1972). Sociocultural variables in the etiology of health disturbances. Dissertation. Groningen.

ALEXANDER, F. (1934). The influence of psychological factors upon gastro-intestinal disturbances. *Psychoanal. Quest.*, **3**, 501.

—— (1950). *Psychosomatic medicine*. Norton, New York.

——, FRENCH, T. M., and PALLOCK, G. H. (1968). *Psychosomatic specificity*. University of Chicago Press, Chicago.

ALSTED, G. (1939). *The changing incidence of peptic ulcer*. Munksgaard, Copenhagen.

BASTIAANS, J. and GROEN, J. J. (1952). Psychosomatische onderzoekingen bij patiënten met Ulcus duodeni vóór en na maagresectie. *Ned. T.v. Geneesk.*, **96**, 2329.

BEAUMONT, W. (1833). *Experiments and observations on the gastric juice and the physiology of digestion*, p. 87 Allen, Plattsburg.

BOBER, H. and SCHRÖDER, H. (1956). Die Magen Kranken im Betrieb. *f. Arbeits Med.*, **6**, 49.

BYKOV, K. M. and KURZIN, L. T. (1954). *Die Kortikoviszerale pathogenese der Ulkus Krankheit*. V.E.B. Verlag, Berlin.

BRADY, J. V. (1958). Ulcers in executive monkeys. *Scient. Amer.*, **199**, 95.

CANNON, W. B. (1909). Emotional states and the function of the alimentary canal. *Am. J. Med. Sci.*, **137**, 480.

—— (1929). *Bodily changes in pain, hunger, fear and rage* (2nd edn). Appleton and Company, New York.

CRUVEILHIER, J. (1829–35): *Atlas d'anatomie pathologique du corps humain*. Paris.

CUSHING, H. (1932). Peptic ulcer and the interbrain. *Surg. Gynec. Obstet.*, **55**, 1.

DAVIS, R. C. and BERRY, F. (1971). Gastro-intestinal reactions during a noise avoidance task, quoted by Yager and Weiner (1971).

DOLL, R. and JONES, F. A. (1951). Occupational factors in the aetiology of gastric and duodenal ulcers with an estimate of their incidence in the general population. *Med. Res. Council Spec. Rep. Ser. No. 276*, His Majesty's Stationery Office, London.

—— and —— (1958). Smoking and peptic ulcer. *Schweiz. Z. allg. Path.*, **21**, 309–13.

DRAPER, G. and McGRAW, R. B. (1927). Studies in human constitution, the psychological panel. *Am. J. Med. Sci.*, **174**, 299.

—— and TOURAINE, G. A. (1932). The man-environment unit and peptic ulcer. *Arch. intern. Med.*, **49**, 616.

ELY, N. E. and JOHNSON, M. H. (1966). Emotional responses to peptic ulcer management. *Am. J. Psych.*, **122**, 1362.

FABER, K. (1935). *Gastritis and its consequences*. Munksgraard, Copenhagen.

GLEN, A. I. and COX, A. G. (1968). Psychological factors, operative procedures and results of surgery for duodenal ulcer. *Gut*, **9**, 667.

GOLDBERG, C. M. (1958). *Family influences and psychosomatic illness*. Tavistock Publications, London.

GADOUREK, I. (1965). *Absence and well-being of workers*. van Gorcum, Assen.

GARDELL, B. (1971). Alienation and mental health in the modern industrial environment. In Levi, L. (Ed.): *Society, stress, and disease* (ed. L. Levi), Vol. I, p. 148. Oxford University Press, London (with references on work and mental health in general).

GROEN, J. J. (1947). *De psychopathogenese van ulcus ventriculi et duodeni*. Scheltema and Holkema, Amsterdam.

—— (1971a). The psychosomatic specificity hypothesis for the etiology of peptic ulcer. *Psychother. Psychosomatics*, **19**, 295.

—— (1971b). Social change and psychosomatic disease. In Levi, L. (Ed.) *Society, stress, and disease* (ed. L. Levi), Vol. I, p. 91. Oxford University Press, London.

—— (1974). The challenge of the future. The prevention of psychosomatic disorders. In *Mechanisms in symptom formation* (ed. H. Musaph), p. 283. Karger, Basel.

HALLIDAY, J. L. (1948). *Psychosocial medicine. A study of the sick society*. Norton, New York.

HAMILTON, M. (1950). The personality of dyspeptics. With special reference to gastric and duodenal ulcer. *Brit. J. med. Psychol.*, **23**, 182–98.

JONES, F. A. (1957). Clinical and social problems of peptic ulcer. *Brit. Med. J.*, **I**, 719, 786.

KALK, H. (1943). Ueber kriegsbedingte Änderungen im Verdauungskanal und Kreislauf. *D. Med. W. Sch.*, **69**, 559.

KONJETZNY, G. E. (1930). Die entzündliche Grundlage der peptischen Geschwürsbildung im Magen. *Ergebn. Inn. Med. u. Khk.*, **37**, .

—— (1931). Ursache und Werdegang der Geschwürsbildung im Magen und Duodenum. *Med. Welt*, **20**, 217, 258.

KOUWENAAR, W. P. (1930). Betekenis van het voorkomen van maagzweren in de tropen voor de studie der aetiologie. *Ned. T.v. Geneesk*, **30**, 2321–41.

LEVI, L. (ed.) (1971). Society, stress, and disease, Vol. I. (Psychosocial environment and psychosomatic diseases: introduction), Oxford University Press, London.

LEVY, I. S. (1959). The acute and chronic peptic lesions of the stomach and the duodenum. *Med. Diss. Utrecht*.

—— and FUENTE, A. A. (1963). Postmortem study of gastric and duodenal peptic lesions. *Gut*, **4**, 349.

LICHTENBELT, G. (1912). *Die Ursachen des chronischen Magengeschwürs*. Jena.

LOGAN, W. P. D. and CUSHION, A. A. (1958). *Morbidity statistics from general practice. Studies on medical and population subjects No. 14*. Her Majesty's Stationery Office, London.

McRIOCH, D. (1971). The development of gastro-intestinal lesions in monkeys. In *Society, stress, and disease* (ed. L. Levi), Vol. I, p. 261. Oxford University Press, London.

210

MELTON, G. (1940). Haematemesis and the war. *Lancet*, **i**, 316.

MIRSKY, I. A.: Physiologic, psychologic and social determinants in the etiology of duodenal ulcer. *Amer. J. digest. Dis.*, **3**, 285.

—— (1952). Blood plasma pepsinogen in plasma from normal subjects and patients with duodenal ulcer. *J. Lab. clin. Med.*, **40**, 188.

MITTELMAN, B. and WOLFF, H. G. (1942). Emotions and gastroduodenal function. *Psychosom. Med.*, **4**, 5.

MORRIS, J. N. and TITMUSS, R. M. (1971). Epidemiology of peptic ulcer (quoted by Pflanz (1971)).

PFLANZ, M. (1962). *Sozialer Wandel und Krankheit*. Enke, Stuttgart.

—— (1971). Epidemiological and sociocultural factors in the etiology of duodenal ulcer. *Adv. psychosom. Med.*, **6** [Duodenal ulcer (ed. H. Weiner)] 121–51.

——, ROSENSTEIN, E., and VON UEXKÜLL, TH. (1956). Sociopsychological aspects of peptic ulcer. *J. Psychosom. Res.*, **1**, 68.

PHILIPSEN, H. (1969). Afwezigheid wegens ziekte. Dissertation, Groningen.

PORTER, R. W. (1958). Gastroduodenal lesions in behavioral conditioned monkeys. *Psychosom. Med.*, **20**, 379.

REXED, B. (1971). Synopsis of the general discussion: what to prevent and how. In *Society, stress and disease* (ed. L. Levi), Vol. I, p. 467. Oxford University Press, London.

RUESCH, J. (1948). *Duodenal ulcer, a sociopsychological study of naval personnel and civilians*. University of California Press.

SALLSTRÖM, T. (1945). The ulcer and wartime. *Acta Med. Scand.*, **120**, 288.

SMELL, W. P. and CAY, E. L. (1973). Emotional aspects of peptic ulcer surgery. In *Emotional factors in gastro-intestinal disease* (ed. A. E. Lindner). Excerpta Medica, Amsterdam.

SPICER, C. C., STEWART, D. N., and WINDSOR, D. M. (1942). Perforated peptic ulcer during heavy air raids. *Lancet*, **i**, 259.

——, ——, —— (1944). *Lancet*, **i**, 14.

SUSSER, M. (1961). Environmental factors and peptic ulcer. *The Practitioner*, **186**, 302.

—— (1967). Causes of peptic ulcer. *J. chron. Dis.*, **20**, 435.

—— and STEIN, Z. (1962). Civilization and peptic ulcer. *The Lancet*, **i**, 115.

TALMA, S. (1889). Onderzoekingen over Ulcus Ventriculi Simplex. *Ned. T. v. Geneesk.*, **25**, 669.

—— (1890). Untersuchungen über Ulcus Ventriculi Simplex, Gastromalacia und Ileus. *Zeitschr. Klin. Med.*, **17**, 10.

—— (1895). De indicaties tot maagoperaties. *Ned. T. v. Geneesk.*, **31**, 824.

THOROUGHMAN, J. C., PASCAL, G. R., JENKINS, W. O., and CRETCHER, J. C. (1964). Psychological factors predictive of surgical success in patients with intreatable duodenal ulcer. *Psychosom. Med.*, **26**, 618.

——, ——, ——, and —— (1966), *Psychosom. Med.*, **28**, 207.

——, ——, ——, and —— (1967). *Psychosom. Med.*, **29**, 273.

VAN DER HEIDE, C. (1940). Study of mechanisms in two cases of peptic ulcer. *Psychosom. Med.*, **2**, 398.

VAN IJZEREN, W. (1901) De pathogenese van de chronische maagzweer. *Ned. T. v. Geneesk.*, **37**, 478.

VAN NIEUWENHUYZEN, M. G. (1961). Peroon en Milieu van de Ulcuslijder. Dissertation, Utrecht.

VERTIN, P. G. (1954). Bedrijfsgeneeskundige Aspecten van Ulcus Pepticum. Dissertation, Groningen.

VIRCHOW, R. (1853). Historisches, Kritisches und Positives zur Lehre der Unterleibsaffektionen. *Virch. Arch.*, **5**, 362.

VON BERGMANN, G. (1913). Ulcus duodeni und Vegetatives Nervensystem. *Berl. Klin. Wo. schr.*, **50**, 2374.

—— (1936). *Funktionelle Pathologie*. Berlin.

WEINER, H. (1971). Duodenal ulcer. *Advan. psychosom. Med.*, **6**.

—— (1973). The interrelationship of emotional and physiological factors in peptic ulcer disease. In *Emotional factors in gastro-intestinal disease* (ed. A. E. Lindner). Excerpta Medica, Amsterdam.

WESTPHAL, K. (1914). Untersuchung zur Frage der nervösen Entstehung peptischer Ulcera. *D. Arch. f. klin. Med.*, **114**, 327.

—— and KETSCH, G. (1913). Das neurotische Ulcus duodeni. *Mitt. a.d. Grenzgeb. Med. u. Chir.*, **26**, 391.

WEYEL, J. (1974a). Effect of social security in an affluent society on sickness behaviour. In *Mechanisms in symptom formation* (ed. H. Musaphl), p. 272. Karger, Basel.

—— (1974b). De invloed van Sociale Zekerheid in een Maatschappij van Overvloed op Ziektegedrag. *T. Sociale Geneesk.*, **52**, 209.

WOLF, S. (1965). *The stomach*. Oxford University Press, New York.

—— (1971). Patterns of social adjustment and disease. In *Society, stress, and disease* (ed. L. Levi), Vol. I., Oxford University Press, London.

—— and WOLFF, H. G. (1943). *Human gastric function*. Oxford University Press, London.

DE WOLFF, C. J. (1972). *Arbeid in Organisaties* (contains most of the important references to modern psychological industrial management). Kluwer, Deventer.

WRETMARK, G. (1953). Peptic ulcer individual, study in heredity, physique and personality. *Acta psychiat. neurol. Scand. Suppl.* **84**.

YAGER, J. and WEINER, H. (1971). Observations in man. *Adv. psychosom. Med.* **6**, 40.

28. PSYCHIATRIC AND PERSONALITY ASPECTS OF THE WORK CAPACITY OF PSYCHOSOMATIC PATIENTS

V. P. BELOV

INTRODUCTION

The major problems of clinical medicine, physiology, and social psychology are defined by the questions of cause-and-effect relations between somatic pathology, individual psychological peculiarities, and neuropsychic disorders. One of these problems is directly concerned with pathogenesis, the matter and dynamics of neuropsychic disturbances constituting the psychiatric aspect of somatic diseases. In the narrow sense of the word, borderline mental anomalies and psychotic syndromes, the formation and dynamics of which are inseparably linked with the progress of internal diseases, can be recognized as somatogenic.

However, the somatopsychic aspects are only one side of the problem. The other side concerns the role played by mental pathology in the origin of visceral somatic disturbances. Affective disorders, such as feelings of emotional strain, anxiety, depression, or annoyance and anger, are considered an important part of the pathogenesis of the so-called psychosomatic diseases (for example, stomach ulcer and unspecific ulcerated colitis). The structure and development of neuropsychic disturbances in the course of these diseases are determined by the action of various factors. The peculiarities of their combinations would some time or other directly affect not only the role functions and the system of social contacts but also the work capacity of patients.

Directly connected with the stated problem are contemporary notions about the correlation of the functional and the organic, the evaluation of the role of somatic pathology in the origin of neuroses, and the understanding and delimitation of the criteria of pathological development of personality as the expression of an anomalous character that has taken shape in the course of psychosomatic disease.

The examination of the problem of psychosomatic interrelations requires at the very least a concise description of specific correlated questions. In our opinion these should necessarily include:

(1) Neurosis and viscero-vegetative disorders of a neurotic nature;

(2) Neuroses of organs;

(3) Correlation of the functional and the organic;

(4) Psychosomatic diseases.

NEUROSES

Neuroses are dynamic examples of borderline mental pathology, a variant of a psychogenic reaction. In this case the disorders are of a partial nature and the clinical picture of neurotic disturbances reflects the contents of a psychic trauma, while the awareness of illness with its phenomena characterized by an element of estrangement and a sensation of internal lack of freedom remains (Kerbikov 1900). An emotional tension inherent in conditions unfavourable for a patient constitutes one of the major factors that provoke an attack of neurotic derangement.

From the standpoint of time parameters, the criteria of neurosis that apply to such integrative and social levels of consciousness as a critical attitude towards the symptoms of the disease and serious consideration of its discord with the principles of the personality, do not always apply. Perhaps the concept of a pathogenically significant degree of mental trauma should be recognized more adequately in the examination of conditions bringing about neurotic disorders. This mental trauma assumes the quality of an aetiological factor of neurosis only if there has been situational–psychological and somatic predisposition. Therefore even the same mental trauma affects the same patient in different ways depending on his mental and somatic state at the moment of traumatizing.

Neurotic disturbances change the character of relations between the patient and his environment. The stimuli that have been indifferent prior to the illness become pathogenic. This results in the creation of prerequisites for the repetition and fixation of pathological (anomalous, in the broader sense) forms of responding. However, the clinical dynamics of neuroses cannot be reduced only to reactive forms which are immediately conditioned by concrete psychotraumatizing influences.

Mechanisms of syndrome formation should not be considered an exceptional and unique phenomenon peculiar to the given case. They take the form of a derivative of active complex factors, including those which mediate the phylogenetic common character of metabolism of neural tissue and the physiological fundamentals of cerebration. Other factors define the primary differentiation and dynamics of neurotic disorders. Hereditary and congenital features of the nervous system as well as didactic, psychological, situational factors and different pathogenic influences throughout all stages of ontogenesis play a certain part ere. These factors serve as the cause of individual differences in the manifestation and feeling of neurotic symptoms.

To a certain extent it can be said that a mental trauma results in neurosis and determines the pattern of feelings, while hereditary, congenital, and acquired peculiarities of a mental individuality add clinically specific character to the neurotic syndrome. If this correlation is considered in the reverse order, i.e. from the aspect of psychopathological structure of neurosis, it can be acknowledged that the picture of psychogenic reaction reflects the degree of maturity and the synchronization of the mind as a whole or in respect to its separate parts.

Vegetative-diencephalic and visceral disorders

These form an integral part of the clinical picture of neuroses and in a number of cases they come to the fore and prove to be the most structural and expressive component of neurotic states. This used to underlie numerous ideas concerning the character, content, and even nosological classifications of the disorders which were described recently as vegetative neurosis, vegetative dystonia or disfunctions, vegetosis, vegetopathy, vegetative nervous syndrome, etc.

At present few people doubt that vegetative neuroses are a historical category but all the so-called general neuroses and mononeuroses are characterized by more or less distinct viscerovegatative and diencephalic disorders — sometimes diffuse, sometimes accentuated mainly in one or another system of internal organs.

Functional pathology of the diencephalic–hypothalamic region plays a significant part in the formation of a sequence of mechanisms that is interconnected in the process of development of neurotic reactions. These interrelations are concentrated around the principal dynamic link, which is represented by the apparatus of adaptation activity and human phylogenetic self-protection against pathogenic conditions in particular (Ivanov-Smolensky 1965).

In this case the cause-and-effect relation proves to be complex. It is determined by functional and morphological features and by the significance of subcortical and cortical structures for the preservation and development of the apparatuses defining human biological and social adaptation. Neurosomatic activities, equilibration, and environmental adjustment are mainly controlled by the cortex (corticopyramidal and corticoextrapyramidal). At the same time the cerebral cortex is an anatomic substratum of human social and work activities. However, in practice the fixing of habits of socially significant behaviour depends to a great extent on the synchronism and interrelation of work of different cerebral zones. A synchronism in the development of functional systems responsible for the formation of certain components of mental individuality may cause disharmony and anomaly of personality with painful responses to the action of ordinary and commonly indifferent stimuli, including those of a situational and psychological nature.

ORGAN NEUROSES

Viscerovegetative disorders may assume a distinct reflex character. This can be explained by the fact that in addition to chronic forms there are paroxysmal forms of diencephalic disorders that are combined with the action of both elementary and complex environmental stimuli addressed to a single analyser. The dysfunction of those sections of the diencephalo–hypophysal region that constitute an anatomic substratum of the limbic system (McLean's 'visceral brain') predetermines to a considerable degree the appearance of neurotic reactions accentuated on viscerovegetative disorders and commonly known as neuroses of organs.

The problems of aetiology, pathogenesis, and terminological independence of neuroses of organs are the subject of lively discussions by internists, neuropathologists, psychiatrists, and psychologists. In the 1930s the problem of organ neuroses was widely reflected in the works of G. Bergmann, the founder of the theory of functional pathology, who disapproved of the term 'neurosis of organ' on the whole, or, to be more accurate, the concept of 'reine Organneurose' which was commonly used at that time. Bergmann considered it unlikely that there were diseases that were related solely to the nervous system of the stomach, for example, and thus caused 'pure neurosis' of that organ.

At present many authors are studying the nature of preferential visceral affections in the course of neurotic disturbances with regard to a number of factors. Particular importance is attached to acquired or constitutional deficiency of any organ; to the coincidence of a mental trauma with intensified activities of one or another part of the viscerovegetative system; to the relation of an organ function to the mental content of a pathogenic experience; to the degree and character of the injury of central innervation mechanisms which partly control several functional systems; to the formation of a conditioned reflex to an external signal that was previously directed to a pathological point in the corticovisceral connection; to the fixation of vegetative–somatic manifestations of emotional reactions, originating under the influence of mental traumas.

The concept of local corticovisceral disturbances comes from acknowledging the fact that general neurosis as a prolonged, chronically progressing disorder of higher nervous activity creates the conditions for the appearance of functional and organic injuries in one or another visceral system which is characterized by locally increased sensitivity.

CORRELATION OF THE FUNCTIONAL AND THE ORGANIC

The problem of organ neurosis is linked with the development and present state of different concepts

213

which are meant to explicate the character of inter-relations between the functional and the organic, between the psychogenic and the structural–morpho-logical, between neurosis and anatomical visceral affection. In other words the problem concerns psychosomatic interrelations, the meaning of which is interpreted differently, proceeding from diverse trends of psychiatry and general medicine.

According to Myasishchev (1900) the role of a neuro-psychic factor is not identical in neuroses and in the progress of internal diseases. General neuroses and psychosomatic diseases, represented mainly by system neuroses, in practice differ from one another. A psychogenic somatic disease with symptoms common to both of the above constitutes a selective injury of one system.

Attempts to give a universal prescription for the explanation of the nature of different diseases and mechanical utilization of empirical examples applied to the wide problem of psychosomatic pathology often result in a sceptical or even negative attitude towards the former ideas or fashionable concepts.

In the USSR the traditions of integrative clinical assessment of a patient and the recognition of the leading role of reflex mechanisms in pathology reflect one of the major aspects of the concept of psychosomatic inter-relations. In that case, the term 'psychosomatic' implies that diverse circumstances of social, occupational, and family life have an impact on the personality, are endured in accordance with individual experience, and arouse psychogenic, i.e. reactive, conditions accompanied by pronounced viscerovegetative disorders of a functional or organofunctional type.

PSYCHOSOMATIC DISEASES

In international medical and socio-psychological literature the psychosomatic concept that took shape in the 1930s leads to a certain approach to the examination of clinical data and tends to oppose the one-sided interpretation of a disease as 'organ pathology'. This concept emphasizes the idea of body integrity, the paramount significance of peculiarities of personality, and the patient's basic affective characteristics as playing major roles in the dynamics of any pathological process.

In recent times the overwhelming majority of the supporters of this trend have adhered in their starting points to Freud's notion of the energy of primitive impulses. The energetic nature of forced-out impulses would find its further expression in roundabout ways by provoking clinical syndromes symbolizing allegorically the inhibited effect that aroused them.

From that point of view the clinical manifestation of a somatic disease is considered to be a symbolic expression of an unresolved emotional conflict, a form of specific protective device, a result produced by mental strain on a certain organ, and it is regarded as the transformation of that strain into a bodily symptom.

The psychosomatic approach applies mainly to the diseases progressing in connection with psycho traumatizing effects, i.e. Selye psychological stress. The affect causing the bodily changes which are known a excessive tension appears as a link between mental an somatic spheres. The most frequent affects are anguish anxiety, and depression expressed in neurovegetative endocrine, and motor reactions as well as in the feeling c fear which is a subjective perception of 'danger'. A specific and stereotyped character of reactions is distinctive feature of psychosomatic diseases notwith standing the fact that the nature of pathogenic factor ('stressors') may be rather diverse.

Repeated or continuous disturbances of a function of any organ as a result of the action of psychological stres may eventually lead to irreversible changes in the livin being, or in other words to a psychosomatic disease. I this concept the problem of 'vulnerability' and 'choice o organ', i.e. the problem of a specific and definit psychosomatic disease, is a stumbling-block.

Various theories underlying the psychosomatic concept

It is the different understandings of the mechanisms o visceral affection and the concrete sources of psycho genic reactions that mainly account for the fact that th general concept of psychosomatic medicine splits int numerous hypotheses that tend to squeeze the dialectica problem of psychogenesis into the narrow bounds o 'pathological substance'.

At present the psychosomatic concept, in the opinio of many authors (Bassin 1962; Kimball 1970; Kurtsin 1973; Lipowski 1970; Morozov and Lebedinsky 1972; V M. Morozov 1961; Tsaregorodtsev and Shingarov 1972 does not represent a clearly outlined trend though i possesses a doctrine which constitutes in a way it theoretical foundation. The ranks of its supporter include both those who try to throw off the dogmas tha have considerably influenced the psychosomatic trend and those who are still adhering to these orthodo traditions and deepening them.

The psychoanalytical concept is not always uniforml and equally reflected in psychosomatic medicine Lisitsin (1965) distinguishes two major trends in it: (1 psychoanalytical, and (2) theoretical concepts with th application of achievements of modern natural scienc (the role and significance of the reticular formation o the brain, Selye's (1973) theory of a common adaptatio syndrome, the work of Gellhorn and Loofborougl (1966) on the role of hypothalamus and sympathopara sympathetic equilibrium in emotional processe attempts to apply certain theses of Pavlov's refle theory, etc.).

Strategic aims of the psychosomatic trend can only be attained through all-round studies of the physiological endocrino-metabolic, and psychological reactions tha appear in response to influences of the natural and socia environment, principally in response to those influence which are directed to the mechanisms of the adaptatio syndrome. In the last two or three years these ideas hav found their representation in the works of Argüelles *et al.* (1972), Curtis (1972), Yegorkova *et al.* (1971), Kimball (1970), Lipowski (1970), Mason (1970) and Ursova (1973).

The psychosomatic concept, in the opinion of Mason (1970), still remains more of a collection of numerous clinical observations and case histories than a guide to action. The amazing paradox of modern biology, the author continues, consists in the fact that there is not yet a sufficiently organized and established science of integrative physiology, that is, a science which might serve as the basis of psychosomatic medicine.

One of the most significant objectives of psychosomatic medicine, as stressed by Lipowski (1970), is to identify a chain of events interconnecting perception, thoughts, and feelings on the one hand, and physiological changes on the other. Furthermore, it is necessary to ascertain how a change in physiological functions of organs is perceived and evaluated by an individual and what effect it produces upon his cognitive, emotional, and psycho-motor activities.

Of special practical importance is the study of inter-relations of these processes and their influence on the development, progress, and sequellae of a disease. In this connection one should refer to the original view-point of Levi (1972) that it is the intensity, and not the quality, of physiological reactions to psychosocial stimuli that constitutes the basic correlative of Selye stress.

Contemporary scientific publications expounding researches in the field of psychosomatic medicine con-sider a number of essentials which are undoubtedly interpreted in different ways but are still aimed at solving problems of the immediate or near future.

Psychosomatic illness viewed as self-inflicted
First and foremost it is necessary to emphasize critical analysis and revaluation of the concepts which defined the content of the first stage of development in the psychosomatic trend (1930–55), in particular Dunbar's conception of personality specificity and Alexander's concept of specific conflict.

As asserted by Buchner, the emphasis in these cases is shifted from the causes of disease to their meaning, arising from which, pathological bodily disturbances are regarded as freely chosen conditions of human existence. This eventually leads to the submission that a human being 'makes' his illnesses himself. Illness turns out to be the price man has to pay for the personality he embodies. Moreover, the types of personalities estab-lished by psychosomatics are static and many-sided, while the overwhelming majority of 'specific' situations typical for the genesis of certain diseases suggest the meaning common to all mankind, which casts doubt on their pathogenicity.

As stated by L. I. Lipowski (1970), the viewpoint that existed for a long time in psychosomatic medicine and which was based on the assumption that an organic disease was a means of expressing subconscious conflicts and effects, is rather a tenet than a verified scientific hypothesis. The psychosomatic theory, the author adds, is no longer a continuation of psychoanalysis. We live at a time when the role of emotions is increasing and they are being expressed in the conscious sphere more and more openly but this does not reduce the gravity of serious vegetative disorders and diseases. The Soviet psychologist V. N. Myasishchev (published in Russian) says that the deeper the awareness of a pathological factor in its pathological and psychotraumatizing action, the more severe its effect in terms of the vocational, socio-economic, and everyday consequences for a patient and his relatives.

Adaptation and defence mechanisms
The growing purposefulness of the study of mechanisms of adaptation and psychological defence cultivated by an individual in response to the action of stressing factors is the positive aspect of the many-sided and complex pro-cess of critical analysis of psychoanalytic and existential attitudes in psychosomatics. In accordance with V. V. Kovalyov's (1972) opinion, active and passive adapta-tion reactions are more or less characteristic of all chronic somatic patients. They include various com-pensatory reactions (e.g. heightened interest in intel-lectual studies, artificial limitation of contacts, disposition to day-dreaming, etc.). L. L. Rokhlin (1972) is justified in singling out not only a personality component in the structure of such reactions but also a pattern of public response emerging around one or another disease and accompanied by prevalent notions about it.

Regarding psychosomatic diseases as a disturbance of failing integrative mechanisms, L. W. Mason (1970) lays emphasis on the necessity of scrutinizing methods of psychological defence in the broad sense and of defining these methods as a number of mechanisms for preven-tion, reduction, or counteracting of emotional experiences.

Jallade (1971) believes that a psychosomatic disease is one of the particular examples of defence process that should be studied in a wider group along with neurotic and psychotic processes. While emphasizing the neces-sity of drawing physiological and psychological research together, Knapp (1970) thinks, however, that neither stress nor defence properties can be considered stable exponents of emotional reactions of the human organism and, therefore, that they should rather be studied jointly as a part of the extensive psychosocial sphere of psycho-somatic medicine.

Need for more clinical research into psychosomatic illness
However, such a broad deductive attitude cannot be an alternative to the accumulation of empirical data obtained experimentally or by comparing clinical evidence and aimed at disclosing the character of correlations between the action of socio-psychological stimuli on the one hand, and personality reaction, psychoendocrinous, humoural, and physiological changes, on the other. Lately the objects and results of

this type of research have found expression in the works of Mason (1970), Curtis (1972), Lipowski (1970), Argüelles *et al.* (1972), Fröberg *et al.* (1970), Brock (1972), and Hittmair (1970).

Formulating one of the aims of the researches carried out in the period 1962–5, Levi (1972) asserts that Selye's concept must be regarded as a working hypothesis which requires evaluation and re-evaluation with the use of refined methods. That concept does not necessarily prescribe an unconditional acceptance of the idea of 'non-specificity'. The system of evidence evolves by the successive development of hypotheses in respect of the fact that a particular reaction of the human organism appears:

(a) In a relatively diverse number of situations;
(b) In response to a relatively diverse number of stimuli;
(c) In response to 'any stimulus'.

As a result of the experiments conducted, the author obtained confirmation that the psychosocial stimuli of short-term or moderate duration make for the change in sympathicomedullary activity, probably in the form of a component of a phylogenetically old, unspecific reaction picture, i.e. 'Selye stress'.

Parallel with the expansion of the range of researches connected with the study of physiological and bio-chemical components of the reactions caused by emotiogenic forces, the quest continues for a rational answer to various aspects of this problem from the standpoint of the psychological, personality, and social contents of psychosomatic conceptions. In addition to the authors already referred to, I should mention here Platonov (1972), Myasishchev (1967, 1972), Gefter and Ivanov (1972), G. Condron (1971), Wan (1971), Wardwell (1973), Paykel and Prusoff (1971), Horowitz (1973), and G. Schwöbel (1971).

Questioning the necessity of transcultural studies of the stress theory, Lazarus (1966) writes about the validity of the recognition of a sociological stress caused by various social cataclysms and catastrophic events. In examining personality factors the author focuses his attention on

(1) Motivation characteristics of an individual;
(2) System of attitudes (*ustanovka*) that co-ordinates the relations with the environment;
(3) Intellectual capabilities, educational level, and aptitude for conceptual thinking.

Growing consideration is being given to the study of the psychological problem of a vocational stress and, in particular, to the estimation of the correlated stress and work capacity (Wolff 1968; Nitsch 1973; Adum 1971; Pincherle 1972). Attention is drawn to the realistic attitude of Nitsch (1973), who recognizes the practical significance of the stress theory proceeding from prevention, a sound approach to, and elimination of

stresses as the basic condition for the organization of labour. The author is quite optimistic when he asserts that a stress is not only a consequence but a basis of vocational activity, i.e. it is simultaneously a consequence and condition of man's participation in socially useful labour. In the end he arrives at a general formula that conveys the dialectic idea of the biosocial unity of the human being, namely a stress is not only dangerous for life but is also an indispensable condition for existence. A stress is a taste of life, Selye (1973) writes; life is based on human comprehension of reaction to stress undergoing continuous changes. This compre-hension proves to be the only path that takes us out of the jungle of conflicting thoughts.

In conclusion it should be said that factual scientific data and generalizations obtained while solving clinical, physiological, and socio-psychological aspects of the problem will be of great significance for the progress of the psychosomatic trend in medicine. They disclose, for instance, the part played by a mental factor in the emergence and course of certain somatic diseases, reveal endocrinous–metabolic and physiological mechanisms of negative emotions (psychological stress) as well as psychogenic forms of viscerosomatic pathology linked with a personality reaction representing in that case an important element of pathogenesis of functional and organic disorders.

CHARACTER VARIATIONS AMONG PATIENTS WITH ULCERS OR ULCERATIVE COLITIS

No existing conception postulating the idea of somatic integrity can deny the role of personality features and the subjective significance of psychotraumatizing effects in the origin of many somatic diseases. However, of similar importance is the study of correlations between psychic and somatic pathology, psychiatric evaluation of psychoneurological disturbances developing in the course of the principal disease and also precise linking of mental pathology and personality reactions to the modified family and social status in the framework of factors resulting in reduced work capacity and failure of social adjustment mechanisms. It is in this context that we have studied stomach and duodenal ulcer and unspecific chronic ulcerated colitis.

For the last 12 years 316 patients have been under dynamic supervision, 104 of them with ulcerated colitis.

Ulcer and ulcerated colitis affect patients with different characters; their personality features cannot be squeezed into the Procrustean bed of a concept of a definite character type. With a great degree of conven-tionality, the common features of these patients' neuro-psychic structure might be represented by heightened uneasiness and irritability, extreme social commitment, and pronounced sense of duty. The total number of cases was subdivided into several character variants with intermediate forms in between.

The first character variant

The most typical feature for the first variant (91 cases) was prompt adjustment to the conditions of social and vocational activities. They are basically orderly and purposeful people who see their capacities in proper perspective and perform their functions conscientiously. Within reasonable limits they take care of their prestige and value their reputation as a skilled and honest experts. They have little trouble in maintaining old contacts and setting up new ones but almost always keep their distance and rarely exploit their acquaintances for their purely time-serving benefits. Being energetic and active, these people often display creative initiative, they willingly join in public activities, devoting plenty of strength and time to them. As a rule, they are organizers in their collectives, heads and leaders by virtue of their characters.

Placed in work conditions they look orderly, work efficiently, easily stand physical strain, insomnia, and other mishaps. In their work they are notable for rapidity and dexterity, there is no mercantile narrow-mindedness in their attitude towards wages. They are reasonably economical and sometimes even indifferent to money. Stinginess is alien to them. They speak of careless and lazy workers with contempt or condescending indifference.

They accept life's misfortunes as something fated and inevitable. Their struggle against various hardships is active and purposeful but without rancour, morose discontent, or panic confusion. Their compassion is sincere with no traces of affectation, hypocritical tearfulness, and melodrama. These people have respect for their families, value fellowship of friends or business-like contacts with fellow workers; they are thoughtful and sympathetic, they try to avoid conflict situations and can reach a compromise settlement. However, in their estimation of moral and ethical aspects of behaviour they show intolerance, extreme peremptoriness, refusing sometimes to be indulgent to the faults of their acquaintances and fellow workers. But this personality feature never grows into exaggerated moralizing. These people do not take offence at a joke, they possess a sense of humour, and can get on even with those who are very scrupulous in their choice of friends. Their emotional reactions to psychotraumatizing effects are characterized by vividness, expressiveness, and pithiness; and the content and manifestation of the reactions are more likely to reflect discontent and resentment than anxiety and agitation.

Some of these persons are notable for their jovial and amiable disposition and for good-natured and elated moods. They do not go deeply enough into relations between people, which accounts for their one-sided evaluation of many facets of vocational and family conflict situations from positions of narrow personal interpretation of social behaviour categories. If they actively participate in domestic or labour conflicts they often take the stand of 'advocates of a just settlement, reasonable approach, and immediate elimination of defects'. However, such behaviour is a somewhat hypertrophic but objective reaction to actions of people who permitted themselves to take gross administrative measures or arrived at a wrong decision.

The second character variant

The patients included in the group of the second variant (85 cases), with all the variety of their professional activities as well as of their intelligence, educational, and social levels, were united by personality features of which the most essential are pronounced obligingness, high sense of duty, somewhat exaggerated adherence to moral and ethical standards, anxious attitude towards work and working programmes, emotional unsteadiness, and impatience. They are easily kindled by an idea but rarely persist in carrying out the adopted decision. Their reaction to life's misfortunes assumes an oversensitive or even pathological character, with frequent emergence of disappointment accompanied by depressed and irritable mood and by taking to heart ideas of little value. Displaying anxious conscientiousness, these people spend disproportionately much effort and time even on the fulfilment of ordinary work to the detriment of their health and repose. In their relations with those around them they are sometimes harsh, unrestrained, and straightforwardly formal and sometimes superfluously sensitive and tiresome. Up to a point their hot temper and irritability are camouflaged by correct social and ethical personality orientation.

Despite emotional syntony and seemingly easy readjustment from one form of activity to another, these people are characterized by inertness and one-sided attachment, insufficient operativeness, and even rigidity in evaluations, labour activities, and modes of behaviour. They are uncompromising to what in their opinion describes a person negatively and criticize people for their lack of principles with undisguised indignation, implicating by this the change in their attitude in respect to a certain person, a group of persons, an object of spiritual value, an ideal, or a social institution. The restoration of contacts between people who have previously been on bad terms with each other provokes their naïve surprise. Sometimes they realize that a conflict situation which they have created for some reason or other is quite artificial but still they are not resolute enough to admit pettiness of their 'struggle for reasons of principles'.

Within the framework of the same variant one can consider cases with the features of heightened impressionability, vulnerability, and touchiness. Shyness, inability to actively and consistently uphold one's interests, implicit observance of formal demands, altruistic content of personality trends and labour motives logically supplement these signs. These patients can be easily confused, they feel ill at ease in acute situations. Failures give rise to a painful reaction, often accompanied by a sense of inferiority. Of some of them it can be said that they are subtle and mild by nature, with pronounced traits of inhibition. On encountering life's predicaments they are easily provoked to irritation, intractability, petty captiousness, and stubbornness. All this testifies to the fact that their social adjustment mechanisms are not sufficiently stable and firm; sometimes they are rather fragile while the character, the form, and the degree of manifestation of mental disharmony in some cases approximate or meet the criteria of anomalous asthenic personality.

Under the influence of emotiogenic stresses and conflict situations, especially in combination with the action of harmful somatic symptoms, borderline mental disturbances characterized by excessive irritability, worried expectation, and anxiety appear. Owing to the mental features typical of these individuals, they have difficulties in enduring psychotraumatizing experiences and emotional strain.

The third character variant

The third variant (61 cases) was represented by patients who could be ranked with a category of straightforward, uncompromising justice-seekers, harsh and exacting 'champions of justice', captious moralists, primitively narrow-minded lovers of 'truth and principle'. They cherish their prestige and keep jealous watch that their authority should not be undermined either in social or family life. In a concrete psychological situation they frequently display selfishness, stubbornness saturated with affection, irritability, and negativistic attitude to disciplinary requirements of 'superiors', which is given as a formal reason for conflict with management and compulsory change of workplace.

As a matter of fact the described typology of individuality manifests itself in its exaggerated form in explosive epileptoid characters with their affectiveness, explosiveness, fits of irritability and rage, exceptional diligence and industry, slavish attachment to belongings, pedantry, fruitless questing for justice, and sanctimonious struggle for high moral standards. Extreme demands in respect to their associates and petty fault-finding make them tiresome and importunate.

The standing of these people in working collectives took different forms. In some cases they appeared to be 'punctual functionaries' and good workers, skilful and able experts with detailed knowledge of their jobs, highly trained specialists, people filled with elevated sense of duty and social consciousness. In other cases these people were at the bottom of grave conflicts not only in their microgroups but also in large collectives of fellow workers. They constantly brought an element of rigidity and ill will into mutual relations between people, groundlessly accused managers of the institution of red tape and poor knowledge of their duties, started heated quarrels on insignificant occasions, intensifying the emotional content of such conflicts by continuous insinuations and insults. Some of these patients shifted the entire weight of their feelings on to their jobs, showing extraordinary diligence and industry.

Exaggerated and grotesque forms of the above-mentioned personality structure quite often resulted in

failure of social adjustment mechanisms and more or less stable pathological reactions to life's adversities. In general this group embraced patients with the symptoms of epileptoid character and inclinations toward paranoia formations. In eleven cases the point involved anomaly of personality of explosive epileptoid stamp, while nine suffered from epilepsy.

The fourth character variant

The people included in the fourth variant (39 cases) are notable for emotiveness with an inclination towards maxims and fervid worship of rather questionable idols. Their characteristic features involve spontaneity and frankness, an overt manner of giving opinions and evaluations, prompt and sometimes impulsive decision making, undisguised yearning to be in the spotlight and to dictate one's demands. These personality traits are organically supplemented by irritability and impatience.

Egoism is not infrequently coupled with inconsistency, and inability to build up any harmonious system of mutual relations with relatives, friends, and strangers. The circumstances limiting an immediate bent for pleasure are hardly taken into account; everything that interferes with instant fulfilment of wishes is straightforwardly and abruptly rejected. Sometimes simple motives and naïve desire to stand one's ground in face of public opinion are the basis of this. These persons prefer the ideas of the *avant-garde*, they are inclined to brilliant and resounding roles. Parallel with this, heightened suggestibility and imitativeness are found in similar cases. The patients get tired, with frequent mood fluctuations; their relations with people around them are built up on an unstable basis of emotional contact but at the same time their belief in ideals and their formally trusting attitude towards people remain.

The frequent combination of heightened suggestibility and suspiciousness may seem paradoxical on the face of it. The peculiarity of such a combination may be explained by asynchrony of personality, where spontaneity and straightforward reaction to imperative tone and meaning of speech remain at the same time as a timid and distrustful attitude to new people and situations acquires a hypertrophic tone. Sometimes such patients disguise themselves in the make-up of 'partisans of justice' and 'protectors of the weak', trying to show by their behaviour comprehension of man's spiritual world and high principles of humanism.

Some of these persons, possessing a lively temperament and jovial disposition, lead a care-free, untroubled life; they easily change jobs, frequently move from one place to another, 'enjoy their life' without discovering their vocations as a rule. The women usually prove to be poor housekeepers, unskilful in carrying out household work; they thoughtlessly and unpractically waste money on delicacies and sweets, taking no care to provide the family with food each day, and to buy in stores. The men devote little attention to he upbringing of their children, look for 'easy' money, nd sometimes become chronic alcoholics.

Individual peculiarities of some patients (33 cases) ould not be consigned to any one variant, while in seven ases serious neuropsychic diseases (oligophrenia, raumatic or epileptic dementia, schizophrenia) were •bserved.

Discussion of the character variants

n summarizing the findings of clinico-psychological xamination of the composition of cases it should be noted that the differentiation of the above-mentioned personality variants is to a certain extent schematic. Such classification is possible by virtue of correct accentuation of the essential and most expressive features of the personality, which constitute its sociopsychological ndividuality.

One pole of this characterological scale was occupied by basically harmonious individuals with sufficiently stable mechanisms of social and labour adjustment. The other pole was taken up by patients whose personality structure was to a certain degree defined by traits in the epileptoid or hysterical range.

The central part of the scale was represented by a less homogeneous group. Those cases were united by similar or even allied mental peculiarities that made up a kind of link, imparting a definite degree of structure and often a qualitative originality of the entire personality to the chain of individual forms. The hypersocial direction of motives and actions, a high level of claims, heightened irritability and anxiety, weak stability of social adaptation mechanisms, disposition to psychogenic reactions (stressful ones in the broad sense) projected to the foreground.

From the standpoint of the established notions used in clinical psychiatry, the entire composition of the patients could be subdivided into three basic categories. The first one embraced harmonious individuals whose character peculiarities could be considered in the framework of psychological evaluations (156 cases).

For understanding the neuropsychic structure of the patients in the second category (128 cases), Leonhard's theses on individuals with 'accentuated personality features', Gannushkin's work on latent psychopaths, or W. Bayer's work on threatened structures of personality are useful; Kahn called them discordantly normal people, while Luxenburger characterized them as 'people of external norm'. On the whole the social adjustment mechanisms of these people in the pre-morbid stage (i.e. prior to emergence of a somatic disease) turned out to be intact.

Social maladjustment and personality disharmony are a distinctive feature of the patients of the third category (32 cases). Without dwelling on the comparison of different opinions it can nevertheless be maintained that in a given situation, the point can be applied to psychopathic and anomalous structures.

CORRELATIONS BETWEEN SOMATIC DISEASE AND PERSONALITY DISORDERS LEADING TO REDUCTION OF WORK AND SOCIAL ACTIVITIES OF ULCER PATIENTS

In order to arrive at an understanding of the role of different factors in reducing the labour and social activities of individuals who suffer from ulcer or unspecific ulcerated colitis, it is necessary to consider the most typical interrelations of somatic disease and personality reactions to situational-somatogenic (stressor) effects. These interrelations are multiple in type and can form a dynamic and structural unity within the limits of different variants.

The first correlation

A distinctive feature of the first variant (26 cases) is a vivid manifestation of a somatic disease against a background of psychogenic psychosis. Generally these were depressive and melancholy states that developed after a severe bereavement. As a rule, mental disturbances in such cases were liable to further development. The functions of the principal mechanisms which galvanized that process were performed by situational–somatogenic effects and constitutional (including anomalous) personality features that, so to say, paved the way for pathogenic reactions and for the fixation of psychogenic disorders under the influence of endocrinometabolic and vegetative components of reactive psychosis. This combination of pathogenic factors and the neuropsychic disorders caused by them appears to be essential for chronically progressing visceral disease. Such a correlation of causative factors creates favourable conditions for the pathological development of personality.

The second correlation

For the second variant (184 cases) it was somatopsychic interrelations that proved to be most typical of the first stage of progressing stomach ulcer and ulcerative colitis. The sequence of causative factors, if their clinical aspect is considered, testifies to the fact that originally a somatic disease emerges and is then followed by the development of somatogenic or reactive mental disturbances. The latter are chiefly represented by experiences of alarm, anxiety, inward tension, and an acute feeling of helplessness. In a majority of cases the disorders did not overstep the limits of neurotic syndrome.

Somatogenic psychic asthenia was of great significance since here it assumed the role of a basic determinant of the course and development of neuropsychic disturbances. However, it should be said that for a significant proportion of these patients the dynamics of such disturbances were of a qualitative nature, although transient alarm and moods of wistful melancholy appear with exacerbation of somatic disease.

In other instances (37 cases) asthenic syndrome turned out to be one of the mechanisms of pathological development of personality. Hypochondriac phenomena, fear of death from malignant tumour, as well as symptoms of vasovegetative dystonia were quite significant. Later the hypochondriac alarm acquired monothematic contents. Anxiety, introversion, and low spirits prevail in the patients' behaviour. Annoyed discontent, heightened sensitivity, a wish to shut oneself off from every obstacle to a contemplative and measured life, frequently project to the foreground.

The emergence of new psychogenic reactions and the development of previous ones are caused by coarsening of premorbid personality features, as well as by the fact that the stimuli that had previously been indifferent acquired pathogenic quality. Neurasthenic features become intensive in the structure of personality. To a great extent this is promoted by the fixation of pathological interconnections of somatic and neuro-psychic disturbances, and also by the formation of a diencephalic syndrome with stable forms of chronic and paroxysmal disorders. In such cases one is justified in referring to a neurotic development of personality with predominating phenomena of asthenic stamp.

Although the attempts to emphasize the features of one or another composition of patients are rather relative, one can nevertheless say that restrained social contacts, egoistical change of interests, and reduction of level of social claims proved more typical of patients who suffered from ulcerative colitis than of those who suffered from stomach ulcer.

The process became more intense if surgical therapy failed to produce the desired result. The bulk of this group was composed of premorbidly adjusted, orderly persons and patients with traits of hypersociality and heightened annoyance.

The third correlation
The third variant (67 cases) combines some features of the first two but possesses its own peculiarities. In these cases the appearance of objective and typical signs of somatic disease was preceded by a vivid picture of chronic neuropsychic disturbances and viscerovegetative disorders of functional character. This was caused by psychotraumatizing situations which, by their contents and peculiarities of psychological effect, are related to two large categories: (1) conflict situations, and (2) situations of forced emotional isolation (Lakossina 1970).

Phenomena of irritated weakness as well as emotional disorders in the form of low spirits, uneasiness, and melancholy are essential in the structure of psychogenic disturbances. Thus, emotional overstrain and repeated or permanent conflicts turned into a generator of that particular form of pathological development of personality which at present is described sometimes as neurotic depression or depressive development of personality, sometimes as 'depression of exhaustion' or asthenic depression. The clinical dynamics of illness passed through a stage of 'somatic complaints', consisting in pathologic sensations from the heart and gastrointestinal tract. At first they would be characterized as a viscerovegetative component of neurotic reactions. Then they acquired an autonomous quality, though the connection with the changes in the mental states of patients remained in one form or another.

With the emergence of stomach ulcer or ulcerative colitis, there was a relatively brief concentration of personality reactions and somatogenic-situational disturbances. The depressive syndrome lost clinical independence, fears became fragmentary and changeable, and premorbid features of personality acquired a brutal and one-sided character. The asthenic kernel was mainly strengthened elements of hypersociality were losing their expressiveness and gradually supplanted by sensitivity, weak will, and annoyed impatience. Eventually this led to the formation of those forms of borderline mental pathology that belong to a collective form of neurotic (pathological) development of personality. This variant was chiefly represented by patients with symptoms of heightened uneasiness and constitutional asthenia.

An asthenic variant of neurotic development correlated, as a rule, with continuously recurrent and painful progress of somatic disease, with persistent diencephalic dissociations and a pronounced picture of physical and mental asthenia. A close interconnection of somatic and mental disturbances was an essential factor. A recurrent exacerbation was often observed during intense family clashes, divorce suits, performance of an important and urgent task, conflict with the management of an enterprise, etc. Objective manifestations and the internal picture of the illness attracted attention owing to the diversity and vividness of symptoms expressiveness and lability of experiences; rapid changes of mood; the emotion-filled content of complaints; the outwardly accentuated dramatic nature of physical sufferings with the active purpose of contemplating sensations of pain.

While estimating in this connection certain facets of the psychosomatic conception, attention ought to be drawn to the discrepancy and groundlessness of the hypothesis of 'replacement', where pathological bodily disturbances are recognized as freely chosen states of human existence. First, stomach and duodenum ulcer and ulcerative colitis appear as a result of different pathogenic effects and are accompanied by diverse neuropsychic disturbances. Second, symptoms characteristic of neurotic depression, such as 'dull melancholy', low spirits, patients' worsened feelings in the morning, tearfulness, taking 'refuge in work', remain for a lengthy period. Third, alongside the above-mentioned, the clinical picture of disease is complicated by polymorphous neurotic reactions and characterological disturbances which are based on the process of accentuation of premorbid personality features (sensitivity, scrupulousness, paranoidal features). It is the asthenic kernel that mainly becomes hypertrophic in the process, whereas hypersociality is constantly losing its energy potential and gradually being supplanted by reactions of refusal and annoyed impatience.

The fourth correlation
Finally, the last variant of correlations between ulcerative colitis, on the one hand and neuropsychic disturbances, on the other, is basically represented by forms of constitutional development. Somatogenic asthenia was not of independent significance here; in fact, that syndrome was abortive in character in a majority of cases.

The dynamics of borderline mental disorders were defined by personality reactions which acquired increasingly grosser forms in the course of somatic disease. The disease, with its characteristic complex of situational–somatogenic effects, revealed, so to speak, the pathological facade of the patients, whereas neurotic disturbances took a modest place in the structure of mental disorders. This group embraced 39 cases. The contents of the above-mentioned forms of mental pathology involved explosive (excitable), hysterical, and litigiously querulent variants of development, with reactive symptoms emerging at some stages. The appearance of these symptoms was facilitated as pathological changes of personality intensified.

Thus, the adduced comparisons reflect the diversity and different phases of participation of genetic, constitutional, situational–environmental, and personality–psychological factors in the origin, manifestation, and further progress of psychosomatic disease. Any illness, as an antithesis to health, changes the work capacity of man and limits his freedom to perform social functions.

SOCIAL CONSEQUENCES OF PSYCHOSOMATIC DISEASE

An illness that results in a reduction or loss of work capacity is at the same time a cause of upsetting social relations and social adjustment. This thesis has particular implications for psychosomatic diseases, which emerge, as repeatedly emphasized, in some way or other in connection with the influence of psychological stress.

In any given case the dynamics of disease and the state of work capacity are determined not only by the character and seriousness of somatic pathology but also by mental disturbances in their integrative and universal sense.

Essentially, in the course of prolonged and un-favourable progress of stomach and duodenum ulcer or ulcerative colitis that required surgical intervention, every other patient became disabled and for many years ahead (or for good) leaves the sphere of socially useful labour activity.

In addition, it is necessary to accentuate the significant and factual aspects of the circumstances which are not registered among the traditional indications of health but which exert a considerable influence upon work capacity of people with prognostically favourable forms

of illnesses. The point is that there are such deviations from the norm that do not lead to a cessation of man's labour activity but reduce his potentialities. Biological, social, and psychological factors, composing an unbroken unity of interrelations of an individual and natural–social environment, have a 'perturbing' influence on the mechanisms of the patient's adaptation activity. It cannot but affect the state of health and the level of work capacity, although in this case the person does not quit his labour activities.

Mental and somatic consequences of these 'perturbations' that proceed without an obvious and, therefore, a frequently unregistered reduction of work capacity are evidently deposited on the general groundwork of the endocrinous–metabolic processes that upset health.

Satisfactory work capacity vital to health
Social values, including work capacity, mediate in an invalid's health, so that work capacity is an active principle in respect to health. It is hardly possible to conceive a harmonious and synchronous development of personality, 'health for health's sake', without realized work capacity. From this point of view health determines the needs which, if satisfied, create the prerequisites for the preservation and restoration of health. It is these needs that work capacity applies to and the efficient use of which ensures the preservation of health and its restoration after illness. The reduction of work capacity and especially its complete loss leads to psychological and economic damage for every patient and for the entire society. Any illness that upsets work capacity constitutes a socially significant phenomenon. From this derives the importance of work capacity as a requisite for the social value of health.

Different reactions to loss of work capacity
Realizing his position in society by means of role functions and the system of social relations, man proceeds first and foremost from an *a priori* premiss about a sufficiently high level of his work capacity. Categories of work capacity and health are perceived in the patient's mind from a different standpoint. If we disregard numerous variants with a particular meaning, the psychological contents of these values may be expressed by the following two formulas. A serious and acutely progressing somatic disease becomes a subject of logical constructions, interpretations, alarm, and experiences: emotions and thoughts are concentrated around manifestations and attributes of the disease as a natural expression of sufferings that cause corresponding or hypertrophic fears for life. In this situation the loss of work capacity is interpreted as a natural development of events and it cannot therefore be a main source of psychological stress for the patient himself.

In the case of chronic or continuously recurring somatic disease, an individual reacts to the reduction or loss of work capacity in a different way. During many months or years of psychological struggle against the disease, an individually significant system of adjustment reactions that limit the contents of alarm and fears applicable to present-day tasks has been worked out. The patient takes some measure or other to remove physical sufferings, weakness, or discomfort, since he is aware of the origin and character of these disorders. This does not mean that adjustment reactions take standard and unified forms, and in the pattern of psychosomatic correlations they are always filled with rational contents. Psychiatric clinicians know various types of experiences of diseases which are either limited by the framework of psychological forms, or take the form of pathological psychogenic syndromes (anxiously-depressive, hypochondriacal, hysteroid, etc.). Now it is necessary to emphasize the other side of the problem.

In the prolonged course of a somatic disease the role of a psychotraumatizing factor is assumed by the patient's social disadaptation, one of the main reasons for this being the reduction or loss or work capacity. For a long time a socially orientated individual regards the new situation as a temporary episode in his life, as an inevitable and fated ordeal that has a beginning and end. Later this position is replaced by ideas of valuelessness, with experiences of emotional strain, alarm, and annoyed discontent.

The patient finds himself ensnared by permanent psychological stress, which accounts for personality reactions becoming more acute and for a further development of psychogenic neuromental disturbances. Such a stress structure has a special significance for the dynamics of psychosomatic disease since a combination of neurotic disorders and organo-functional pathology on the part of the gastrointestinal tract is a typical variant here, as shown by the example of patients suffering from stomach and duodenum ulcer and ulcerative colitis. There is enough reason to accentuate a special role of experiences generated in the patient's mind by the establishment of the fact of disablement and the associated narrowing or change of the system of social stereotypes. In fact the loss or reduction of work capacity, parallel with other reasons, proves to be an important pathogenic factor which facilitates the development of previous mental disorders and the appearance of new ones. As a result, neurotic disturbances and personality reaction variants are subjected to evolutive dynamics in the form of mediated expressions of an internal mechanism of pathological (and in particular, neurotic) development of personality.

Inadequacy of adaptation and psychological defence mechanisms in psychosomatic illness

In ordinary conditions that are defined as a norm, adaptable tendencies towards stress effects are displayed in the contents of personality reactions, which eventually result in the reduction of reactivity and the relaxation of body strain provoked by superpowerful stimuli.

Personality plasticity, i.e. capacity for adjustment in respect to excessive strain, is manifested in this relaxation. This personality feature in a generalized form is a reflection of lability as the fundamental quality of the central nervous system. There are several dynamically connected levels of adjustment to external effects, their actuality being conditioned by different states of the human body.

Under conditions of continuously recurrent progress of stomach and duodenum ulcer or ulcerated colitis which are doubtlessly accompanied by a limitation of social contacts, by a change of dynamic stereotype, and by a reduction (loss) of work capacity, the reactions that have previously been adequate acquire an excessive or pathological character. This sensitized excitability becomes very obvious when the patient finds himself in a situation where failures tend to build up and prospects become more limited. The emotional vividness and pithiness of perceptions make them quite significant for the given conditions, reducing their dependence on the contents of past experience. The acts of perception turn out to be superfluously narrow and insufficiently accurate. These peculiarities are distinctly displayed in a one-sided or even illusory perception of conflict situations.

Accelerated tempos of social life and labour activities that constitute the essence and content of the age of technological revolution require not only high efficiency and tension in work but also a rational attitude towards psychotraumatizing effects, so that a conflict experience can be localized in time to prevent switching of mechanisms of somatovegetative components of reaction. Such forms of psychological defence proved to be imperfect in the presence of somatic suffering and upset work capacity. First, there was an increasingly close relation between somatic and mental disorders which was concretely expressed, for example, in the psychogenic origin of relapses of somatic and, in particular, painful symptoms. Second, provoked and spontaneous confusions of mood appeared more often. Third, chronic and fit-like vegetativediencephalic disturbances became more and more significant in the structure of pathological phenomena. Fourth, conflict experiences accompanied by growing anxiety, emotional strain, discontent, and even aggressive fantasies easily emerged in accordance with mechanisms of actualization of previous images. The process of 'unwinding reminiscences' went with the intensification and expansion of the sphere of negative characteristics in relation to the central figure of the conflict. Frequently only minor or even positive parts of some situation or other originally emerged in patients' minds. But the mechanism of similar and contiguous associations promptly led them to reproduce just those conflict experiences which were chiefly linked with family failures, ruin of hopes for consolidation of role functions, limitation of social contacts, and progressive physical suffering.

Intense flights of the imagination carry patients' minds away to the sphere of complicated and unreal situations where personality does not always occupy the most important place but occupies sometimes the role of a martyr or hero, sometimes that of an avenger or preacher. Emotions accompany, so to say, the swift

...ovement of images and promote the complication of ...heir contents by attaching now a dynamic, now an ...lmost immobile, inert character to them.

One patient aptly called this phenomenon psycho-...ogical self-flogging. At the same time it should be ...mphasized that patients with impaired work capacity ...asily develop a sensation of 'vulnerability' and a ...athological reaction to the restriction of work and social ...anding.

Current occupational activities are carried out at times ...ith enthusiasm, impatiently, in jerks, and at times just ...ominally, forcedly, with frequent mistakes. Under the ...fluence of an unexpected stimulus or an extraneous ...ause some urgent, pressing work can be put aside even ...ough this causes direct and appreciable damage to a ...rge labour collective.

PERSONALITY CHANGES RESULTING FROM PSYCHOSOMATIC ILLNESS

...iscrepancy of personality attitudes (sociability), actual ...apacities (impaired work capacity), and tendencies to ...mit the more strenuous and complicated social contacts ...ade up on the whole a distinctive feature of the group ...f patients who suffered from stomach and duodenum ...lcer. These social and psychological parameters defined ...e personality conflict of patients who suffered from ...lcerative colitis to a lesser degree.

Those patients take ideas of inferiority close to heart, ...ey seek to maintain contacts among themselves, as if ...pporting the structure of a clan, and often find ...emselves devoid of intent to take the initiative or to act ...eyond the sphere of wishes of a leader chosen by them. ...hey avoid doing things that require an effective ...eorganization of the programme and contents of work ...nd rarely experience a feeling of significance and ...nportance of their occupational activities.

The availability of sensitized experiences leads in ...ome way or other to the reconstruction of personality ...'end according to the type of introversion, fixation on ...gnals that mainly bear negative information. Prevailing ...ntroversion cannot but affect general activity, resulting ...1 a narrowing of the range of requirements and the level ...f claims and at the same time leading to an intensi-...cation of irritable weakness.

A more or less consecutive movement of situational–...omatogenic and characterological disturbances can be ...bserved in such cases:

(1) Irritable weakness together with cancerophobic thoughts and anxiously temporizing mood;
(2) Sensitivity and inclination for paranoia with the presence of transient or stable hypochondriac formations;
(3) 'Congelation' of neurotic symptoms and patho-logical reactions with relatively distinct delimitation of syndromic features, annoyed impatience, anxiety; depressiveness, biased attitude towards one's associates, etc.

Thus, the point concerns the criteria of pathological (neurotic) development of personality which should be understood, in accordance with Kerbikov's (1955, 1962) view, as one of the stages in the formation of acquired character pathology. Neurotic development combines the features of neurosis and personality anomaly when the whole patient's life appears to be unsuccessful, rather than a certain life situation.

Neurotic development not only becomes apparent in clashes with extraordinary and psychotraumatizing circumstances but is manifested spontaneously as well, i.e. it turns into a peculiarity of responding to relatively invariable everyday stimuli of the environment. The basic mechanism is really a dynamic complication of situational–somatogenic disorders, with gradual singling-out and 'congelation' of the central syndromic link that determines a clinical variant of this form of border line pathology.

This process actually results in a disharmonious personality change when one of the previously indistinct features acquires hypertrophic acuteness and becomes a sort of dominant in the changed personality structure. Strict single-mindedness is reflected in a selective attitude towards perceived phenomena, with collective single-mindedness replaced by egocentric, narrowed isolation. The existence of a deep epicentre of uneasiness inevitably leads to failures and frustrations, which furthers the intensification of an introverted attitude and heightens sensitivity to stress effects. Even sharp words with a manager may arouse a prolonged pathological reaction (depression, anger, alarm) that constitutes a subjective state, actualized in behaviour but maturing long before the given occasion.

The sharp narrowing of the range of active motives creates the premises for the emergence of an original conflict between 'obligation' and 'desire'. The preservation of a certain range of responsibilities which do not correspond to the desire leads to inward com-pulsion, outwardly expressed by activities with little efficiency but inwardly accompanied by excessive strain. As a result the entire complex of collectively directed activities loses its dominant motivation and yields to individualistic, purely personal motives.

Thus, there are enough reasons to speak of an inter-related chain of events representing psychiatric and socio-psychological aspects of the problem of psycho-somatic diseases. Progressing against a background of mental health or against that of acute and chronic neuropsychic disturbances, stomach and duodenum ulcer or ulcerated colitis appear to be direct causes of somatogenic and situational-psychogenic disturbances that pave the way for the formation of personality disharmony, i.e. pathological development of per-sonality. An important role of a psychotraumatizing factor is played by a complex of circumstances linked with the impairment of work capacity and the narrowing of social contacts. Psychosomatic illness, progressing as a result of different pathogenic agents and peculiarities of homeostasis, eventually proves to be a reason for the

223

reduction (loss) of work capacity and for stable mental disturbances which in turn galvanize the progress of somatic pathology and the limitation of social contacts. The general law of cyclic recurrence finds here its regrettable corroboration.

CONCLUSIONS

1. Stomach (and duodenum) ulcer and unspecific ulcerative colitis affect patients with different personality structures; therefore it is baseless to speak about a universal or specific type of personality.

2. In addition to harmonious, socially adjusted individuals, the observed patients include persons with sharpened streaks ('accentuated', according to K. Leonhard) and anomalous personalities (psychopaths in the traditional sense).

3. While rejecting the idea of the universal personality structure, it is necessary to emphasize that different variants and combinations of heightened uneasiness, irritability, and hypersociality were essential features of patients' mentality.

4. Somatic illness progresses, as a rule, against a background of emotional strain, neurasthenic neurosis, neurotic depression, or reactive psychosis.

5. One of the particular variants of the dynamics of pathological phenomena consists in the following stages: (1) vegetative–diencephalic disturbances as an essential correlate of general neurotic disorders, (2) a stage of 'somatic complaints' that was considered within the framework of neurotic development of personality, (3) increasingly precise accentuation of one or another zone of the gastrointestinal tract, (4) organofunctional pathology as a clinical form of psychosomatic illness.

6. Somatic illness and its socio-psychological consequences are a source of various but constant stressful influences.

7. In the course of continuously recurrent, chronic somatic disease, intensification, 'congelation', and dynamic complication of previous border line mental disturbances or newly emerged ones take place in the form of a reflection of the inward mechanisms of pathological (neurotic, in particular) development of personality.

8. The reduction (loss) of work capacity accompanied by the narrowing sphere of social contacts is a source of conflict experiences and one of the fundamental mechanisms that intensify the process of pathological development of personality.

9. The chain of cause-and-effect relations between somatic pathology, neuropsychic disturbances, and reduction (loss) of work capacity in its socio-economic expession bears a complex cyclic character. Influenced by stressful effects, various links of this chain are of major significance and impart a dynamic character to different forms of pathology.

REFERENCES

ADUM, O. (1971). *Oboljenja saobracajuin radnika Glasnik* Belgrade, **20**(1), 39–46.

ARGÜELLES, A. E., MARTINEZ, M. A., HOFFMAN, C., ORTIZ, G. A., and CHEKHERDEMIAN, M. (1972). Corticoadrenal and adrenergic overactivity and hyperlipidemia in prolonged emotional stress. *Hormones*, **3**, 167–74.

BASSIN, F. V. (1962). *Consciousness and 'the unconscious'*. Moscow (in Russian).

BOYLE, B. P. and COOMBS, R. H. (1971). Personality profiles related to emotional stress in the initial year of medical training. *J. med. Educ.*, **10**, 882–8.

BROCK, J. F. (1972). Nature, nurture and stress in health and disease. *Lancet*, **i**, 701–4.

BYKOV, K. M. and KURTSIN, I. T. (1960). *Cortico-visceral pathology*. Leningrad (in Russian).

CONDRAU, G. (1971). Psychosomatische Krankheit als soziales Problem. *Ther. Umschau*, **6**, 364–72.

CURTIS, G. C. (1972). Psychosomatics and chronobiology: possible implications of neuroendocrine rhythms. *Psychosom. med.*, **34**, 235–56.

DAVIDENKOV, S. N. (1963). *Neurosis*, Leningrad (in Russian).

FRÖBERG, J., KARLSSON, C. G., and LEVI, L. (1970). Conditions of work: psychological and endocrine stress reactions. *Arch. environm. Hlth.*, **21**(6), 789–97.

GEFTER, A. I. and IVANOV, N. V. (1972). On the place of the psychic factor in etiology, pathogenesis and clinical aspects of myocardic infarcts. In *On the role of the psychic factor in the appearance, course and treatment of somatic diseases*, pp. 87–94. Moscow (in Russian).

GELLHORN, E. and LOOFBOURROW, G. N. (1966). *Emotions and emotional disorder*. Moscow (in Russian).

HITTMAIR, A. (1970). Funktionelle Krankheiten als Teil der Zivilisationskrankheiten. *Vitalstoffe Zivil.-Krankh.*, **15**(6), 210–12.

HOROWITZ, M. J. (1973). Cognitive response to erotic and stressful films. *Arch. G. Psych.*, **1**, 81–6.

IVANOV-SMOLENSKY, A. G. (1965). *Interaction of experimental and clinical cerebro-pathophysiology*. Moscow (in Russian).

JALLADE, S. (1971). Medicine psychosomatique, mythes et réalité. *Lyon med.*, **225**, 1057–63.

KERBIKOV, O. V. (1955). *Lectures in psychiatry*. Moscow (in Russian).

KERBIKOV, O. V. (1962). *The clinical dynamics of psychopathy and neurosis*. Moscow (in Russian).

KIMBALL, C. P. (1970). Conceptual developments in psychosomatic medicine: 1939–1969. *Ann. intern. Med.*, **73**, 307–16.

KNAPP, P. H. (1970). The psychosomatic field. *Psychosom. med.*, **32**, 425–31.

KOVALYOV, V. V. (1972). Personality and personality disorders in somatical diseases. In *On the role of the psychic factor in the appearance, course, and treatment of somatic disease*. pp. 102–14. Moscow (in Russian).

KURTSIN, I. T. (1973). *Theoretical discoveries in psychosomatic medicine*. Leningrad (in Russian).

LAKOSSINA, N. D. (1970). *Clinical variants of neurotic development*. Moscow (in Russian).

LAZARUS, R. S. (1966). *Psychological stress and the coping process*. New York

LEVI, L. (1972). Stress and distress in response to psychosocial stimuli. *Acta med. scand.*, *Suppl.*, **528**.

LIPOWSKI, L. I. (1970). New perspectives in psychosomatic medicine. *Can. psychiat. Ass. J.*, **15**, 515–25.

LISITSIN YU P. (1965). On present psychosomatics and their importance in medical sciences. In *Methodological problems in diagnostics*, pp. 63–90. Moscow (in Russian).

MASON, J. W. (1970). Strategy in psychosomatic research. *Psychosom. Med.*, **14**, 427–39.

MOROZOV, V. M. (1961). *On present trends in foreign psychiatry and sources of their ideas*. Moscow (in Russian).

—— and LEBEDINSKY, M. S. (1972). Relationship between psyche and psychosomatics in somatic diseases, and our tasks. In *On the role of the psychic factor in the appearance, course and treatment of somatic disease*, pp. 5–22. Moscow (in Russian).

MYASISHCHEV, V. N. (1967). Systematic neurosis and somatogenic neuropsychiatric diseases. In *The second all-Russian Workshop of Neuropathologists and Psychiatrists*, pp. 367–9. Moscow (in Russian).

—— (1972). Psychology and medicine. In *On the role of the psychic factor in the appearance, course and treatment of somatic disease*, pp. 41–6. Moscow (in Russian).

NITSCH, I. R. (1973). Industrielle Beanspruchung als psychologisches Problem. *Die Rehabilitation*, **2**, 68–77.

PAYKEL, E. S. and PRUSOFF (1971). Scaling of life events. *Arch. gen. Psychiatry*, **4**, 340–7.

PINCHERLE, G. (1972). Fitness for work. *Proc. roy. Soc. Med.*, **4**, 321–4.

PLATONOV, K. K. (1972). Personal approach in understanding the psychosomatic interaction. In *On the role of the psychic factor in the appearance, course and treatment of somatic disease*, pp. 47–55. Moscow (in Russian).

ROKHLIN, L. L. (1972). The psychic factor in endocrine disease. In *On the role of the psychic factor in the appearance, course and treatment of somatic disease*, pp. 120–34 (in Russian).

SCHWÖBEL, G. (1971). Psychosomatische Medizin, ihre Bedeutung für die Gesundheit von Familien und auf die Sozialmedizin ausgerichteten therapeutischen Methoden. *Ther. Umschau*, **28**(6), 397–403.

SELYE, H. (1973). On stress and the executive. *Executive Health*, **9**.

TSAREGORODTSEV, G. I. and SHINGAROV, G. H. (1972). Some philosophical aspects of psychosomatic problems. In *On the role of the psychic factor in the appearance, course and treatment of somatic disease*, pp. 56–75. Moscow (in Russian).

URSOVA, L. G. (1973). 'Psychopathology of myocardial infarction', doctoral dissertation, University of Moscow (in Russian).

WAN, T. (1971). Status stress and morbidity: a sociological investigation of selected categories of work-limiting chronic conditions. *J. chron. Dis.*, **7**(8), 453–68.

WARDWELL, W. J. (1973). A study of stress and coronary heart disease in an urban population. *Bull. N. Y. Acad. Med.*, **6**, 521–31.

WOLFF, H. G. (1968). *Stress and disease*. Springfield.

YEGORKOVA, A. S., KOLODYAZHNY, S. F., KOROVIN, K. F., SEVEROVOSTOKOVA, V. I., STABROVSKY, E. M., and TARABRINA, N. V. (1971). Experimental, psychological and biochemical research in studies of mental stress of nervous diseases. In *Clinico-psychological character research*, pp. 202–5. Leningrad (in Russian).

29. WORKING SITUATIONS AND PSYCHOPHYSIOLOGICAL PATHOLOGY — A SYSTEMS APPROACH

SAMUEL A. CORSON and ELIZABETH O'LEARY CORSON

UNBRIDLED REDUCTIONIST TECHNOLOGY — AN EXERCISE IN REDUCTIO AD ABSURDUM

In sorrow shalt thou eat . . .
In the sweat of thy face shalt thou eat bread

[From *Genesis* 3: 17–18]

Even in the meanest sort of Labour, the whole soul of a man is composed into a kind of real harmony the instant he sets himself to work.

[From *Past and present Book* III, Ch. 11, by Thomas Carlyle.]

Work in its broadest sense is an essential ingredient in the life of all animals. In essence, work is a manifestation of the operation of the basic twin instincts (drives) of self-preservation and species perpetuation. Even the simplest unicellular organisms must engage in food-seeking activities. In animals with sexual forms of reproduction, work includes mate-seeking and nest-building tasks.

It is instructive to note that rats and pigeons, when offered a choice between freely available food (free-loading) and work (bar-pressing for food), show a preference for working for their food rather than free-loading (Carder and Berkowitz 1970; Jensen 1963; Neuringer 1969, 1970; Singh 1970).

In some animals (e.g., squirrels, many social insects) work also involves gathering and storing food for future use. In man, work is involved not only with the problems of providing food and shelter for current and future use for himself but also for future generations. Work also involves the modification of hostile environments, so as to make them habitable and pleasant. As was so elegantly pointed out by Dubos (1973), man has achieved a 'creative transformation of the earth', so as to endow it with a 'humanized charm'.

It may be more than a mere linguistic coincidence that in the Hebrew language the same word 'Avodah' means 'work' as well as 'worship' or 'prayer'.

Since work is a natural biological phenomenon, it *per se* cannot be considered to be stressful. On the contrary, work, like any positive biological drive, can be a source of self-fulfilment, satisfaction, and joy, even when it is accompanied by 'the sweat of thy face'.

It was when work became institutionalized, with a master and hired labour (or slave) arrangement, that some types of work became for some individuals also a source of grief and a host of negative emotions. The Industrial Revolution, although it increased the pro-

ductivity of a labourer on the whole, turned out to be in many instances more of a curse than a blessing to the workers. The cities of nineteenth century industrial England were appropriately referred to as condominiums of 'grandeur and filth' (Kermode 1974). In describing Belfast, Kermode quotes a succinct poem by Sybil Baker:

Belfasts's a famous northern town,
Ships and linen its occupation;
And the workers have a riot on
The slightest provocation

Victorian industrial England built grandiose municipal centres and elegant private mansions. At the same time, it condensed the workers into filthy crowded slums and channelled untreated sewage into the rivers, thus managing to pollute its own nest. For example, during the summer of 1858 the unbearable stench from the Thames River forced the suspension of the deliberations of the House of Commons (Dyos and Wolff 1974).

Twentieth century technology has continued and intensified the dichotomy between, on the one hand, the tremendous increase in the productivity of labour and the hoped-for happiness and self-fulfilment that technology could bring to the individual and, on the other hand, the reality of alienation, frustration, and social disorganization we are witnessing. The self-defeating, dehumanizing aspects of the way we have been using technology are evidenced in the fact that, at least in the United States, most of our cities have become centres of physio-chemical and psychological stress from which many are trying to escape into suburbs. In turn, many suburbs are eventually converted into new slums.

THE REDUCTIONIST VERSUS THE SYSTEMS APPROACH IN SCIENCE AND TECHNOLOGY

It is the thesis of this essay that one of the major factors contributing to the dehumanizing and stress-inducing aspects of our working life patterns is the persistence of an exclusively reductionist approach in the orientation and management of our technological and scientific activities.

Webster's dictionary defines reductionism as 'A procedure or theory of reducing complex data or phenomena to simple terms; especially: oversimplification'. This approach is based on the assumption that any given phenomenon or event can be considered as a closed system involving linear cause–effect relationships.

It is this reductionist philosophy that underlies the development of the scientific method and the various scientific disciplines and eventually made possible the development of technology. One is therefore not justified in disparaging reductionism *per se* or denying the validity of science or of the scientific method and turning to counterculture anti-intellectualism or anti-scientific mysticism (see Roszak 1969).

The problem with Roszak's counterculture anti-scientific analysis is that he fails to see the distinction between exclusively reductionist and dehumanized technology (or technocracy) and humanistic systems-approach science, such as is well articulated by Commoner (1972). Roszak also fails to appreciate the importance of the *scientific method* as an essential prerequisite for solving problems or for maintaining the framework of an enlightened (as contrasted with a bigoted) society. By a strange twist of logic Roszak ridicules Jacob Bronowski's statement that 'Men have asked for freedom, justice, and respect precisely as the scientific spirit has spread among them' (Roszak 1969, p. 300). Similarly, Roszak misinterprets the substance, the logic, and the spirit of the writings of the great humanistic scientist Norbert Wiener. On page 294 Roszak states:

Norbert Wiener's *The Human Use of Human Beings* (Boston: Houghton Mifflin, 1950) established the concept of "cybernetics" and worked out one of the key propositions of technocratic managerialism: namely, that man and social life generally are so much communications apparatus. Along the lines of this unfortunate metaphor we arrive at all sorts of commonplace contemporary idiocies which small minds are now busily elaborating into a *Weltanschauung*, such as that a photoelectric cell is a "sense organ," that feedback is "proprioception," that computers have "memories," can "learn," "teach," "make decisions," and "create." Despite Wiener's intelligent forebodings about the potential abuses of cybernation (see his tenth chapter), the book is a painful example of how a scientist of great conscience contributes in spite of himself to the degradation of human personality.

By the same logic one may as well accuse the inventors of the alphabet and printing technology as being responsible for the Nazi anti-Semitic decrees because without an alphabet and the printing press these decrees could not have been printed. By the same token, how would Roszak's books be printed and distributed without the printing and publishing technologies?

The main trouble with reductionist science and technology is the failure to appreciate the limitations of the reductionist approach and to recognize the fact that in nature there are no closed systems. As was so elegantly pointed out by Weiss (1970, p. 17), all systems should be considered as 'open systems', since everything in the universe is interrelated in non-linear complex patterns.

This failure to recognize the *limitations* and pitfalls of an exclusively reductionist approach (divested of a value system) is chiefly responsible for the distressing, noxious aspects of our working environment. It has led to polluted, disjointed megacities. The distinguished English economist, Walter Bagehot (1826–77) compared London to a newspaper: 'Everything is there, and everything is disconnected.' In agriculture, reductionism resulted in an injudicious excessive use of insecticides and pesticides which in turn led to ecologic disaster and the poisoning of the very foods we are trying to produce (see Rachel Carson 1962). The food industry added insult to injury by over-purifying our foods and incorporating into them toxic food additives. In the United States, the automobile industry mindlessly overproduced and largely substituted polluting, accident-prone, energy-wasting automobiles for relatively clean, energy-efficient, and safe railroad transportation.

The reductionist approach reached its acme of absurdity and social irresponsibility in building costly, awesome military instruments of destruction and overkill, in extensive testing of atomic and hydrogen bombs, and in using technological, remote-control warfare and systematic defoliation of forests and destruction of crops. It is a case of poetic retribution that these defoliating agents used in the Vietnam war have turned out to be carcinogenic and have thus afflicted with cancer some of the innocent Americans involved in dispersal of these defoliants.

The chemical reductionist technology managed to substitute polluting, ecologically destructive detergents for relatively benign biodegradable soaps. It foisted on the public non-biodegradable, often toxic, plastics as substitutes for nontoxic biodegradable natural fibres. As pointed out by Commoner (1972), 'the same technological changes that have created the environmental crisis have reduced the efficiency with which we use fuel'.

The fiasco of producing non-biodegradable polluting detergents illustrates one of the major defects of a rigidly reductionist technology which operates in isolation from other scientific disciplines and from social considerations. By the time technology was producing non-biodegradable detergents (consisting of branched-chain molecules) biochemists had already demonstrated that branched-chain molecules resist enzymatic degradation by bacterial action. Thus, this ecological insult and costly commercial venture could have been prevented by interdisciplinary communication and by a humanistic orientation.

Commoner cites many examples of disastrous environmental and health-endangering results of reductionist technology. One of these is worth citing here. In the 1950s, polyvinyl chloride plastic materials were introduced and eventually widely used in the automobile industry and in many other areas, including the storage of blood and blood substitutes used for transfusions in patients. It eventually turned out that the plasticizers in the polyvinyl tubing leached out into the stored blood and often led to serious medical complications in the patients receiving that blood (e.g., so called 'shock lung'). It also was discovered that one of the plastic additives (phthalic anhydride) is also a constituent of thalidomide, a well known teratogenic compound.

Yet all the examples of environmental technological insults do not justify the argument against technology or science *per se*, but only against a rigidly narrow reductionist technology not oriented towards humanistic aims and devoid of moral principles and common sense.

Technology should not rush headlong into producing new gadgets or new organic chemicals just because technology finds it possible and profitable to do so. As stated so succinctly by Press (1978), (the director of the Office of Science and Technology Policy in Washington, D.C.), 'We face great environmental challenges. . . . One of the most important of these has become dealing with the numerous toxic substances and other chemicals we introduce into our environment, workplaces, and consumer production. We live in a sea of chemicals.' According to Press, some 63 000 chemicals are currently in use in the United States. Press reports that the Chemical Abstract Service computer registry includes 4 039 907 chemical entities, while the number of entries is now growing at the rate of 6000 per week. Would reductionist technology consider it a mortal sin if one were to suggest a temporary moratorium on the introduction of new organic chemicals until a systematic evaluation is made of the environmental and health impacts a new compound may have?

Perhaps one of the attributes of rigid reductionist science and technology—its identification of science with absolute certainty—may have contributed to a large extent to the current waves of anti-science and anti-intellectualism. Yet, science is nothing but a problem-solving enterprise and represents the very antithesis of dogmatism. As expressed by Bronowski (1973), pp. 353–74,

There is no absolute knowledge. And those who claim it, whether they are scientists or dogmatists, open the door to tragedy. All information is imperfect. We have to treat it with humility. . . . We are always at the brink of the known. . . . Every judgment in science stands on the edge of error.

Bronowski (p. 334) recalls that Niels Bohr used to begin his lecture courses by saying to his students: 'Every sentence that I utter should be regarded by you not as an assertion but as a question'.

The contrast between reductionist certainty and a systems science humility is well illustrated in an exchange between B. F. Skinner and Carl R. Rogers (as paraphrased in Wann 1964, pp. 139–40):

The discussion has treated modern science as though "it had no real certainty, no notion of how it might be sure of anything". Skinner would argue that the "physical scientists are, indeed, at sea", not because they lack "scientific sophistication", but because they lack "psychological sophistication, particularly the implications of a science of behavior for epistemology". Much that has been written by physical scientists and mathematicians about thinking and intellectual processes is "ridiculously elementary" and "simple minded."

He thinks the position developed in *Verbal Behavior* could be applied profitably to the "analysis of scientific methodology". Not only Goedel's Theorem but "*all paradoxes can be cleared up from a behavioral point of view*". While "the physical sciences badly need a scientific epistemology," psychology does not "need the present muddle in the physical sciences."

To which Dr. Rogers retorted:

In view of Dr. Skinner's remarks, I shall modify an earlier statement of mine about scientific certitude. I will say that it seems to me [that] science does not lead to certitude, except in the case of Dr. Skinner.

In medical practice, reductionism led to serious therapeutic errors, such as injudicious use of surgical procedures, e.g., overuse of hysterectomies and tonsil-lectomies (Rodgers 1975), frontal lobotomy, and excessive reliance on drug therapy, especially in the treatment of psychopathology.

Preston (1978) in a paper appropriately entitled 'Operating in the dark' summarized data on many surgical operations 'performed without evidence that they are either beneficial or safe'. Among such reductionist surgical manoeuvers, Preston lists: 'freezing of the stomach to cure ulcers', a variety of coronary surgery procedures which eventually proved worthless or harmful, including coronary bypass surgery. Preston states that 'in 1977 approximately 70 000 (coronary bypass) operations were peformed in more than 600 hospitals in the US.' Preston further states, 'To date, with only one exception—for a rare condition—the controlled studies show no prolongation of life or reduction of heart attacks for patients who underwent this surgery, as compared to treatment with conventional nonsurgical therapy.' Regarding heart transplantation surgery, Preston has this to say: 'with no evidence of long-term success in animal testing, this procedure was initiated with unprecedented public and professional acclaim, only to slowly drop from favor because of poor results.'

Thalidomide teratogenesis is probably one of the best known examples of reductionist iatrogenic medicine, but there are many other examples. The National Cancer Institute recently distributed a leaflet entitled: *Were you or your daughter born after 1940? Did your mother take a drug during pregnancy to avoid miscarriage?* The reference, of course, is to Diethylstilbesterol which turned out to be carcinogenic to many of the daughters of the mothers who received this drug. Tardive dyskinesia, an irreversible neurological disorder, resulting from long-term administration of large doses of phenothiazines, is another example of reductionist medicine that failed to take into account the multifactorial effects of drugs and constitutional differences in reactions to external chemical agents.

Many examples could be cited for reductionist approaches in biomedical research which eventually may ad to disastrous therapeutic errors. Suffice it to cite ere two recent reports. One such experiment involves e surgical removal of the lower third of the small testine where most of the exogenous cholesterol is sorbed. This surgical bypass (devised by an American eart Association Established Investigator), performed rabbits and humans, did lead to a lowering of blood olesterol. That this operation (in addition to presenting a surgical and anaesthetic stressor) may ad to various nutritional biochemical disorders is not entioned in the report (*Heart Research Newsletter* 65).

A more ambitious and expensive direct reductionist slaught on serum cholesterol was reported by the nited States Coronary Drug Project Research Group 975) (see also Marx 1975). This study, conducted der the auspices of the National Heart and Lung stitute at a cost of $40 million, involved 55 clinical ntres and included 8300 men who had suffered from e or more myocardial infarcts. This project consisted f testing the efficacy of five drugs known to lower blood olesterol. Three of the drugs studied had to be scontinued before the projected completion of the rogramme because of serious toxic effects and excess ortality rates as compared to the placebo groups.

The 1975 report described the data obtained with two rugs: niacin and clofibrate. These drugs did produce a wering of serum cholesterol, on the average less than) per cent, about the same percentage of lowering as at reported for dietary restriction of cholesterol and fat take. The presumed justification for this ambitious, sky, and expensive drug project is that allegedly not all atients stick to their diets.

In any case, in spite of the decrease of serum choles-rol, there was no significant decrease in mortality as ompared to the placebo groups of patients. The drug gimens also had many side-effects, some relatively inor (e.g., decrease in libido, skin problems, bdominal pain, frequent urination, excessive sweating, ecrease in appetite) and some major (e.g., cardiac rrhythmias, gastrointestinal problems, abnormal blood hemistry findings).

An integrative (common sense) systems approach ould have suggested a number of considerations that ould have saved the patients and the experimenters a lot f trouble and also saved the expenditure of already mited research funds:

(1) Serum cholesterol is only one of the risk factors in coronary disease and is in a sense part of the final common pathway in the interaction of many factors, including psychosocial factors, regular physical activity, various drugs, smoking, etc.

(2) Attempts to lower serum cholesterol by means of drugs not only do not attack the overall problem of metabolic derailment but also add insult to injury by introducing foreign agents which may further disturb the body's regulating homeostatic mechanisms.

(3) A holistic approach to a sensible and acceptable dietary regimen would include not merely limitations on caloric and cholesterol and fat intakes, but also a more radical shift from 'fast'. highly refined, and additive-rich (junk) foods to tasty, natural, less refined foods, such as protein-rich legumes, a variety of whole grain cereals, and fresh fruits and vegetables. Such natural foods are more likely to be found in student co-operative stores than in hospital or university dietary departments.

The concept of the General Systems Theory (G.S.T.) was introduced apparently quite independently by von Bertalanffy in 1948 (see von Bertalanffy, 1969) at about the same time Norbert Wiener (1948) published his monograph *Cybernetics.*

As formulated by von Bertalanffy, the G.S.T. concerns itself 'with properties and principles of "wholes" or systems in general, irrespective of their particular nature and the nature of their components' (von Bertalanffy 1969). The quest for the development of the G.S.T. was based on the recognition that the biological, behavioural, and social sciences are not amenable to the mechanistic approach used in the physical sciences.

Cybernetics can be considered as a particular subdivision of the General Systems Theory. Cybernetics, as formulated by Wiener (1948), deals with the study of methods of control and communication common to living systems and mechanical communication systems and devices.

In cybernetic terms living organisms can be defined as possessing the following characteristics:

(1) They are goal-directed systems, i.e., they engage in activities designed to maintain optimization of functions and ensure survival of the individual and the species.

(2) They incorporate in their structure receptors (sensors) designed for the reception of information from changes occurring in the internal and external environments.

(3) They possess reliable channels for informing the controlling centres regarding internal or external environmental changes, or regarding the efficacy of any of the activities of the organism designed to maintain optimization of function or homeostasis (feedback).

(4) They possess control centres for receiving, storing, and evaluating the feedback information and initiating appropriate adaptive activities.

(5) The control centres exhibit adaptive plasticity, so that they can develop anticipatory responses to changing environmental signals signifying biological positive or negative events.

(6) Changes in patterns of configuration of matter may lead to the acquisition of new qualitative properties not possessed by the components of the system or by the more simple configuration

patterns. The development of more complex neural configurations in the cerebral cortex of man and the concurrent development of neural and motor substrates for speech and abstract thinking endowed man with *qualitative properties* strongly differentiating him from lower mammals not possessing the 'second signal system' (Pavlov 1940, 1954).

Thus, while a laboratory rat or pigeon might do well without 'freedom and dignity' (Skinner 1971), man possesses neural structures and a complex behavioural repertoire which make such mechanistic existence intolerable.

Actually, the development of the G.S.T. was presaged by theoretical formulations by several biologists in different countries. Probably the most definitive approach to a systems view of living organisms was developed in the mid-nineteenth century by the Russian school of physiology represented by Sechenov (1863) and Botkin (see Corson 1957; Corson and Corson 1975, 1976) who formulated the theory of 'nervism' or the neurogenic theory. In this paper *The reflex of purpose* Pavlov (1916) clearly delineated living organisms as goal-directed integrated systems.

One of Pavlov's most brilliant students, Peter K. Anokhin, as early as 1935 clearly foreshadowed the development of the G.S.T. by demonstrating the operation of the principles of feedback or, as Anokhin (1974) referred to it, 'return afferentation' in living organisms. A distinguished student of Anokhin, K. V. Sudakov (1971), expanded Anokhin's concept of functional systems to the investigation of biological motivations and their role in psychobiological adaptation.

Walter B. Cannon's (1929) formulation of the principles of physiological homeostasis and Selye's (1971) development of the stress concept represented significant contributions to the elucidation of an integrative holistic approach to biomedical problems.

The unitary systems concept was clearly developed by Barukh (Benedictus) Spinoza as early as 1663 in a critique of Cartesian mechanistic rationalism (see Elwes 1883; Spinoza (H. H. Briton, translator) 1905). In one of his letters, Spinoza presents his systems concept as follows (see Wolf 1928):

Suppose that a parasitic worm living in the bloodstream tried to make sense of its surroundings: from the point of view of the worm, each drop of blood would appear as an independent whole and not as a part of a total system. The worm would not recognize that each drop behaves as it does in virtue of the nature of the bloodstream as a whole. But in fact the nature of the blood can be understood only in the context of a larger system in which blood, lymph, and other fluids interact; and this system in turn is a part of a still larger whole. If we men begin with the bodies that surround us in nature and treat them as independent wholes, the relation between which is contingent and given, then we shall be in error precisely as the worm is in error. We must graps the system as a whole before

we can hope to grasp the nature of the part, since the nature the part is determined by its role in the total system.

Norbert Wiener (1948) extended the principles cybernetics to the analysis of social interactions. particular, Wiener pointed out the importance of viabl feedback channels in maintaining social homeostasis Nevertheless, reductionism has to this day remained th dominant driving force in our biomedical, socia economic, and technological activities.

An instructive example of the way a fractiona reductionist approach can lead to erroneous conclusior in psychophysiological research is represented by th controversy regarding the clinical efficacy of mepro bamate, an axiolytic drug (minor tranquillizer). In 195′ a conference was convened by the New York Academ of Sciences on *Meprobamate and other agents used mental disturbances* (see Gerard 1957).

In reviewing the dramatic discrepancy between th many favourable clinical reports on meprobamate and number of negative laboratory studies on this drug Gerard (1957), in his usual elegant and succinct manne summarized the situation as follows:

On the one hand, laboratory studies indicate that meprobamat is quite inert; on the other hand, a great number of takers seer to experience some benefit, and clinical reports included i these pages—many seemingly well controlled and convincir enough as reported—indicate a definite action. From this, on must conclude either that the experimenters have not yet foun the right thing to test—which would not be surprising, since w are dealing with agents active on the nuances of complex huma behavior for which it is difficult to find electrical or chemic: indicators, either in the laboratory or in the patient—or els that the clinical impressions are wrong . . . I doubt that th latter is the case, especially because of the genuine awareness c the problem of controls that exists today among the bette clinicians and laboratory workers handling these problems.

Our studies on the effects of meprobamate on do models of anxiety (Corson, 1966a,b; Corson and Corso 1967, 1969) have demonstrated that Gerard hit the na on the head. The laboratory workers indeed failed to te: the drug on clinically relevant parameters.

We suspect that the main reason why the laborator workers found meprobamate to be inert was that the were testing the drug on normal animals. In our studie on normal dogs, meprobamate, in therapeutic dose: had no measurable influence on behavioural or physio logic variables, such as heart rate, respiration, or ren; function. However, in dogs with experimental anxiety meprobamate exhibited remarkably normalizing effect by *inhibiting conditional visceral responses to an aversiv environment, without significantly affecting conditiona classical motor defence reflexes or conditiono discriminated avoidance or escape responses.* Th laboratory workers who reported that meprobanmat was inert were in error not only because they studied th effects of this drug on normal animals, *but also becaus they used a reductionist approach and recorded onl conditional avoidance or escape responses.*

We previously reported (Corson *et al.* 1936) the case of a dog which exhibited a highly selective aggressive behaviour toward one kennel attendant who had apparently abused the dog before this animal was acquired by our laboratory. When this dog was on a chronic meprobamate dosage that inhibited all conditional visceral responses to an aversive environment, the aggressive attacks on the attendant were just as easily provoked and as well directed as they had been before the dog was treated with meprobamate. *It is this selective action on exaggerated conditional visceral reactions that endows anxiolytic drugs with their useful therapeutic properties.* Thus, a systems approach made it possible to bridge the gap between basic research and clinical practice.

One of the major factors contributing to the persistence of a rigid reductionist fractionated approach in biomedical and psychological research and practice is the persistence of the mind–body and nature–nurture dichotomy orientation. In medical research and practice this led to the establishment of two opposing 'camps': the mechanistic medical model and the mechanistic behaviourist model. Thus, psychosomatic medicine which represented an attempt to develop a unitary model of health and disease gradually became a sort of medical specialty instead of serving as an integrative unifying principle in all of medical research and practice. As pointed out by Engel (1977), the biomedical model of disease 'leaves no room within its framework for the social, psychological and behavioral dimensions of illness'. Engel proposes a biopsychosocial model which would permit an integrative holistic approach in health maintenance.

It is instructive to note that although Virchow (1858) may be considered as one of the major proponents of the mechanistic localistic cellular theory of disease, in his later years Virchow emphasized the importance of psychosocial and economic factors in the maintenance of optimal health and prevention of disease, and he referred to medicine as a social science (see Virchow 1958).

One of the reasons for the popularity of Laetrile therapy among cancer patients (in spite of lack of scientific verification of its therapeutic efficacy) may be the failure of many physicians to take into account the role of emotional factors in the course of cancer or other diseases. When a patient is told that he has a 'terminal disease' (and perhaps with a funereal voice of finality and hopelessness) this may well become for the patient a self-fulfilling prophecy and may lead to the development of what has been referred to by Seligman (1975) as learned helplessness, and aggravation of the disease processes.

In contrast, the purveyors of Laetrile tell the patients with a voice of confidence and reassurance that a cure is possible. Whether the purveyors' statements of reassurance are honest or fraudulent, in many cases a powerful placebo effect may have a favourable influence on the course of the disease. Since spontaneous remissions do occur occasionally, it would appear to be the better part of a wisdom to offer psychological support and reassurance and not to contribute to the development of a state of helplessness and despair by telling the patient that he has a terminal disease.

Also, in the course of developing reliable clinical testing of the alleged therapeutic efficacy of Laetrile, it would be imperative for the physicians and staff involved in the tests to exhibit a positive encouraging attitude to the patients receiving the Laetrile, as well as to those receiving the placebo.

In a recent interview, Hans Selye (1978), while discussing his optimistic philosophy of life based on scientific principles, related the following incident about himself:

Being the descendant of several generations of dedicated physicians, I was told as I grew up that hard work is both an obligation and, if approached in the right spirit, a pleasure. . . . This same attitude helped me very much a few years ago, when my doctor told me I had cancer and only a few months to live. I refused to retreat from life in desperation, or to rail at fate, and was determined to keep living and working without worrying about my end. And although I can't prove it, perhaps this attitude helped my body combat the stress of my disease, since as you see, I am still ticking today—and, I might add, ticking quite well.

One good indication of the fact that Selye is still ticking perfectly and creatively is the flourishing of the International Institute of Stress Research recently organized by Selye who is now 71 years young.

DISTRESS FACTORS IN WORKING ENVIRONMENTS DOMINATED BY A REDUCTIONIST PHILOSOPHY

> Ah, the glory of the day's work,
> Whether with hand or brain! I have tried
> To exalt the present and the real
> To reach the average man the glory of his
> daily work or trade.
> [From Walt Whitman]

In the last section we presented an outline of attributes of living organisms. In this section we shall examine the failure of the mechanistic reductionist approach to take into account the psychobiological needs of working people.

Mechanistic working arrangements: lack of job satisfaction

Probably one of the most essential needs for mental, emotional, and physical well-being is the possession of a goal and the feeling that one's work has some meaning and some social usefulness and personal fulfilment. In contrast to mechanistic 'animalistic' behaviourism, Pavlov (1916) expressed his evaluation of this unique human characteristic in his paper *The reflex of purpose*:

The Reflex of Purpose (goal reflex) has great vital significance; it represents the basic form of vital energy in every one of us . . .

231

all of life, all its improvements, all its culture is achieved through the reflex of purpose, is achieved only by those individuals who strive to reach this or that life goal which they placed before themselves. . . . In contrast, life ceases to be attractive as soon as the purpose disappears. Do we not often read in the notes left by suicide victims that they ended their life because it was purposeless.

The working atmosphere in large assembly-line industrial enterprises and business conglomerates is certainly not conducive to offering the workers a feeling that what they are doing has some meaning. In assembly-line factories all the worker sees is the meaningless, monotonous, repetitive operations, often performed at break-neck speed unrelated to the physical or psychological capacity of the individual worker. This distress is compounded further in industries dedicated to the production of means of destruction or of products which tend to pollute the very environment in which the worker lives.

The reorganization of assembly-line production arrangements into units that will offer the worker an opportunity for developing a pride in his performance may go a long way toward minimizing the distress associated with robot-type factories.

The Saab–Scania automobile factory in a Stockholm suburb introduced in 1969 a group assembly arrangement wherein teams of three workers assemble a complete engine. Each team determines how the work should be divided and how fast the work should be done. The Saab Company officials claimed that with the introduction of the team assembly system there was less absenteeism and less employee turnover than with a conventional production line (*New York Times* 1974, 1975).

Nevertheless, following a visit by six American automobile workers at the Saab factory in 1974 for a period of four weeks, only one of these workers expressed a preference for the Swedish system. The other five American workers preferred the monotonous traditional production line, stating that the Swedish system demands more concentration.

This points out the importance of individual differences in work preferences and the person–environment fit pointed out by French (1973) and French *et al.* (1974) and the need for vocational counselling. It is possible that the traditional American assembly-line system has selectively attracted workers who prefer monotony and boredom. In any case, a better controlled study of the Saab system is needed, to include a larger and more representative number of American workers and a longer period of time in the Swedish factory, in order to avoid the complicating factor of 'culture shock'.

Lack of viable feedback and sensitive response channels
Another important source of psychophysiological distress is the lack of viable feedback and response channels in many industrial enterprises and even in educational institutions. The growing self-perpetuating bureau-cracies often become self-serving instead of serving the needs of the institutions and their individual constituents. In a previous publication (Corson 1971a) we pointed out that this lack of effective feedback and response channels makes it difficult to correct errors and to maintain social homeostasis and stability. The individuals within these enterprises feel helpless, become alienated, and may develop psychopathological disturbances characteristic for individuals who feel trapped and unable to develop control of their situation. We postulate that psychopathology is likely to result not from mere exposure to hard work or being faced with difficult problems. Rather, *it is the exposure to no-solution problems* (or the development of a conviction or feeling that the problems are insoluble), i.e., *the inability to achieve an adaptive consummatory response, that leads to psychophysiological and/or behavioural disturbances.*

We previously reported marked and persistent psychophysiologcal visceral disturbances in certain types of dogs exposed to Pavlovian conditioning with aversive reinforcement. These psychophysiological disorders disappeared or became markedly ameliorated when the same dogs were permitted in a different environment to develop discriminated conditional avoidance responses, in spite of the fact that the same aversive stimuli were used for reinforcement (Corson 1971b; Corson *et al.* 1970a,b; Corson and Corson 1976).

A great deal of confusion has arisen in the literature because the concepts of stress and of anxiety have been given different meanings. In particular, both stress and anxiety have been used to denote both biologically positive and biologically negative phenomena. It would be helpful if the term 'stress' were to be restricted to the definition proposed by Selye, the originator of the concept of stress, namely: 'the nonspecific responses of the organism to any demand made upon it'. The set of reactions of an individual exposed to unavoidable nociceptive stimuli or situations wherein the individual cannot develop adaptive coping mechanisms should be referred to as *distress*. Lennart Levi (1971, 1973) and Hans Selye (1971) have attempted to make such a distinction.

The term 'anxiety' has caused even more confusion because it has been used to denote both psychopathology as well as positive motivation for achievement of biologically useful goals. Mowrer (1939) for example stated:

Anxiety is a learned response, occurring to signals (conditioned stimuli) that are premonitory . . . (to) situations of injury or pain . . . anxiety is thus basically anticipatory in nature and has thus great biological utility in that it adaptively motivates living organisms to deal with traumatic events in advance of their actual occurrence. . . . Anxiety, i.e., mere anticipation of actual organic need or injury, may effectively motivate human beings.

It appears to us that it serves no useful purpose to confuse anxiety with biological drive or motivation. The studies of Cattell (1964) and Cattell and Scheier (1961),

ing factor analysis techniques, demonstrated that
ere is only one type of anxiety and that it never serves
a motivational drive, but on the contrary always
uses an impairment of performance.

Our data suggest that it is exposure to *unavoidable
ressors* or *insoluble problems* that may lead to the
velopment of a state of anxiety in *organisms with
certain constitutional make-up*.

In cybernetic terms, anxiety may be considered a
ronic information deficit. Exposure to new stimuli
ways leads to a temporary information deficit which
n be detected in the central nervous system as
ectrical desynchronization, particularly in the
ppocampus. Anokhin (1974) postulated the operation
the central nervous system of a series of feedback
ops which eventually include an 'action acceptor'
volving the hippocampus and frontal areas of the
rebral cortex. The operation of this action acceptor
ads to the development of integrated somatic-
havioural and visceral-endocrine adaptive responses,
which point the hippocampal electrical desynchro-
zation disappears. The information deficit is thus
iminated and the animal develops what Pavlov (1903,
28, 1954) referred to as a 'dynamic stereotype'. When
organism is repeatedly exposed to unavoidable
ychological stressors under conditions where an
aptive consummatory response cannot be achieved,
en Anokhin's action acceptor would continue to signal
d a chronic information deficit would develop, thus
ading to a persistent 'emotional dominant' as described
Simonov (1965). This animal would then simulate
me aspects of the psychopathological conditions of
xiety and frustration.

The fact that the psychovisceral reactions of some of
ur dogs exposed to Pavlovian reinforcement with
ociceptive stimuli were markedly ameliorated when the
nimals were permitted to develop discriminated
voidance responses supported the proposition that it is
e inability to cope with stressors that provokes anxiety
nd psychopathology. This is in accordance with the
iews expressed so elegantly by Lazarus (1966, 1967).
lowrer and Viek (1948) reported that rats subjected to
navoidable shock (uncontrollable shock) exhibited a
reater degree of conditioned suppression than rats
ocked but permitted to escape.

Our experimental data on the therapeutic function of
eveloping control over stressful situations appear to be
t variance with the reports of Brady (1958) and Brady *et
l.* (1958) regarding the development of gastrointestinal
lcers in the so-called 'executive' monkeys who allegedly
ad control over the aversive stimuli. However, the
esign of the experiments by Brady *et al.* is such that the
o-called 'executive' monkeys were *actually not in
ontrol of the situation. Their situation was more like that
f galley slaves being driven by a merciless whip.* The
rady experimental design was such that in order to
void unsignalled powerful shocks the 'executive'
onkey had to press a lever *every 20 seconds for 6 hours
n and 6 hours off every 24 hours for a period of 6–7*

weeks. Such a schedule represents a rather severe form
of exposure to exhausting physical and psychological
stressors and may be comparable to an extreme form of
speed-up on a factory assembly line or a chain gang. By
contrast, in our experimental design, the reinforcement
schedule in the operant room was of the type which
permitted relatively easy mastery. The intervals between
signalled electrocutaneous reinforcement were one
minute. Moreover, the total period of presentation of
stimuli in both the Pavlovian aversive room and in the
operant room was only 20 minutes during a two-hour
experiment.

Moreover, the so-called 'executive' monkeys were
selected on the basis of being high avoidance responders.
Such a biased selection may have resulted in the
assignment of 'executive' roles to monkeys with high
emotionality and a constitutional predisposition to
psychovisceral disorders, such as ulcerations (see
Seligman 1975, pp. 41–2). Since the 'executive' monkeys
were highly efficient compulsive avoidance bar pressers,
the yoked monkeys rarely received any shocks at all and,
therefore, should not have been expected to develop
psychopathological disorders.

Weiss (1971a,b,c) repeated the Brady experiment on
rats using a triadic design ('executive', helpless, and no
shock conditions). The 'executive' rats showed far fewer
and less severe ulcerations than the yoked animals which
had no control over the occurrence of shocks. The
importance of developing control over situations was
pointed out in elegant studies by Masserman (1943,
1971) in his studies on experimental neurosis in
monkeys.

The importance of unavoidable psychological stress and
of frustration in the development of psychosomatic
disturbances was pointed out in the admirable studies of
Stewart Wolf *et al.* (1948) on human subjects. These
authors reported the case of a patient who actually left
the interview office to beat up the person he resented.
His resting diastolic pressure during the interview was
110 mm. After his return from this rather uninhibited
physical aggression, his diastolic pressure decreased to
85 mm.

Stewart Wolf and co-workers (1955) in an elegant
study concluded that the hypertensive patients were
generally 'fundamentally driving and often hostile, but
not able fully to commit or assert themselves'. These
authors also had the impression that 'freer or more
fearless self-assertion, brought about by a variety of
devices, has been associated among our subjects with a
short or long-lasting lowering of arterial pressure'.

Hambling (1959) reported cases of hypertensive
patients who exhibited marked elevation of diastolic
blood pressure whenever they were faced with a
frustrating situation that was beyond their control. The
same patients remained normotensive in stressful
situations which permitted them appropriate response
outlets.

Lundberg and Frankenhaeuser (1978) (see also
Frankenhaeuser and Lundberg 1977) reported a series of

233

well controlled experiments on two groups of university students exposed to white noise while performing mental arithmetic. One group had the option of deciding the level of noise intensity they wished to accept (Condition Control group (C)). The yoked partners had to accept the same noise level as the C students (NC group). The authors concluded that 'subjective and physiological arousal was lower when the subjects were permitted to exert control over noise intensity than when they lacked control'. The authors also reported that there were considerable interindividual differences.

On the basis of many elegant laboratory and field studies, Frankenhaeuser (1977) concluded that 'a moderately varied flow of stimuli and events, opportunities to engage in psychologically meaningful activities and to exercise personal control over external conditions, may be considered key components in the quality-of-life concept'.

The lack of effective feedback and sensitive response channels and the resultant alienation and psychopathology become more prominent the larger the institution. Because during the past several decades industrial and business institutions have tended to conglomerate (especially in the United States), the problems of maintaining viable communication in our working places have become progressively more complex. Even secondary and higher educational institutions have become victims of the drive to become bigger, on the questionable assumption that 'bigger means better'. This unlimited growth in size has been true particularly for many state universities in the USA, which seem to have developed all the deficiencies of a socialist economy without its benefits.

The need to limit the size of universities was recognized by the Robins report (see Gallant and Prothero 1972) which recommended the founding of new universities and expanding of regional colleges so as to keep the enrolment of all institutions below 10 000.

It appears that in order to minimize psychopathology and social disorganization in large working institutions it would be necessary to decentralize the institutions into smaller semi-autonomous subunits and to broaden decision-making processes, so as to involve as many of the workers as possible.

That such broadening of responsibility and authority is possible and desirable, not only in educational institutions but also in factories, has been demonstrated in the United States by at least two industries, the American Brake Shoe Company, and more recently by the Harman International Industries.

William B. Given, Jr. (1949), President of the American Brake Shoe Company, published the results of such decentralized management in a book appropriately entitled *Bottom up management*. In essence, the philosophy of this type of management can be summarized by the following statement by Given:

Lately businessmen have come to realize that the success and progress of an enterprise is the sum-total of the success and progress of its people. The management that fails to stimula their wholehearted interest and loyalty, and fully utilize th ideas and initiative . . . is shortchanging itself, its stockholde and the public it serves. . . . Gradually a philosophy maximum freedom in management began to evolve, and found ourselves moving farther and farther away from t conventional top-down techniques of management.

It would be of great interest to compare the incidence various forms of psychopathology in such a 'Bottom management' enterprise with that in the tradition centralized autocratic institutions.

The programme on management democratization the Harman International Industries (HII) was initiate in 1943 by its President, Sidney Harman.† In a person communication, Dr. Harman (1976b) wrote that he w convinced 'that if a program of human development w to grow within the factories, such a program would ha to begin at the highest levels of management . . . or fa the likelihood, if not the certainty, that it will destroyed there.'

The Harman International Industries employ abo 4000 people in 13 manufacturing plants locate principally in the United States, but also in Englan Scotland, and Germany. The programme in share management began in 1973 in the Automotive Divisio Plant at Bolivar, Tennessee, eventually leading to tl establishment of an *ad hoc* 'working committee consisting of five members each from the manageme and the United Automobile Workers. The 'workin committee' identified the following four operatin principles for the shared management experimen These principles state that the worker:

(1) Must feel secure about his job and be free fro fear and anxiety concerning his health, safet income and future;
(2) Must feel fairness in his treatment;
(3) Must feel that his needs are respected and that I can develop his individual capabilities to tl fullest;
(4) Must have a say in the decisions that affect hin starting with the job itself.

During the life of the programme, a fifth and cruci principle evolved; that is, that in any social enterprise tl parties must respect each other's differing roles. In shor there must be a sense of mutual respect and trust.

According to Dr. Harman's testimony at the Sena Hearings (1976a), this programme has had a dramat favourable effect on the attitudes of the workers towar their jobs and the factory. The programme had als resulted in a significant increase in productivity, th submission by workers of many useful innovativ suggestions, and the development of a cost-saving sharing programme in which both the management an the union are involved.

†Dr. Harman served as the Undersecretary of Commerce in the Cart administration.

234

The need for enlightened industrial management, for broadening decision-making responsibilities, and for improving the psychosocial environment in industrial and business institutions has been demonstrated in a series of careful studies by Bakke (1946, 1958) at the Labour and Management Centre at Yale University. Bakke referred to such management–labour interactions as 'antagonistic co-operation'.

Lack of job security. The stress of unemployment

Another important factor contributing to the development of anxiety and psychophysiological distress is the problem of job security. What is needed in all working places is a system of economic security comparable to tenure provisions in some of our best academic institutions.

In order to maintain optimal health, a worker should be assured that as long as he is willing and able to do his best in a job, that job will be made secure for the worker. This is not to be confused with the advocacy of assuring a pay cheque to anyone in an enterprise regardless of the willingness of the worker to meet his work obligations to the best of his ability. A policy offering job security coupled with a 'bottom-up management' arrangement and appropriate educational measures is likely to lead to more positive attitudes on the part of the employees than a fear-inducing policy of job insecurity. In essence, it is a choice between using positive reinforcement methods and negative punishment-type reinforcement.

Bakke (1940, 1969) in an extensive series of studies of unemployed workers, came to the conclusion that what the majority of the unemployed workers wanted most was not merely income but a job, 'to perform in a *socially respected* role: to be a producer . . . a fellow his mates look to . . . a man who never lets his family down, the good father of successful kids . . . obtaining an *increasing measure of control* over one's own affairs'. When asked whether the workers would prefer high but irregular wages or lower but regular wages, 90 per cent of the unemployed workers voted unhesitatingly for the latter.

That punishment-type reinforcement may lead to psychopathological manifestations in certain individuals has been demonstrated in our experiments on low adaptation (antidiuretic) dogs (Corson and Corson 1976). These dogs exhibited highly generalized, almost inextinguishable psychovisceral turmoil to the entire conditioning room where electrocutaneous reinforcement was used. In contrast, the same dogs developed highly discriminated adaptive reactions when positive food reinforcement (rewards) were used. Hearst (1960) in a series of experiments on monkeys reported that with electrocutaneous reinforcement, the responses were generalized, poorly discriminated, and nonadaptive. In contrast, in the same monkeys with food reward reinforcement, the responses were well discriminated. Hearst suggests that these results

'. . . may have relevance to clinical descriptions of hypersensitivity and seeming irrationality under conditions of strong anxiety; an 'anxious' patient may respond strongly to stimuli which are only remotely similar to an original anxiety-provoking stimulus. There are experimental data from studies of human beings which also show a greater than normal amount of stimulus generalization in subjects who are highly anxious or even schizophrenic, or who are made anxious experimentally.'

The psychophysiologic effects of involuntary unemployment are likely to be much more severe than mere punishment for nonperformance. The anxiety associated with unemployment is comparable to random punishment or exposure to no-solution problems. Bakke (1940) reports many behavioural and psychophysiological disorders in workers during long periods of unemployment:

(a) disruption in family harmony and transformation of formerly co-operative family interactions into maladaptive quarrels and mutual recriminations;
(b) the loss of ambitions and the development of a feeling of helplessness and loss of self-esteem;
(c) severe insomnia in many cases. The workers 'report that they lie awake staring into the dark wondering what they are going to do. They used to be able to arrive at their decisions during the day, they said, but now where there are so many of them to make and they are so impossible to make, they just can't get it all done, and they lie awake thinking. Then in the morning they are tired and cranky, and the chances for arguments are increased. Lack of rest must in the end make its effect on health evident.'

Thirty faculty members and students associated with the American Studies Program (1975) of the State University of New York at Buffalo conducted interviews in 1975 with 80 unemployed workers in that city. In 1975 the unemployment rate in Buffalo was 10·3 per cent, but the total percentage of the unemployed and underemployed in that city may be as high as 60 per cent of the labour force. Here are some case histories reported by the American Studies Program, State University of New York (SUNY) at Buffalo (1975).

Rosie W. 27 years old, unemployed and on welfare, shares a small apartment with her daughter, 6, and another woman, and is about to be evicted. 'You go looking for a job . . . 50% of the time there is not a job anyway . . . I was an administrative assistant at a community center . . . an employment coach on a Federal program . . . I've said I never wanted to work in any plant. I wish I could get a plant job now . . . and the welfare system. Isn't that a design to fail? I have a child, and she's part of me. She sees me doing nothing . . . depressed, worried, sometimes crying. I mean, I try . . . I do love her . . . but with all the pressure, sometimes I can't even talk to her . . . I think it's going to affect her emotionally. I went to school with her and the teacher said, 'she's a good, bright child, but she's so sad. Why?' 'Because that's all we got in our home. Sadness. No hope. No future' . . . What I'd like to know, really, is what am I supposed to do with my life?'

Ron B. Ron received his M.S. in aerospace engineering. 'I applied to about 50 engineering firms, and I was interviewed by

235

only two. Since that time, I've been delivering furniture for a living'.

F.P.H. Wire cutter, 55, unemployed since 1972 when the Sylvania plant closed. He had been with Sylvania for 31 years. 'I feel as though we got the short end of the stick'.

L.H. Concrete finisher, 28; in the unemployment line. 'There's going to be a lot of stealing, a lot of mugging . . . People are going to get tired of coming down here and standing in line . . . And when they finally get unemployment (pay) a person, say, only gets $45 or $50 a week might have 3 or 4 children; before a man's going to see his children and his family go hungry, it seems he's going to go out there and do something'.

Ann E. C. Waitress, 50, in the unemployment line. 'I've always had a job, so I didn't realize it was this bad . . . I tell them I've been a waitress for 30 years and it does not make an impression. They're just not hiring. I've gone up and down Main Street . . . There is just no hope. That's why I came down here. I figure it doesn't look like I'm going to get anything. I want to work; I like working; it's just a way of life with me . . . Right now, I'd take anything, just to have a job'.

A factor closely related to job security is job satisfaction, which, among other things, involves appropriate vocational placement. In an enlightened enterprise, provision should be made for continuing vocational guidance and, when necessary, appropriate retraining programmes, so as to ensure optimal utilization of the potentialities of the workers.

Lack of attention to aesthetic and psychological needs of workers in the design of work places

A factor often overlooked in relation to occupational health is the aesthetic environment and architectural design of work places. These designs often fail to take into account the psychological needs of workers. A good example of such dehumanized designs is the building of large edifices without windows. Paradoxically, such windowless structures were built only recently for a school of biological sciences and for student dormitories in one large American state university.

Many, if not most, factories and business structures are drab and uninviting and certainly do not contribute to emotional well-being. This, incidentally, appears to be the case also for some scientific institutions and many hospitals. A description of the drabness of hospitals by a student of Botkin, the physician Manassein (1876), would apply to many hospitals and business and industrial enterprises in this day:

In this respect most hospitals and clinics present a very unhappy picture with their unfriendly, uniform wards and their dull monotonous daily routines. Such shameful conditions in our hospitals, in my opinion, are no less harmful to the patients than all the other errors in regard to hygienic and dietetic arrangements, because of which many patients perish, not because of their diseases, but because of their hospitals.

In such hospital environments

the thoughts of patients have nothing to concentrate on . . . they are therefore invariably centered around their own

pains. . . . The first concern of a physician who understands significance of psychic influences should be with the need fo more cozy appearance of the wards. In this respect, flov arrangements, birds in cages, wall pictures, aquaria, and forth, would help us, without interfering with hygie requirements of cleanliness and simplicity, to a large exten remove that uniform dishearteningly deadly character wh reflects itself at present from almost every hospital, from bare walls, the monotonous uniforms and rows of be . . .

PSYCHOSOCIAL STRESS IN MEDICAL EDUCATION

In one pan of the balance, put the pharmacopoeias of the wor all the editions from Diocorides to the last issue of the Uni States Dispensatory; heap them on the scales as did Euripi his books in the celebrated contest in the *Frogs*; in the other the simple faith with which from the days of the Pharaohs u now the children of men have swallowed the mixtures th works describe, and the bulky tomes will kick the beam. It is *aurum potabile*, the touchstone of success in medicine. Galen says, confidence and hope do more than physic— cures most in whom most are confident.'
[Osler 1974, p. 259]

One day in July, 1975, two physicians, Cyril and Stew Marcus (identical twins), were discovered dead, victi of barbiturate addiction (Cohen 1977). Shocking as su an event is, it is even more distressing to learn that dr addiction and suicides are more common among phy cians than among the rest of the population. It appe that each year the equivalent of a graduating class of average medical school commit suicide (Breo 1978a, According to Bressler (quoted by Cohen 1977), suicide highest among physicians during the first few years practice. It appears that, paradoxically, physicians ha a suicide rate twice that of the population they are tryi to keep healthy.

Thomas (1976, 1977), in a follow-up study of Joh Hopkins University Medical students, reported that in cohort of 1337 medical students from the classes 1948–64, there were 1248 graduates and 89 no graduates. In a follow-up study of the cohorts, 3·1 p cent of the graduates and 11·2 per cent of the no graduates have died prematurely. Thomas concludes: is a sobering fact that more than 10 per cent of t medical students in the Johns Hopkins cohort failed reach their full potential as physicians'.

That this malady of the healing profession is phenomenon of longstanding is suggested by Thom reference to an essay by Paget which appeared in S Bartholomew's Hospital Reports for 1869. In tracing t careers of 1000 of 1226 former medical students, only per cent were living and active as physicians; 13 per ce of the entering medical students were dead within years.

On the basis of these studies, Thomas concludes 'th psychological stamina is of vital importance to t entering medical student if he or she is to reach the go

236

f becoming a sound physician.' She quotes Paget that the personal character, the very nature, the will must be strong if the student is to survive the rigors of medical school, residency training, and the practice and teaching of medicine'.

No mention is made of the possibility that something may be wrong with the patterns of medical training that may contribute to stress-associated morbidity and mortality. As formulated by Lennart Levi (1971).

Much of today's medical activity is concerned with the diseases induced by man's present environment and by his unsuccessful adaptation to it. Much less attention is paid to 'the *inhuman* actor', by which is meant environmental conditions, often arising from modern civilization, that induce disturbances of a medical and/or social nature even in a perfectly normal biological organism.

Is it possible that the present highly regimented, stress-inducing methods of training medical students and hospital residents may contribute to dehumanizing future physicians and driving some of them to drug dependence and suicide?

Recently we saw a newspaper item regarding the demand by a group of hospital residents for a 72-hour week. This was indeed a strange demand in a country where some labour unions are discussing seriously the need for a 30-hour week.

It turns out that the average work load of residents (e.g., in departments of internal medicine and family medicine) runs somewhere between 86 and 110 hours per week. In addition, 4 to 5 times per month in many teaching hospitals interns and residents may work continuously through a 24- to 36-hour shift.

Dennis Breo (1978a) describes

An intern's personal story: 'I guess it's best to be a little brash, to see an internship simply as a means to an end. Not to let it affect you personally. I guess I'm just too sensitive. But I think of these patients as my responsibility. I've been working for 110 hours a week. It never varies . . . Every other day I'm on call. That's a hard day. I work through all night. Oh, I may be able to snatch two or three hours of sleep by intermittently napping. Then I go right through the next day until 7 that night. A 36-hour shift. Absolutely senseless. I just feel drained. It's a deadening experience. Just chipping away at you . . . There is little time for a personal life . . . The little things finally got me. I just became incapacitated by frustration.'

A paediatric resident in a metropolitan public hospital in a group session with a child psychologist says:

It's been a month since I've seen my husband on a weekend. Mary (another woman resident) and I took our internship here and we started out being known as the 'sunshine girls'. Not any more. You get a little bitter. There's no excuse for having to work 12 straight hours and not learn a goddamn thing. The acute care we give is excellent, but preventive services are nil.

A male resident puts it in a nutshell: 'We need to cut the hours in half, double the staff . . . The administrators are all unmitigated—(unprintable).'

According to Dennis Breo, Dr. Ken Peters, a third-year resident in internal medicine, is helping to prepare a 'survivors manual' for young physicians. 'Physicians in training', says Dr. Peters, 'often feel depressed and unsupported . . . We need to pull together data on sleep deprivation studies—how efficiently can a resident read ECGs, for example, when he's been up all night . . . What we need to get away from is this idea on the part of older doctors that a residence should be a little like a fraternity hell week . . . Surgical residents are afraid to take the educational leave they're entitled to because to do so would just increase the work load on their peers'.

Dr. Peters relates that his own internship was particularly rough. 'I know my wife suffered because I couldn't spend much time with her. I found myself taking some of my frustrations out on my patients.'

Becoming a physician is 'dehumanizing' process is the title of an article by Kimball (1974) a psychiatrist at the University of Chicago School of Medicine:

Medical schools have become exercises in stereotyped rituals—despite compulsive rearrangement of the curriculum . . . the learning that occurs is so often passive, the teaching frequently dogmatic and always authoritarian. Little humility abounds . . . Despite our emphasis on 'scientific' medicine, few physicians learn to think as scientists, in an open-ended process. Rather the 19th century model of medicine is directed at achieving closure.

Dr. Kimball points out that little or no attention is paid by the faculty or administration to the students' or residents'

feeling of frustration, anxiety, anger, impotence, hostility, compassion . . . the lengthy period of almost total dependence on authority . . . the inhumaneness of the teaching hospital . . . the absence of integrated behavioral science, the feelings of detachment and isolation from classmates as well as instructors.

The mechanistic dehumanized approach to patient care was exemplified for us by an occurrence on a medical ward related to us by a second year resident. It seems that this resident was 'caught' holding the hand of an anxiety-ridden patient. The chief resident pitched into the resident by stating that 'it is your job to pay attention to the patient's electrolyte balance and not to hold his hand'. Apparently, it never occurred to this chief resident that alleviation of anxiety and reassurance may have some influence on metabolic processes (see also Crane 1974).

It is a sad commentary on the state of physician training in our hospitals that interns and residents have been driven to seek collective bargaining arrangements (see Sullivan 1978).

The long work hours, coupled with an authoritarian system of teaching and supervision, and superimposed on the frustration encountered by interns and residents in facing the suffering of patients while being sleep-deprived—all these factors militate against the ability to learn or to develop attitudes of compassion and caring.

These heavy work schedules violate well known principles of learning theory. Even in dogs, Pavlov (1903, 1940) observed that exposure to too strong or too frequent stimuli leads to the disappearance of well established conditional reflexes and the development of what Pavlov referred to as 'transmarginal inhibition'. Pavlov further described the development of neurotic manifestations in dogs exposed to frustrating situations. In our own studies on dogs, we have observed the development of several psychopathological disorders in certain types of dogs exposed to too intense or too frequent scheduling of Pavlovian conditioning experiments (Corson and Corson 1975, 1977; Corson *et al.* 1963).

The current disarray in the state of medical care and medical education in the United States is perhaps epitomized by a title of a recent monograph, *Doing better and feeling worse* edited by Knowles (1977). It is perhaps a good omen for the eventual improvement of medical care and education that the contributions to this important volume include a number of highly competent medical as well as nonmedical authorities in the health care areas, such as Lewis Thomas, David E. Rogers, Julius B. Richmond, David and Beatrix Hamburg, Donald Frederickson, Leon Eisenberg, etc. Whether these published deliberations may lead to substantial reforms in medical education and health care remains to be seen.

Ironically, the current reductionist approach in medical education and practice can be traced to the pioneering efforts of a nonmedical broadly oriented educator, Abraham Flexner, the author of the famous Flexner Report (see Pattishall 1977). The major thrust of the Flexner report was directed toward the need for more scientific and educationally sound training of physicians and the need for affiliation of medical schools with universities. Unfortunately, the scientific orientation initiated by the Flexner report turned out to be a highly reductionist and fractionated approach to medical education and the practice of medicine and the gradual decrease in emphasis on the humanistic and integrative aspects of medicine. In essence, medical education and practice were based on dualistic concepts, with the physician being concerned primarily with treating the body as though human beings are inanimate objects not subject to psychological and emotional influences.

What is needed in medical education and care is not less science, but the addition to reductionist science of an integrative holistic approach in medical schools, hospitals, and physicians' offices. Unless such a reorientation takes place, there is a danger that American people may be driven more and more towards medical nihilism, as exemplified by Illich (1976) or to quacks and charlatans and dubious enterprises on the lunatic fringes of various self-appointed commercialized 'healers'.

An anti-science attitude even crept into a headline in the American Medical News in an article written by David Rogers, president of the Robert Wood Johnson Foundation (see Rogers 1974). In this article Dr. Rogers states:

As physicians, we must have first-class scientific technology at our command, but to be fully effective we also need to become much better managers of illness and much better deliverers of sensitive humanistic support to those we care for.

We must not let our search for better scientific ways to deal with disease distract us from what I believe must be our central focus—that of medicine as a caring profession that can improve the quality of life for those to whom we minister.

The headline for the article (obviously not written by Dr. Rogers) read: 'Illness must be understood not in scientific but in human terms.' Reading the entire article indicates that Dr. Rogers was not advocating the abdication of medicine from science or the scientific method. In essence he advocated a humanistic systems-oriented scientific approach to health care.

The trouble with the current stress-inducing system of medical education and residency training is that it would tend to:

(a) Weed out the most sensitive, creative, and humanistic physicians;
(b) Develop in those who remain in training a cynical attitude, callousness, and insensitivity to human needs and suffering;
(c) Enhance extreme competitive tendencies and promote commercialization of medical care;
(d) Perpetuate the dominance of mechanistic reductionist tendencies in academic medicine since the most sensitive and questioning students get turned off by the unresponsive political machine of academic rigidity;
(e) Enhance possibilities for the commission of iatrogenic errors by hospital residents and practising physicians.

The volume on *Primary health care in industrialized nations* edited by Burrell and Sheps (1978) offers a comprehensive definition and overview of primary health care and of the importance of integrating biomedical, behavioural, and psychosocial factors in medical education and health care delivery. Of particular interest in regard to medical education are the erudite and stimulating presentations by Pellegrino (pp. 227–30), Sidel (pp. 188–97), and Engel (pp. 169–81).

Engel (pp. 169–81) presents convincing arguments for the need to introduce the principles of a biopsychosocial model into medical education, with emphasis on the patient and not merely on disease. He questions the wisdom of the adversary atmosphere created by the notion that 'the diagnosis and treatment of disease should be the responsibility of physicians while the care of the patient and maintenance of health may be delegated to other health providers'. Engel states that some nurses attempt to play the role of protector of the patient from the 'cold, insensitive' physician, pointing out that this concern is based on the 'false premise that cience and humanism are somehow in opposition'.

Sidel (pp. 188–97) concludes that 'only a community-based and community-controlled health care system, devoted in large measure to promoting equity, employment, community stability, and community development and not to narrow professional or technical interests, can produce the changes that we need'.

Pellegrino (pp. 227–30) suggests the development of 'a special track leading to primary care which differs from preparation for specialist care'.

Unfortunately, there apparently was no direct input from hospital residents, interns, or medical students, so that the dehumanizing stress-inducing regimen of medical education is likely to make it difficult, if not impossible, to develop the changes suggested by the participants in the Conference or Primary Health Care. After all, it is the type of physicians we train that will have the major influence on the kind of health care we will get, including the health of those whose mission it is to provide health care.

PSYCHOSOCIAL STRESS IN ACADEMIC INSTITUTIONS

But man, proud man
Drest in a little brief authority,
Most ignorant of what he's most assured,
His glassy essence, like an angry ape,
Plays such fantastic tricks before high
heaven
As make the angels weep.

Shakespeare: *Measure for measure*, II, 2]

There is a dearth of information on the psychosocial environment in academic institutions in general, and research laboratories, in particular. Caplan *et al.* (1975) included scientists and professors in their extensive studies on job demands and worker health. According to these authors, 'scientists were chosen to represent a group which was low in stress and low in risk of coronary heart disease'. This report also states that 'the most satisfied occupations are professors, family physicians, white collar supervisors, police, and air traffic controllers at small sites. Scientists had the lowest blood pressure of the eight occupations measured'.

We were unable to find in this publication what kind of scientists or professors were studied and what institutional connections they had. The statement about family physicians is in contrast to the studies reported by C. Thomas (1976, 1977) and others discussed in the previous section, indicating high morbidity and mortality in physicians.

Sorri *et al.* (1976) reported on stress in the academic world in Finland. They list several factors involved in the production of stress, among which are:

(a) The availability of a very limited number of tenured positions. Thus, the bulk of academic personnel are exposed to economic insecurity, adversary relationships with their colleagues and superiors, and the development of a low self-esteem and depression in the face of non-reappointment or failure to secure a tenured position. This latter fact is particularly stressful since 'when a person takes to research, this means selecting a career which will narrow down his possibilities of choosing his place in society, since returning from research work to a more practical fields is often difficult'.

(b) Forced age-related retirement, even if accompanied by an adequate pension. These authors point out that 'work plays such an important part in the individual's personal life that his retirement on a pension is liable to lead to a serious identity crisis and even to dejection'.

Research scientists in American universities

It is generally agreed that the function of a university is transmission and development of knowledge, culture, aesthetics, and humanistic values by providing 'an atmosphere within which the critical spirit can flourish. . . . Its essential bias is in favour of unencumbered criticism' (Shoben 1970, pp. 695–7).

Free enquiry and free interplay of ideas are essential to a stable, viable social organization. This is the essence of academic freedom, the preservation of which requires that decision-making processes in a university ought to be decentralized to include faculty, as well as students, and all the strata of the public whom the university is supposed to serve.

The exact opposite has been taking place in many American academic institutions, especially state universities. These universities are governed by a board of trustees usually appointed by the governor, who in many cases may have little idea of the nature and functions of an academic institution. Similarly, his appointees generally have little appreciation or understanding of what it is that makes a university tick.

These trustees appoint a president, generally without real faculty input, although there is usually a pretence of such input by the appointment of a search committee, whose function is to search but not to find, and certainly not to appoint.

The president appoints the deans who in turn appoint chairpersons for the departments, all this without any real faculty or student input before, or during, the tenure of these administrators. It is essentially an autocratic set-up in violation of all principles of a democratic system or of a well-managed business.

The members of the board of trustees are usually well-to-do business people who have neither the training, experience, time, nor inclination to manage a university. The president, thus, remains essentially the *de facto* 'Tsar' of the institution, as long as he does not jeopardize the business interests or the particular preferences of the trustees.

According to Epstein (1970) state university board members are:

mainly business and professional men with substantial incomes, and they are not young . . . Although overwhelmingly college or university graduates, often with law, medical or other advanced degrees, they are seldom professional educators . . . Neither are they faculty members from other institutions . . . In this respect, state university boards differ from those private college boards that have included, notably in recent years, members belonging to the educational community itself, often alumni who haved become administrators or professors at other institutions. A similar membership for public university boards would not be impossible.

The deans and chairpersons in a public university generally serve 'at the pleasure' of the president, and thus represent the wishes and whims of the president, rather than representing the needs of the faculty, or the students, or the university as a whole, or, for that matter, the needs of the people whose taxes support the institution. In essence, at many universities there are no viable grievance procedures, few or no means of correcting or preventing errors, and no legitimate means whereby faculty or students can participate in a recall of a university administration or of the board of trustees.

No truly democratic government could long survive with such a 'no feedback' type of administration, nor could any business enterprise with this type of autocratic management long endure. In a free enterprise economy corrective measures would come from stockholders and/or the market place.

In the case of a state university, such corrective measures are lacking. Thus, a state university is perhaps the only institution in a free enterprise economy that seems to have many of the disadvantages of a dictatorial socialist economy without any of its benefits.

It has been said that the human mind is remarkable for being able to resist new ideas and for holding tenaciously to stereotypes. It is remarkable that for all these years, in the United States in a society where federal, state, and local governments are elected periodically by the people and are subject to public scrutiny and recall, that in the same country, academic institutions (and particularly state universities) should have remained as bastions of undemocratic, unresponsive management.

Stephen R. Graubard (1970) in a preface to the *Daedalus* issue of 'Rights and responsibilities: the universities' dilemma', written during the period of student unrest, stated:

The students (and the universities dare not disclaim or repudiate them) challenge some of the most deeply-held beliefs of the society; they remind the society of promises once made; they raise questions about rights and responsibilities, and insist that *authority can be made legitimate again only if it accedes to the founding principles of the nation* [italics ours].

In the same issue of *Daedalus*, Robert S. Morison, a distinguished neurophysiologist and university administrator, recognizes that 'the pursuit of academic freedom requires that decision-making in a university be decentralized.' Nevertheless, Morison advocates that overall academic policy remain largely with the administration and trustees.

The reasons given by Morison for such a recommendation are:

(a) A possible conflict of interests if faculty members vote on budgetary matters;
(b) Faculty members lack qualities required by legislators: 'tolerance of ambiguity, the ability to compromise, a desire to get on with the job, and a nice sense of the possible';
(c) 'The administration, and especially the president, is in a way uniquely concerned with the welfare of the university as a whole'.

Our argument is not to abolish the office of the university president or the institution of the board of trustees, but to make the administration and the trustees accountable to those whose activities are essential for the functioning of a university (i.e., the faculty and students) and to develop effective feedback and sensitive response channels, so as to permit optimal functioning and social stability in the university community. If a private enterprise involving, on the one hand, profit-oriented owners and stockholders and, on the other hand, workers who are in an adversary position of trying to secure a greater share of the profits—if such a privately owned business (such as Harman International Industries) can devise effective mechanisms for sharing decision-making processes—why should not a non-profit public university be able to broaden its decision-making base so as to develop co-operative, rather than adversary, relationships with the entire university community, including faculty, non-academic personnel, and students?

One of the factors contributing to the inefficient and stress-inducing management in public universities is the progressive (perhaps we should say 'regressive') increase in the size of these institutions during the past several decades. Some of these universities have 50 000 or more students. This tends to create a huge, often self-serving, faceless and inefficient bureaucracy, mountains of paperwork, and a tremendous waste of taxpayers' funds. Under these conditions, even the most competent and highly motivated administrators tend to become cut off from the real tasks of the university and may become cynical and/or frustrated, thus creating a vicious dehumanizing and demoralizing cycle and creating an atmosphere inimical to intellectual and aesthetic growth.

One can cite numerous examples of economic waste and senseless activities which do not promote the interests of the university or the public as a result of a bulky administration lacking in effective feedback channels. In the face of decreasing budgets for research and teaching, one observes expensive periodic replacement of intact doors, floors, ceilings, and furniture. Without consultation with faculty, laboratories are being dismantled, often against the expressed wishes of faculty. In one large public university, the administration sent in a 'demolishing crew' that wrecked, in a few days, a highly sophisticated biobehavioural laboratory that took about a decade of hard work and many multidisciplinary talents and large sums of public money to design and build. Reasoned supplications by the scientists who developed the laboratory and by many clinical colleagues were not only of no avail, but did not even merit a courteous response, to say nothing of a reasonable explanation or an attempt at indicating a willingness at least to listen.

The same administration continued for years to badger a scientist to remove a colony of dogs (used for longitudinal biobehavioural psychosocial stress studies) from kennels adjoining the conditioning and physiological laboratories to a central animal holding facility in another building. As would be obvious to any elementary student of behavioural sciences, such a move would undercut any possibilities for behavioural control of the dog colony. It would expose experimental animals to a variety of unpredictable and uncontrollable psychosocial and physical stimuli, including extreme weather conditions in transit to the laboratory building, and would invalidate the entire research programme. Needless to say, the administration eventually succeeded in removing these animals and in abolishing the interdisciplinary psychobiological and psychophysiological studies. The administration also succeeded in making it impossible to secure psychophysiological, behavioural, neuroendocrine, and genetic data associated with ageing changes in these animals. Many of these dogs had been studied for about a decade before the colony was disbanded.

In a carefully researched paper, Gallant and Prothero (1972) attempt to present an analogy between cell growth and institutional growth, pointing out the principle of size optimization. Although

cells exist in a variety of sizes, each size representing an optimization to one or another set of constraints, yet there are upper bounds. There are no cells the size of basketballs because essential metabolic functions are limited by the surface-to-volume ratio. In the case of the university, no grand theory of education is needed in order to identify dysfunctions of growth that affect essential activities (for example, the diffusion of individuals through, in, and out of the university) or that affect all activities (for example, overall morale). Balanced against these dysfunctions are such advantages of growth as economy, the achievement of a critical mass, and flexibility in staffing.

However, the analysis by these authors of 'data from the California system indicates that unit costs of education decline very little above a size of 10 000 or 15 000 students . . . at the same time, the dysfunctions attendant on growth become steadily more severe'.

In the case of universities 'already well into the dysfunctional size range' these authors suggest either the establishment of a new university or the decentralization of the existing university into two or more campuses. Gallant and Prothero conclude: 'Returning to the natural world, we note that cells do not grow indefinitely. Instead they divide'.

We suggest another even simpler way of achieving the benefits of decentralization and that is to broaden decision-making processes by permitting more autonomy to different colleges and departments within the university and increasing faculty–student participation in decision-making. Many functions could easily be decentralized and performed more efficiently and with less cost. For example, with every appointment of ancillary personnel, one gets involved with the tremendous red tape of a college personnel office, then a central all-university personnel office with all the attendant paper-polluting manoeuvres and costly delays. If the funds come from a research grant, the appointment is also channelled through the research foundation. Such appointments could more easily be processed locally by every college. Records of such appointments could, of course, be maintained in a central office, but there would be a saving of time and paperwork.

Similarly, why is it necessary for every order of equipment and supplies to go through the numerous delaying stages of a centralized purchasing department, when it would be more efficient and less costly for every department or even every laboratory to order these items directly from the supplier?

Under such a decentralized system, not only would university functions be performed more efficiently, but it would also save financial resources by making it unnecessary to organize huge bureaucractic superstructures and thus cut down the expense of maintaining a paper-pollution machinery. These funds thus saved could be used for research, education, and service.

Tenure, stress, and obligatory retirement in academia

A story was circulated some years ago in academic circles about a speech made by the president of the University of Chicago wherein he advocated the abolition of tenure for university professors in order to keep the professors on their toes. In this way, the president suggested, professors are less likely to rest on their laurels. It is alleged that the late Professor A. J. Carlson, one of America's most distinguished physiologists, quipped: 'Mr. President, you are confusing the anatomy; you must have meant that to abolish tenure would keep the professors on their knees'.

Professorial tenure is probably one of the most important factors that has contributed to the maintenance of the university as a centre for intellectual stimulation, the preservation of free expression and open discussion of unpopular and controversial issues, and the preservation of the rights of dissidents.

The argument that tenure may contribute to the protection in academic institutions of lazy nonproductive professors and the accumulation of 'dead wood' rests on the false assumption that excellence can be achieved by negative reinforcement and anxietyengendered insecurity. As mentioned earlier, anxiety is not conducive to achievement and should not be confused with drive and motivation. The latter could best be achieved by providing an intellectual atmosphere conducive to scholarship and excellence in the performance of all academic tasks.

The stress of the young untenured members of the

faculty described by Sorri *et al.* (1976) for Finnish universities also holds for American academic institutions. It may be argued that perhaps *all members* of the university faculty should be tenured, i.e. they should feel secure in their positions as long as they perform their duties to the best of their abilities. One might argue for a brief (e.g., one year) probationary period. Perhaps the weeding out of individuals unsuited for academic teaching or research positions should take place in the graduate schools before they are awarded advanced degrees.

In a humanistic society, students unfit for academic positions should be properly counselled and offered systematic vocational guidance, so that each person could find a suitable occupational niche in society. The same approach ought to be used with young members of the faculty who may be found unsuited for a particular academic task. In a civilized affluent society, forced unemployment should not be an acceptable phenomenon, and certainly not for individuals with extensive training. Such an approach to tenure and academic excellence would go a long way in eliminating psychological stress and associated psychopathological and social disorders.

The presence in each department of many competent non-tenured young faculty members, the fact that only a limited number of them may become tenured, creates an unwholesome stressful situation of unprincipled rivalry, intrigue, paranoia, backbiting, and 'toadyism' to superiors. The 'publish or perish' dictum as a major precondition for tenure is often counterproductive to scholarly achievements and encourages superficial research, hasty publication of poorly substantiated data, and in many cases, the pursuit of trivia embroidered with pompous, jargonistic verbosity.

Thus, a promotion system presumably designed to ensure academic excellence actually would appear to promote mediocrity and hinder the creative processes of faculty members because the system is based primarily on the utilization of negative reinforcement methods.

When the United States recently passed a law eliminating obligatory retirement at age 65, college professors were exempted from that law, in part due to the insistence of a number of college presidents. The argument was that the presence of a large number of tenured professors represents an obstacle to the promotion of younger faculty members to tenured positions. This argument is based on the assumption of genetic egalitarianism and neglects to take into account constitutional differences in maturation and ageing rates. As stated by Botwinic (1975), 'However great may be the differences among young adults in their behavioral and physiological functioning, the differences among old adults are greater; this appears to be true in most all areas of function'.

Whereas some individuals may need to retire at the age of 65 (or even earlier), others may continue to function effectively, well above the age of 65. One can cite many examples of individuals who continued to do creative work long after the age of 65. Bernard Baruch at 76 became the United States representative to the Atomic Energy Commission of the United Nations, and formulated the Baruch Proposals for international control of atomic energy. Morris Fishbein at 83 was still writing for publication up to 10 000 words per week and continued to edit *Medical World News.* Benjamin Franklin at 84 wrote his masterful appeal to Congress for the abolition of slavery. Oliver Wendell Holmes wrote a biography of Emerson at 75. Marl Menninger, a distinguished psychiatrist, at age 80 established in Chicago a centre for the study of juvenile delinquency. I. P. Pavlov at 76 organized a neurological and psychiatric clinic at the Institute of Physiology and continued to publish extensively on the application of his basic conditioning studies to psychiatric problems. At the age of 86 he was president of the International Congress of Physiological Sciences. Giuseppi Verdi wrote *Falstaff* and *Othello* after the age of 74.

Think of the immense loss of creative talent that could result from obligatory retirement at age 65. The faculty, students, and administrators lose the important ingredients of a matured talent: wisdom, the accumulation of many skills, and the mellowness that could contribute to balanced judgement and a humanistic atmosphere on the campuses.

One can sympathize with university administrators in their heroic attempts to balance the budget in the face of declining appropriations and declining student enrolment. But one would like to see university presidents take the leadership in 'thinking the unthinkable' and take the long-range view of what is needed for the preservation of a stable, just, and viable social order. According to a report prepared by Sivard (1977), for the Rockefeller Foundation and four other sponsors, the annual world military expenditures for 1975 reached *$324 billion* and are estimated to have been about $350 billion in 1976. Throughout the world an estimated 60 million people are paid through military budgets. *It costs an average of $14 800 per year to maintain one soldier.* Would it not make good sense to offer tenured positions to the deserving untenured faculty members not at the expense of retiring, competent, mature, tenured faculty members but rather at the expense of a few less soldiers? To paraphrase Gilbert and Sullivan, 'they never will be missed.'

In the face of increasing unemployment, there is talk about our government providing funds for public works. This involves the creation of a new bureaucracy and often, the creation of make-believe work. During the 'great' depression in the United States in the 1930s, President Roosevelt, faced with mass unemployment and public disquietude, created the Works Progress Administration (WPA). This act certainly served as a great turning point in reversing the increasing economic and social disorganization and political unrest. Eventually, it is alleged, the WPA was faced with the problem of finding work for the employees on WPA funds. A story was being circulated during that period that many highly educated individuals were engaged in raking leaves until no more leaves were available; whereupon, the director of the leaf-raking project sent a telegram to Washington which read: 'Send more leaves!' Would it not make more sense to offer tenured positions to competent faculty members than to have to resort eventually to public works projects?

Stress of research workers in academic institutions

History is dominated by two types of minds. The history of human suffering is dotted with the names of men of willpower and ambition, who make wars, build empires which then collapse, leaving behind only destruction and misery. The history of human progress is the story of a relatively small number of creative people, creative in art, sciences, or any other human endeavor. As progress, in the past, depended on them, so it will in the future, and the fate of any nation depends, to a great extent, on the question: How far does it produce creative minds.

[Szent-György: 1962].

Scientists in universities require for optimal functioning:

(a) Sufficient funding;
(b) Assurance of continuity of a research programme;
(c) An academic atmosphere conducive to creative research.

Most, if not all, university administrators proclaim their intense interest in promoting research. Unfortunately, in many cases, this interest is not really in the promotion of research *per se*, but in securing outside research funding and especially indirect costs. The assumption appears to be that it is not the universities' responsibility to support research activities. Therefore, when research is conducted at the university, the scientist is expected not only to find his own funding, but also to procure so-called 'overhead' or indirect costs.

Thus, the research scientist is obliged to spend much time and energy in 'grantsmanship' activities and is thus diverted from utilizing his talents and energy for creative research. The responsibility for securing research funding ought to be that of the university administration.

During the past several decades the bulk of research funding in the United States came from federal sources, such as the National Institutes of Health and the National Science Foundation. One of the major stimuli for the federal support of scientific research came from the launching of the Soviet Sputnik.

It would appear that after the novelty of space competition wore off, there has been a progressive decline in federal and state research funding, particularly for basic research. Many other factors have contributed to the decline in financial support for research,

Quite apart from the general decline in federal funds for research, scientists are also faced with problems associated with the way research funds are awarded. The system of awarding research grants has recently been geared primarily to short-term support for specific projects, often for periods as short as two years. This prevents planning of research strategies, and assembling and training of research personnel. In particular, this makes it impossible to conduct longitudinal studies. The renewal of a research grant is unpredictable and does not appear to be necessarily related to the accomplishments of the scientists.

Such a system of haphazard 'on and off' research support is not only wasteful of talent, but is also wasteful in economic terms. The termination of a research grant often leads to the dispersal of effective research teams. Often highly sophisticated and expensive instrumentation remains unused and eventually may deteriorate and become obsolete. If the same scientists eventually secure another research grant, a great deal of time, energy, and funding may be wasted in attempting to purchase and design new instrumentation, assemble a new research team, and train new technical assistants. Such an unpredictable system of research support is comparable to a system of random punishment and may be conducive to the development of various psychopathological manifestations.

In a report released by the National Board of the National Science Foundation (1978), serious concern was expressed about the 'health of the university science establishment'. The report emphasized that 'basic research is long-term and needs continuity of funding. "Stop-and-go" funding does not insure a continuing high-quality scientific capability.' (see also Roark 1978).

Shanin (1978) presented an analysis of data on the continuing decline in research support in the United States compiled by the National Science Foundation. Several items from that analysis should be a cause for concern. If one compares the number of scientists and engineers engaged in research and development (R and D per 10 000 population), that number has been declining in the United States beginning in about 1970, whereas that number in Japan, West Germany, and the Soviet Union has been rising steadily. The rise has been particularly spectacular in the Soviet Union.

Another item that catches one's attention is the fact that whereas the United States government spends approximately 64 per cent of its R and D outlay on defence and space-related work, the Japanese government spends only 8 per cent of its outlay on defence and space research.

During the past decade or so, one of us (S.A.C.) has had the opportunity to observe the comparative types of support for basic research in the neurosciences in the United States and the Soviet Union. This did not involve a systematic study of research support in the Soviet Union, but it did involve systematic monitoring of psychophysiologic and neurophysiologic research in several institutions and laboratories engaged in research closely related to our own. One is impressed with *the stability of research support which enables the Soviet scientists to plan their research activities on a long-term basis.* This support is not only continuing but it has been increasing progressively every few years. Our Soviet colleagues have been able to maintain and expand their research teams. In contrast to our research scientists, our Soviet colleagues have been able to maintain the same technical assistants and even the same animal caretakers for many years. In fact, knowing the American reputation for efficiency, our Soviet colleagues have found it difficult to comprehend our inefficient and wasteful way of haphazard support for scientific research.

Another source of psychological stress for research scientists is the operation of the peer review system. This system is designed for the purpose of assuring scientific objectivity and fairness in the evaluation of research grant applications. This system has been functioning reasonably well as long as ample research funds were allocated by the Federal government. When these funds have become scarce, many scientists had the impression that the fairness and objectivity were not always there. Mehl (1975), former Deputy Director of the Division of Biological and Medical Sciences, National Science Foundation, outlines some of the concerns of the scientific community as follows:

One criticism has been that peer review is self-serving in the sense that people question the objectivity of scientists in making recommendations to provide government funds to support other scientists. . . . A somewhat different view is that it is self-serving for a small in-house group of scientists. It has been characterized as a system by which scientists at a small group of universities review each other's grants and assure that they will be well funded at the expense of those outside the privileged circle. Other criticisms have been that the system does not encourage innovative research or that which challenges accepted paradigms; that the bases on which decisions are reached are excessively secret and do not permit an adequate rebuttal by those proposing research; that the system is manipulated by program managers to support the decisions they wish to make; or that the system results in grants that are an obvious waste of tax monies. . . . Reviewers, and particularly panel members, constitute an in-group serving their own interests rather than the community at large. . . . The review process is cloaked in excessive secrecy which may serve to hide incompetent reviewing or the incompetence of agency staff. While the members of study sections and advisory panels is a matter of public record, the identity of those providing specific reviews and the identity of letter reviewers is not revealed. Although program staff provides feedback on declined proposals to investigators in order to provide some basis for revising a proposal, some investigators find this adequate. They would prefer to have access to verbatim comments of reviewers in full and, in view of the time required to prepare a revised proposal and have it cycled through the review procedure again, to be able to respond to adverse comment developed in the first review before a final decision is made.

Garb (1974) called attention to some rather disturbing aspects of the peer review system:

(1) The use of secret dossiers, euphemistically called 'pink sheets' should be abolished. For each scientist who applies for an NIH grant, a secret dossier is kept on file at NIH. This dossier contains the unedited comments of each study section that has ever reviewed the scientist's applications. The scientist himself is not permitted to see his dossier, and has no way to correct misstatements about himself. These dossiers are reviewed by subsequent study sections, so that a severely derogatory comment by a previous reviewer, whether correct or not, can ruin a scientist's chance of getting an NIH grant. Although these dossiers are supposed to be used only as background for reviewing a current grant application, I have learned that sometimes, surreptitiously, they are used for other purposes as well. It is difficult to reconcile these practices either with basic American values or with the concept of scientific freedom.

(2) At present, a retiring member of a study section is invited to suggest the name of his successor. Obviously, this leads to inbreeding and the formation of cliques. It counters the purpose of rotation of study section members. A retiring study section member should be forbidden to suggest his successor.

(3) The choice of study section members should be decided by a democratic process. At present, they are appointed on the recommendation of executive secretaries. As a result, the term 'peer review' has become incorrect and misleading. A true peer review system would involve election of study section members by the scientists who are working in the field. Each scientist might be allowed to choose the study section for whose members he wishes to vote. Then, a secret ballot could decide the election of study section members. There are drawbacks to this, as to any other democratic procedure, but I think they are less than those attending the present undemocratic system.

In 1975 an NIH Grants Peer Review Study Team was appointed. The report of this team was published in two volumes which are available at the National Institutes of Health, Bethesda, Maryland 20014, U.S.A. These reports contain several important recommendations the implementation of which may lead to an increase in objectivity and fairness in the awarding of research grants.

Three problems, however, appear to remain unsolved. One is the problem of inadequate federal funds for research, and particularly for basic research. The second problem relates to the lack of long-term funding, so as to afford continuity of basic research programmes and especially of those dealing with longitudinal studies. In particular, studies on the behavioural and physiological effects of psychosocial stressors are more meaningful and clinically relevant in longitudinal studies.

The third problem relates to predominance of a mechanistic reductionist approach in the evaluation of research grant applications, the insistence on detailed spelling out of methods and sequences of experimental procedures and detailed descriptions of statistical evaluation methods. Such requirements of detailed outlines of research procedures may be suitable for some types of applied technological research. In contrast, such requirements are inimical to creative basic research which involves charting a course in 'terra incognita'.

This point was perhaps best stated by the Nobel laureate, Albert Szent-Györgyi (1974):

Research means going out into the unknown, which demands a pioneering spirit. This spirit is now strangled by the way in which the main federal biomedical granting agency, the

National Institutes of Health, distributes its grants. The unknown is the unknown because one does not know what is there. If one knows what one will do and find in it, then it is not research any more and is not worth doing. The NIH wants detailed projects, wants the applicants to tell exactly what they will do and find during the tenure of their grants, which excludes unexpected discoveries on which progress depends. . . . Nobody can really judge the value of another fellow's project. Projects are nonsense. I don't think that any of the great discoveries were ever made by projects. They were made by intuition. . . . The foundation of science is honesty. The present granting method is so much at variance with the basic ideas of science that it has to breed dishonesty, forcing scientists into devious ways. One of the widely applied practices is to do work and then present results as a project and report later that all predictions were verified. . . . I have been, myself, unable to secure a grant and am unable to believe that the thousands of applicants who got grants were all that much better scientists. I am not applying any more, having made it a rule to take no more than three kicks in the pants by anyone. I do not think that the rejection of scientists who have contributed to science is a great encouragement to young scientists. I also want to remain free to turn in whatever direction my research demands.

If one looks up the history of any of the major discoveries, one can readily see how constricting a detailed research procedures outline could be for any creative work. Would Otto Loewi have had to include in a grant application a description of the dream he had about a method which enabled him to discover the *'Vagusstoff'*? Or would Banting and Best (see Best 1964) have had to describe in advance all the steps and the serendipitous insights which eventually enabled them to discover and isolate insulin?

Perhaps the most useful suggestion one could offer to any research granting agency is the advice offered by Cowan (1972) on the role of a science administrator: 'His role is to create an environment that nourishes scientific creativity.'

SOME SUGGESTIONS FOR THE DESIGN OF LABORATORY EXPERIMENTS TO SIMULATE THE EFFECT OF PSYCHO-SOCIAL FACTORS IN WORKING LIFE

1. *Recognition of constitutional differences in responses to emotional stimuli.* In comparing the psychophysiological effects of stimulated work situations, one should take into consideration constitutional differences of the experimental subjects. Averaging psychophysiological data may give results which have no relationship to the emotional reactions of real individuals (Corson *et al.* 1970b; Corson 1971b; Corson and Corson 1971).
2. *Acute versus longitudinal experiments.* One should be careful in drawing conclusions regarding psychophysiological reactions in working life from experiments involving a single exposure to stressful situations. Longitudinal studies may offer results much more closely related to psychophysiological effects encountered in real working environments.
3. *The need to study patterns of psychoendocrine and psychophysiological reactions.* Our studies (Corson *et al.* 1970a,b; Corson 1971b) and those from other laboratories demonstrate the importance of concurrent measurements of many physiological, endocrine, and biochemical parameters in order to determine the *patterns of adaptive* psychophysiological reactions and the mechanisms of transformation of these adaptive reactions into maladaptive patterns. McCleary (1954) reported, for example, that changes in heart rate afford 'a very dubious measure of anxiety'. Lacey and Lacey (1962) suggested that emotions might correlate with *patterns of autonomic responses.*

In particular, in studying psychoendocrine responses, it is unwise to attempt to draw conclusions on the basis of measuring one or two hormonal responses. As was pointed out by Houssay (1957), 'In the whole organism one hormone never works alone. . . . If we study any function we find that it does not depend on one hormone, but on a balance between hormones acting together or in a consecutive way'. Endocrines also act in a manner comparable to reciprocal inhibition, so that the 'state of any given metabolic activity at any given moment must be . . . a resultant of the varying balance between multiple cooperating and opposing hormonal influences' (Mason 1968, p. 796).

One of the reasons for the neglect of an integrated approach in psychoendocrinology (in addition to the persistence of reductionist orientation) is that such investigations require substantial long-term financial support. As pointed out by Mason (1968, pp. 805–6),

Hormone assay methods . . . require considerable laboratory space, superior technical skill, and scrupulous and consistently painstaking care. . . . Practical problems involving not only cost, space, and personnel but also quality control and supervisory management techniques multiply rapidly as establishment of a larger battery of hormone assay methods is attempted. Considerably higher space–investigator and technician–investigator ratios are required than conventionally prevail in most medical research centres at the present time.

What is urgently needed in psychophysiology is an integrated interdisciplinary research programme involving concurrent measurements not only of endocrine patterns but also of patterns of physiological and behavioural responses, including electrophysiological correlates.

Finally, a systems approach implies that any conclusions drawn from laboratory experiments need to be tested in actual field conditions in order to avoid simplistic reductionist recommendations.

AMERICAN STUDIES PROGRAM, SUNY AT BUFFALO (1975). Down and out in America. *New York Times Magazine*, 9 Feb. 1975, pp. 9–11, 30–35.

ANOKHIN, P. K. (1935). Problema tsentra i periferii v sovremennoi fiziologii nervnoi deyatel'nosti [The problem of centre and periphery in modern physiology of nervous activity]. In *Problema tsentra i periferii fiziologii nervnoi deyatel'nosti* [The Problem of centre and periphery in the physiology of nervous activity] (ed. P. K. Anokhin), pp. 1–70. Gorki, Gosizdat [in Russian].

—— (1974). Biology and neurophysiology of the conditioned reflex and its role in adaptive behavior. Samuel A. Corson, scientific and translation ed. In *International series of monographs on cerebrovisceral and behavioral physiology and conditioned reflexes* (ed. S. A. Corson), Vol. 3. Pergamon Press, Oxford and New York.

BAGEHOT, W. (1872). *Physics and politics.* [Quoted in Kermode (1974), p. 6].

BAKKE, E. W. (1940). *Citizens without work: a study of the effects of unemployment upon the workers' social relations and practices.* Yale University Press, New Haven, Connecticut.

—— (1946). *Mutual survival: the goal of unions and management.* Harper and Brothers, New York and London. (2nd edn., revised and enlarged '20 years after 1st' (1966). Archon Books, Hamden, Conn.).

—— (1958). Mutual survival after twelve years. In *Proceedings of the eleventh annual meeting of the Industrial Relations Research Association,* pp. 2–18.

—— (1969). *The unemployed worker: a study of the task of making a living without a job.* Archon Books, Hamden, Conn. (Reprinted from Bakke 1940).

BEST, C. H. (1964). How we discovered insulin. *Reader's Digest,* March 1964.

BOTWINICK, J. (1975). Behavioral processes. In *Ageing* (eds. S. Gershone and A. Raskin), Vol. 2, pp. 1–98. Raven Press, New York.

BRADY, J. V. (1958). Ulcers in "executive" monkeys. *Sci. Amer.,* **199,** 95–100.

——, PORTER, R. W. CONRAD, D. G., and MASON, J. W. (1958). Avoidance behavior and the development of gastroduodenal ulcers. *J. exp. Anal. Behav.,* **1,** 69–72.

BREO, D. (1978a). Out to the edge of despair . . . and back. *Amer. med. News,* 5 May 1978, pp. 7–8.

—— (1978b). Residents struggle to cope with stress. *Amer. med. News,* 5 May 1978, pp. 7–8.

BRONOWSKI, J. (1973). *The ascent of man.* Little, Brown and Co., Boston.

BURRELL, D. and SHEPS, C. G. (Eds.) (1978). Primary health care in industrialized nations. *Anns. N.Y. Acad. Sci.* **310,** 1–274.

CANNON, W. B. (1929). Organization for physiological homeostasis. *Physiol. rev.* **9,** 397.

CAPLAN, R. D., COBB, S., FRENCH, J. R. P., Jr., VAN HARRISON, R., and PINNEAU, S. R., Jr. (1975). *Job demands and worker health.* U.S. Department of Health, Education, and Welfare/Superintendent of Documents, U.S. Government Printing Office, Washington, D.C. 20402.

CARDER, B. and BERKOWITZ, K. (1970). Rats' preference for earned in comparison with free food. *Science,* **167** (392), 1273–4.

CARSON, R. (1962). *Silent spring.* Fawcett, Greenwich, Conn.

CATTELL, R. B. (1964). Psychological definition and measurement of anxiety. *J. Neuropsychiat.,* **5,** 396–402.

—— and SCHEIER, I. H. (1961). *The meaning and measuremen of neuroticism and anxiety.* The Ronald Press Co., New York.

COHEN, D. (1977). When the magic runs out for doctors. *Psychology Today,* July 1977, pp. 26–7.

COMMONER, B. (1972). *The closing circle.* Bantam Books, New York.

CORONARY DRUG PROJECT RESEARCH GROUP (1975). Clofibrate an hiacin in coronary heart disease. *J. Amer. med. Assoc.,* **231** (4), 360–81.

CORSON, S. A. (1957). Review of *S.P. Botkin and the neurogenic theory of medicine* by F. R. Borodulin. *Science,* **125** (3257), 75–7.

—— (1966a). Conditioning of water and electrolyte excretion. In *Endocrines and the central nervous system.* Research Publication Association of Nervous and Mental Disorders, Vol. 43, pp. 140–99. Williams and Wilkins, Baltimore.

—— (1966b). Neuroendocrine and behavioral response patterns to psychologic stress and the problem of the target tissue in cerebrovisceral pathology. Proc. Conference on Psychophysiological Aspects of Cancer. *Ann. N.Y. Acad. Sci.,* **125** (Art. 3), 890–918.

—— (1971a). The lack of feedback in today's societies—a psychosocial stressor. In *Society, stress and disease* (ed. L. Levi), Vol. 1, pp. 181–9. Oxford University Press, London.

—— (1971b). Pavlovian and operant conditioning techniques in the study of psychosocial and biological relationships. In *Society, stress and disease* (ed. L. Levi), Vol. 1, pp. 7–21. Oxford University Press, London.

—— and CORSON, E. O'LEARY (1967). Pavlovian conditioning as a method for studying the mechanisms of action of minor tranquilizers. In *Neuro-psycho-pharmacology* (ed. H. Brill, J. O. Cole, P. Denikers, H. Hippius, and P. B. Bradley). Excerpta Medica International Congress Series No. 129, pp. 857–78.

—— and —— (1969). The effects of psychotropic drugs on conditioning of water and electrolyte excretion: experimental research and clinical implications. In *Psychotropic drugs in internal medicine* (ed. A. Pletscher and A. Marino). Excerpta Med. Int. Congr. Ser. No. **182,** 147–64.

—— and —— (1971). Psychosocial influences on renal function—implications for human pathophysiology. In *Society, stress and disease* (ed. L. Levi), Vol. 1, pp. 338–51. Oxford University Press, London.

—— and —— (1975). Cerebrovisceral physiology and pathophysiology and psychosomatic medicine. *Totus Homo,* **6** (1–3), 85–123.

—— and —— (1976). Constitutional differences in physiologic adaptation to stress and distress. *Psychopathology of human adaptation* (ed. George Serban), pp. 77–94. Plenum Press, New York.

—— and —— (1977). Comparative psychosomatic reactions to unavoidable and avoidable stressors; the problem of developing control over stressful situations. *Psychosom. Med.,* **39** (1), 56.

—— and —— (1978). Psychologic influences on drug action. *Fed. Proc.,* **37** (3), 617.

——, ——, HAJEK, J., HAJKOVA, M., and KIRILCUK, V. (1970a). Studies on psychophysiologic individuality. *Activitas Nervosa Super.,* **12** (2), 174–5.

——, —— and KIRILCUK, V. (1970b). Individual differences in respiratory responses of dogs to psychologic stress and Anokhin's formulation of the functional system as a unit of biological adaptation. *Int. J. Psychobiol.,* **1**(1), 1–12.

—, —, and ENGLAND, S. J. M. (1963). The influence of meprobamate on conditioned and unconditioned visceral and motor defense responses. In *Psychopharmacological methods* (eds. Z. Votava, M. Horrath, and O. Vinar), pp. 244–55. Pergamon Press, London and New York.

COWAN, T. A. (1972). Paradoxes of science administration. *Science*, 177 (4053), 964–6.

CRANE, L. M. (1974). Schools 'dehumanizing' (Letter to the editor), *Amer. med. News*, 17(48), 5, 9 Dec., 1974.

DUBOS, RENE J. (1973). Humanizing the earth. *Science*, 179 (4075), 769–72.

DYOS, H. J. and WOLFF, M. (Eds.) (1974). *The Victorian city: images and realities*. Routledge and Kegan Paul, Boston (2 Vols.).

ELWES, R. H. M. (Translator) (1883). *The chief works of Spinoza* (2 Vols.), pp. 1955, 1966. London, New York. Vol. 1, 1955; Vol. 2, 1956.

ENGEL, G. L. (1977). The need for a new medical model: a challenge for biomedicine. *Science*, 196(4286), 129–36.

EPSTEIN, L. D. (1970). State authority and state universities. In *Rights and responsibilities: the university's dilemma* (ed. S. R. Graubard), *Daedalus*, 99 (3), 700–12.

FRANKENHAEUSER, M. (1977). Quality of life: criteria for behavioral adjustment. *Int. J. Psychol.*, 12 (2), 99–110.

— and LUNDBERG, U. (1977). The influence of cognitive set on performance and arousal under different noise levels. *Motivation and Emotion*, 1 (2), 139–49.

FRENCH, J. R. P., Jr. (1973). Person role fit. *Occup. mental Health*, 3 (1), 15–20.

—, RODGERS, W., and COBB, S. (1974). Adjustment as person-environment fit. In *Coping and adaptation* (eds. G. V. Coelho, D. A. Hamburg, and J. E. Adams). Basic Books, New York.

GALLANT, J. A. and PROTHERO, J. W. (1972). Weight-watching at the university: the consequences of growth. *Science*, 175 (4020), 381–8.

GARB, S. (1974). Letter. *Fed. Proc.*, 33 (4), 1030.

GERARD, R. W. (1975). Concluding remarks. In Meprobamate and other agents used in mental disturbances. *Ann. N.Y. Acad. Sci.*, 67 (Art. 10), 885–94.

GIVEN, W. B., Jr. (1949). *Bottom-up management. People working together*. Harper and Brothers, New York.

GRAUBARD, S. R. (Ed.) (1970). Preface to the issue Rights and responsibilities: the university's dilemma. *Daedalus*, 99 (3), v–xiv.

HAMBLING, J. (1959). Essential hypertension. In *The nature of stress disorder*, pp. 17–33. Thomas, Springfield, Ill.

HARMAN, S. (1976a). Statement of Sidney Harman, Ph.D., board chairman and chief executive officer of Harman International Industries, Lake Success, Long Island, N.Y. In *Changing patterns of work in America, 1976: hearings on examination of alternative working hours and arrangements*, pp. 279–304. (94th Congress, 2nd sess., 7 and 8 April 1976). U.S. Government Printing Office, Washington, D.C.

HARMAN, S. (1976b). Personal communication.

HEARST, E. (1960). Simultaneous generalization gradients of appetitive and aversive behavior. *Science*, 132 (3441), 1769–70.

Heart Research Newsletter (1965). Operation on small intestine may help lower cholesterol levels. *Heart Research Newsletter*, 10 (3), 3–4. American Heart Association, New York.

HOUSSAY, B. A. (1975). *Hormonal regulation of energy metabolism*. Thomas, Springfield, Illinois.

ILLICH, I. (1976). *Medical nemesis: the expropriation of health*. Pantheon, New York.

JENSEN, G. D. (1963). Preference for bar-pressing over "free loading" as a function of the number of rewarded presses. *J. exp. Psychol.*, 65, 451–4.

KERMODE, F. (1974). Grandeur and filth. *N.Y. Rev. Books*, 21 (9), 6–12.

KIMBALL, C. P. (1974). Becoming a physician is a 'dehumanizing' process. *Amer. med. News*, 23 Sept. 1974, p. 21.

KNOWLES, J. H. (Ed.) (1977). Doing better and feeling worse. Health in the United States. *Daedalus*, 106 (1).

LACEY, J. I. and LACEY, B. C. (1962). The law of initial value in the longitudinal study of autonomic constitution: reproducibility of autonomic responses and response patterns over a four-year interval. *Ann. N.Y. Acad. Sci.*, 98 (Art. 4), 1257–90; 1322–6.

LAZARUS, R. (1966). *Psychological stress and the coping process*. McGraw-Hill, Inc., New York.

— (1967). Cognitive and personality factors underlying threat and coping. In *Psychological stress* (eds. M. H. Appley and R. Trumbull), pp. 151–81. Appleton-Century-Croft, New York.

LEVI, L. (1971). The human factor—and the inhuman. In *Society, stress and disease* (ed. L. Levi), Vol. 1. Oxford University Press, London.

— (1973). Stress, distress and psychosocial stimuli. *Occup. Mental Health*, 3 (3), 2–10. Also in *Occupational stress* (ed. A. McLean), pp. 31–46. Thomas, Springfield, Ill.

LUNDBERG, U. and FRANKENHAEUSER, M. (1978). Psychophysiological reactions to noise as modified by personal control over noise intensity. *Biol. Psychol.*, 6, 51–9.

MANASSEIN, V. A. (1876). *Materialy dlya voprosa ob etiologicheskom i terapevticheskom znachenii psikhicheskikh vliyanii* [Material on the problem of the aetiologic and therapeutic importance of psychic influences]. St. Petersburg. (In Russian).

MARX, J. L. (1975). Coronary project: negative results. *Science*, 187 (4176), 526.

MASON, J. W. (1968). Organization of the multiple endocrine responses to avoidance in the monkey. *Psychosom. Med.*, 30 (5), Part 2, 774–90.

MASSERMAN, J. H. (1943). *Behavior and neurosis*. University of Chicago Press.

— (1971). The principle of uncertainty in neurotigenesis. In *Experimental psychopathology* (ed. H. D. Kimmel). Academic Press, New York.

McCLEARY, R. A. (1954). Measurement of experimental anxiety in the rat: an attempt. *J. genet. Psychol.*, 84, 95–108.

MEHL, J. W. (1975). Peer review reviewed. *Fed. Proc.* (Public Affairs), 34 (9), i–iv.

MOWRER, O. H. (1939). A stimulus-response analysis of anxiety and its role as a reinforcing agent. *Psychol. Rev.*, 46, 553–65.

— and VIEK, P. (1948). An experimental analogue of fear from a sense of helplessness. *J. abnorm. Soc. Psychol.*, 43, 193–200.

NATIONAL SCIENCE BOARD, NATIONAL SCIENCE FOUNDATION (1978). *Basic research in the Mission Agencies* (Stock No. 038-000-00365-8). U.S. Government Printing Office, Washington, D.C.

NEURINGER, A. (1969). Animals respond for food in the presence of free food. *Science*, 166, 399–401.

— (1970). Pigeons respond to produce periods in which rewards are independent of responding. *J. exp. Anal. Behav.*, 19, 39–54.

New York Times (1974). 5 of 6 U.S. auto workers dislike Swedish system. *N.Y. Times*, 24 Dec., 1974, pp. 25, 31.

New York Times (1975). Even in Sweden, U.S. workers find

drudgery. *N.Y. Times*, 5 Jan. 1975, Sec. E, p. 11.

New York Times (1977). Concern voiced on cuts in mental-health funds. *N.Y. Times*, 27 Mar. 1977.

OSLER, W. (1974). *Medicine in the nineteenth century*, p. 259. Acquanimitas, The Blakiston Co.

PATTISHALL, E. G., Jr. (1977). The role of social and behavioral sciences in medical education: implications for preventive and/or community medicine. In *The behavioral sciences and preventive medicine. Opportunities and dilemmas* (ed. R. L. Kane). Fogarty International Center Series on the Teaching of Preventive Medicine, Vol. 4. DHEW Publication No. (NIH) 76–878, pp. 169–77.

PAVLOV, I. P. (1903). Experimental psychology and psychopathology in animals. In (I. P. Pavlov) *Lectures on conditioned reflexes* (ed. and transl. W. H. Gantt), Vol. 1 (1928). International Publishers, New York, 1976, pp. 47–60.

—— (1916). Refleks tseli [The reflex of purpose]. In *Dvadtsatiletnii opyt ob"ektivnogo izucheniya vysshei nervnoi deyatel'nosti (povedeniya) zhivotnykh. Uslovnye refleksy* [Twenty Years of experience in the objective study of the higher nervous activity behavior of animals. Conditioned reflexes], pp. 197–201. Medgiz, Moscow. (1951). (In Russian).

—— (1928). *Lectures on conditioned reflexes* (ed. and trans. W. Horsley Gantt). International Publishers Co., Inc., New York. (Fifth printing, 1963).

—— (1940). *Polnoe sobranie trudov* [Complete Works], Vol. 1. AN SSSR, Moscow–Leningrad. (In Russian).

—— (1954). *O tipakh vysshei nervnoi deyatel'nosti i eksperimental'nykh nevrozakh* [Types of higher nervous activity and experimental neuroses] (ed. P. S. Kupalov), Medgiz, Moscow. (In Russian).

PRESS, F. (1978). Science and technology: the road ahead. *Science*, **200** (4343), 737–41.

PRESTON, T. A. (1978). Operating in the dark. *The Sciences*, **18** (8), 21–3.

ROARK, A. C. (1978). U.S. science policies seen thwarting univesities' basic-research effort. *Chronicle higher Educ.*, **7** (1), 9.

RODGERS, J. (1975). Rush to surgery. *N.Y. Times Mag.*, 21 Sept. 1975, pp. 34–42.

ROGERS, D. E. (1974). Illness must be understood not in scientific but in human terms. *Amer. med. News*, 23 Sept. 1974, p. 21.

ROSZAK, T. (1969). *The making of a counter culture. Reflections on the technocratic society and its youthful opposition.* Doubleday and Co. Garden City, N.Y.

SECHENOV, I. M. (1863). Refleksy golovnogo mozga [Reflexes of the brain]. *Med. vestn.* [Medical bulletin] **47**, 461–84 and **48**, 493–512. In English in Sechenov, I. (1956). *Selected physiological and psychological works.* Foreign Languages Publishing House, Moscow.

SELIGMAN, M. E/P. (1975). *Helplessness: on depression, development and death.* W. H. Freeman and Co., San Francisco.

SELYE, H. (1971). The evolution of the stress concept—stress and cardiovascular disease. In *Society, stress and disease* (ed. L. Levi), Vol. 1. Oxford University Press, London.

—— (1978). On the real benefits of eustress. Interview by Lawrence Cherry. *Psychology Today*, Mar 1978, pp. 60–70.

SHANIN, M. M. (1978). R & D expenditures in the United States. *Science*, **200** (4348), 1334–6.

SHOBEN, E. J., Jr. (1970). Cultural criticism and the American college (ed. S. R. Graubard). *Daedalus*, **99** (3), 676–99.

SIMONOV, P. V. (1965). O roli emotsii v prisposobitel'noi povedenii zhivykh sistem [The role of emotions in adaptiv behavior of living systems]. *Vop. psikhol.* [Problems c Psychology], **114**, 75–84. (In Russian).

SINGH, D. (1970). Preference for bar pressing to obtain rewar over free-loading in rats and children. *J. comp. Physio Psychol.*, **73**, 320–7.

SIVARD, R. L. (1977). *World military and social expenditure* WMSE Publications, Leesburg, Va.

SKINNER, B. F. (1971). *Beyond freedom and dignity.* Alfred A Knopf, New York.

SORRI, P., ACHTÉ, K., and VARILO, E. (1976). Work and stres in the academic world. *Psychiat. Fenn.*, pp. 195–200.

SPINOZA, B. (Barukh) (1905). *The principles of Descarte. philosophy* (transl. H. H. Briton), Chicago.

SUDAKOV, K. V. (1971). *Biologicheskie motivatsii* [Biologic. Motivations]. Meditsina, Moscow (In Russian).

SULLIVAN, R. (1978). Interns and residents at hospitals hope t get collective bargaining. *N.Y. Times*, 19 Mar., 1978, p. 42.

SZENT-GYÖRGYI, A. (1962). On scientific creativity *Perspectives Biol. Med.*, **5** (2), 173, 178.

—— (1974). Research grants. In *Perspectives Biol. Med.*, **1** (1), 41–3.

THOMAS, C. B. (1976). What becomes of medical students; th dark side. *Johns Hopk. med. J.*, **138**, 185–95.

—— (1977). *Habits of nervous tension: clues to the huma condition.* The Precursors Study, The Johns Hopkir University School of Medicine, Baltimore, Md.

VIRCHOW, R. (1858). *Die Cellularpathologie.*

—— (1958). *Disease, life and man, selected essays* (trans. H Rather). Stanford University Press.

VON BERTALANFFY, L. (1969). *General system theory Foundations, development, applications.* Braziller, Nev York.

WANN, T. W. (Ed.) (1964, 1965). Paraphrase of discussion. I *Behaviorism and phenomenology. Contrasting bases fc modern psychology* (Rice University Semicentennial Series pp. 139–40. Chicago & London, The University of Chicag Press, Chicago and London.

WEISS, J. M. (1971a). Effects of coping behavior in differen warning signal conditions on stress pathology in rats. *. comp. Physiol. Psychol.*, **77**, 1.

—— (1971b). Effects of punishing the coping respons (conflict) on stress pathology in rats. *J. comp. Physio Psychol.*, **77**, 14.

—— (1971c). Effects of coping behavior with and without feedback signal on stress pathology in rats. *J. comp. Physio Psychol.*, **77**, 22.

WEISS, P. A. (1970). The living system: determinism stratified In *Beyond reductionism. New perspectives in the life science* (ed. A. Koestler and J. R. Smythies), pp. 3–55. (Th Alpback Symposium 1968). The Macmillan Co., New York (First published in Great Britain in 1969 by Hutchinson an Co.).

WIENER, N. (1948). *Cybernetics.* John Wiley and Sons, Nev York.

WOLF, A. (translator) (1928). *Correspondence of Spinoza* London.

WOLF, S., CARDON, P. V., Jr., SHEPARD, E. M., and WOLFF, H G. (1955). *Life stress and essential hypertension.* Th Williams and Wilkins Co., Baltimore, Md.

——, PFEIFFER, J. B., RIPLEY, H. S., WINTER, O. S., anc WOLFF, H. G. (1948). Hypertension as a reaction pattern t stress: summary of experimental data on variations in bloo pressure and renal flow. *Ann. int. Med.*, **29**, 1056–76.

30. IMPACT OF SOCIAL AND INDUSTRIAL CHANGES ON PSYCHOPATHOLOGY: A VIEW OF STRESS FROM THE STANDPOINT OF MACRO SOCIETAL TRENDS

M. HARVEY BRENNER

INTRODUCTION

A logical, if not ideal, approach to the examination of the possible impact of life stresses on illness is through the use of historical data on major aspects of societal change. Indeed, virtually all of the major types of life stress can be seen to have social trends of their own—e.g., rates of financial loss, unemployment, illness, mortality, birth, migration, marriage, divorce, separation, criminal aggression, etc. The confluence of such trends over time, with a greater or lesser intensity, should therefore produce greater stress. Thus, if stress phenomena increase the risk of morbidity or mortality either directly as agents of disease (Selye 1956; Levi 1972) or by increasing susceptibility (or reducing immunity) (Cassel 1970; Kaplan *et al.* 1977; Moss 1973), then we should be able to observe such intercorrelations historically, and quantitatively. There is a technology which is now about twenty years old that can handle the principal methodological problems encountered in multivariate time series analysis (Johnston 1963; Christ 1966; Griliches 1974).

The clinical researcher who is unfamiliar with these techniques may well wonder how such 'highly individualized' factors as life changes or specific stress reactions can be analysed using macro-level historical data. In fact, however, from the purely methodological standpoint macro-level historical analysis is at least an equally efficient method, as compared with micro-analysis, and frequently is the only method suitable for the analysis of social stresses and their possible consequences for illness.

Problems in using individual analysis in stress research

Perhaps the principal methodological problem in stress research that is encountered at the individual level of analysis is the lack of a means to discriminate the alleged causal variable from its effect. The implication is that it becomes exceedingly difficult to ascertain:

(a) The direction of the relation;
(b) Whether the relation is spurious (due to unobserved relations with a third, and truly causal, variable);
(c) Whether the variables are not symptomatic of the same pathological process.

The most dramatic example of these methodological problems at the individual level of analysis is found in studies of stress which use low socio-economic status as a stress indicator. Theoretically, the lower an individual's socio-economic position:

1. The more exposed he is to deleterious life changes—especially involving economic instability and losses;
2. The less protected he is because of comparatively low financial or human support resources (Bendix and Lipset 1966).

The theory has been supported by empirical evidence that there is a statistically reliable inverse relationship between socio-economic status and the prevalence of mental disorder. This finding has been the single most consistent empirical regularity in the field of psychiatric epidemiology for more than forty years (Dohrenwend and Dohrenwend 1969).

The difficulty has been that alternative hypotheses to the stress formulation could be raised so as to suggest that the relationship actually ran in the opposite direction. Thus, a previous situation of mental disorder might result in diminished competence in the economic sphere. One famous formulation of this thesis maintained that the reason the mentally ill tended to be of lower socio-economic status is that they 'drifted downward' in status as a result of earlier mental disorder (Reid 1961; Dohrenwend 1966). This interpretation has itself been impossible to sustain at the individual level of analysis even where there were findings that the mentally ill of lower socio-economic status had in fact fallen in social status (Dunham and Srinivasan 1966). This finding supports the stress hypothesis at least equally well because from the stress perspective it is that very loss of status that may have precipitated the currently observed mental disorder.

The only solution to this type of problem is to examine situations, as independent variables, which are not under the influence of the subjects. In stress research at the individual level, very few of such circumstances exist. Typically, then, when it is observed that illness tends to follow a period of several life changes or stresses, it is difficult to determine whether the factor(s) which precipitated the illness condition—e.g., a psychopathologic mental state—also precipitated the life changes (e.g., financial loss).

These problems of the direction or existence of causal relations at the individual level of analysis are compounded further by a lack of control for factors which ordinarily influence morbidity or morality due to specific causes. Since the person is put at risk to coronary disease, for example, by smoking, overweight, high levels of serum cholesterol, among other factors (Lilienfeld and Gifford 1966), proper epidemiological procedure requires that these be controlled if we wish to observe the impact of additional factors, including life changes, on coronary morbidity or mortality.

Such controls are very rarely applied in stress research because samples are usually too small to cope with the gathering of data on life changes as well as on risk factors that would apply to the manifold outcomes of stress ranging from the acute infectious disorders and accidents to the chronic diseases, mental disorders, and social pathologies.

There are surely no perfect research designs which are inherently free of all problems of validity and reliability. Yet, for these problems, multivariate time series methods using aggregated (or macroscopic) data do provide a way out of the causal trap and also allow us to control for the coincidence of multiple trends.

MACROSCOPIC HISTORICAL APPROACHES IN STRESS RESEARCH

Effects of adverse economic changes on health

Mental health. It is precisely the time series approach at the macro-level that permitted a solution to the chicken–egg question posed by the socio-economic status–mental illness relationship. It was necessary to find a situation where changes in the economic situation of persons affected by income and employment losses could not, in turn, be influenced by those persons. Such a situation exists at the macro-level, and the employment rate was selected as the independent variable. The research question was, then, to what extent are changes in the employment rate associated with changes in first admissions to mental hospitals. Theoretically, if the stress formulations used in socio-economic status–mental illness research were correct, then a reduction in status for a population average should be associated with increased first admissions. it was found that for at least 127 years in New York State first admissions to mental hospitals were inversely related to the rate of employment (Brenner 1973a).

It was not possible to interpret this relationship as indicating the influence of mental disorder (or hospitalization) on the employment rate because the hospitalization, as compared with the employment rate for the state, was infinitesimally small. This is obviously because severe pathological phenomena are comparatively rare in a population compared to the number earning incomes subject to inflation or to the unemployed, for that matter. Moreover, a variety of tests indicated that it was precisely those who lost the most income, whose social roles were the most seriously affected (e.g., married males), and who were living in counties which were the worst hit by unemployment changes, who were also the most readily hospitalized during economic downturns.

These findings, published in *Mental illness and the economy* (Brenner 1973a) strongly supported the thesis of a causal inverse relationship, based on economic stress, between changes in socio-economic status and the level of mental disorder. Nevertheless, these findings, based on first admissions to mental hospitals, left unclear to what extent—if at all—intolerance of mental disorder, rather than psychiatric symptoms alone, were precipitated by economic stresses. It thus became useful to work with indicators of pathology which would ideally not be contaminated by factors associated with administrative dispositions or changes in family or community behaviour (Figs. 30.1, 30.2, and 30.3).

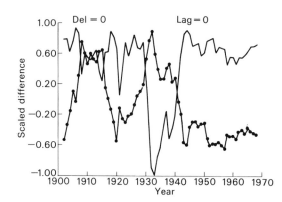

FIG. 30.1. Graphic analysis of the relation between the United States suicide mortality rate (●—●—●) and the United States employment rate (inverted unemployment rate) (———), 1902–70. (Scaled difference: both series are scaled for viewing such that the greatest amplitude from the arithmetic mean of each series, which is set equal to zero, has been normalized to + 1·00 if positive, or – 1·00 if negative. Del = 0: long-term trends subtracted from the mortality series.)

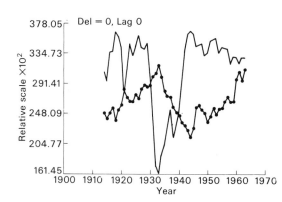

FIG. 30.2. Graphic analysis of the relation between the United States homicide mortality rate (●—●—●) of white males aged 25–9 and the employment rate (inverted unemployment rate) (———), 1912–65. (Scaled difference: both series are scaled for viewing such that the greatest amplitude from the arithmetic mean of each series, which is set equal to zero, has been normalized to + 1·00 if positive, or – 1·00 if negative. Del = long-term trends subtracted from the mortality series.)

250

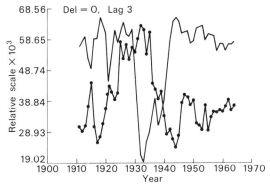

FIG. 30.3 Graphic analysis of the relation between the United States circulatory system disease mortality rate (●—●—●) of non-white males aged 35–9 at a lag of three years and the employment rate (inverted unemployment rate (inverted unemployment rate) (———), 1912–65. (Scaled difference: both series are scaled for viewing such that the greatest amplitude from the arithmetic mean of each series, which is set equal to zero, has been normalized to + 1·00 if positive, or –1·00 if negative. Del = 0: long-term trends subtracted from the mortality series.)

Cardio-vascular mortality. A logical choice appeared to be found in the area of cardio-vascular mortality. There had been substantial theoretical speculation and a body of empirical evidence which linked cardio-vascular illness to stressful events. (Ostfeld *et al.* 1964; Syme *et al.* 1964, 1965; Wardwell *et al.* 1964; Smith 1967; Cassel 1967; Marks 1967; Croog *et al.* 1968; Hinkle *et al.* 1968). The predicted relationship was found between adverse changes in the economy, as indicated by the unemployment rate, and various subdiagnoses of cardio-vascular disease mortality including coronary artery disease. The peak of the average mortality reaction occurred at approximately two years after the peak in the unemployment rate (Brenner 1971a). These findings on approximate lag time correspond well with those obtained by Holmes and Rahe (Rahe *et al.* 1964; Theorell and Rahe 1974; Rahe and Romo 1974; Holmes and Masuda 1974) in their examination of the cumulative effect of life event changes on the onset of subsequent pathology associated with various chronic diseases.

Cirrhosis of the liver. A second study, using similar hypotheses and methodology, found that trends in mortality rates associated with cirrhosis of the liver also tended to peak approximately two years after a peak in unemployment (Brenner 1975). In that case, the multiple regression analysis also revealed that the long-term trend in cirrhosis mortality was positively associated with the growth in real *per capita* disposable income. The same study also indicated that short-term increases in *per capita* consumption of alcohol tended to increase during economic downturns, as did arrests and trials for the crime of intoxication during automobile driving and first admissions to mental hospitals in the United States with a diagnosis related to alcohol abuse.

Infant mortality rates. In a subsequent study, infant mortality rates in the United States were found to be related to economic recessions, as indicated by the unemployment rate, with a lag of from one to two years of the peak average mortality behind the peak of unemployment (Brenner 1973b). The original hypothesis of this study specified that as a result of material deprivation or lack of medical care, in addition to psychological stress, economic decline would be associated with elevated infant mortality rates. It was suggested that the stresses of economic loss might result in maternal cardiovascular illness or in smoking or abuse of alcohol on the part of pregnant women—which are established risk factors in infant mortality.

Criminal aggression. A final group of studies, which followed from the original research on mental disorder as related to economic change, were concerned with the problem of criminal aggression. Beginning with New York State (Brenner 1971b) and finally involving the United States, Canada, England and Wales, and Scotland (Brenner 1976 a, b), economic changes were studied in relation to crimes known to the police, trials, convictions, and imprisonment for each of several crimes against persons (murder, manslaughter, forced rape, robbery) and property (embezzlement, fraud, arson, burglary, larceny). Adverse changes in employment and income were associated with increases in rates of all these crimes, controlling for the effects of urbanization, demographic changes, and changes in criminal justice system activity.

Multiple economic and socio-demographic indicators of economic change

It was subsequently recognized that a single major indicator of intermediate and short-term fluctuations in the entire economy was inadequate—and certainly inadequate to express the full extent of economic stress even where it originated at the national level. Not only were such factors as inflation thought to have possible stressful consequences, but income (real—i.e., in constant dollars), welfare, and education were thought to be important ameliorators of economic loss. In addition, questions were raised as to the more nearly precise timing of the lag in pathological reactions to changes in economic indicators. For example, increased pathology related to recession could appear to the naked eye—especially without multivariate controls—to occur as a result of the subsequent economic upturn if the lag were in the range of 2–4 years (Thomas 1925; Eyer 1977).

The need for more sophisticated analysis to take into account multiple economic and socio-demographic indicators became quite pragmatic when the Joint Economic Committee of the United States Congress requested that estimates be made of the amount of increased pathology that would follow from increased unemployment or the maintenance of it at a high level. In order to deal with this problem it was necessary to control for the effects of those economic and socio-demographic factors which ordinarily influence the pathological phenomena in question. Also, it was crucial to know over how long a span of time the deleterious effect of unemployment might precipitate an increased incidence of pathology. It was not sufficient, therefore, to estimate the average or peak lag interval, but rather the entire span over which the elevated rates of pathology would occur.

The final predictive equation
The predictive equation that was finally set up included the unemployment rate, the inflation rate, real *per capita* personal income, and demographic variables relating to each of the specific types of pathology. The dependent variables or indices of pathology involved the general areas of physical health, mental health, and criminal aggression. The conception, therefore, was that no single type of indicator, such as depression, or heart disease, would serve as a proper measure of the pathological impact of economic life stress. Rather, specific indicators relating to mental disorder and physical morbidity and mortality—involving both acute and chronic problems—would have to be involved. Also, illegal activities involving both violence and property should be included. The following indices of stress outcome were therefore used, based on the United States as a whole: first admissions to mental hospitals by sex and age; total mortality by sex, race, and age; suicide by sex and age; homicide by sex and age; cardio-vascular-renal disease mortality by sex and age; cirrhosis of the liver mortality by sex and age; and imprisonment by age.

A sample of the resulting predictive multiple regression equations, and measures of the goodness of fit of these equations to each major type of pathology, are shown in Table 30.1. It is clear that in Table 30.1 in all cases the unemployment rate is significantly positively associated with increases in each pathology over a five-year period following the first year of impact of an increased unemployment rate. In other words, we allow the cumulative effect of increased pathology within a six-year period to be taken into account. The assumption was that the impact of major economic stresses may occur over each of several years, with the more nearly acute reactions (e.g., mental hospitalization, imprisonment, suicide, homicide) predominating during the first three years and the more nearly chronic reactions (e.g., cardio-vascular-renal disease, cirrhosis, and total mortality) predominating during the second three years.

The same procedure of estimating the five-year distributed lag of pathology to changes in the economic indicator was used in the case of *per capita* income and inflation. Table 30.1 shows that while significant relationships were found for *per capita* income and inflation, the overall results were less stable, predictable, and interpretable than was the case with the unemployment rate.

From these equations it was possible to estimate the historical impact, from 1940 to 1974, of a 1 per cent increase in the unemployment rate on the various pathological indices (Table 30.2).

RAPID ECONOMIC GROWTH VERSUS UNEMPLOYMENT AS SOURCES OF ECONOMIC LIFE STRESS

In the multivariate equations described above, each of the sources of economic life stress—decreased income inflation, and unemployment—are understood to be unidirectional in their impact on pathology. Their impact, in other words, is conceived as entirely deleterious. This view is traditional with respect to the literature on low socio-economic status as a risk factor in mental disorder, morbidity and mortality, and criminal aggression. Indeed, the idea that only deleterious changes provoke pathological reaction has been traditional 'common sense' as well as the professional behavioural science view.

The formulation of Selye (1956) went a considerable distance to change these traditional perspectives and suggested that the phenomenon of change itself—beyond the capacities of the organism to adapt—is the critical precipitant of pathology. This formulation has been the guiding concept to a large number of researchers into the stress-producing potential of different types of life changes. For example, in summarizing the theoretical orientation of many researchers in this field, Levi (1972) indicates that the highest stress levels are usually found at the extremes of the stimulation continuum and thus deprivation or excess of almost any influence is provocative of stress.

However, the research evidence from studies on mental disorder (Mueller *et al.* 1977), especially depression (Paykel 1974), and criminal behaviour (Gersten *et al.* 1974), show clearly that life changes viewed as undesirable showed considerably greater potency to provoke pathological responses. The weight of the evidence, when one includes traditional research pioneered by Holmes and Rahe (1967) (see also Holmes and Masuda 1974 and Rabkin and Struening 1976) and dealing in large measure with chronic physical illnesses (Gunderson and Rahe 1974), is that while all significant life changes are potential stressors, undesirable changes are predictive of higher stress levels.

If this perspective is correct, then we should observe that economic recession should show more severe and longer lasting pathological effects than periods of rapid economic growth, but that the periods of growth themselves, while desirable overall, nevertheless are stressful. A related issue, which the stress literature does not deal with systematically, is that of the interrelation among life changes. The guiding hypothesis of the formulation in the present study is that deleterious life changes in particular are capable of producing stresses which in turn lead to other life changes and stresses. This interaction among stresses we shall label the *principle of acceleration* of stress. An example would be the loss of a job which may lead to financial disruption, marital and parent–child strains and possibly the break-up of family, possible loss of friendships which were occupation-related, and the securing of a new job and at a lower status, with the

TABLE 30.1

Multiple regression equations of national economic indices on selected mortality rates, United States

Dependent variable	Years	Intercept	Time trend	Log time trends	Per capita income	Unemployment rate	Inflation rate	R^2	F	D.W.
General mortality rate[1] (Lag 0–5)[3]										
(1) Mortality rate total whites	1940–74	96·2			-0·53E-2 (1·92)*	0·62 (5·05)*	0·87 (2·96)*	0·89	21·9*	1·93
(2) Mortality rate total non-whites	1940–74	136·4			-0·32E-1 (6·55)*	1·68 (6·95)*	2·83 (5·16)*	0·96	74·1*	1·67
(3) Mortality rate LT 1 whites	1940–74	497·7			-0·24 (7·06)*	12·65 (8·01)*	3·59 (5·44)*	0·97	98·6*	2·11
(4) Mortality rate LT 1 non-whites	1940–74	936·2			-0·43 (10·48)*	17·74 (10·69)*	30·77 (6·49)*	0·99	199·6*	2·40
(5) Mortality rate 75–84 whites	1940–74	1141·0			-0·22 (7·59)*	10·39 (7·02)*	17·56 (5·20)*	0·97	103·8*	2·47
(6) Mortality rate 75–84 non-whites	1940–74	767·1			-0·93E-1 (2·07)*	15·45 (6·96)*	14·80 (2·91)*	0·84	14·8*	2·36
(7) Cardio-vascular disease mortality rate[2] (lag 1–4)[4]	1945–73	537·7			-0·33E-1 (2·49)*	5·46 (2·62)*	-0·04 (0·37)	0·85	11·8*	2·89
(8) Cardio-vascular disease mortality rate[2] (lag 1–4)[4]	1940–73	-2836·8	-17·8 (4·70)*	1077·0 (4·76)*		2·35 (1·83)*	1·04 (0·78)	0·74	6·50*	2·36
(9) Cardio-vascular disease mortality rate[2] (lag 1–4)[4]	1945–73	-843·8	-7·5 (1·43)+	436·3 (1·35)+		6·15 (3·17)*	-1·10 (0·74)	0·79	6·70*	2·02
(10) Cirrhosis mortality rate[2] (lag 0–5)[3]	1940–73	-0·2			0·65E-2 (8·99)*	0·14 (4·21)*	0·16E-3 (0·01)	0·98	114·4*	1·65
(11) Cirrhosis mortality rate[2] (lag 0–5)[3]	1945–73	-0·2			0·63E-2 (8·81)*	0·12 (3·62)*	0·29E-1 (0·37)	0·98	114·4*	1·82

Table 30.1 (continued)

253

Table 30.1 (continued)

Dependent variable	Years	Intercept	Time trend	Log time trends	Dummy constant or trend	Other trends	Per capita income	Unemployment rate	Inflation rate	R^2	F	D.W.
(12) Suicide rate[1] (lag 0–5)[3]	1940–73	6.34					0.90E-3 (1.50)†	0.42 (14.23)*	0.27 (4.23)*	0.91	26.2*	1.80
(13) Suicide rate[1] (lag 0–5)[3]	1945–73	6.38					0.11E-2 (2.17)*	0.40 (17.30)*	0.25 (4.70)*	0.95	40.9*	2.35
(14) Suicide rate[1] (lag 0–5)[3]	1940–73	-0.62		2.08 (3.63)*				0.43 (12.51)*	0.31 (6.68)*	0.87	25.3*	2.03
(15) Homicide rate[1] (lag 0–5)[3]	1940–73	-7.60			DT 1967–74[5] 0.14E-1 (3.90)*	TJ[7] 0.30 (3.16)*	0.16E-2 (1.56)†	0.10 (2.38)*	0.11 (0.92)	0.99	115.6*	2.29
(16) Homicide rate[1] TJ[7] (lag 0–5)[3]	1940–73	1.02	0.65E-1 (5.30)*		DT 1967–74[5] 0.18 (3.79)*			0.54 (5.00)*	0.84 (5.30)*	0.94	47.0*	1.88
(17) Imprisonment rate[1] (minus 1942–45) (lag 0–2)[4]	1935–65	-577.90	-3.18 (3.14)*	195.5 (3.48)*		TJ[7]		1.59 (5.92)*	0.64 (3.35)*	0.76	10.4*	1.87
(18) Imprisonment rate[1] (minus 1942–45) (lag 0–2)[4]	1935–73	-594.50	-2.55 (2.38)*	180.9 (2.93)*	DC 1967–71[6] -8.36 (8.33)*	1.31 (4.27)*		1.52 (5.60)*	0.57 (3.07)*	0.90	23.9*	1.90
(19) Mental hospital admission rate LT 65[1] (minus 1942–45) (lag 0–5)[3]	1940–71	-77.70					0.55E-1 (9.78)*	3.39 (9.58)*	1.78 (2.58)*	0.96	60.0*	1.52
(20) Mental hospital admission rate LT 65[1] (lag 0–5)[3]	1940–71	-70.00					0.49E-1 (8.69)	3.11 (8.92)*	2.19 (3.21)*	0.97	63.4*	1.85

[1] Per 10 000 population.
[2] Per 100 000 population.
[3] Second degree polynomial distributed lag equation.
[4] Ordinary least squares equation.
[5] 'Dummy' trend.
[6] 'Dummy' constant.
[7] TJ: percent of total male population who are ages 15–29.
†0.10 Level of significance. $t = 1.31$; $F = 1.89$
*0.05 Level of significance. $t = 1.71$; $F = 2.28$
*0.01 Level of significance. $t = 2.49$; $F = 3.21$
*0.001 Level of significance. $t = 3.45$; $F = 4.71$
't' values are in parenthesis

TABLE 30.2

Estimates of the total effects of 1 per cent changes in unemployment rates sustained over a six-year period on the incidence of social trauma (based on the populations of 1970 and 1965)

Measures of social trauma	Incidence of pathology related to 1 per cent increase in unemployment based on 1970 population	Incidence of pathology related to 1 per cent increase in unemployment based on 1965 population	Total incidence of pathology, 1965	Incidence of pathology in 1965 related to 1 per cent increase in unemployment, 1960–65 as a proportion of total 1965 pathology
(1)	(2)	(3)	(4)	(5)=(3)÷(4)
Total mortality	36 887	35 042	1 828 000	0·019
whites				
males	12 360	11 866	911 000	0·013
females	16 534	15 709	695 000	0·023
Non-whites				
males	3829	3599	125 000	0·028
females	4161	3911	98 000	0·040
Cardio-vascular mortality	20 240	19 228	1 000 787	0·019
Cirrhosis of liver mortality	495	470	24 715	0·019
Suicide	920	874	21 507	0·041
Homicide	648	616	10 712	0·057
State mental hospital first admissions*	4227	4045	117 483	0·034
males	3058	2935	68 917	0·043
females	1169	1110	48 566	0·23
State prison admissions	3340	2952	74 724	0·040

Estimates are derived from equation types in Table 30.1 as follows: Total mortality classified by sex and race—eqs (1)–(6); Cardio-vascular mortality—eq (9); cirrhosis of liver mortality—eq (10); suicide—eq (14); homicide—eq (16); mental hospital admissions—eq (19); state prison admissions—eq (17).
*Only includes individuals under 65 years of age.

requirement of moving to a home in a new area in order to manage the job. In this formulation, the more undesirable the life change, the greater the probability of additional life changes (or stressors).

Short-term stress effects as a result of rapid economic growth

This principle of stress acceleration which can be observed in the life of a single person should not be confused with that of the 'contagion', or *multiplier*, effect of one person's stresses upon another's. Examples of the latter principle can be seen in the stress of each member of an entire family in the financial and status loss of a head of household. We therefore come to the proposition in this case that while rapid economic growth carries with it short-term stressful effects, based on what may appear to be desirable life changes, the impact of economic recession—based almost entirely on undesirable effects—carries a considerably more stressful impact over a much extended span of time.

A more detailed and incisive examination of the relation between economic change and pathology allows us to test this proposition. We can isolate the impact of long-term economic development from that of rapid economic growth periods because economic growth usually occurs in spurts of 1–3 years and is followed by periods of pause or recession, during which growth usually slows or actually declines a little (Mitchell 1951; Moore 1961). We isolate the long-term, smooth, economic development trend from the rapid growth periods by fitting an exponential trend to the real *per capita* income data. The exponential fit then represents the long-term trend of economic development and the residuals represent the abrupt periods of rapid economic growth and pause. We can also isolate the very short-term 'random' fluctuations in real *per capita* income by calculating the annual changes in that series.

Since there is only a moderate and unstable correlation over time between unemployment rates and *per capita* income in any of the forms:

(a) Long-term exponential trend:
(b) Residuals from the exponential trend;
(c) Annual changes,

we can add each of these components in *per capita* income trends to a prediction equation in which unemployment is also an independent variable. Such an equation is ideally suited to discriminate the differential impact on pathologies of rapid economic growth as compared with unemployment, very short-term income losses (annual changes in *per capita* income), and the long-term trend of economic development.

Further, since the impact of inflation on the pathological indices was observed to be highly unstable, it is useful to determine whether our predictive equation actually requires a separate variable for inflation—especially considering that we have already controlled for inflation by using real *per capita* income (i.e., in constant dollars). Finally, in view of recent work showing the importance of educational level to health (Silver 1972), and the probable contribution of welfare and social security and related health care benefits, it is prudent to control for trends which would measure them.

The principal hypothesis is that rapid economic growth as well as unemployment will be positively related to pathology. Since it is argued that economic growth will have only a short-term pathological effect, we do not require a distributed lag measure for this variable. On the other hand, we continue to suggest that the unemployment rate will show a distributed lag effect of from zero to five years on pathology. All the other independent variables in the predictive equation—the exponential trend of economic growth, welfare (i.e., the per cent of government spending which is allocated to welfare and social security (including health) payments)—except for annual changes in *per capita* income, are considered without lagged effects. Since, however, the annual changes in *per capita* income series has virtually no trend (i.e., zero auto-correlation), one year of lag has been added to the measurement procedure.

Pathological effects of rapid economic growth
The findings (Table 30.3) support the principal hypothesis that rapid economic growth as well as unem-

ployment and short-term income loss are significantly related to the pathological indices. In this test only mortality data in general and for specific causes generally associated with psychosocial stress are used, including suicide, homicide, cardio-vascular disease, and cirrhosis of the liver. It can also be seen (Table 30.3) that the statistical significance of the lag of mortality rates by cause to changes in the unemployment rate varies by cause of death. Thus, the theoretically slower reacting chronic diseases, indicated by cardio-vascular mortality, cirrhosis mortality, and total mortality, often require that the lag estimate of average impact begin with the second year and end in the fifth. The theoretically 'quick' reacting causes of death, such as suicide and homicide, require that the lag structure include the early years 0,1 and indeed the predominant impact is seen during those years. The implication of these findings is that, as hypothesized, while both rapid economic growth and unemployment are positively related to pathology, the impact of unemployment lasts for several additional years, particularly for the chronic illnesses. These findings further explain why it has appeared to some observers using only graphic techniques or simple correlation (i.e., not using multivariate procedures) (Thomas 1925; Eyer 1977) that the heaviest incidence of increased mortality occurs during upswings in the 'economic cycle'.

These findings, therefore, support the position of the majority of researchers in the field that undesirable events are likely to produce far greater stress reactions than are desirable ones. Yet, the thesis is also supported that apparently 'desirable' events (or groups of events) such as are involved in rapid economic growth are also provocative of pathology. We must infer, then, that the totality of changes, rather than only the undesirable ones, are the more appropriately used in a complete index of economic life stress.

'Undesirable' features of 'desirable' life changes
It is also possible, however, that researchers working with 'life change' data have made far too fine a distinction between 'desirable' and 'undesirable' events. In fact, it is perfectly possible that all major life changes, whether inherently agreeable or disagreeable, may possess undesirable features. In the examples of agreeable cases, of marriage, birth of a child, and job promotion, each of these life transitions may involve very substantially increased responsibilities for which a certain proportion of individuals may be unprepared. The unprepared persons then stand a substantial risk of role-failure. We may say, in a rather straightforward manner, that it is entirely likely that when marriage, childbirth, and job promotion are associated with stress, it is because of anxiety over—if not the actuality of—failure. In general, then, probably all 'desirable' life changes are potentially stressful to the extent that they carry the risk of failure—in which case, of course, they are in fact undesirable.

In terms of the present study, rapid economic growth

Table 30.3

Multiple regression equations of national economic indices on selected pathological indices, United States

Dependent variable	Period (unempl. lags)	Constant							R²	F	D-W
Total Mortality Rates	1940–73 (unempl. lags 2–5)	137·06** (5·92)	−0·03 (−0·22)	−0·04** (−2·95)	−0·02+ (−1·65)	0·01* (2·29)	−0·6E-2 (−0·73)	0·60** (4·72)	0·94	38·17**	2·38
	1940–73 (unempl. lags 0–5)	113·13** (3·85)	0·16 (0·81)	−0·04** (−3·29)	−0·01 (−0·51)	0·5E-2 (0·84)	−0·76 (0·89)	0·54** (3·21)	0·94	40·34**	2·55
Suicide Mortality Rates	1940–73 (unempl. lags 2–5)	−24·85+ (−1·59)	−0·01* (−2·43)	34·49** (3·08)	0·02* (1·98)	−0·2E-2 (−1·13)	−0·6E-2* (−2·26)	0·20** (5·13)	0·87	15·69**	1·96
	1940–73 (unempl. lags 0–5)	−6·27 (−0·47)	−0·9E-3** (−2·70)	23·32* (2·52)	0·6E-2 (0·88)	0·5E-4 (0·03)	−0·3E-2 (1·27)	0·28** (7·56)	0·91	27·55**	2·06
Homicide Mortality Rates	1940–73 (unempl. lags 2–5)	0·38 (0·04)	0·7E-3 (0·26)	38·08** (5·11)	−0·5E-2 (−0·86)	0·4E-2** (3·03)	−0·8E-2** (−4·33)	0·06* (2·27)	0·98	100·95**	1·36
	1940–73 (unempl. lags 0–5)	−4·97 (−0·43)	−0·4E-3 (−0·13)	42·45** (5·25)	−0·2E-2 (−0·34)	0·3E-2 (2·25)	−0·6E-2** (−3·26)	0·07* (2·23)	0·97	97·69**	1·59
Cardio-vascular Mortality Rates	1950–73 (unempl. lags 2–5)	388·6** (11·92)	24·10** (5·91)		−0·80** (−5·56)	0·28** (2·74)	−0·21+ (−1·94)	18·17** (2·62)	0·87	13·63**	2·90
	1950–73 (unempl. lags 0–5)	367·17** (11·56)	21·62** (5·25)		−0·68** (−5·14)	0·16* (2·30)	−0·17+ (−1·40)	8·79** (2·35)	0·86	10·08**	2·57
Cirrhosis Mortality Rates	1940–73 (unempl. lags 2–5)	1·82 (0·25)	−0·03+ (−1·49)	−0·39E-2 (−0·29)	0·48E-2** (7·93)	0·01* (2·15)	−0·01** (−5·16)	0·19** (4·82)	0·98	119·78**	1·43
	1940–73 (unempl. lags 0–5)	0·25 (0·26)	0·66E-1+ (1·49)	−0·1E-2 (−0·29)	0·61E-2** (7·93)	0·5E-2* (2·15)	−0·01** (−4·44)	0·09 (1·30)	0·98	117·09**	1·57

might on the surface be thought of as inherently desirable. It involves new jobs, promotions, increased real income, and is associated with higher marriage and birth rates (Brenner 1971b; Thomas 1925; Eyer 1977). However, since nearly all of these changes involve potential anxieties over fulfilment of new responsibilities, for a certain proportion of persons who are anxious or who actually fail, they may be extremely undesirable.

How then can we practically distinguish between relatively 'desirable' and 'undesirable' events? First, by the *probability* of failure (or maladaptation), and second, by the extent to which *other life changes may follow*. In such a formulation death or serious illness of a husband would be considered extremely grave because of loss of job, income, and family status as well as the need of the wife to manage the family affairs, possibly take a job (or a new job), perhaps move to another residence, and so on. Major undesirable life changes, then, are inherently correlated with other life changes in an almost epidemic fashion.

This feature of the interrelation of life changes, which we have previously in this article called the 'acceleration principle' of stress, is especially important in understanding the lag of several years over which mortality increases with respect to a major undesirable life change such as unemployment. Not only must the unemployed person encounter the short-term disruption to finances, family, social network, and work life, but he encounters an entirely new set of stressful life changes when re-employed. First, it is probable that the re-employed individual will be at a lower position than was previously held; thus, despite a new job this situation really indicates downward mobility, with loss of work status, income, and social position. Second, the implications of the downward mobility for family and social relations need to be considered, as well as the possible move of residence associated with the job change.

SUMMARY

We have endeavoured to show that major economic life changes, as basic stressors, are associated with severe pathology in the areas of mental and physical health and criminal aggression. The hypotheses underlying the studies involved are that the number and magnitude of life changes which disrupt patterns of social organization are generative of stress. The observation was made that the pathological impact of life changes can often be more easily observed on the macro, or societal, level of analysis than on the individual level. Several factors contribute to the special utility of stress research when conducted at the macro level. Most critical is that a *continuous scale over time* can be constructed of the occurrence of any particular life change as it affects a population in terms of rates (e.g., unemployment, migration, divorce, illness, or birth rates). The confluence of high rates of stressful events can then, through applied regression analysis over time, be tested with respect to relations with pathological indicators. In this way, quite sophisticated causal models can be investigated, including simultaneous, reciprocal, and detailed multivariate causation.

Additionally important contributions of time series analysis with macrohistorical data are that they permit the use of large population aggregates so as to allow controls for multiple sources of causation which may be important in disease epidemiology but minimally related to stress. Finally, these techniques permit a clearer resolution of issues of direction of causation that have proven nearly intractable in stress research using socio-economic status or life changes as independent variables.

The use of some of these time series techniques has been reviewed with respect to the pathological impact of major economic changes such as unemployment rates and changes in *per capita* income. In the present paper, data were utilized to examine the question of whether major economic changes in general, rather than only undesirable ones, were associated with mortality rates for stress-sensitive causes. It was found that in most instances, these sources of mortality responded both to rapid economic growth and to increased unemployment. The response to unemployment, however, was both more intense and occurred over a considerably longer period (at least five years for unemployment as compared with one year for rapid economic growth).

Conclusions

We conclude, therefore, that abrupt economic changes, regardless of direction, are stress provoking, but that undesirable changes such as unemployment and income loss are substantially more generative of pathology. Thus, these macroscopic analyses confirm the importance of the overall stressful nature of extremely high stimulation, as in the formulations of Selye (1956) and Levi (1972), or put another way, of a large number of stressful events, as in the Holmes and Rahe (1967) scheme. These analyses are also consistent with the findings of Paykel (1974), Mueller *et al.* (1977), Gersten *et al.* (1974), and others who argue that undesirable changes are more stress-provoking than desirable ones. The findings in this paper suggest that the undesirable events are not only inherently more stressful, but have further implications for additional life stresses subsequent to the initial major event.

The findings of this study are also highly consistent with those of an earlier period of stress research when the emphasis was on the impact of discrete categories of stressful phenomena. Indeed, the framework of national economic change, as described in this study, provides additional insights into, and interpretations of, those studies. Two of the more important categories of these stressful events include rapid social change and acculturation (e.g. Syme *et al.* 1965; Smith 1967; Marks 1967; Wolff 1968; Scotch 1960; Scotch and Geiger 1963), associated in this study with rapid economic growth, and unemployment (e.g. Friedmann 1961; Cobb *et al.* 1966; Ferman 1964), associated here with recession. The largest group of studies bearing on the stresses of working life, however, concern work pressures, including overload (e.g. Friedmann *et al.* 1958; Pepitone 1967; Russek 1965), and work satisfaction (e.g. Palmore 1969; Sales and House 1971; Gross 1970). We have discussed earlier the work stresses of economic expansion, or rapid economic growth, as based largely on the relative deprivation of those who benefit least—and particularly compounded in the cases of those who had recently experienced a major loss of socio-economic status.

The stress of *work* during periods of economic contraction, however, is considerably more severe than during economic expansion. The basic reason for this is that work pressures are substantially increased, and work satisfactions substantially decreased during the contraction phases of economic activity. Work pressures are increased because, first, purchasing power has declined and the employee or executive must work harder in order to earn his accustomed salary or wage. Second, there is a considerably heightened level of competition among firms in the same industry for the consumers' decreased purchasing power, often to the point that financial survival of the enterprise is at stake. Third, there is competition by employees and executives in the same firm over retention of jobs and use of declining resources in a shrinking market for the firm's goods or services. Fourth, there are increased demands on the employees from different supervisory sources in the firm to respond to a variety of needs which, under conditions of threat to the survival of the enterprise, have become particularly urgent.

These four sources of work pressure and overload represent part of the cost side of the equation which bears on work satisfaction. The other side of this equation, the remuneration or benefit side, is also damaged. Not only is income reduced and the threat of job loss present, but relations with supervisors and work peers become strained, and the extent to which the worker is valued in the society—i.e., in light of public response through 'effective demand' for his labour—is reduced. To put this position more generally, since economic activity in a given enterprise is constantly in a dynamic state—i.e., either in expansion or contraction, the extent to which work life is stressful will depend on the resources of the firm and the public demand for the goods and services it offers on the market. Thus, work pressures will be comparatively great and satisfactions comparatively low in the enterprise which is both (1) on the average at a relatively low level of economic success and (2) highly unstable in its economic performance.

REFERENCES

BENDIX and LIPSET (Ed.) (1966). *Class, status, and power: social stratification in comparative perspective.* (2nd edn). Free Press, New York.

BRENNER, M. H. (1971a). Economic changes and heart diseases mortality. *Amer. J. publ. Hlth*, **61**, 606–11.

—— (1971b). *Time series analysis of the relationships between selected economic and social indicators*, Vols. I and II. National Technical Information Service, Springfield, Virginia.

—— (1973a). *Mental illness and the economy.* Harvard University Press, Cambridge, Mass.

—— (1973b). Fetal, infant and maternal mortality during periods of economic instability. *Int. J. Hlth Serv.*, **3** (2), 145–59.

—— (1975). Trends in alcohol consumption and associated illnesses. *Amer. J. publ. Hlth*, **65**, 1279–92.

—— (1976a). *Estimating the social costs of national economic policy: implications for mental and physical health and criminal aggression.* Joint Economic Committee of the U.S. Congress, Washington, D.C.

—— (1976b). Effects of the economy on criminal behavior and the administration of criminal justice in the United States, Canada, England and Wales, and Scotland. In *Economic crises and crime: correlations between the state of the economy, deviance and the control of deviance.* United Nations Social Defense Research Institute, Rome.

CASSEL, J. (1967). Factors involving sociocultural incongruity and change: appraisal and implications for theoretical development. In Social stress and cardiovascular disease (ed. S. L. Syme and L. G. Reader). *Milbank Men. Fund. Quart.*, **45**, 41–5.

—— (1970). Physical illness in response to stress. In *Social stress* (ed. S. Levine and N. A. Scotch), pp. 189–209. Aldine, Chicago.

CHRIST C. (1966). *Econometric models and methods.* Wiley, New York.

COBB, S., KASL, S. V., BROOKS, G. W., and CONNELLY, W. E. (1966). The health of people changing jobs: a description of a longitudinal study. *Amer. J. publ. Hlth*, **56**, 1476–81.

CROOG, S. H., LEVINE, S., and LURIE, Z. F. (1968). The heart patient and the recovery process: a review of the directions of research on social and psychological factors. *Soc. Sci. Med.*, **2**, 111–64.

DOHRENWEND, B. S. and DOHRENWEND, B. P. (1969). *Social status and psychological disorder.* Wiley, New York.

DOHRENWEND, B. P. (1966). Social status and psychological disorder: an issue of substance and an issue of method. *Amer. soc. Rev.*, **31**, 14–34.

DUNHAM, H. W. and SRINIVASAN, P. (1966). A research note on diagnosed mental illness and social class. *Sociol. Rev.*, **31** (2), 223–7.

EYER, J. (1977). Prosperity as a cause of death. *Int. J. Hlth Serv.*, **7** (1), 125–50.

FERMAN, L. (1964). Sociological perspectives in unemployment research. In *Blue collar world* (ed. A. Shostak and W. Gomberg). Prentice-Hall, Englewood Cliffs, New Jersey.

FRIEDMAN, M., ROSENMAN, R. H., and CARROLL, V. (1958). Changes in the serum cholesterol and blood clotting time of men subject to cyclic variation of occupational stress. *Circulat.*, **18**, 852–61.

FRIEDMANN, G. (1961). *The anatomy of work*, pp. 126, 128. Free Press, New York.

GERSTEN, J. C., LANGNER, T. S., EISENBERG, J. G., and ORZECK, L. (1974). Child behavior and life events: undesirable change or change per se. In *Stressful life events: their nature and effects* (ed. B. S. Dohrenwend and B. P. Dohrenwend), pp. 159–70. Wiley, New York.

GRILICHES, Z. (1974). Errors in variables and other unobservables. *Econometrica*, **42**, 971–98.

GROSS, E. (1970). Work organization and stress. In *Social stress* (ed. S. Levine and N. A. Scotch), pp. 54–110 (especially pp. 78–92). Aldine, Chicago.

GUNDERSON, E. K. and RAHE, R. H. (1974). *Life stress and illness*. Thomas, Springfield, Illinois.

HINKLE, L. D., WHITNEY, L. H., LEHMAN, E. W., DUNN, J., BENJAMIN, B., KING, R., PLAKUN, A., and FLEHINGER, R. (1968). Occupation, education, and coronary heart disease. *Science*, **161**, 238–46.

HOLMES, T. H. and RAHE, R. H. (1967). The social readjustment rating scale. *J. psychosom. Res.*, **11**, 213–8.

— and MASUDA, M. N. (1974). Life change and illness susceptibility. In *Stressful life events: their nature and effects* (ed. B. S. Dohrenwend and B. P. Dohrenwend), pp. 45–79. Wiley, New York.

JOHNSTON, J. (1963). *Econometric methods*. McGraw-Hill, New York.

KAPLAN, B. H., CASSEL, J., and GORE, S. (1977). Social support and health. *Med. Care*, Suppl. 15, 47–58.

LEVI, L. (1972). Stress and distress in response to psychosocial stimuli. *Acta Med. Scand. Suppl.* **528**, 191. (Simultaneously published in book form by Pergamon Press, Oxford, 1972).

LILIENFELD, A. M. and GIFFORD, A. J. (Eds) (1966). *Chronic diseases and public health*. Johns Hopkins University Press, Baltimore.

MARKS, R. B. (1967). Factors involving social and demographic characteristics; a review of empirical findings. In *Social stress and cardiovascular disease* (ed. S. L. Syme and L. G. Reeder). *Milbank Mem. Fund Quart.*, **45**, 51–108.

MITCHELL, W. C. (1951). *What happens during business cycles: a progress report*. National Bureau of Economic Research, New York.

MOORE, G. H. (Ed.) (1961). *Business cycle indicators* (2 Vols.). Princeton University Press, Princeton, New Jersey.

MOSS, G. E. (1973). *Illness, stress and social interaction: the dynamics of social resonation*. Wiley, New York.

MUELLER, D. P., EDWARDS, D. W., and YARVIS, R. M. (1977). Stressful life events and psychiatric symptomatology: change or undesirability? *J. Hlth soc. Behav.*, **18**, 307–17.

OSTFELD, A. M., LEBOVITS, B. A., SHEKELLE, R. B., and PAUL, O. (1964). A prospective study of the relationship between personality and coronary heart disease. *J. chron. Dis.*, **17**, 265–76.

PALMORE, E. (1969). Predicting longevity: a follow-up controlling for age. *Gerontol*.

PAYKEL, E. S. (1974). Recent life events and clinical depression. In *Life stress and illness* (ed. E. K. Gunderson and R. H. Rahe), pp. 134–63. Thomas, Springfield, Illinois.

PEPITONE, A. (1967). Self, social environment, and stress. In *Psychological stress* (ed. M. H. Appley and D. Trumbull). Appleton-Century-Crofts, New York.

RABKIN, J. G. and STRUENING, E. L. (1976). Life events, stress and illness. *Science*, **194**, 1013–20.

RAHE, R. H. and ROMO, M. (1974). Recent life changes and the onset of myocardial infarction and coronary death in Helsinki. In *Life stress and illness* (ed. E. K. Gunderson and R. H. Rahe), pp. 105–20. Thomas, Springfield, Illinois.

——, MEYER, M., SMITH, M., KJAER, G., and HOLMES, T. H. (1964). Social stress and illness onset. *J. psychosom. Res.*, **8**, 35–44.

REID, D. D. (1961). Precipitating proximal factors in the occurrence of mental disorders: epidemiological evidence. *Milbank Mem. Fund Quart.*, **39**, 227–48.

RUSSEK, H. I. (1965). Stress, tobacco, and coronary heart disease in North American professional groups. *J. Amer. med. Assoc.*, **192**, 89–94.

SALES, S. M. and HOUSE, J. (1971). Job dissatisfaction as a possible risk factor in coronary heart disease. *J. chron. Dis.*, **23**, 867–73.

SCOTCH, N. A. (1960). A preliminary report on the relation of socio-cultural factors to hypertension among the Zulu. *Ann. N.Y. Acad. Sci.*, **84**, 1000–9.

—— and GEIGER, H. J. (1963). The epidemiology of essential hypertension. A review with special attention to psychologic and sociocultural factors. II. psychologic and sociocultural factors in etiology. *J. chron. Dis.*, **16**, 1183–1213.

SELYE, H. (1956). *The stress of life*. McGraw-Hill, New York.

SILVER, M. (1972). An economic analysis of spatial variations in mortality rates by race and sex. In *Essays in the economics of health and medical care* (ed. V. R. Fuchs), pp. 161–227. Columbia University Press, New York.

SMITH, T. (1967). Factors involving sociocultural incongruity and change: a review of empirical findings. In *Social stress and cardiovascular disease* (ed. S. L. Syme and L. G. Reeder). *Milbank Mem. Fund Quart.*, **45**, 23–38.

SYME, S. L., HYMAN, M. M., and ENTERLINE, P. E. (1964). Some social and cultural factors associated with the occurrence of coronary heart disease. *J. chron. Dis.*, **17**, 227–89.

——, BORHANI, N. O., and BUECHLEY, R. W. (1965). Cultural mobility and coronary heart disease in an urban area. *Amer. J. Epidemiol.*, **82**, 334–46.

THEORELL, T. and RAHE, R. H. (1974). Psychosocial characteristics of subjects with myocardial infarction in Stockholm. In *Life stress and illness* (ed. E. K. Gunderson and R. H. Rahe), pp. 90–104. Thomas, Springfield, Illinois.

THOMAS, D. S. (1925). *Social aspects of the business cycle*. Routledge, London and Dutton, New York.

WARDWELL, W. I., HYMAN, M. M., and BAHNSON, C. B. (1964). Stress and coronary heart disease in three field studies. *J. chron. Dis.*, **17**, 73–84.

WOLFF, H. G. (1968). *Stress and disease* (2nd edn) (revised and ed. S. Wolf and H. Goodell). Thomas, Springfield, Illinois.

SESSION 4

Health protection and promotion through psychosocial factors

31. STRESS WITHOUT DISTRESS IN WORKING LIFE

HANS SELYE

am very grateful for the opportunity to contribute to this volume, which is to explore the convergence of society, stress, and disease in the domain of working life. I remember that in 1970, at a symposium held under the auspices of the World Health Organization (Selye 1971a), I was allowed to suggest to some of the world's leading experts on psychosocial health factors the definition of stress as *the non-specific response of the organism to any demand made upon it*. This formulation certainly includes any type of work.

Since our own research over the past four decades was especially concerned with this topic, I am very gratified to note that the stress theory helps to provide an exploratory framework not only for medical science as such but also for the study and amelioration of social conditions. This ongoing series of psychosocial symposia surely reflects the importance which has been attached to this approach. Nevertheless, I am certain you would all agree that, as yet, we have seen but a shadow of the promise.

Working life is an especially fruitful area for stress research since it is thickly interwoven with stress factors — and I feel that eventually it will be recognized that the overwhelming majority of problems involving vocational motivation and performance can be reduced to improper handling of stress. It is already a matter of widespread concern that our factories and offices are filled with bored and resentful men and women who have been made to feel less important than the machines they operate. For the most part, they drift into their jobs by accident, remain there through inertia, and accumulate frustrations which make them likely candidates for what we have called 'diseases of adaptation'.

For me personally, the topic of this volume is particularly timely since I have recently completed a book entitled *Stress without distress* (Selye 1974), which attempts to prescribe a code of behaviour based on scientific principles rather than tradition, superstition, or blind subservience to the commands of an unquestionable authority. Besides offering guidelines for handling the stresses of everyday working life, it summarizes close to 40 years of laboratory research, including many new observations that have been made since I addressed the World Health Organization symposium in Stockholm on 17 April, 1970 (Selye 1971a).

This time I should like to explain my views not as an expert on the morphology or biochemistry of stress reactions, but merely as a citizen who is worried about what stress is doing to our society. I can claim no expertise in politics and sociology, though this is the kind of talent that would be needed now. We must find men who can translate the lessons of the laboratory into a code of behaviour. It seems to me that a way of life based on the understanding of man's response to the stress of constant change is the only road that leads out of the jungle of conflicting thoughts about right and wrong, justice and injustice that has confused our sense of values.

It is said that ours is a particularly difficult period of history characterized by wars, revolutions, terror, and destructiveness. Almost every day, newspapers report acts of wanton lawlessness and cruelty: hijackings, drug abuse, and bombs which destroy innocent people. These acts are usually ascribed to the loss of any generally acceptable purpose to life and work, leaving man with the frantic urge to express himself and to attract attention by no matter what means.

I do not think that this sad state of affairs is much more characteristic of our period than of any other; there have always been terrible wars, revolutions, and crime. These have been born out of the suffering and despair caused by overwork or the lack of anything worth doing, which incites revolt and spasmodic efforts to break away from it all at any cost in order to reach some more satisfying style of life.

Throughout the centuries, all sorts of suggestions have been made about how to achieve peace and happiness through technical or political advances, rises in living standards, more rigorous law enforcement, or strict adherence to the commands of a particular religion. Yet history has proven, over and over again, that none of these means is reliably efficacious. To my mind, what man really needs is more natural ideals than those which presently guide him. It seems to me that the rules which act so efficiently at the level of cells and organs could also be the basis of a natural philosophy of life and conduct with respect to the various problems that man must face every day. We are all the children of nature and cannot go wrong by following her laws in conjunction with whatever additional ideals or convictions may guide us.

HORMONES AND RESISTANCE

Ever since 1936, when we noticed that the animal organism responds with a stereotyped homeostatic reaction to any kind of stress, my colleagues and I have been interested in the possibility of preventing or curing various diseases by 'stress hormones', that is, substances the body produces in an effort to treat itself during emergencies. Between 1936 and about 1960, most of these works centred around the use of glucocorticoids whose main effect is to diminish potentially harmful and excessive reactions to injury (e.g., excessive inflammation). More recently, it became evident that an entirely different group of hormones, the 'catatoxic steroids', are often even more potent in maintaining homeostasis, but they do so by actually destroying pathogens, usually through enzymatic degradation.

It has long been recognized that steroid hormones participate in the regulation of growth, reproduction, and general metabolism; yet, it is only in the course of the last four decades that we became aware of their participation in diverse non-specific adaptive reactions, particularly in the maintenance of the body's resistance to stress.

It is not too difficult to imagine that, as a consequence of their special chemical activities, hormones can produce specific biological responses, such as an increase in the BMR, vasoconstriction, or lactation. Although we still know very little about the intimate mechanism of these reactions, there is no reason to doubt that it is closely related to that of selective drug actions in general. Presumably, as a consequence of their specific molecular configuration, different hormones—like drugs—possess specific affinities only for certain receptor sites, or 'target organs', which consequently respond to them selectively. In all these cases, a particular agent acts upon a particular receptor, inducing it to execute only the function that it was built to perform.

It is difficult to visualize, however, how a hormone could carry the message of simply 'improving resistance' against virtually any disturbance throughout the body. And yet that is essentially what the adaptive hormones appear to do. Of course, the qualifying term 'virtually' restricts the number of agents against which hormones can offer resistance; but the more this field is being explored, the more do we realize how impressively large this number is.

The most instructive recent advance in the understanding of adaptive hormone action was the realization that several steroids can increase non-specific resistance through very different mechanisms. In this connection, it has been found convenient to classify the adaptive steroids into two main groups which control essentially dissimilar defensive processes:

1. *Syntoxic steroids* (from '*syn*' = together) are essentially tissue tranquilizers in that they create a state of passive tolerance which permits a kind of symbiosis with the pathogen.
2. *Catatoxic steroids* (from '*kata*' = against) actively attack the pathogen, usually by accelerating its metabolic degradation.

Sometimes, the same molecule is endowed with both types of properties; yet these effects are certainly not interdependent since many steroids possess exclusively syntoxic or exclusively catatoxic potencies.

Both types of compounds are widely used in daily practice for the treatment of various specific morbid conditions; yet, few physicians give much thought to the mechanisms which explain the efficacy of steroids in so many and diverse disease states, that is, their non-specific effects. It may be opportune, therefore, to review here the basic research that led to this pharmacological classification.

SYNTOXIC STEROIDS

The fact that syntoxic, antiphlogistic hormones suppress inflammation without destroying the causative irritant was first demonstrated using the granuloma-pouch technique. About 25 cc of air was injected under the skin of a rat to form a subcutaneous sack into which croton oil was then introduced as a local irritant. This caused considerable inflammation with granuloma and exudate formation in normal but not in cortisone-treated animals. Yet, the croton oil removed from such an irresponsive air sack of a hormone-treated animal still retained all its power to produce inflammation when it was injected into a non-pretreated animal.

The systemic action of the syntoxic steroids is mainly of the 'life-maintaining corticoid' type. These hormones are particularly efficient in restoring the non-specific stress resistance of adrenal-deficient organisms to normal, but then a plateau is reached above which tolerance cannot be raised easily. Only in some instances (e.g., damage due to endotoxins, inflammatory irritants, immune reactions) do the syntoxic glucocorticoids increase tolerance far above normal because, here, 'disease' is primarily due to active morbid reactions of the tissues, not to direct tissue damage by the exogenous aggressor. Thus, endotoxin shock is thought to be caused mainly by the liberation of enzymes normally sequestered in certain organelles of the cell (the lysosomes), whereas inflammation and various pathogenic immune reactions (allergy, anaphylaxis, homograft rejection) represent excessive responses of the body to different types of irritation.

Osteolathyrism is an experimental disease model of little concern to the practising physician, but it should be mentioned here because of its historic importance in the clarification of syntoxic steroid actions. In rats fed a sweet pea *(lathyrus odoratus)* diet, the bones become unusually sensitive to local stress; they react to virtually any type of injury (even to traction at the insertion site of muscle tendons) with excessive and deforming tissue proliferation. Hence, animals kept on this pea diet (or treated with certain aminonitriles which represent its active ingredients) develop osteoma-like giant exostoses at sites of tendon insertions and around fractures. This exaggerated tissue response is decisively influenced by hormones; it can be totally suppressed by antiphlogistic steroids, such as cortisone, cortisol, or triamcinolone, and is greatly aggravated by the prophlogistic somatotrophic hormone (STH). Indeed, the latter is quite indispensable for the development of osteolathyrism since

he disease fails to occur on lathyrogenic diets after
hypophysectomy (which removes the source of endogenous STH) but develops even in the absence of the
pituitary if physiological amounts of exogenous STH are
administered. Incidentally, this latter observation shows
that the endocrine regulation of reactivity to local stress
is not limited to the steroids since STH belongs to the
polypeptide type of hormones. Finally, it must be
remembered that some protective hormone actions are
based on specific pharmacological antagonisms between
steroids and toxic substances (e.g., mineralocorticoid-
induced potassium tolerance, glucocorticoid-induced
insulin tolerance). Here the basic mechanism is more
specific but also syntoxic since, again, homeostasis is
achieved by adjusting the body's reaction to the
damaging agent, not by destroying the latter.

CATATOXIC STEROIDS

The catatoxic steroids act primarily by inducing aggressive reactions which inactivate toxic substances (e.g., by
accelerating their metabolic degradation). They not only
restore a deficient resistance to normal (as do the
glucocorticoids after adrenalectomy) but are capable of
raising it far above the norm.

Among the great variety of catatoxic effects recently
observed are the virtually complete suppression by
ethylestrenol, spironolactone, and related steroids of:

1. Barbiturate or steroid anesthesia;
2. The gastro-intestinal ulcers produced by indomethacin over-dosage;
3. The generalized calcinosis characteristic of intoxication with large amounts of vitamin-D derivatives
   (particularly dihydrotachysterol);
4. The cardiac damage caused by excessive amounts
   of digitoxin;
5. The muscular paralysis induced by mephenesin or
   meprobamate;
6. The disturbance in blood coagulation elicited by
   phenindione;
7. The adrenal necrosis induced by certain carcinogenic hydrocarbons;
8. The mortality that normally follows severe poisoning with various pesticides, cycloheximide,
   colchicine, and many other drugs.

This broad spectrum of protective effects against so
many agents, widely differing in their chemical structure
and the type of damage they produce, clearly shows that
the actions of catatoxic steroids are not specific.
Occasionally, acceleration of drug-metabolism defeats
its purpose, because the products of metabolic degradation are more toxic than the original poison which was to
be inactivated. Yet the response, though actually
harmful, is still catatoxic since it attacks the toxic
aggressor. For similar reasons, we speak of allergy and
anaphylaxis as 'immune reactions', although they
actually produce damage.

OVERLAPS

There are many overlaps between syntoxic and catatoxic
steroid actions. Thus, stimulation of inflammation may
lead to topical degradation of the irritant by enzyme
activation in the inflammatory focus; furthermore,
under certain circumstances, the primarily syntoxic
glucocorticoids (e.g., dexamethasone) may also enhance
the hepatic detoxication of barbiturates. Yet, the distinction between these two categories appears to be as
justified as, say, the distinction between glucocorticoids
and mineralocorticoids, because, despite some overlaps,
individual steroids usually act predominantly by eliciting one or the other reaction form.

Furthermore, available evidence suggests that the two
types of defence are mediated through essentially distinct biochemical mechanisms. For example, as stated
above, homeostatic reactions to endotoxins or inflammatory irritants appear to depend upon the stabilization
of membranes which isolate toxic enzymes that are preformed within the cell. Thereby, they protect against
damage resulting from a kind of auto-intoxication by
natural substances liberated under the influence of an
aggressor. Conversely, many catatoxic hormones have
been shown to induce 'multipurpose' (that is relatively
non-specific) microsomal liver enzymes which destroy
many endogenous or exogenous toxic substances. Yet,
without further evidence, it would be hazardous to
ascribe all catatoxic actions to the same mechanism.

Not all catatoxic steroids induce enzymes against the
same set of substrates; for example, certain steroids
inactivate digitoxin but not indomethacin or vice versa;
others inactivate both these drugs. There is evidence also
that some catatoxic steroids induce drug-metabolizing
enzymes in extrahepatic tissue. Finally, spironolactone
offers an extraordinary degree of protection against
systemic intoxication with corrosive sublimate ($HgCl_2$),
presumably by synthesis rather than degradation
because the sulphur-containing group of this steroid
forms non-toxic compounds with mercury.

GENERAL CLASSIFICATION

On the basis of this survey, it seems reasonable to classify
the physiological and pharmacological actions of steroids
as shown in Fig. 31.1.

The important effects upon growth, reproduction,
and metabolism are mentioned here only because no
classification of steroids would be complete without
them. However, in this chapter we have dealt exclusively with the non-specific adaptive functions of these
extremely versatile compounds which perform so many
and varied tasks in health and disease.

One of the cardinal questions that faces us now is to
show whether the endogenous secretion of catatoxic
steroids can be increased as a defensive measure in
response to need, just as corticoid production rises under
conditions of stress. We have no proof of this, but many

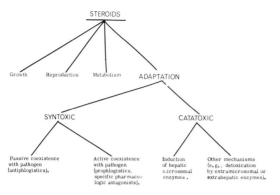

FIG. 31.1. A classification of the physiological and pharmacological actions of steroids.

of the catatoxic steroids are natural products that might thus be made available.

HOMEOSTASIS AND HETEROSTASIS

In recent years, the discovery of the important role played by hepatic microsomal enzyme induction in defence against certain toxicants led to the development of a new field of pharmacology designated 'xenobiochemistry' and defined as the 'biochemistry of foreign organic compounds' (Williams 1959). This science is concerned with the fate of 'xenobiotics' (from the Greek *xenos* and *bios* for 'stranger to life'), that is, compounds which are foreign to the metabolic network of the organism (Mason *et al.* 1965).

At first, the term xenobiochemistry appeared to be a particularly suitable label for the new approach, because both the toxicants and the inducers of their biodegradation were foreign to the body. (Most of the initial work was performed with barbiturates, polycyclic hydrocarbons, insecticides, etc.). Brodie and his co-workers (1955), who probably did more for the development of this field than any other group of investigators, came to the conclusion that presumably the defensive enzyme systems 'are not essential to the normal economy of the body, but operate primarily against the toxic influences of foreign compounds that gain access to the body from the alimentary tract'.

The large number of investigators and the fast-growing literature dealing with problems in this field have recently prompted the founding of a special journal under the name *Xenobiotics*. Yet, nowadays, hardly anyone doubts that neither the substrates nor the inducers of such defensive enzymes need be foreign to the body's economy (Conney 1967). Of course, in the case of poisons completely foreign to the organism, any amount in the body is excessive and hence 'foreign', whereas normal body constituents become 'foreign' only if their concentration greatly exceeds physiological levels. Thus, various hormones and hormone derivatives can protect against both exogenous and endogenous

damaging substances, catatoxically by inducing enzyme capable of accelerating their biodegradation, or syn toxically by increasing tissue resistance to them (Sely 1971b). Among the most important natural compound amenable to catatoxic or syntoxic defence are: steroi hormones, bile acids, bile pigments, fat-soluble vitamin inflammatory mediators (histamine, serotonin, prosta glandins), and so forth, all of which are either mad within the body or absorbed from the diet as essentia physiological ingredients of living matter.

The salient feature of these adaptive mechanisms i therefore not that they attack only substances foreign t the body but that they establish a new equilibriun between the body and an unusually high level of th potential pathogen, either by destroying the exces (catatoxic action) or by making tissues tolerant to i (syntoxic action).

When such an abnormal equilibrium must be estab lished to protect against potential pathogens, I propos to speak of *heterostasis* (*heteros* = other; *stasis* = fixity as the establishment of a new steady state by exogenou (pharmacologic) stimulation of adaptive mechanism through the development and maintenance or dorman defensive tissue reactions (Selye 1973). In a sense, thi would be the counterpart of homeostasis (*homoios* = like) which has been defined as the maintenance of normal steady state by means of endogenous (physic logical) responses. In heterostasis, as in homeostasis, th fixity of the *'milieu intérieur'* is not absolute. Bot Claude Bernard (1878–9) and Walter B. Cannon (1926 have clearly realized that in order to maintain a state c relative stability the body cannot remain completel inert but must answer each stimulus with an appropriat counter-stimulus to maintain equilibrium. However, i homeostasis, this equilibrium is maintained with smal fluctuations near the physiological level, whereas i heterostasis unusual defence reactions are mobilized t permit resistance to unusual aggression. Furthermore, i general, homeostasis, unlike heterostasis, depends upo rapidly developing and vanishing readjustments although—as in all biological classifications—transitiona types are common.

Of course, both homeostatic and heterostatic read tions, though usually of defensive value, may be worth less or even harmful under certain circumstances. Thi can be illustrated by the following examples: (1) In pre disposed individuals, excessive neuroendocrine 'emer gency reactions' may precipitate a cardio-vascula accident. (2) Antibody formation can result in anaphy laxis or allergy; indeed, even phagocytosis can offer suitable milieu to certain organisms and protect then against blood-borne antimicrobials (e.g., in a tubercle (3) Defensive syntoxic hormones can interfere with th encapsulation and destruction of micro-organisms b suppressing useful inflammatory or immunological reac tions. Similarly, by accelerating the biotransformation o relatively innocuous compounds, catatoxic steroids ca enhance the production of highly pathogenic metabolites.

The most salient difference between homeostasis an

terostasis is that the former maintains the normal
eady state by physiological reactions, whereas the
tter 'resets the thermostat' to maintain a higher state of
efence by artificial exogenous intervention. Hetero-
asis can be accomplished by exogenous administration
f natural (e.g., hormones) or artificial (e.g., bar-
turates) substances capable of inducing responses of
is kind. Furthermore, the heterostatic reactions may
e syntoxic (e.g., corticoids, anti-inflammatory drugs),
ermitting co-existence with potential pathogens by
voking responses which make our tissues indifferent to
ertain potentially pathogenic stimuli. Thus, they
appress excessive inflammatory reactions which
epresent the very essence of some diseases. However,
ey may also be catatoxic (e.g., some anabolic
ormones, barbiturates, insecticides) if they enhance
rug-metabolizing enzyme activity and thereby
ccelerate the biodegradation of potential pathogens.
he most potent catatoxic substance known to date is
regnenolone-16-carbonitrile (PCN); this is a close
elative of the naturally occurring pregnenolone and yet
n artificial compound in that it is produced synthetically
y the introduction of a carbonitrile group into its
atural congener.

Thus, the concept of heterostasis includes both syn-
oxic and catatoxic reactions induced by natural or
rtificial exogenous compounds. On the other hand, it
xcludes all therapeutic measures which act directly (or
oassively') not by stimulating the body's own adaptive
apacities. For example, (1) Antidotes, which act
irectly upon potential pathogens (e.g., buffers that
eutralize acids, chemicals which inactivate poisons by
irectly combining with them, antimicrobial agents).
2) All forms of substitution therapy (e.g., vitamin C for
curvy, corticoids for Addison's disease, transplanted or
rtificial kidneys for renal failure) which merely
epresent chemical or mechanical prostheses. (3) The
blation of diseased tissues (infected parts, tumors).
4) Passive 'shielding' (e.g., by lead screens against
X-rays, receptor blockade against drugs, competition for
substrate).

Thus, the types of adaptation, which depend upon
ctive participation of the body, are: homeostatic—
a) syntoxic, (b) catatoxic.

This list comprises all active defence reactions
rrespective of their nervous, immunological, phagocytic,
r hormonal mediation. It can be incorporated into a
eneral classification of adaptive mechanisms, whether
he 'milieu intérieur' participates actively or passively, as
ummarized in Fig. 31.2.

Adaptability is probably the most distinctive characteristic of
fe. In maintaining the independence and individuality of
atural units, none of the great forces of inanimate matter are
s successful as that alertness to change which we designate as
fe—and the loss of which is death. Indeed, there is perhaps
ven a certain parallelism between the degree of aliveness and
he extent of adaptability in every animal—in every man (Selye
950).

SYNTOXIC AND CATATOXIC BEHAVIOUR

The great laws that regulate defence of living beings
against stressors of any kind are essentially the same at all
levels of life, from individual cells to people and even
societies of man. Our own research is concerned with
defence against aggressors within the body, such as toxic
chemicals produced by our organism or introduced into
it. But what about *defence against assaults by other
people?*

Suppose you encounter a drunk who showers you
with insults, but is obviously far too severely intoxicated
to be dangerous; the most efficient response is a 'syntoxic' one: you merely ignore him and nothing will
happen. However, if you take an aggressive 'catatoxic'
attitude, you start arguing with him and get angry. Sub-
consciously you prepare for a fight by a rise in blood
pressure, pulse rate, nervous tension, etc. In this case,
the result may be catastrophic. In a coronary candidate,
this reaction to fight may suffice to cause a fatal
myocardial infarction, in a man with cerebral arteriosclerosis a stroke. The apparent pathogen—here the
drunk—did not even touch you. So who was the cause of
your death? You were. This is biological suicide by
choosing the wrong defensive reaction. On the other
hand, if a homicidal maniac comes at you with a dagger
ready to kill you, the only possible attitude is 'catatoxic'; you must try to disarm him, even at the risk
of self-inflicted damage by the mobilization of your own
defence mechanisms. So, when it comes to interpersonal
defence reactions, three possibilities exist: (1) the syntoxic, which ignores the enemy and puts up with him
without trying to attack him; (2) the catatoxic, which

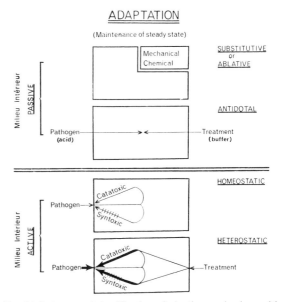

FIG. 31.2. A general classification of adaptive mechanisms with
the *milieu intérieur* participating actively (bottom) and
passively (top).

results in a fight; and (3) flight, an attempt to escape from the enemy without either putting up with him or trying to destroy him. This last possibility obviously does not exist in the fight against poisons inside our body.

These remarks on interpersonal relations gave us the first inkling of the close connections that exist between adaptive and defensive reactions on a cellular level within the organism, and between different people or even groups of people.

At first sight, it is odd that the laws governing life's responses at such different levels as a cell, a whole person, or even a nation should be so essentially similar. Yet, this type of uniformity is true of all *great laws of nature.* For example, in the inanimate world, arrangement of matter and energy in orbits, circulating around a centre, is quite characteristic of the largest celestial bodies as well as of individual atoms. Why is it that on these opposite levels of the smallest and the largest, the satellites circling a huge planet and the minute electrons around an atomic nucleus, should go around in orbits?

We find comparable similarities in the great laws governing living matter. Countless phenomena run in cycles, such as the periodically recurring needs for food, water, sleep, sexual activity. Damage is unavoidable unless each cycle runs its full course.

In terms of controllable human conduct, interference with the fulfilment and completion of man's natural drives leads to as much distress as the forced prolongation and intensification of any activity beyond the desired level. Ignoring these rules leads to frustration, fatigue, and exhaustion which can progress to a mental or physical breakdown.

In formulating a natural code of behaviour, these thoughts are of fundamental importance. We must not only understand the deep-rooted biological need for the completion and fulfilment of our aspirations, but we must also know how to handle these in harmony with our particular inherited capacities. Not everybody is born with the same amount of adaptation energy.

WORK—A BIOLOGICAL NECESSITY

Most people consider their work to be their primary function in life. For the man or woman of action, one of the most difficult things to bear is enforced inactivity during prolonged hospitalization or after retirement. Any code of behaviour founded on biological laws must therefore recognize that work as such is a basic necessity of living matter, especially work whose fruits can be accumulated. Just as our muscles become flabby and degenerate if not used, so our brain slips into chaos and confusion, unless we constantly use it for some work that seems worthwhile to us. The average person thinks he works for economic security or social status, but at the end of a most successful business career when he finally achieves this, there remains nothing to fight for–no hope for progress, only the boredom of assured monotony. The question is not whether we should or should not

work, but what kind of work suits us best.

The Western world is being racked by the insatiable demand for less work and more pay. In practice, the urgency of the clamour for improvement does not depend so much upon the number of working hours or the salaries earned as upon the degree of dissatisfaction with life. We could do much—and at little cost—by fighting this dissatisfaction. Many people suffer because they have no particular taste for anything, no hunger for achievement. These—not those who earn little—are the true paupers of mankind. What they need more than money is guidance.

If man has no more incentive to work out his role as *homo faber,* he is likely to see destructive, revolutionary outlets to relieve his basic need for self-assertive activity. He may be able to solve his age-old problem of having to live by the sweat of his brow, but the fatal enemy of all Utopias is boredom. What we shall have to do after technology makes most 'useful work' redundant is to invent new occupations. It will require a full-scale effort to teach 'play professions'—the arts, philosophy, crafts, science—to the public at large; there is no limit to how much man can work on the perfection of his own self and on giving pleasure to others.

'EARN THY NEIGHBOUR'S LOVE'

Each person must find a way to relieve his pent-up energy without creating conflicts with his fellow men. Such an approach not only ensures peace of mind but also earns the goodwill, respect, and even love of our fellow men, the highest degree of security, the most noble 'status symbol' to which man can aspire.

This philosophy of hoarding a wealth of respect and friendship is merely one reflection of the deep-rooted instinct of man and animals to collect. It is as characteristic of ants, bees, squirrels, and beavers as of the capitalist who collects money to put away in the bank. The same impulsive drives entire human societies to amass a system of roads, telephones, cities, fortifications that strike them as useful means of accumulating the ingredients of future security and comfort.

In man, this urge first manifests itself when children start to amass match boxes, shells, or stickers; it continues when adults gather stamps or coins. The natural drive for collecting is certainly not an artificial indoctrinated tradition. By collecting certain things, you acquire status and security in you community. The guideline of earning love merely attempts to direct the hoarding instinct towards what I consider the most permanent and valuable commodity that man can collect: a huge capital of good will which protects him against personal attacks by his fellow men.

To live literally by the Biblical command of 'Love thy neighbour as thyself' only leads to guilt feelings, because it cannot be reconciled with the laws of objective science. Whether we like it or not, egoism is an inescapable characteristic of all living beings. But we can continue to

nefit by the wisdom of this time-honoured maxim if, in
e light of modern biological research, we merely re-
ord it. Let our guide for conduct be the motto: 'Earn
y neighbour's love' (Selye 1974, 1976).

SUMMARY

he great laws of nature that regulate defence of living
ings against stressors of any kind are essentially the
me at all levels of life, from individual cells to entire
complex human organisms and even societies of men. It
helps a great deal to understand the fundamental
advantages and disadvantages of 'catatoxic' and
'syntoxic' attitudes by studying the biological basis of
self-preservation as reflected in syntoxic and catatoxic
chemical mechanisms. When applied to everyday
problems, this understanding should lead to choices
most likely to provide us with pleasant stress of fulfilment and victory, thereby avoiding the self-destructive
distress of failure and frustration.

REFERENCES

ERNARD, C. (1878–9). *Leçons sur les phénomènes de la vie
communs animaux et aux végétaux.* Paris.

RODIE, B. B., AXELROD, J., COOPER, J. R., GAUDETTE, L.,
LA DU, B. N., MITOMA, C., and UDENFRIEND, S. (1955).
Detoxication of drugs and other foreign compounds by liver
microsomes. *Science,* **121**, 603–4.

ANNON, W. B. (1926). In *À Charles Richet: ses amis, ses
collègues, ses élèves* (ed. A. Pettit), Paris.

ONNEY, A. H. (1967). Pharmacological implications of microsomal enzyme induction. *Pharmacol. Rev.,* **19**, 317–66.

ASON, H. S., NORTH, J. C., and VANNESTE, M. (1965).
Microsomal mixed-function oxidations: the metabolism of
xenobiotics, *Fed. Proc.,* **24**, 1172–80.

SELYE, H. (1950). *Stress,* Montreal.

——, (1971a). The evolution of the stress concept. Stress and
cardiovascular disease. In *Society, stress and disease* (ed. L.
Levi), Vol. 1, pp. 299–311. London.

——, (1971b), *Hormones and resistance.* Heidelberg.

——, (1973). Homeostasis and heterostasis. *Perspect. Biol.
Med.,* **16**, 441–5.

——, (1974). *Stress without distress.* New York.

——, (1976). *Stress in health and disease.* Reading, Massachusetts.

WILLIAMS, R. T. (1959). *Detoxication mechanisms: the
metabolism and detoxication of drugs, toxic substances and
other organic compounds* (Second edition). New York.

32. THERAPEUTIC AND PREVENTIVE OCCUPATIONAL MENTAL HEALTH ACTIVITIES IN INDUSTRIALIZED SOCIETIES

ALAN A. McLEAN

Occupational mental health and therefore its attendant activities, may be defined in several ways. In the narrowest sense this area is concerned solely with the psychiatrically ill worker whose symptoms interfere with his effective functioning on the job. This is the purest clinical concept of the field. In a broader sense, occupational mental health is concerned with thought, feeling, and behaviour—both healthy and unhealthy—as it occurs in the work organization or as it relates to the performance of a job. In this larger context the field deals with factors in the work environment which support mentally healthy behaviour as well as those which may be involved in triggering the development of symptoms of emotional disturbance.

Over the years the literature of occupational mental health has increased in breadth, scope, and content. Through it, the clinician has contributed a great deal to our understanding of the individual's motivation for work, his suitability for various occupational roles, and the influence of work on his physical and mental health (Lapinsky 1965).

The volume of sophisticated study from the behavioural sciences is equally great in its contribution to our understanding of work groups, interaction patterns at work, job satisfaction, employee attitudes and morale, and of the corporate subculture in which the individual functions. From all this work one might conclude that if there is such a field as occupational mental health at all, it cuts across and through occupational medicine; social, clinical, and industrial psychology; cultural anthropology; social psychiatry; and psychiatry proper. An indication of this may be obtained from a listing of the subject matter most frequently cited in a partially annotated bibliography published by the National Clearinghouse for Mental Health Information (NIMH 1965): accidents; absenteeism; alcoholism; the executive, his role and psychopathology; industrial health and occupational medicine; organized labour and the unions; leadership and supervision; motivation and incentives; specific occupations. Also, industrial mental health programmes; occupational roles and status; the relationship between specific personality variables and the work setting; specific psychiatric illnesses as they relate to the job (traumatic neurosis, psychosomatic reactions, and organic brain syndromes are most often discussed); rehabilitation of physically and psychiatrically disabled; psychodynamics of personality functioning in relation to work; the roles of psychiatrist, psychologist, industrial physician, and behavioural scientist; the meaning of work; and the structure, function, and environment of the work organization.

Occupational mental health programmes, then, are concerned with both the psychiatrically ill employee and with factors in the work environment which stimulate mentally health behaviour. This chapter will trace historical influences which have contributed to present practices and discuss current activities in some industrialized societies.

HISTORICAL REVIEW

In the first issue (1917) of the journal *Mental Hygiene* Herman Adler, previously chief of staff of the Boston Psychopathic Hospital, reported on patients for whom unemployment had been a serious problem (Adler 1917). Males between the ages of 25 and 55 were grouped into three classifications: 'paranoid personalities', 'inadequate personalities', and the 'emotionally unstable'. Three years later Mary Jarrett reported a follow-up of this same group, observing that 75 per cent were successfully adjusted from an occupational point of view (Jarrett 1920). Few articles appearing in the literature prior to Adler's 1917 report could properly be included in the emerging field of industrial or occupational psychiatry. Both his work and Jarrett's appear to have resulted from the stimulus of E. E. Southard, Director of the Boston Psychopathic Hospital and Professor of Neuropathology at Harvard.

In 1919 Southard was asked by the Engineering Foundation of New York to investigate emotional problems among workers. Working with a clinical team that included a social worker and a psychologist, he found that '62 per cent of more than 4000 cases reached the discharged status through traits of social incompetence rather than occupational incompetence' (Jarrett 1920). These statistics are still quoted today as a valid representation of a continuing industrial pattern.

The following year Southard (1920) commented as follows:

Industrial medicine exists, industrial psychiatry ought to exist . . . I think that we will have a place in the routine of industrial management not as a permanent staff member (except in very large firms and business systems) but as consultants. The function of this occasional consultant would be preventative rather than curative of the general condition of unrest.

Thus was set down in Boston some 55 years ago an operating philosophy for the occupational mental health professional.

1920–9

The first 'Review of industrial psychiatry' in the *American Journal of Psychiatry* in April, 19

Sherman), summarized the literature to date, defined the field, and traced its development. Mandel Sherman, its author, considered the psychiatrist's rightful area of concern to be the 'individual's adjustment to the situation as a whole'. The psychiatrist also is said to 'attempt to forestall maladjustments by aiding in developing interests and incentives'.

At the conclusion of his first review of the field Sherman said that among the various methods of industrial psychiatry, the most successful procedure used to aid the individual in adjusting to industry had been one which attempted to analyse the total situation—the early life history, the social situation, the worker's motives and incentives, in addition to the immediate difficulties at work. 'Classification of maladjusted individuals into types or groups has been of little help.' His final plea was for vocational guidance during the formative years to obviate many later industrial maladjustments.

The year 1922 saw the introduction of the first full-time psychiatrist in an American business organization of which we have a full description: Lydia Giberson was employed by the Metropolitan Life Insurance Company (Giberson 1936). In 1924 a mental health service was introduced at the R. H. Macy department store. V. V. Anderson (1944) summarized this programme in the first book of industrial psychiatry. In a paper at the eightieth annual meeting of the American Psychiatric Association, also in 1924, Osnato (1925) discussed current concepts of the industrial neuroses, by which he meant post-traumatic reactions. His primary concern was in distinguishing between 'malingerers and hysterics'.

In the 1920s the greatest stimulus to the study of industry as a social organization came from Professor Mayo. Psychiatrists then and now acknowledge his influence on their thinking about the individual and his environment. Professor Mayo became interested in studies on fatigue and monotony at the Harvard Physiology Laboratory. In 1923 he was asked to investigate high labour turnover in a textile mill. He noted that with the introduction of rest periods for workers in monotonous jobs, morale rose and labour turnover decreased.

In 1924 Mayo and his associates undertook a study of working conditions at the Hawthorne Plant of the Western Electric Company in Chicago. In several years of study at this location, 20 000 employees were interviewed and small experimental groups of workers intensively observed as changes were made in their work situation. These studies demonstrated the tremendous importance of human interaction as an integral part of the work situation, and that dissatisfactions arising in or out of the plant become entwined, influencing each other, and affecting work production. Mayo's classic volume, *The human problems of an industrial civilization* (1934), describes this work, as does the book *Management and the Worker* by Roethlisberger and Dickson (1939).

The Hawthorne studies concluded that an industrial enterprise has two functions: economic and social.

Production output was felt to be a form of 'social' behaviour, and all the activity of a plant may be viewed as an interaction of structure, culture, and personality. If any one of these variables is altered, change must occur in the other two. Reactions to stress on the part of individual employees arise when there is resistance to change, when there are faulty control and communications systems, and in the adjustments of the individual worker to his structure at work (Miller and Form 1951).

During the First World War a series of papers from the Industrial Fatigue Research Board in England began to focus attention on the psychological components of industrial accidents (Greenwood 1918), on fatigue, and on psychiatric illness in the work setting (Culpin and Smith 1930). Little mention was made of these studies in American literature until some two decades later. Basic concepts of accident proneness and our first indications of the prevalence of psychiatric disorder in an industrial population came from this work.

The applications of psychiatry to industry in this country during the 1930s are well described in Rennie, *et al.'s* 1947 paper, 'Toward industrial mental health: an historical review'.

1930–9

The depression years were characterized by quiescence in the field; even the annual review was dropped from the *American Journal of Psychiatry*. The major clinical activities were those of Giberson (1936, 1939, 1940) and Burling (1939, 1942), the only psychiatrists operating full-time programmes. Some interest continued to be shown by industrial medicine (Culpin 1936). Mayo's work, which continued well into this decade, was the most significant research of the period.

1940–9

The Second World War had tremendous impact upon clinical applications of the psychiatrist, and to a lesser degree the clinical psychologist, in industry. Concepts of psycho-analytic psychology were introduced and applied. Expectations of industry were high, perhaps unrealistically so, and to a certain extent psychiatry and psychology were 'oversold'. Yet during the war years greater and more sophisticated applications in the mold of Southard, Sherman, and White could be seen (Brody 1945a, b; Ling 1945; Lott 1946; McLean and Taylor 1958).

Of the many documents produced during these years, three will illustrate the pattern of activity during the early 1940s. In a 1943 editorial in the *American Journal of Psychiatry*, C. Macfie Campbell stated that the war had 'swept the psychiatrist out of his hospital wards and his administrative routine'. It was to be hoped, he said, that the psychiatrist would continue 'devoting more attention to that portion of social living which occupies the major portion of an individual's life—his job'.

In 1943 Rosenbaum and Romano discussed workers in the defence industry. They pointed to the need for industrial physicians to concern themselves with the recognition of emotional factors underlying behaviour, which so frequently resulted in inferior output, high sickness rates, high labour turnover, and absenteeism— 'of prime importance under wartime conditions which cannot countenance impaired efficiency'.

Among the many mental health programmes in wartime industry, those concerning the Oak Ridge, Tennessee Industrial community subsequently received major attention (Burlingame 1946, 1947, 1948, 1949). With available psychiatric assistance, primarily through 'emotional first-aid stations', a minimum of on-the-job treatment resulted in conspicuous on-the-job improvement. As in publications prior to the war, psychiatrists outlining their wartime experiences noted that the causes of emotional disturbance in industry lie primarily in the individual or in the home or non-work social surroundings, rather than in the job situation.

Following the war, with the sharp cutback in defence industries which had employed psychiatrists, many industrial mental health programmes came to a halt. Interest in the rehabilitation of the psychiatrically handicapped veteran gave impetus to the development of civilian programmes such as that at Eastman Kodak Company. Successful application of psychiatric skills in the armed forces during the war stimulated the interest of several psychiatrists to broaden their scope of practice and to include preventive concepts born of their experiences in the service.

In the United States, the federal government initiated the Vocational Rehabilitation Act Amendments of 1943 and the Office of Vocational Rehabilitation. Stimulus was given to the training of clinical psychologists in greater numbers, primarily in programmes of the Veterans Administration. Many were subsequently to work in industry.

Roffey Park was established by British industry immediately after the war as an industrial rehabilitation centre for 'neurosis cases'. During the next decade 8000 cases were treated. In the introduction to the volume describing this work, Ling (1945) states that 'Maladjustment to work has been a major factor in the ill health of many of these men and women'. At the Central Institute of Psychiatry in Moscow, Melekhov and his associates also dealt specifically with psychoneurotic Second World War patients. An article by Melekhov outlining the rehabilitation of these patients appeared in *Occupational Therapy and Rehabilitation* in 1947.

In the United States problems of workmen's compensation were receiving increasing attention, since the courts had by then ruled a wide variety of illnesses, including psychiatric, were compensable. Coronary infarcts occurring on the job following occupational stress, hypertension, cancer, and tuberculosis activated by employment, suicide caused by job-related depression, and 'paralysis by fright' had all been awarded claims. This trend has in the 1960s received closer atten-

tion as awards increase for psychiatric disability unrelated to physical accident (Lesser 1967).

The first fellowship programme for training psychiatrists for work in industry was announced in 1948. Under a grant from the Carnegie Corporation, and under the direction of Leighton and Burling, seven psychiatrists were eventually trained at Cornell University's New York State School of Industrial and Labour Relations (Burling and Longaker 1955). The late 1940s also saw the publication of books by Tredgold (1950), Ling (1955), Brodman (1947), and Rennie *et al.* (1950). These and other monographs focused professional interest on the role of the psychiatrist in industry.

Along with continuing concern for the effects of the emotionally disturbed employee on his work environment and the early recognition and treatment of his symptoms came increased attention by psychiatrists for specific problems such as alcoholism, accidents, psychosomatic reactions, the aging worker, the executive and his emotional problems, emphasis on techniques of management education, and the structuring of the work environment. These areas were receiving increasing attention from several of the behavioural science disciplines during the same period.

Labour union interest in the field did not appear *de novo* but took place against a background of several decades of interest by individuals and groups in the labour movement. As far back as 1944 Clayton W. Fountain of the United Auto Workers addressed the American Psychiatric Association of 'Labour's place in an industrial mental health program'. While confirming the interest of the unions in the workers' mental health, he stated that to be acceptable to labour, any programme developed must not be paternalistic, nor should it be used to undermine the grievance procedure or in any other way subvert the union movement (Fountain 1945). These cautions continue to influence labour's attitude toward industrial mental health programmes and have resulted in few programmes being developed under joint sponsorship. Where a company has successfully established a programme that avoids these pitfalls, the union will often work with it in close collaboration, but formal participation is avoided.

1950–60

From the Tavistock Clinic in London came the first volume of the Glacier Metal Company studies, led by Jaques (1952). Both the methodology and the research results of this pilot application of psycho-analytic concepts to organization behaviour had considerable influence on the development of subsequent programmes. Jaques's later concepts of equitable wage payment based on the time span of responsibility inherent in any job were mainly published in the late 1950s and in the 1960s but had their roots in the earlier work (1947, 1951, 1956). The reactions of the management of the Glacier Metal Company were subsequently reported by the chairman of its board of directors, Wilfred Brown (1960).

Kalinowsky's psychiatric study of war veterans in Germany (1950), Pokorny and Moore's 'Neuroses and compensation' (1953), Burling *et al.'s* volume on the hospital (1956), Ross's excellent psychiatric text for the industrial physician (1956), and the Group for the Advancement of Psychiatry's definitive statement on the role of the psychiatrist in industry (1951) are but a few representative samples of United States publications.

During these same first few years of the 1950s Mindus conducted a 6-month survey of industrial psychiatry in Great Britain, the United States, and Canada for the World Health Organization and later developed his own concept of industrial psychiatry (1955). The survey resulted in the most extensive report on programmatic activities in the field (1952). The author visited plants, universities, institutions, agencies, and union facilities, summarizing his observations and relating them to prior experiences in the Scandinavian countries. National committees in the United States included those of the American Psychiatric Association—which served as a clearinghouse of information and represented the official professional viewpoint—the Group for the Advancement of Psychiatry, which continued to evaluate current developments in the field, and, while less active at this time, those of the American Medical Association and the Industrial Medical Association.

This period saw concern for management and executive education with more formalized techniques than previously existed. Laughlin's (1954 a, b; Laughlin and Hall 1951) work with government executives, lectures and seminars sponsored by individual companies and by community agencies such as local mental health associations, and 'sensitivity training' as exemplified by programmes of the National Training Laboratories received considerable attention from psychiatry. A psycho-analytic view of work and employment (Pederson-Krag 1955), significant research on industrial accidents (Schulzinger 1956), and concern with executive mental health, with labour union programmes, and with the rehabilitation of the previously hospitalized psychiatric patient were all subjects of discussion.

Training for psychiatrists, industrial physicians, and executives expanded, particularly with the stimulus of the Menninger Foundation and an enlarging number of other sponsoring agencies including the University of Cincinnati, Cornell University, the National Association for Mental Health, and the American Psychiatric Association. Interest on the part of the lay and business press in industrial mental health programmes became heavier with feature articles in papers such as the *Wall Street Journal*, syndicated stories by a writer for the Associated Press, and articles in *Business Week*, *Fortune*, and the *Saturday Evening Post*.

New full-time psychiatric programmes were begun at International Business Machines Corporation, American Fore Insurance Group, the Metropolitan Life Insurance Company, and elsewhere. At Metropolitan, Giberson, now reporting to an executive vice-president, was no longer associated with the medical department where a psychiatrist was added. With the death of Walter Woodward, the programme at American Cyanamid was discontinued in favour of outside psychiatric consultations. The short-lived programme at General Electric Company in Cincinnati was discontinued in favour of a part-time consultant. James Conant, a clinical psychologist, was added to the medical staff of the General Electric Company at Hanford, Washington, to concentrate of a full-time basis. Research activities under Ross at the University of Cincinnati and Levinson at the Menninger Foundation were instituted.

Books included McLean and Taylor's *Mental health in industry* (1958) and Menninger and Levinson's *Human understanding in industry* (1957). By this time articles and monographs concerning the psychiatrist and clinical psychologist in industry, and publications by them and others about mental health problems in the world of work were issued frequently. The majority of citations in a recent bibliographic definition of occupational mental health, which included nearly 2000 items, appeared during the late 1950s and early 1960s (NIMH 1965). In 1956 Collins, consulting psychiatrist and neurologist for Eastman Kodak Company, assumed responsibility for the annual reviews of occupational psychiatry. He included major contributions and developments in this area at home and abroad (1956, 1959, 1960, 1961a, 1962). Alcoholism, automation, absenteeism, rehabilitation, research, post-traumatic neurotic reactions, the psychological fulfilment of the individual in the work setting, the ever-present, generally descriptive discussions of psychiatric applications in business and industry—these were frequent concerns in the literature.

In 1957 labour movement interest in mental health crystallized around the formation of the National Institute of Labour Education, an organization under the joint directorship of union leaders and mental health professionals. The purpose of this group was to stimulate research and programme development in the area of labour and mental health. As part of this programme two documents (Morrow *et al.* 1959; Reiff and Scribner 1963) have been published to serve as guides to interested professionals.

Mental health care did not appear in union-sponsored insurance programmes until 1959 when Retail Clerks Local 770 in Los Angeles obtained a contract providing funds for psychiatric services. Since that time a number of other programmes have appeared. There has generally been something innovative about each of them. An early one was established by the United Mine Workers of America, which contracted with a private mental hospital in Virginia to serve their members and dependants through a programme of travelling clinics. As the demand for service grew, these clinics became permanent establishments in several communities, partly supported by a retainer from the United Mine Workers and partly from fees from non-union patients (Morrow *et al.* 1959).

1960–70

The first half of the 1960s was marked by continuing

growth and expansion of interest in the field. On the international level a worldwide interest in the mental health implications of the industrial setting was evident in the content of papers read at the Fourteenth International Congress on Occupational Health held in Madrid in 1963. More than 40 presentations were concerned with the psychological problems of the industrial environment. The 1964 annual meeting of the World Federation for Mental Health, held in Berne, had its entire programme devoted to mental health in industry. The First International Congress on Social Psychiatry in London in 1964 included many formal presentations on this topic.

In the United States surveys indicated more than 200 psychiatrists and 150 clinical psychologists active in industry. New professional organizations were created, including the Occupational Psychiatry Group and the Centre for Occupational Mental Health. The former, in New York City, consists of 75 industrial medical directors and psychiatrists who meet five times a year for formal discussions followed by a social hour and dinner. The latter, a non-profit organization, was incorporated in 1963 to collect and disseminate data in the field and develop research and educational programmes and services for the expanding activities of those interested in occupational mental health. It is now a part of Cornell University's Department of Psychiatry.

Significant events in the early 1960s included the omission of the word 'physically' from the title of the President's Committee on the Handicapped, with its subsequent emphasis on the 'mentally restored' and mentally retarded worker. Legal implications from the Carter vs. General Motors case (Waters 1962), where a psychosis was held compensable in the absence of specific physical or psychological trauma, stimulated increased psychiatric attention to matters of workmen's compensation.

In the programme area, new activities continued to develop and old ones to grow. In the universities these ranged in focus from the pure behavioural science research activities of the Institute for Social Research of the University of Michigan (French et al. 1962) through the studies on job satisfactions and psychological growth of Herzberg at Western Reserve University (Herzberg and Hamlin 1963; Herzberg et al. 1959) to the clinical analysis of the organization and application of group dynamics by Argyris (1957, 1960) at Yale.

Under the leadership of Levinson, the Division of Industrial Mental Health of the Menninger Foundation conducted research on the relationship between man and the organization and operated a fellowship programme for psychiatrists in industrial psychiatry and an educational programme for industrial physicians and executives (Levinson et al. 1962).

Industry itself developed a full range of programmes from part-time outside consultants to full-time staff personnel. Their activities might be based on the medical departments or personnel departments or they might report directly to a senior executive. Their work might consist of straightforward clinical evaluation or treatment with varying regard to the circumstance of the work setting, of clinical consultation, education, training, policy consultation, research, or a combination of these; the last arrangement was most common with those spending a major part of their time in the work setting.

Journal articles and books varied in their content from psychodynamic speculations to precise engineering studies of man–machine relationships. Many writers continued the earlier trend of exhorting and directing others to develop better mental health programmes or to become interested in psychiatric problems. Carefully executed clinical research continued to be rare and not often seen in the literature. However, many clinical programmes of fair sophistication have not seen the light of the printed page, the feeling of some companies being that conduct of clinical programmes and the results of behavioural science research within the organization are properly proprietary. Additional reluctance stemmed from professionals conducting such programmes who feel that outlines of their activities are not proper subjects for the scientific literature. And of course many journals discourage such purely descriptive articles in favour of those reporting research results. It is fair to say that the literature does not accurately represent the level of activity in the field.

In the periodical literature, in addition to the occasional individual papers, special sections relating to occupational mental health are appearing from time to time. The greater portion of one issue of *Industrial Medicine and Surgery* (June, 1963) was devoted to 'The worker in the new industrial environment', while a previous issue dealt extensively with 'Emotional problems of executives' (May, 1963), and one complete issue was concerned with 'The impact of psychiatry on American management' (November, 1962).

This decade also produced a number of major publications covering all aspects of occupational mental health. On the clinical side there is a textbook by Collins (1961b). The American Medical Association issued a guide for employability after psychiatric illness (Howe and Wolman 1962). Levinson's *Emotional health in the world of work* appeared in early 1964 to aid executives' understanding of behaviour, and the American Psychiatric Association's Committee on Occupational Psychiatry issued *The mentally ill employee,* a management-oriented guide, in early 1965. Research publications include monographs by Levinson and associates (1962), by the staff of the Institute for Social Research of the University of Michigan (French et al. 1962) and a volume *Mental health of the industrial worker* by Kornhauser (1965). A unique publication is a study of industrial mental health by a group of Harvard Business School graduate students, entitled *The legacy of neglect* (Ferguson et al. 1965).

Publication of a regular newsletter in occupational psychiatry was undertaken by the American Psychiatric Association's Committee on Occupational Psychiatry in 1960. This was superseded in 1965 by *Occupational*

Mental Health Notes, an information bulletin prepared at and issued by the National Clearinghouse for Mental Health Information and containing abstracts of all recent publications in the field.

1970–

In the early 1970s (at least in the United States) there has been a broadening in the areas of interest of those concerned with preventive and therapeutic activities in occupational mental health. Although there continues a literature describing clinical programmes and the role of mental health practitioners in work organizations, there is increasing interest in specific problems such as drug abuse and occupational stress and in more diffuse issues such as the quality of working life. Among clinicians, those in occupational medicine have generally developed a greater level of sophistication in dealing with the emotionally disturbed employee. There appears to be no great increase in the number of psychiatrists and clinical psychologists acting as consultants to medical departments.

In the United States the Occupational Safety and Health Act of 1970 stimulated the development of an increasingly large bureaucracy to monitor health and safety practices but the focus initially has been on the physical environment, on safety standards, and on toxicology. Very little stimulus came from this legislation to foster the expansion of occupational mental health activities. In Great Britain the Robens report, 'Safety and health at work', was presented to Parliament in July 1972. Here again the emphasis is on the administration of occupational safety and health programmes with very little reference to psychological health.

Representative of the interest in occupational stress were volumes edited by Levi (1972), Kearns (1973) and McLean (1974). In addition articles by Levinson (1973), Margolis and Kroes (1974), Kahn (1973), Cobb (1973), and French (1973) address different facets of the topic. These are merely illustrative of wide ranging interest in psychosocial aspects of this ill-defined field.

Drug abuse as an occupational health problem emerged in the late 1960s in the United States as a key issue. Particularly in metropolitan centres, a marked rise in the number of applicants and employees whose use of drugs interfered with employment paralleled increasing national concern with the abuse of 'controlled substances'. In the early 1970s a literature burgeoned, seemingly over-night, directed at general audiences, at management, and at the health professions. A single publisher of scientific and professional literature (Thomas) listed twenty-seven new books in 1972 on drug abuse and in 1973 published two with the same title (*Drug abuse in industry*). By mid-1970 most major employers in the New York City area, at least, had developed guidelines for the employment of persons who were addicted and innumerable conferences had directed the attention of medical directors and corporate management to the problems of work adaptation of the drug-abuser (see Stewart 1970 and McLean and Goldstone 1972).

Meanwhile literature concerned with programmatic implications was enhanced by publications of Collins (1969) and McLean (1970). The quarterly *Occupational Mental Health* published by the Centre for Occupational Mental Health at Cornell began in 1970, replacing the federal publication, *Occupational Mental Health Notes*. Carrying abstracts of relevant documents, original articles, and news germane to the field, its contents in the first three volumes reflect the increasing concern with drugs, stress, and issues such as the employment of the disadvantaged, rehabilitation of psychiatric casualty, social change, aging, and job satisfaction.

The initial interest of the World Health Organization led to a committee of temporary advisers preparing a brief report to frame recommendations for occupational mental health programmes (WHO Temporary Advisers 1972).

Illustrative of clinical approaches to work organizations are, at the one extreme, those of the Industrial Social Welfare Centre of Columbia University (Weiner *et al.* 1973) and, at the other, Levinson's *Organizational diagnosis* (1972). The former describes a pioneering mental health programme for labour union members in New York City; the latter describes application of the individual clinical evaluation format to the work organization itself. Each is innovative in its own way; each may be described as 'hard core' occupational mental health in the United States today.

Considerable attention was focused on issues concerning the quality of working life in the early 1970s. Although thought by some to be peripheral to the health of workers, others (I among them) would suggest that factors in a work environment which encourage healthy behaviour or which moderate feelings of anxiety or depression or withdrawal are a very real concern to the field. An interest in work quality issues, particularly among social scientists is reflected in a burgeoning literature illustrated by a major annotated bibliography (Taylor *et al.* 1973). The introduction to this volume states,

The past several years have seen an increasingly widespread and intense interest in the idea of quality of working life as evidenced by significant recent demonstration of growing governmental and public awareness, such as the following: Senate hearings that led to the first bill in recent years (S.3196) to fund the study of worker alienation and pursue further research on ways to reduce it; the Ford Foundation's sponsorship of an international social scientists' conference on quality of working life; the mass media's recognition of and publicity about quality of working life and effects of ongoing research and action projects; and efforts by business, government, and social science to come to grips with the issues.

A major stimulus to the current level of concern about these issues came in the form of a special task force to the Secretary of Health, Education, and Welfare in December 1972. The name of the task force and its subsequent report was *Work in America*. During an intensive one-year's study thirty-nine papers commissioned in a large group of consultants helped the group focus their materials. The authors conclude in part:

Because work is central to the lives of so many Americans, either the absence of work or employment in meaningless work is creating an increasingly intolerable situation. The human costs of this state of affairs are manifested in worker alienation, alcoholism, drug addiction and other symptoms of poor mental health. Moreover, much of our tax money is expended in an effort to compensate for problems with at least a part of their genesis in the world of work. A large part of the staggering national bill in areas of crime and delinquency, mental and physical health, manpower and welfare are generated in our national policies and attitude toward work. Likewise, industry is paying for a continued attachment to Tayloristic practices through low worker productivity and high rates of sabotage, absenteeism, and turnover. Unions are paying through the faltering loyalty of a young membership that is increasingly concerned about the occurrent disinterest of its leadership in problems of job satisfaction. Most important, there are high costs of lost opportunities to encourage citizen participation: the discontent of women, minorities, blue collar workers, youth, and older adults would be considerably less were these Americans to have an active role in the decisions in the work place that most directly affect their lives.

The above represents fully half of the brief concluding chapter. Secretary of Health, Education, and Welfare 1972)

SUMMARY

This chapter samples activities in the field of occupational mental health in the United States in an historical context. It obviously represents my biases, my interests, and associations. In no way is it intended to be inclusive in some ways it offers a definition of our field of concern.

At least two themes seem to emerge. Perhaps the most significant is that relatively little progress has been made over the past fifty years in the most developed countries—progress, that is, toward enhancing the mental health of employee population. There has been a great deal of churning; the numbers of clinicians employed in occupational settings is relatively high—but only relative to the very few who pioneered these efforts in the 1920s and 1930s. And the actual service functions have not kept pace with the expansion seen in clinical sciences elsewhere.

There are many more social scientists actively studying the world of work than there are clinicians and here perhaps we can acknowledge some modest strides in understanding the many forces operative upon an employee and his work organization. Many of these insights however relate but tangentially to health and few are acknowledged by the clinicians.

A second theme may not be so clear. That is, the literature of the social sciences is generally unfamiliar to the clinicians and vice versa. For that matter, among many of the same disciplines there is surprisingly little international communication, particularly across language barriers. How many English-speaking readers for instance are aware of Haruhara's work in Tokyo or the work of Bogganovich in the Soviet Union in the prevention of emotional disturbances among production line workers? Serious communication gaps exist; if anything they widen as greater knowledge and experience is developed but not transmitted. It is for this reason that seminars such as those which produced this volume are of such tremendous value.

REFERENCES

ADLER, H. M. (1917). Unemployment and personality. *Ment. Hyg.*, **1**, 16.

American Psychiatric Association Committee on Occupational Psychiatry (1965). *The mentally ill employee: his treatment and rehabilitation. A guide for management.* New York.

ANDERSON, V. B. (1944). Psychiatry in industry. *Amer. J. Psychiat.*, **100**, 134.

ARGYRIS, C. (1957). *Personality and organization.* New York.

——, (1960). *Understanding organizational behavior.* Homewood, Illinois.

BRODMAN, K. (1947). *Man at work—the supervisor and his people.* Chicago, Illinois.

BRODY, M. (1945a). Dynamics of mental hygiene in industry. *Indust. Med.*, **14**, 760.

——, (1945b). Neuropsychiatry and placement of industrial workers. *Conn. Med.*, **9**, 84.

BROWN, W. (1960). *Exploration in management.* New York.

BURLING, T. (1939). Personality and the economic situation. *Amer. J. Orthopsychiat.*, **9**, 616.

——, (1942). The role of the professionally trained mental hygienist in business. *Amer. J. Orthopsychiat.*, **11**, 48.

——, LENTZ, E. M., and WILSON, R. N. (1956). *The give and take in hospitals.* New York.

——, and LONGAKER, W. (1955). Training for industrial psychiatry. *Amer. J. Psychiat.*, **111**, 493.

BURLINGAME, C. C. (1946). Psychiatry in industry. *Amer. J. Psychiat.*, **103**, 549.

——, (1947). Psychiatry in industry. *Amer. J. Psychiat.*, **104**, 493.

——, (1948). Psychiatry in industry. *Amer. J. Psychiat.*, **105**, 538.

——, (1949). Psychiatry in industry. *Amer. J. Psychiat.*, **106**, 520.

CAMPBELL, C. M. (1943). The psychiatrist and industrial organization. *Amer. J. Psychiat.*, **100**, 286.

COBB, S. (1973). Role responsibility: the differentiation of a concept. *Occupational Mental Health*, **3**, (1).

COLLINS, R. T. (1956). Industrial psychiatry. *Amer. J. Psychiat.*, **112**, 546.

——, (1957). Industrial psychiatry. *Amer. J. Psychiat.*, **113**, 633.

——, (1958). Industrial psychiatry. *Amer. J. Psychiat.*, **114**, 627.

——, (1959). Industrial psychiatry. *Amer. J. Psychiat.*, **115**, 630.

——, (1960). Occupational psychiatry. *Amer. J. Psychiat.*, **116**, 608.

——, (1961a). Occupational psychiatry. *Amer. J. Psychiat.*,

117, 605.

——, (1962). Occupational psychiatry. *Amer. J. Psychiat.*, **118**, 604.

——, (1961b). *A manual of neurology and psychiatry in occupational medicine.* New York.

——, (ed.) (1969). *Occupational psychiatry.* Boston, Massachusetts.

Culpin, M. (1936). Psychological disorders in industry: symposium on industrial medicine. *Practitioner*, **137**, 324.

——, and Smith, M. (1930). *The nervous temperament.* Government Publications—Medical Research Council, Industrial Health Research Board, Report No. 61. His Majesty's Stationery Office, London.

Ferguson, C. A., Fersing, J. E., Allen, A. T., Baugh, N. P., Gilmore, G. A., Humphrey, J. W., McConnell, F. E., Mitchell, J. W., Sauer, J. W., and Scott, T. J. (1965). *The legacy of neglect: an appraisal of the implications of emotional disturbances in the business environment.* Fort Worth, Texas.

Fountain, C. W. (1945). Labor's place in an industrial mental health program. *Ment. Hyg.*, **29**, 95.

French, J. R. P. (1973). Person role fit. *Occupational Mental Health* **3** (1).

——, Kahn, R. L., and Mann, F. C. (eds.) (1962). Work, health and satisfaction. *J. Soc. Issues*, **18**, 1.

Giberson, L. G. (1936). Psychiatry in industry. *Personnel J.* **15**, 91.

——, (1939). Emotional first-aid stations. *Personnel J.* **16**, 1.

——, (1940). Pitfalls in industry for the psychiatrist. *Med. Wom. J.*, **45**, 144.

Greenwood, M. (1918). *A report on the cause of wastage of labour in munition factories.* Government Publications–Medical Research Council. His Majesty's Stationery Office, London.

Group for the Advancement of Psychiatry, Committee on Psychiatry in Industry (1951). *The application of psychiatry to industry.* (GAP Report No. 20), New York.

Herzberg, F., and Hamlin, R. M. (1963). The motivation-hygiene concept of psychotherapy. *Ment. Hyg.*, **45**, 384.

——, Mausner, B., and Synderman, B. (1959). *The motiviation to work.* New York.

Howe, H. F. and Wolman, W. (1962). Guide for evaluating employability after psychiatric illness. *J. Amer. Med. Assoc.*, **181**, 1086.

Jaques, E. (1947). Some principles of organization of a social therapeutic institution. *J. Soc. Issues*, **3**, 4.

——, (1951). Standard earning progression curves. *Human Relations* **11**, 167.

——, (1952). *The changing culture of a factory.* New York.

——, (1956). *Measurement of responsibility,* Cambridge, Massachusetts.

Jarrett, M. C. (1920). The mental hygiene of industry. Report of progress on work undertaken under the Engineering Foundation of New York City, *Mental Hyg.*, **4**, 867.

Kahn, R. L. (1973). Conflict, ambiguity and overload: three elements of job stress. *Occupational Mental Health*, **3**, (1).

Kalinowsky, L. B. (1950). Problems of war neuroses in the light of experience in other countries. *Amer. J. Psychiat.*, **107**, 340.

Kearns, J. L. (1973). *Stress in industry.* London.

Kornhauser, A. (1965). *Mental health of the industrial worker.* New York.

Lapinsky, E. (1965). The future of health in industry. *Indust. Med. Surg.*, **34**, 71.

Laughlin, H. P. (1954a). An approach to executive development: Five years' experience with analytically oriented groups of executives. *Dis. Nerv. Syst.*, **15**, 12.

——, (1954b). Seminars with executives on human relations in the United States Government. *Int. J. Group Psychother.*, **4**, 165.

——, and Hall, M. (1951). Psychiatry for executives: An experiment in the use of group analysis to improve relationships in an organization. *Amer. J. Psychiat.*, **107**, 493.

Lesser, P. J. (1967). The legal viewpoint. In *To Work is human* (ed. A. McLean), Chapter 8. New York.

Levi, L (1972). *Stress and distress in response to psychosocial stimuli.* Oxford.

Levinson, H. (1964). *Emotional health: in the world of work.* New York.

——, (1972). *Organizational diagnosis.* Cambridge, Massachusetts.

——, (1973). A psychoanalytic view of occupational stress. *Occupational Mental Health*, **3** (2).

——, Price, C. R., Munden, K. J., Mandl, H. J., and Solley, C. M. (1962). *Men, management and mental health.* Cambridge, Massachusetts.

Ling, T. M. (1945). Roffey Park Rehabilitation Centre. *Lancet*, **i**, 283.

——, (ed.) (1955). *Mental health and human relations in industry.* New York.

Lott, G. M. (1946). Emotional first-aid stations in industry. *Industr. Med.*, **15**, 419.

Margolis, B. K. and Kroes, W. H. (1974). Occupational stress and strain. In *Occupational stress* (ed. A. A. McLean), p. 15. Springfield, Illinois.

Mayo, E. (1934). *The human problems of an industrial civilization.* New York.

McLean, A. (ed.) (1970). *Mental health and work organizations.* Chicago, Illinois.

——, (ed.) (1974). *Occupational stress.* Springfield, Illinois.

—— and Goldstone, S. (1972). Occupational outcome for treated heroin addicts. *Occupational Mental Health*, **2** (3).

—— and Taylor, G. C. (1958). *Mental health in industry.* New York.

Melekhov, D. E. (1947). Rehabilitation of psychoneurotic World War II patients in the U.S.S.R. *Occup. Therapy*, **26**, 388.

Menninger, W. C. and Levinson, H. (1957). *Human understanding in industry: a guide for supervisors.* Chicago.

Miller, D. C. and Form, W. H. (1951). *Industrial sociology.* New York.

Mindus, E. (1952). *Industrial psychiatry in Great Britain, the United States, and Canada. A report to the World Health Organization.* Stockholm.

——, (1955). Outlines of a concept of industrial psychiatry. *Bull. WHO*, **13**, 561.

Morrow, J. K., King, J. P., Chiles, D. D., and Painter, T. E. (1959). The bituminous coal country: A psychiatric frontier. *W. Virginia Med. J.*, **55**, 164.

National Institute of Mental Health: Selected Bibliography on Occupational Mental Health (Public Health Service Publication No. 1338) (1965). Bethesda, Maryland.

Osnato, M. (1925). Industrial neuroses. *Amer. J. Psychiat.*, **82**, 117.

Pederson-Krag, G. (1955). *Personality factors in work and employment.* New York.

Pokorny, A. D. and Moore, F. J. (1953). Neuroses and compensation. *A.M.A. Arch. Industr. Hyg.*, **8**, 547.

Reiff, R. and Scribner, S. (1963). *Issues in the New National Mental Health Program relating to labor and low-income groups: Report No. 1.* National Institute of Labor Education, New York.

Rennie, T. A. C., Burling, T., and Woodward, L. E. (1950).

Vocational rehabilitation of psychiatric patients. New York.
—— SWACKHAMER, G., and WOODWARD, L. E. (1947). Toward industrial mental health: An historical review. *Ment. Hyg.,* **31,** 66.

ROBENS, LORD (1972). *Safety and health at work, report of the Committee 1970–72.* Her Majesty's Stationery Office, London.

ROETHLISBERGER, F. J. and DICKSON, W. J. (1939). *Management and the worker.* Cambridge, Massachusetts.

ROSENBAUM, M. and ROMANO, J. (1943). Psychiatric casualties among defense workers. *Amer. J. Psychiat.,* **100,** 314.

ROSS, W. D. (1956). *Practical psychiatry for industrial physicians.* Springfield, Illinois.

SCHULZINGER, M. S. (1956). *The accident syndrome.* Springfield, Illinois.

Secretary of Health, Education, and Welfare, Report of a Special Task Force to (1972). *Work in America.* Cambridge, Massachusetts.

SHERMAN, M. (1927). A review of industrial psychiatry. *Amer. J. Psychiat.,* **83,** 701.

SOUTHARD, E. E. (1920). The modern specialist in unrest: a place for the psychiatrist in industry. *Ment. Hyg.,* **4,** 550.

STEWART, W. W. (ed.) (1970). *Drug abuse in industry.* Miami, Florida.

TAYLOR, J. C., LANDY, J., LEVINE, M., and KAMATH, D. R. (1973). *The quality of working life: an annotated bibliography.* Los Angeles, California.

TREDGOLD, R. F. (1950). *Human relations in modern industry.* New York.

WATERS, T. C. (1962). Mental illness: Is it compensable? *Arch. Environ. Health,* **5,** 178.

WEINER, H., AKABAS, S. and SOMMER, J. (1973). *Mental health care in the world of work.* New York.

WHO Temporary Advisors (1972). *Occupational mental health-report of a meeting.* Geneva.

33. AUTONOMY AND PARTICIPATION AT WORK

BERTIL GARDELL

THEORETICAL ASPECTS AND DEFINITION

The question of the relationships between job design and job involvement and their bearing on industrial democracy has been highlighted by the experiments with 'automonous groups' that have been conducted in Norway by Thorsrud (Thorsrud and Emery 1969). One of the fundamental ideas here seems to be that an active orientation towards working life and the demand for worker participation in company affairs are generally favoured by autonomy and the right to determine activities in one's own job. Hypotheses to this effect have also been formulated by Dahlström (1969). In a study of the human condition in large-scale, highly mechanized industry in Sweden the most important finding was that at work places where production technology and organization restrict the individual's say in his own job performance there arises a passive, alienative type of adjustment that stresses the instrumentality of work. In other words, the job is valued only as a means for the satisfaction of needs via different forms of consumption. The work itself is considered trivial and uninteresting, which in our terminology means that it will be assigned a low needs-satisfying value (Gardell 1971a). The findings also show that these feelings of alienation go together with generally lower life satisfactions, with lower self-confidence, and with a higher degree of anxiety. Given the value judgements implicit in the study, we hold these relationships to indicate that the alienative adjustment model makes a poor mechanism for resolving conflicts between the efficiency demanded by the industrial production system and the individual's need for autonomy and the full realization of his human resources.

It is now relevant to ask: Does the passive, alienative adjustment model, and the lower self-confidence that flows from it, also lower aspirations to influence decisions in the firm ('participative management')? In other words, we want to know whether the prospects for involving broader groups in the work organization's decision-making processes—and hence in a change of their own situation in the job world—are influenced by production technology and work design and by the interest or lack of interest in work that is generated thereby. The experiments made by Thorsrud and his colleagues in Norway have apparently not been evaluated from this aspect, even though he operates with a hypothesis of this nature; on the contrary, Thorsrud seems to have confined himself to certain attempts to evaluate the connection between increased autonomy on the one hand and work commitment and productivity on the other. The foregoing also seems to hold true of most experiments with job enrichment and other types of organizational changes that strive towards greater autonomy, but, in contrast with Thorsrud's work, these experiments have usually not been fitted into the larger perspective of industrial democracy. However, the experience gained to date—including our own findings—suggest that increased autonomy is accompanied by increased interest in work, from which it follows that these studies can be held to have confirmed Stage 1 of the hypothesis.

Our research material affords certain opportunities to study the relationship in a non-experimental situation between objectively existing differences as regards autonomy at work, job involvement, and aspirations to influence, both for the individual and for the employees as a group. Consequently it would be possible to test the second stage of the hypothesis, namely that increased autonomy plus related greater commitment to work and increased self-confidence will intensify aspirations to exercise personal influence not only over decisions affecting the immediate job but also over higher-level decisions relating to the firm's management, finances, technological advance, etc. The assumption we are going to test is schematically summarized in Fig. 33.1.

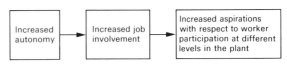

FIG. 33.1. A model relating autonomy at work, job involvement, and aspiration to influence.

Even if one can never be quite confident about the meaning of cross-sectional relationships, we feel that there are certain methodological advantages in testing the assumption of a relationship between autonomy at work and aspirations to decision-making influence in a non-experimental situation, since then we need not be apprehensive that any experimental effect will make it hard to interpret the relationship obtained. This risk of unintended experimental effects will always arise in a planned change situation, especially if the changes involve such sensitive issues as worker participation in management decisions. At the same time, of course, it is only by means of real-life experiments or changes that ideas can be subjected to practical application and testing. We feel that it may be easier to evaluate such experiments by having access at the same time to data from non-experimental situations and that our study may be able to further understanding of how production technology affects the potentialities for getting broader groups committed to greater involvement in the decision processes of the employing firm.

Adapting a terminology introduced by Dahlström (1969, pp. 50–60), we have tried to uphold two distinctions. The first concerns the form of influence or participation, where we distinguish between (a) direct decision-making influence for oneself i.e. *personal level,* and (b) decision-making influence for the employees as a collective, i.e. *group level.* The latter form refers to representative democracy at work places, i.e. to participation of the kind that is looked after by the formal system of industrial relations.† The other distinction concerns the substance of participation, where we distinguish between (a) autonomy over work performance, i.e. *job level*; (b) decision-making influence over the personal work situation i.e. *team/department level*; and (c) decision-making influence over general management policy, i.e. *plant level.*

As to the strength and diffusion of worker demands, we assume that these will vary with the existing opportunities for participation. The picture we therefore envisage is one where personal aspirations to decision-making influence at job and team levels will be more widespread than personal aspirations to influence decisions at plant level. The actual state of affairs, of course, is for the workers to have most to say about doing their own jobs and least about how their company is run, so any aspirations in the latter respect should reasonably be expected to be adjusted to square with this reality. As to aspirations on the part of employees to exercise influence as a collective, we proceed on the following tentative assumption. Since Sweden has long had national agreements on collaboration and worker participation, thereby serving to institutionalize this form of influence in our system of collective bargaining, the individual employees will translate part of their aspirations to influence plant level decision processes to this system of representative democracy. Accordingly we expect personal aspirations to direct influence at plant level to be lower than aspirations to influence the same decision processes through the medium of employee representatives. We assume, however, that such aspirations, both for oneself and for the employees as a group, will intensify with growing autonomy in the individual job. These problems will be dealt with in the next section.

At the same time we expect *the degree of success for representative democracy* to affect the individual worker's aspiration to greater personal influence. This latter problem complex will be discussed later in this chapter.

The opportunities open to us are to proceed from the actual differences among jobs with respect to autonomy, as expressed by our overall measure of job content called

† In this study reference is made to the influence of local union representatives through collective bargaining and through different forms of joint bodies covered by the 1966 National Agreement on Work Councils in Sweden.

'the level of *discretion and skill (D–S level)*' associated with the particular job. This measure contains a series of relevant work characteristics such as the exercise of *discretion* as regards working pace, working method, impact on production quality, etc., and requirements with respect to manual and social *skills.* Measures of job involvement and different aspects of job satisfaction as well as demands for increased worker participation have been collected through questionnaires and interviews with workers in different types of jobs. (For a more detailed description of the D–S level, as well as attitude measures used see Gardell 1971a, p. 150.)

The material is drawn from two paper and pulp plants (process industry) and two metal-working industries with a mixture of mass-production and batch characteristics. Within each industry the two plants belong to the same company and all plants are located in small industrial towns. In all, the sample consists of 33? workers from process industry distributed among 13? different jobs, and 640 metal workers distributed among 128 different jobs.

RELATIONSHIP BETWEEN AUTONOMY AND INVOLVEMENT IN PRESENT WORK AND THE DESIRE FOR MORE DECISION-MAKING INFLUENCE

Our aim in this section will be to test the question that most directly bears upon our main problem, namely whether the degree of autonomy over work performance and its influence on work commitment is related to the individual's aspiration to influence *at job and plant level.* Such an assumption will be found in the experimental studies carried out by Thorsrud and Emery (1969).

It has not been possible in the present study to measure in-depth employee aspirations to participate in different types of decisions. We have measured the aspirations with a couple of direct, generally worded questions by which we sought to obtain an expression for a general emotional readiness or interest in increasing personal influence over decisions at job and plant level. It goes without saying that results based on such simple measuring methods should be interpreted with caution. It is also important to observe that answers to questions of this type are likely to be highly sensitive to the state of opinion in the domain that these questions touch upon.

Data were collected from 1966 to 1968, i.e. before the Swedish debate on work environment and industrial democracy entered a more intensive phase and before the political parties had spelled out a proper policy on these issues. That in itself is all to the good, since the results might otherwise have been influenced by this public debate. Were the same questions to be put today, a different set of responses would probably be obtained. For this reason, any conclusions as to the *absolute level* of the decision-making aspirations that we obtain through our questions should be interpreted with the utmost caution. On the other hand it seems feasible to use the

280

answers to draw *relative* comparisons between groups that diverge in various respects. Our primary interest then is in the *direction* taken by the relationships between job content and aspirations to worker participation in the plant.

Autonomy and aspirations towards increased influence

If we first look at the relationship between *degree of autonomy in present work* and the desire for more personal influence, we can draw upon our job content measure relating to the discretion and skill level of the job (D–S level). The correlations between D–S level of the present job and the desire for more decision-making influence are set out in Table 33.1 by type of industry. Table 33.1 may be read off as follows:

TABLE 33.1

Correlation between D–S level of present job and desire to increase decision-making influence

D–S level of present job	Desire to increase personal influence over decisions at plant level	Desire to increase personal influence over decisions at team/department level
Pulp and paper		
1 Low ($N = 90$)	3·44	2·07
2 Mean ($N = 157$)	3·16	1·82
3 High ($N = 92$)	2·87	1·75
	$p(t)$ 1–3 = 0·000	$p(t)$ 1–3 = 0·024
Engineering industry		
Low ($N = 228$)	3·34	2·20
Mean ($N = 201$)	3·46	2·23
High ($N = 211$)	3·31	2·15
	NS	NS

low values = strong desire to increase decision-making influence.

(1) The desire for greater personal influence at team/department level is more widespread than the desire for personal influence at plant level. This finding is valid for both the industrial types investigated. In an earlier publication we presented figures from five other firms together with those from the firms included in the present study (Gardell 1969, p. 87). This series of responses shows a very uniform picture: 15–35 per cent want to exercise greater influence at plant level, whereas 68–81 per cent would like to have more personal influence over the immediate job situation. The primary concern of workers with matters affecting their own jobs is natural enough, especially when one considers that the firms investigated are of medium or large size. The actual opportunities available to individuals in large organiza-

tions for bringing greater influence to bear on overall management policies are, as we all know, very small. Obviously, this does not preclude the existence of a widespread desire to obtain greater influence *for the employees as a group* over decisions at plant level. Of the workers employed with the forestry and engineering companies we studied, no more than 13–17 per cent are of the opinion that the employees as a group have an adequate say in management decisions; a similar opinion was held by 30–35 per cent of the workers employed in flow-process plants. These figures may be interpreted as signifying the presence of a widespread desire to increase influence in the firm for the employees as a group.

(2) Workers in *pulp and paper mills* who enjoy substantial autonomy (high D–S level) in their present work have *higher* aspirations to greater personal influence over decisions both at plant level and at team/department level. This relationship between job content and demand for increased worker participation is especially clear-cut with respect to demands for participation at plant level.

(3) By contrast, the results from the engineering industry lend no support to these ideas, but then again they do not point to the movement of any correlations in the opposite direction. Although it is hard to say anything with certainty about what the differences among different types of industry might be due to, it seems reasonable to invoke differences of integration and continuity of production, signifying that process workers assigned to skilled tasks are quite unlike their craft-based counterparts in engineering in their dependence on the production flow and their ability to grasp its total structure.

In our sample most of the highly skilled engineering workers are tool-makers and deal with a well-defined task which is more or less detached from the rest of the production flow, from which it may be inferred that they enjoy a higher degree of autonomy over performance compared with the skilled process workers. The latter are brought into a highly integrated production chain, where planning flaws or errors at an earlier stage in the process noticeably affect their ability to perform their own work satisfactorily. It may safely be assumed that not only are the process workers aware of these shortcomings, but that they also have ideas about setting them aright, provided only they are permitted a greater role in the work planning.

We consider that this state of affairs may well explain the higher aspirations to influence over work planning among the process workers, which also makes it reasonable to suggest that these aspirations extend to more general decision processes at plant level because of the more tangible link between these and the process workers' own working situation. Obviously the same kind of link exists in batch manufacturing, but it is not as evident as in a highly integrated flow process. Besides, it appears as though vertical contacts are more pronounced in the process industry, indicating that process workers already have some ingrained habits of communicating face to face with technical experts and line superiors—a fact that no doubt in its turn makes them aspire more to influencing management decisions. Then, too, the skilled process workers—and here they contrast sharply with their counterparts in engineering—can imagine being promoted upwards on the hierarchical ladder (Gardell 1971b, p. 311).

However, any attempt to extend this interpretation would require follow-up analyses of a kind beyond our present means, so we present out interpretation here as no more than an interesting possibility.

Job involvement and aspiration towards increased influence

The second main question in this section is to find out whether subjectively felt job involvement relates in any way to interest in increased decision-making influence. This question becomes relevant in the light of what we know about a generally positive relationship between autonomy and job involvement, and also in the light of the theory that a more widespread interest among workers in participating in management decisions is encouraged by high autonomy, high interest in work, and involvement in problems of the work place. However, we also know that a smaller group reacts to work as interesting and motivating *despite* low autonomy and low D–S level of the job. We shall therefore keep this group separate from the larger group which has a high D–S level and high job involvement. This concurrent breakdown by D–S level and job involvement is shown in Tables 33.2 and 33.3.

The first thing to notice in Tables 33.2 and 33.3 is that both industries contain roughly twice as many individuals in those groups which attach interest to jobs of high D–S level compared with those working in jobs of low D–S level. Second, the tables show—and this is the central point—that *wider aspirations to increased decision-making influence are more common among those individuals who are involved in high D–S level jobs.* This relation holds for both industrial types and for decisions both at team and at plant level. By contrast, a monotonous, unskilled job felt to be interesting and involving does not combine with more elaborate aspira-

tions to increased decision-making influence to such a great extent. In the latter case the attitude to work should probably be interpreted as manifesting generally low aspirations. Hence it is not the attitude to work *per se* that seems to be most crucial: rather, it is not until high involvement can be seen as flowing from greater autonomy and more highly skilled tasks that we can expect a process that also leads to higher aspirations to influence decisions over the immediate job and over management policies.

These findings are important because they stress the necessity of structural changes in work organization and job design for instilling a more active orientation towards decision processes at different levels in the plant. It is not until job involvement has its counterpart in objective properties of job content, here embodied by discretionary factors and skill requirements, that the psychological processes leading to a more active orientation towards higher-level decision processes will be triggered.

At the same time the results show a clearer relationship within the process industry, and it is possible that increased autonomy over the immediate job, unrelated to production as a whole, will not intensify interest in participating in higher-level decision processes to the same extent as when production processes are more integrated. As we see it, these relationships between technology, work content, and aspirations to decision-making influence, both at team and at plant level, deserve attention for purposes of projects seeking to extend industrial democracy.

ASPIRATIONS TO INCREASED COLLECTIVE INFLUENCE AND ITS RELATIONSHIP TO SKILL LEVEL AND AUTONOMY OF TASKS AS WELL AS TO SUCCESS OF REPRESENTATIVE DEMOCRACY AT THE WORKPLACE

When by way of introduction we referred to the system of collective bargaining and the agreements governing industrial relations that have long existed in Sweden, we suggested that the consequence was for the employees to

TABLE 33.2

Desire for increased influence at plant level among groups with high job involvement and low or high D–S level in present work

	Pulp and paper	Engineering
Low D–S level	$N = 26$	$N = 51$
High job involvement	3·46	3·80
High D–S level	$N = 46$	$N = 118$
High job involvement	2·89	3·46

5- point scale; low values = strong desire for increased influence.

TABLE 33.3

Desire for increased influence at team/department level among groups with high job involvement and low or high D–S level in present work

	Pulp and paper	Engineering
Low D–S level	$N = 26$	$N = 51$
High job involvement	2·15	2·94
High D–S level	$N = 46$	$N = 118$
High job involvement	1·80	2·32

5-point scale; low values = strong desire for increased influence express their aspirations to influence over management policies by way of representative democracy in the firms. Given the established forms of collaboration that have long been operating in Swedish working life, it is reasonable to expect that aspirations to influence via the representative system would be higher than aspirations to influence for oneself over higher-level decisions. At the same time it is plausible to imagine:

(1) That the demands of individual employees to greater collective influence over management policies will grow with a higher degree of autonomy over the immediate job in the same way as has been shown earlier for aspirations to increased influence for oneself;
(2) That the degree of success for *representative democracy* in the firm will intensify individual aspirations to *direct democracy,* i.e. increase the aspirations to exercise more personal influence at plant level.

These questions seem to be well worth testing, not least in view of two contentions put forward in the debate on industrial democracy—*first* that increased autonomy at work will lessen the interest in influence by way of representative democracy; and *second* that a successful representative democracy lessens the opportunities for, and hence the aspirations of, individual employees to exercise personal influence in the firm. Obviously we do not lay claim to being able to exhaust these vital issues, but we nevertheless feel that our material opens up some intriguing possibilities.

The first question, i.e. whether demands to increased influence for the employees as a group grow with greater autonomy, was tested with one question put in the pulp and paper industry and three questions put in the engineering industry. Here we proceeded from subjectively perceived decision-making influence, reckoning that those who are unhappy about influence for the employees as a group will express a desire to exercise more such influence. Our hope was that this indirect method of measuring the level of aspirations to collective influence would better reflect the individual's attitude than a more direct question, in which case the answers might well have been biased because of official ideology or made socially desirable for other reasons.

Respondents in both industrial types were asked about influence for the employees at plant level. Two additional questions were put in the engineering industry about employee influence over the firm's future planning and personnel policy. The results may be read from Table 33.4, which for both industrial types shows that aspirations to greater influence at plant level for the workers as a group rise in tandem with rising skill and autonomy in one's own job. The two questions exclusively confined to the engineering industry strengthen the tendency taken by the correlations. Hence it may safely be concluded that there is great interest among the more highly skilled workers in increased collective influence in working life. Our data lend no support to the view that increased autonomy and its related variable, increased job involvement, would *lessen* the interest among individual workers to exercise influence by way of representative democracy.

The central result, however, is that all the correlations found are weak. This suggests that the aspirations to greater influence for the employees as a group essentially derive from other factors, presumably of a more macro

TABLE 33.4

Correlation of D–S level and aspirations for the employees as a group to influence decisions at plant level

	Desires increased collective influence over corporate management in general	Desires increased collective influence over firm's future plans	Desires increased collective influence over firm's personnel policy
Engineering industry D–S level			
Low ($N = 228$)	2·53	2·49	2·50
High ($N = 211$)	2·34	2·26	2·33
	$p(t) = 0·068$ NS	$p(t) = 0·020$	$p(t) = 0·068$ NS
Pulp and paper D–S level			
Low ($N = 90$)	3·00		
High ($N = 92$)	2·62		
	$p(t) = 0·020$		

5-point scale, low values = high aspirations to influence for the employees as a group.

and ideological nature, and are not very much influenced by those psychological motivation mechanisms which are bound up with job content.

As to the second question—whether success for the system of representative democracy in the firm will raise individual aspirations to exercise personal influence at plant level—we elected to test it with reference to the results we obtained in the present study as well as through data collected in five additional firms where the same questions were asked. The matter at issue is whether subjectively perceived success for the employee representatives will increase personal aspirations to influence in the firm; or, conversely, whether successful representative democracy lessens interest in direct democracy.

If we proceed from the ratings of perceived influence, the enterprises in our studies can be divided into three categories: (1) the insurance company; (2) the process industries; and (3) the engineering and forestry companies. These three categories depict a falling scale of perceived success for the representatives of employees in terms of their influence in the firm. For each of these levels of success one can then study the answers to the question about desiring enlarged decision-making influence in the firm for *oneself*. This has been done in Table 33.5, which shows in the main that the different levels of success for the employee representatives are accompanied by commensurate differences of aspirations to increased personal influence. The following tentative inference may be drawn from Table 33.5. In firms where the employees feel that representative democracy gives them relatively great influence (the insurance company and the processing industries), the aspirations to enlarged influence for oneself will be relatively great; whereas in those firms where the employees as a group are felt to exert slight influence (engineering plants and forestry companies), then the demands for personal influence will be weak. In other words, there appears to be no contradiction between a successful representative democracy and aspirations to direct democracy; on the contrary, it may be possible that a strong representative democracy stimulates the individuals to develop aspirations and interest in direct personal participation in decision processes at plant level.

RELATIONSHIPS BETWEEN PERCEIVED INFLUENCE CRITERIA OF JOB SATISFACTION

In the previous sections we have dealt with fairly complex and elusive relationships between technology, job involvement, and aspirations to decision-making influence, and have sought to demonstrate how a more active orientation towards the firm's decision processes is concurrently dependent upon technology and job content and the status of representative democracy. This active orientation towards work deriving from increased autonomy, more highly skilled jobs, and a well-functioning representative democracy is something we regard in two ways: first, as a goal in itself, permitting the expression of greater self-esteem and greater job satisfaction; and second, as a condition to be met before a more wide-spread interest in the firm's decision processes can be developed, which in its turn must necessarily precede the further development of industrial democracy.

It follows that the efforts to develop industrial democracy operate with an assumption that greater influence for the employees will increase job satisfaction. If the trend towards a more democratic working life is to make any sense to the individual employee, it should also be possible for him to see and feel that his day-to-day working conditions are being improved in various respects.

One approach to a study of this assumption is to find out whether persons who differ on the influence criterion also differ in their job satisfaction. Concerning the correlations between *autonomy* over immediate work performance and job satisfaction, these were accounted for at the first WHO Symposium on *Society, stress and disease,* where it was particularly shown that feelings of alienation from work diminished with rising degree of autonomy at work (Gardell 1971a, pp. 155 ff). No equivalent objective measure of decision-making influence at the team/department and plant levels is at our disposal; in this case we shall have to proceed from *subjectively perceived decision-making influence.*

In the present section we propose to take up the question of how perceived decision-making influence at the team/department level and the plant level relates not only to feelings of alienation from work but also to other criteria of job satisfaction. In line with the distinctions drawn in the first section, we shall now distinguish between (1) *perceived personal influence over the immediate work situation* (personal level, team/department level); and (2) *perceived decision-making influence for the employees as a group over general management policies* (group level, plant level). The answers to the questions on perceived decision-making influence were treated to impute satisfactory influence to those who provided any of the 'yes' alternatives and unsatisfactory decision-making influence to those who provided any of the 'no' alternatives. Persons who answered neither 'yes' nor 'no' to the question of whether they felt their influence was large enough were excluded from the analysis. These expressions of perceived decision-making influence formed the independent variable, which was then tested against different criteria of job satisfaction. The results, set out in Figs. 33.2–33.5, may be read as

(1) The facilities for discussing and affecting the immediate work situation are thought to be greater in the engineering industry compared with the pulp and paper industry, which is plausible enough considering the technology and degree of integration embodied in the manufacturing process. However, the differences of

TABLE 33.5

Relation between perceived influence by local union and aspirations to increased personal participation at plant level

	Insurance company N = 280 (per cent)	Pulp and paper I N = 230 (per cent)	Pulp and paper II N = 184 (per cent)	Chemical products N = 87 (per cent)	Engineering plant I N = 255 (per cent)	Engineering plant II N = 398 (per cent)	Forestry company I N = 129 (per cent)	Forestry company II N = 128 (per cent)	Forestry company III N = 118 (per cent)
Thinks local union has sufficient influence at plant level	48	30	33	35	13	15	17	16	16
Interested in increased personal participation at plant level	35	31	27	35	26	22	25	15	20

perceived personal influence over the immediate work situation are related to expressions of job satisfaction in a similar way in both types of industry. Those who feel they already exercise sufficient influence over the immediate work show consistently higher job satisfaction on all criteria (Figs. 33.2 and 33.3).

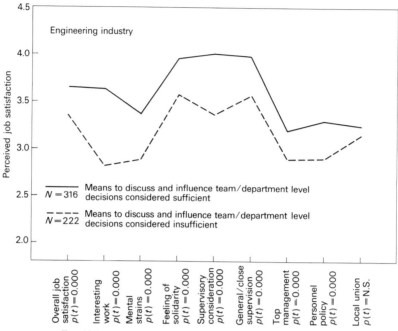

FIG. 33.2. Relation between perceived influence over decisions at team/department level and different criteria of job satisfaction (5-point scale, low values = low job satisfaction).

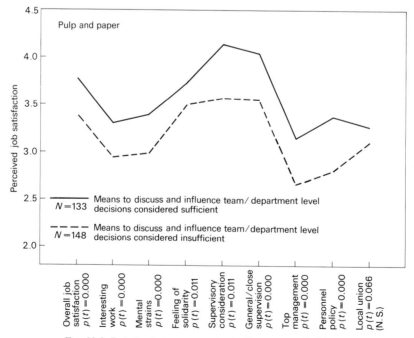

FIG. 33.3. Relation between perceived influence over decisions at team/departmental level and different criteria of job satisfaction (5-point) scale, low values = low job satisfaction.

(2) There is a tendency in both industries for the greatest differences in job satisfaction to lie between groups who feel either 'satisfactory' or 'unsatisfactory' *personal influence over their work situation*. This is linked to their feelings of 'involvement' and their attitudes to foremen and top managers (Figs. 33.2 and 33.3) A reasonable interpretation of this finding is that respondents will tend to react to matters of personal participation in decisions concerning the immediate work situation as being subject to the attitudes held and the methods used by members of line management. Any superior who encourages his subordinates to participate in decision processes is felt to be a good manager. Yet another consequence of these variations in supervisory technique will be for greater personal influence over the immediate work situation to make the work more interesting. It is important to bear this in mind alongside the variations in autonomy conferred by production technology considered in a narrower sense.

(3) The groups who feel that employees do not exercise enough collective influence over corporate management show poorer job satisfaction on all criteria, both in the engineering plants and in the pulp and paper mills. Especially noticeable is the difference of attitude to top management and to the firm's personnel policy, where for both types of industry the critical attitude is decidedly more pronounced in those groups who feel that the employees as a group have too little influence in the firm (Figs. 33.3, 33.4, and 33.5).

(4) In the engineering plants, the feeling of insuf-ficient influence in the firm for its employees is associated with a strongly critical attitude not only to top management but also to the local trade union (Fig. 33.4). A significant difference in this respect also applies to the pulp and paper mills, but it is not of the same magnitude as in the engineering plants (Fig. 33.5). The fact that men who sit on *both sides* of the collective bargaining table are criticized is important, since it connotes feelings of powerlessness not only in relation to the employing firm but also to the trade union, which is supposed to speak for the employees. It should be pointed out that we investigated the engineering plants over a period cover-ing late-1967 and early-1968, i.e. *before* the Swedish economy had recovered from the recession then prevail-ing and *before* the public debate and union activities concerning work environment and industrial democracy had been triggered off. So, it is not likely that any temporary external factors have been operating on our data. The results, rather, should be seen as an expression of a serious trend taking place in organizational life, namely that the individual, when unable to make his voice heard in a satisfactory manner, is coming to look more and more on his trade union as an integral part of the managerial control system as opposed to a represen-tative of the employees.

CONCLUSIONS

The data presented here lend support to the idea that

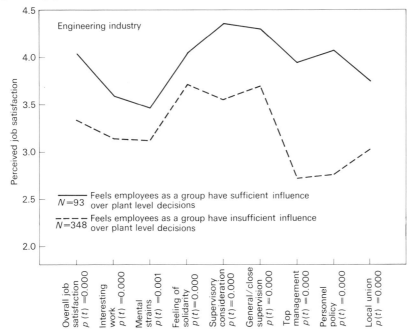

Fig. 33.4. Relation between perceived influence for the employees as a group over decisions at plant level and different criteria of job satisfaction (5-point scale, low values = low job satisfaction).

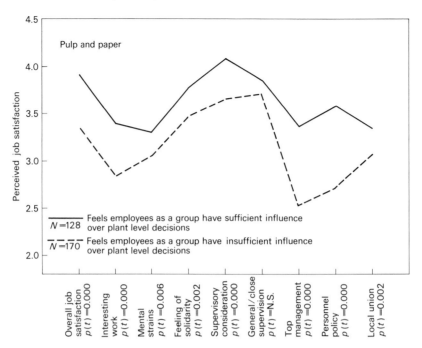

Fig. 33.5. Relation between perceived influence for the employees as a group over decisions at plant level and different criteria of job satisfaction (5-point scale, low values = low job satisfaction).

worker interest in company affairs is favoured by a design of jobs that allows for high autonomy and high demands on skill and co-operation. However, this seems to be more true in integrated production processes, where the socialization of workers is not confined to a craft-based and self-sufficient organization of work. The alienation of mass production workers with repetitive and unskilled tasks seems to imply not only lack of interest in the job *but also a withdrawal from interest in those changes processes that might lead to more autonomous tasks and to increased worker influence in working life*. This is true also for mass production workers who are satisfied with repetitive and unskilled tasks. This is an important observation since it implies that it is not until high involvement can be seen as derived from greater autonomy and more skilled tasks that we can expect a psychological process to start that leads to a more widespread interest for worker participation in higher-level decision-making in working life.

Systems of representative democracy seem incapable by themselves of coping with the powerlessness of individual workers in mass production industry; rather, when they are perceived as not providing the opportunities to influence, they risk being regarded as part of the control system of the plant. On the other hand, there is no inevitable conflict between representative democracy and direct democracy; on the contrary, an effective system of representative democracy or collective bargaining seems to increase the demands among

the workers for personal influence in company matters. The crucial factors, however, in coping with worker alienation seem to be related to technology and job content. Increased autonomy and increased requirements on manual and social skills are not only favourable to job involvement but seem also to favour aspirations towards increased worker participation both at the personal level and for the workers as a group. The system of industrial relations in Sweden is now changing through a new set of laws providing the employees with legal rights to participate in decisions at all levels in the plant. If this development is going to involve the individual workers and carry meaning in their everyday lives, it seems necessary that management and unions involve themselves in a systematic way in the abolition of the 'robot jobs' so prevalent in today's industrial life.

SUMMARY

The interrelationships of job content, job involvement, and worker participation are investigated for process workers, mass production workers, and batch workers on the basis of the hypothesis that demands for worker participation are generally favoured by autonomy and high skill requirements in one's own job. As to demands for increased *personal participation*, the hypothesis is supported in the process industry, but not in the metalworking industry, where high skill demands are found in craft-based batch production. This difference is discussed in terms of integration and continuity in the production process. In both industries it is found that high involvement in repetitive and unskilled tasks is not accompanied by increased demands for participation. As to demands for *worker participation through the system of representative democracy,* these are generally high and tend to increase with increasing autonomy in one's own job. Perceived success for the system of representative democracy leads to increasing demands for personal participation. Perceived worker influence is followed by increased job satisfaction.

REFERENCES

DAHLSTRÖM, E. (1969). *Fördjupad företagsdemokrati* [Towards industrial democracy]. Prisma, Stockholm.

GARDELL, B. (1969). *Skogsarbetarnas arbetsanpassning.* [Job satisfaction and mental health among forest workers]. The Swedish Council for Personnel Administration, Stockholm.

—— (1971a). Technology, alienation and mental health in the modern industrial environment. In *Society, stress and disease* (ed. L. Levi), Vol. I. Oxford University Press, London.

—— (1971b). *Produktionsteknik och arbetsglädje.* [Technology, alienation and mental health]. The Swedish Council for Personnel Administration, Stockholm.

—— (1976). *Arbetsinnehall och livskvalitet* [Job content and quality of life]. Summary and discussion of social science research on man in working life, presented to the 1976 Congress of the Swedish Confederation of Trade Unions. Prisma, Stockholm.

THORSRUD, E. and EMERY, F. (1969). *Mot en ny bedrifts-organisasjon.* Taunus, Oslo.

34. AGES AND STAGES IN OCCUPATIONAL CHOICE

H. LEVINSON

The increasing emphasis on making work more intrinsically important to those who do it has now gone through five major orientations.

The first of these, a pre-scientific orientation still widely practised, is one of trial and error in selection. With limited criteria and little planned effort, organizations choose people to fill certain jobs, and people take jobs which they think will meet their needs. This process is also frequently followed in promotion, transfer, career change directions, and similar activities. It is essentially a winnowing-out process with all of the costly consequences of trial and error.

The second orientation came about with the development of aptitude, skill, and interest testing. This stage is characterized by multidimensional normative inventories which provide gross general information and make it possible to differentiate interests shared by physicians from those shared by executives. These measures, however, are limited by the fact that they cannot differentiate within broad occupational ranges. Though there are measures for sales aptitude, for example, a salesman for IBM might not do equally well as a salesman for Sears Roebuck. Furthermore, such predictors assume that a person will continue to fit the same position over his life span. They are essentially static.

The third orientation, an extension and elaboration of the second, is the use of comprehensive batteries of tests, including those of intelligence, personality, values, situational judgements, and others. This stage arose from efforts to select more carefully, particularly for managerial and executive role. However comprehensive these batteries might be, their outcomes are severely limited. There is no way such batteries can take into account either the climate of the employing organization or the kind of boss to whom a candidate would be reporting; both are crucial to success. Furthermore, the measures themselves are frequently of variable, if not dubious, reliability and validity. Personality tests especially are notoriously poor predictors of occupational success. Thorndike and Hagen (1959) demonstrated that those who did well when placed in the American Air Force on the basis of such batteries, also did well in civilian life where they spontaneously chose different directions.

The fourth major orientation recognizes the importance of social relationships at work and of the informal social structure. This was pioneered in the Hawthorne studies (Roethlisberger and Dixon 1939) and led to a greater understanding of the psychosocial meaning of work as well as the more critical importance of the relationship between superiors and subordinates. This orientation became the forerunner of much of the contemporary consideration of differentiated organizational structures and organizational systems and their impact on people.

The fifth orientation focuses heavily on group processes and the impact of group relationships, group decision-making, socio-technical systems, participative management, and other forms of influence by employees on the way they are supposed to do their work, as well as the nature of their relationship with their companies. In various combinations, activities stemming from these five orientations are currently in vogue. However, new trends are beginning to suggest that they are no longer enough to do an adequate job of fitting person to task and task to person. Rather, we must begin to think of new refinements and new differentiations so that the person–job fit can be viewed as a dynamic, rather than a static process. That is, rather than fitting person to job and letting it go at that, we must begin to think of fitting and refitting and refitting further as both multi-faceted person and tasks change over time.

It is now time to begin to think of the interaction of a number of different forces in the continuous process of facilitating the opportunity for a person to master his work and integrate it as a creative and constructive part of his personality. Among these forces we can now begin to consider are: (1) a person's career stage; (2) age-specific proclivities; (3) stage-specific psychological tasks; (4) crisis-specific psychological needs; (5) value-system behaviours; (6) need-level requirements; and (7) changing organizational adaptive patterns.

This is not an exhaustive list, but it certainly points out the complexity of the task we face when we think about making organizations more congenial to the human beings who work in them. It is my contention that it is not enough to think of the elaboration of the five orientations I have outlined as sufficient to making organizations more human, but rather that we must think of ever more subtle and differentiated efforts or our work will fall far short of both our expectations and desirable outcomes.

MODES OF REFINEMENT

Career stages

If we examine each one of these seven forces, potential avenues of refinement begin to be apparent. For example, if we look at career patterns, it becomes possible to distinguish a phase of early career development from that of mid-career or of late career (Veiga 1973).

In the period of early career development the person is frequently casting about for a direction, a sense of purpose, and an area of specialization. Alternatively he may be building a range of experiences out of which to develop a generalized career position such as that of manager. The early career period is one of trying oneself out, sampling organizations, developing skills, learning political techniques, and developing a reputation. Work assignments during this period should heavily emphasize these multiple activities as contrasted with learning how to conform, how to stand in line for bureaucratic promotional procedures, and marking time in so-called orientation tasks which do nothing to further skills and competence. The young person should have an opportunity to view the whole of an organization before undertaking to work in one or another area. He should be able to test himself, to show what he can do, to develop a sense of competence, usefulness, and being valued.

In mid-career, one presumably has established his own occupational reputation and has acquired competence and skills. In organizations he is often in a position of mediating organizational needs and requirements on one hand, and the demands and problems of early career people on the other. Mid-career is frequently a time of powerful identification with an organization in which one works or with a profession which one practices. It is a time in which one acts on behalf of the organization and represents it both to subordinates and to its various publics. It is the mature action phase of career, one which might be likened to the parental role in the family. Work in this period should involve leadership and supervisory activities, responsibility for other people, and responsibility for representing the organization and acting on its behalf in the sense of mature partnership with the organization.

The third stage is one in which one has developed a historical perspective on his own career experiences and on those of the organization. It is a time when one is no longer competing for position and, therefore, when others can more readily turn to such a person. However, it is also a time of obsolescence when many managers manage on what they once knew. Therefore, while such people may more conveniently be used and use themselves in a role that calls for counselling, political understanding, taking into account their experience with the past and giving more careful attention to selection, they should also be required to be involved in long-range planning and anticipating the future. That requirement will compel them to continue to learn.

These career stages probably will vary in different organizations and among different career paths. It will be difficult to fix permanent beginning and ending points for them. Simultaneously as we move further from a blue-collar work force to a white-collar work force, career phases will become more widespread among the population. It will be increasingly necessary to define specific activities within certain career paths and patterns in organizations and to gear training and development activities to the enhancement of effectiveness during those phases.

Age-specific proclivities

Intertwined between career patterns and stage-specific developmental experiences are age-specific experiences. As yet we know little about them. It has been suggested (Keniston 1965), for example, that the age span from approximately 21 to age 25 is increasingly a time for a moratorium period. While one is defining goals, attaining reputation, acquiring skills, presumably at the same time one is looking sceptically at one's environment and refraining from making formal commitments. It is a time of questioning, juxtaposing academic experiences with those of the real world, re-examining parental values no longer as a student, but now as a mature adult earning his own livelihood, and warily making choices. This suggests that it is unwise to pressure young people to make formal choices or to entice them into sticking with an organization. Rather it might be better to view this period as one of mutual examination—occupational dating so to speak.

In some occupations, such as that of aircraft controller, one reaches a chronological point where one can no longer be as effective balancing multiple responsibilities and continuous, heavy amounts of data input as one previously was. Organic changes which begin to come about at age 55 have significance for such people as railroad engineers. They may have implications for scientists and technicians who are compelled to deal with increasing complexity at a time of decreasing ability. Such age-specific issues will need to be more clearly pinpointed.

Stage-specific psychological tasks

The third major force, that of stage specific tasks, will dovetail with career phases. By stage-specific proclivities I mean those psychological tendencies which have greater force at one stage of development than another and indeed which constitute great internal pressures at that time.

Jaques (1970) points out that the time from early adulthood to mid-life, a period described by Erikson (1959) as the period of intimacy, is also one of greatest creativity, innovative energy, and imagination. It is also a period during which still-maturing people more easily deny their underlying dependency needs, for they see themselves as more instrumental than younger or older people. That is, they are more active, support themselves and often others, and have not yet arrived at that point where they begin to decline physically. Taken together, these forces compel an action orientation. Occupational tasks and training activities should be geared to enabling them to act, particularly in innovative and creative tasks. Organizations should use such people for new ideas, for critical examination of the old, for risk-taking ventures, and for counteracting stultifying processes. The more volatile a market, the greater it depends on style changes or new orientations, the more important it is for the interface between the organization and its environment to be comprised of younger people.

At this point young people need a great deal of supportive supervision which will enable them to act creatively while being protected from the rest of the organization and simultaneously to have impulsive and poorly-thought-through activities reasonably guided and controlled so as to be productive rather than negatively impulsive. Such supervision will have to deal with feelings of intense rivalry, the residues of attempting to establish close adult interpersonal relationships of an enduring kind.

The mid-life period is one in which one reorganizes one's own thinking about oneself. Taking into account his mortality, the individual restructures his value system, shifts emphases in his life activity, and copes with the loss of his growing family (Jacques 1970). He comes to terms with the limitations of his aspirations prescribed by time, experience, life station, and opportunity (Neugarten 1968; Sofer 1970). Middle age, roughly from 35 to 55 is also a time of physical and intellectual decline. It is this period which Erikson (1959) characterizes as the stage of generativity where one begins to be more interested in perpetuating oneself through others. Individuals who do not develop generativity, Erikson says, often begin to indulge themselves as if they were their own one and only child. The task, therefore, in middle age is to free oneself from narcissistic self-indulgence and competitiveness to become instrumental in rearing others.

With the declining average age at which men and women become company presidents, many more people will know earlier in their lives that they are no longer competitive for top management positions. Ideally many should make the shift from a playing role to a coaching role. The psychological work of this period is to not only make that shift but to accept oneself in that new role. A major effort of management training at this point should be to help persons in this age range yield some of their intensely competitive feelings so that they can accept themselves for who they are and what they are and invest themselves in the development of others. Training experiences should include not only skills in coaching and development but also opportunity to freely express the anguish of this role shift which for so many people, particularly men, seems to signify a personal defeat.

The third stage, which Erikson speaks of as a stage of integrity, is a time of consolidation and coming to terms with how one has used one's own life. It is a time when one's own dependency is increasing because of declining physical and intellectual resources (Gutman 1971), when one feels oneself to be less instrumental in the sense of being more self reliant than in earlier periods, and when, ideally, one has acquired judgement and wisdom and one can more carefully weigh innovation in the context of experience. One must deal with gradual detachment from one's personal activities or from the organization with which one has worked while at the same time still being able to make useful contributions to both.

The psychological task of coming to terms with how one has used his own life is a painful one. According to Erikson, it is the time when one must accept one's own and only life cycle and of the people who have become significant to it as something that had to be. People who cannot accept that fact then despair and fear death. For many people, to leave an organization because of age increases their sense of uselessness and worthlessness. Those who have depended on an organization for a working life time now feel bereft at a time when they are increasingly dependent because of their advancing years. Sometimes they feel that their efforts have been useless if, as they leave, so much changes behind them.

The psychological work of this stage requires preparation for shifting from an authoritative and power role to one of consultation, guidance, and wisdom. This is a time when little attention is given to training or support experiences, yet such training for counselling activities and support opportunities for discussing the pain of separation and extremely helpful. Ideally the work people do at this stage contribute to a sense of wholeness, of career integration. Ideally people at this age should be able to see their integrated life experiences as a platform from which others can start.

Crisis-specific psychological needs

Career stages, age-specific proclivities, and stage-specific psychological tasks interrelate to give rise to crisis-specific needs.

Crisis-specific here refers to the crisis of normal development. Some are more environmentally determined, others are more a product of internal psychological processes. For example, for many young people there is a crisis experience around the issues of occupational choice or direction. For both men and women, becoming parents may accentuate this issue. Certainly it accentuates the problem of accepting the dependency of others on them. For the first time they are responsible for the life of someone other than themselves. For many this may have import with respect to the additional burden of accepting the dependency of those whom they must supervise or organizational demands which come in conflict with parental responsibilities. They have a need at this point to understand the nature of the crisis they are experiencing, for support in coping with it, and for avenues of action through which it might be resolved.

Daniel Levinson (1978) has called attention to the crisis experience which occurs in the late 30s around 'becoming one's own man' or BOOM. He points out that the men in his study usually have been guided by a mentor, someone who has taken a personal interest in them and helped them advance their careers. However, at this point in time they seem to be called upon to assert their independence of their mentor and to go their ways, hence the acronym. Their separation from the mentor, the establishment of themselves as their own men, and the reinvigorated pursuit of their own directions combine to make for a powerful emotional experience of crisis proportions.

The BOOM experience is part of the general middle-age crisis, that adaptational struggle coincident upon becoming aware of the fact that life is half over and that one has to evolve new strategies more suitable to a declining organism than to a growing one. The crisis is reflected in the rise of physical symptoms with psychological origins, a peak in the death rate between 35 and 40, confirmation from career paths that one will or will not continue to rise in managerial ranks and the tendency to begin to re-do repetitively in new roles what one had done before rather than to be innovative. There is frequently a shift in values and a tendency to be both more disillusioned and more conservative while at the same time more angry at being displaced by younger competitors.

As with any crisis the middle-age crisis needs open discussion, recognition of its pains and its inevitability, while at the same time evolving modes of coping with it. At work a person in such crisis might have the opportunity to discuss with his superiors what now he would like to do in the organization and what he can most fruitfully do. For example, a highly successful sales executive ultimately made a shift out of an organization into a public service conservation activity. His company could well have used him to handle a whole range of problems like that in his own organization. In another instance, a corporation insisted on over-controlling a high level vice president by ordinary management policies and procedures. When he left they failed to understand his 'lack of ambition'. Many others leave the organization figuratively by remaining depressed, plateauing, and doing minimal work. They need not do so, if careful attention is given to this crisis and steps are taken to turn it to mutual advantage. Developmental programmes for men in this age range should be concentrated largely on retraining, updating, and conceptualizing both the problems and the organization. The psychological time is one of reworking and therefore, the tasks to which they are assigned should be reworking, reorganizing, refining, and restructuring efforts.

The retirement experience for most is a crisis experience. Few people are adequately prepared for it. Most tend to deny it until the last minute and little is done in most organizations to provide transitional activities that might be perpetuated *ad lib* once one has formally left an organization or intensive career activity.

One way to deal with the retirement crisis experience is by helping the prospective retiree establish himself in activities outside the business. Ideally this should be done on a part-time basis beginning, perhaps at age 60. It would be much better if the prospective retiree could undertake an activity on behalf of the organization which would require him to spend more time outside of it and away from his previous regular duties. Ideally this would provide prospective retirees with the opportunity to establish themselves away from the organization and gradually separate from it. It is particularly important that they establish themselves because without membership in the organization they gradually lose their leverage

in the community and are left to doing low-level volunteer work which frequently does not appeal to them. A critical aspect of this experience is the continuous message to the retiree that his work life has indeed been worthwhile, that the company appreciates him, that he still has something to offer, and that he has not wasted his life.

Value system behaviour
Hughes and Flowers (1973), building on a theory of Clare Graves, have delineated seven value systems. These value systems are:

1. Reactive, that is, primitive response to physiological needs.
2. Tribalistic, valuing easy work, friendly people, fair play, and a good boss. Money and supervisory direction are important.
3. Egocentric, which emphasizes good pay and freedom from being tied down.
4. Conformist which values job security, rules and fairness.
5. Manipulative in which there is variety of work, some freewheeling activity, and pay and bonuses based on results. Mastery, power, and political manipulation are important considerations.
6. Sociocentric, where friendly relationships, doing what one likes to do, and working with others to a common goal are important. Material issues are secondary to social contributions.
7. Existential, in which goals and problems are more important than money, prestige, or methodology. The preference here is for continuing challenge, imagination, and initiative.

Determination of which of the value systems various people hold makes it more possible to differentiate employee communications, job design, management systems and procedures, and growth opportunities which fit the needs of people who hold these diverse value structures. Thus, Hughes and Flowers are creating the groundwork for differentiation and refinement of occupational roles and career paths. By doing so they are attempting to specify the intensity and degree to which various kinds of career issues, age- and stage-specific issues and crises will affect one or another group of people.

Need-level requirements
The value system conception ties in nicely with the Maslow (1954) concept of hierarchy of needs which is another way of differentiating occupational role according to the need level of the employee. Maslow classified human needs on five levels, each succeeding need becoming more pressing as the preceding ones were satisfied. In ascending order these are: physiological needs, safety needs, needs for belonging and love, needs for esteem, and needs for self-actualization. Such needs presumably would cut across the developmental pattern

which I outlined earlier in the form of career stages, age-specific proclivities, stage-specific psychological tasks, and crisis-specific psychological needs. While the Maslow concept applies across the board, and complements the value system idea, the latter suggests that various people become fixed at different points along the Maslow continuum. The Maslow conception suggests the possibility of raising the need levels for people who are fixated at various points and thereby presumably freeing them and the organization for more adaptive efforts. While the Hughes and Flowers conception would seem to speak for organizing work around groups differentiated according to values, Maslow points to directions in which movement might take place. For example, conceivably a manager who holds value system (5) – manipulative – might change as a result of experiences in the middle-age crisis to a value system (6) – socio-centric – or a value system (7) – existential. In fact, if such movement were possible and desired by the individual, the company could facilitate his movement in that direction by refining occupational roles which would allow it to take place.

Changing organizational adaptive patterns

Finally, as organizations change rapidly, there are necessarily significant and often radical role shifts in occupational demands. Such role shifts are usually quite stressful. Inasmuch as we are likely to see more frequent reorganization and even more radical demands on people for changes in occupational behaviour, it becomes necessary to continuously delineate and differentiate the new kinds of roles which people are expected to perform on a continuing basis to facilitate the person–job fit.

These roles might be differentiated according to the career stage, the need levels, the value systems they require, and the degree to which they relate to one or another of the dimensions I have outlined. If adaptation is the crucial element in organizational survival, as well as individual mastery, then these criteria for task differentiation, if followed, should enhance that adaptation for both.

Complementing the role differentiation, there must also be adequate structural definition in organizations which gives particular attention to the distribution of power. Without adequate role power a supervisor or manager at any level is not in a position to provide adequate support and authority for those who report to him.

IMPLICATIONS

What are the implications of this thesis?

First, it seems to me that instead of organizing organizations along hierarchical lines and defining jobs according to those lines, it is necessary to begin with the tasks to be done on behalf of the organization. That is, what does the environment require if the organization is to master it

successfully? Reasoning backward from those requirements, what are the tasks to be accomplished and how might the organization go about allocating those tasks under conditions which make both the task and the roles necessary to accomplish them continuously modifiable on the basis of experience?

Second, in the process of continuously reassessing tasks and roles within task requirements, it seems to me that it will be increasingly important to ask: What configuration of the variables I have outlined and others which may be added would characterize, define, and describe the persons most appropriate for the accomplishment of those tasks? That is, what career stage, what age- and stage-specific tasks, what value systems, what need-level requirement, and what organizational adaptive task bring to the fore those feelings, thoughts, and behaviour which are most relevant? There may even be considerable thought given to what kind of tasks are most congenial to people in developmental crisis. For example, it might be most appropriate to assign a person who is not yet fully at mid-career, but who is between 38 and 40, experiencing the need to be his own man with a manipulative value system at the self-actualization level in a company which is decentralizing, to aggressive managerial tasks requiring mobilization of a team of people to solve a critical marketing problem, which requires high risk and promises to pay off handsomely.

Third, there is need for a broad educational effort so that people can better understand career issues, age issues, crisis issues, value issues, hierarchy of need issues, and organizational change requirements so that they may better engage with management in their own career planning, and in continuous renegotiations of their psychological contracts (Levinson *et. al.* 1962).

If people are to think more freely and more frequently about their occupational alternatives and career choices in keeping with changing configurations of needs, inevitably they will be involved in multiple career planning in anticipation of personal, professional, and organizational changes. For that planning to be effective and supported adequately by high-level management, it will be necessary to have upward appraisal systems in which subordinates appraise superiors on the degree to which they are helpful to them in their professional growth and development. Otherwise there will be little pressure on superiors to engage in such discussions. In addition, since all change involves the experience of loss and depressive feelings of varying intensity, it becomes necessary for organizations to evolve modes through which people can talk about their loss and change experiences so that the negative feelings which accompany them do not inhibit their adaptive efforts.

Finally, we will have to develop an increasingly broad appreciation of the meanings of configurations of variables for occupational stress. It is already evident that the core occupational stress is the feeling of guilt people experience for not measuring up to their ego ideals (Levinson 1972). That is, for not doing as well as they ought to be doing in terms of their unconscious and onscious aspirations. The ego ideal is necessarily ffected by career stage, chronological stage, value system, need level, and transitional crises. The closer we ome to understanding these phenomena and planning ork experience around that, the more likely it is that we an make organizations more human.

SUMMARY

as work becomes more sophisticated, increasingly careful attention must be given to the process by which people are placed in jobs. Recognition must be given to a person's career stage, age-specific proclivities, life stage-specific psychological tasks, life-crisis needs, value system behaviours, and need-level requirements in the context of changing organizational adaptive patterns. If work is to be less stressful, then work organizations must give careful attention to the subtle but important psychological processes among their employees and managers, in selection, assignment, and career development.

REFERENCES

ERIKSON, E. H. (1959). Identity and the life cycle. *Psychological Issues*, **1**, (1), 1–171.

GUTMAN, D. (1971). The hunger of old men. *Trans-action*, **9**, 53–66.

HUGHES, C. L. and FLOWERS, V. S. (1973). Shaping personnel strategies to disparate value systems. *Personnel*, **50**, 8–23.

JAQUES, E. (1970). *Work, creativity and social justice*. New York.

KENISTON, K. (1965). *The uncommitted*. New York.

LEVINSON, D. J., DARROW, C. N., KLEIN, E. B., LEVINSON, M. H., and McKEE, B. (1978). *The seasons of a man's life*. New York.

LEVINSON, H. (1972). *Executive stress*. New York.

——, PRICE, C. R., MANDL, H. J., MUNDEN, K. J., and SOLLEY, C. M. (1962). *Men, management and mental health*. Cambridge, Massachusetts

MASLOW, A. H. (1954). *Personality and motivation*. New York.

NEUGARTEN, B. L. (ed.) (1968). *Middle age and aging*. Chicago.

ROETHLISBERGER, F. J. and DIXON, W. J. (1939). *Management and the worker*. Cambridge, Massachusetts.

SOFER, C. (1970). *Men in mid-career*. London.

THORNDIKE, R. L. and HAGEN, E. (1959). *10 000 careers*. New York.

VEIGA, J. F. (1973). The mobile manager at mid-career. *Harvard Business Review*, **51**, 115–19.

35. HEALTH ASPECTS OF WELL-BEING IN WORKPLACES

RICARDO EDSTRÖM

UNION APPROACH TO THE GOVERNMENT

In 1963 the Swedish government was approached by the unions representing the civil servants with a request for better services for personnel welfare in the national administration. There were about 400 000 civil servants in Sweden at that time, including professions like clerks and judges but also railwaymen, postmen, and others.

Behind the request lay the experience of several unions that members often had problems in their working conditions, problems which fell outside the traditional union interests in salaries and job security. The problems were to be taken seriously since they were sometimes threatening to health and well-being. The unions did not consider it their responsibility to acquire the competence needed to investigate these kinds of problems or to give medical or social advice to the members concerned. So they asked the employer, the administration, to provide these facilities. The reaction to this request was positive. The management side also felt the need for better access to medical and social advice to assist directors and personnel departments with personnel problems.

Civil servants in our country have free medical service. That means that they get treatment free of cost when needed. But the physicians in general know very little about working conditions. And the employers' access to medical advice with respect to personnel problems was provided for only formally; it hardly existed in practice.

Adding to the interest on the part of management was the fact that, through negotiations, the unions had managed to raise the salaries for employees on sick leave to almost 95 per cent of the usual pay and absence rates were, if not yet alarming, at least increasing.

The government bill

The government bill (1963:160) stated that the personnel welfare service should include advisory activities directed at employees and their supervisors and other initiatives directed at workplaces for the purposes of reducing maladjustment to work, superiors, and co-workers, increasing well-being, and thereby reducing absenteeism.

Parliament was thus asked to provide the means for a pilot group, consisting of physicians, nurses, social workers, and necessary administrative personnel to establish a model organization for the personnel welfare service in the national administration. The group was to be free to experiment with various forms of internal organization and external service in order to gain the experience necessary to submit a suggestion on the final form for this kind of work.

A PILOT GROUP FOR PERSONNEL WELFARE SERVICE

I was asked to become the first medical adviser to the pilot group, probably because of my background as neurologist with an interest in psychiatry. To me it was a challenge to experiment in preventive psychiatric work.

The group was organized in January 1964. The project lasted until 1 July 1971, that is for seven and a half years. By that time we had grown to about 50 persons, spread out in five subgroups in various parts of the country. Each group consisted of one physician (usually a psychiatrist), about five social workers, and a secretary. The first teams included a nurse each, but, for reasons that will be discussed later, we abandoned the use of nurses in teams formed later. The central administration was kept small; we had an ambition to keep the organization 'flat', that is to avoid a bureaucratic hierarchy. The local teams were headed by 'chairmen' who were to be appointed among the social workers. The physician was to serve primarily as adviser to them. The group was meant to be a 'refuge' and a platform from which to operate in the working premises.

I myself visited each team at least monthly and discussed accumulated problems. At my side I had an administrator taking care of all formalities involving our internal administration. The whole project was led by a board, consisting of representatives of the various personnel unions within the national administration and also of employers' representatives. The board was chaired by a high government official. This joint influence over our activities was essential. It provided us with the credibility we needed. We could work on a neutral, professional basis, without any glances at employer or employee interests. We had no formal power. We had to rely on the quality of our advice to be trusted and perhaps followed.

Objectives and strategies

This fact of course influenced our strategy. We had to prove useful in order to be used. We had to show that we could solve problems that responsible people in the various administrative units had not been able to solve themselves. This led us into a role as 'trouble shooters' before we had really formulated a considered strategy.

The reasons for our existence have already been given. It could be assumed that through ignorance or lack of competence in behavioural sciences, a lot of unnecessary suffering might be engendered in places of work. It could be further assumed that if we showed the responsible parties how to handle personnel problems better, or how to avoid them, this unnecessary suffering might be reduced. This was our simple philosophy to begin with.

Thus, the teams were to start with a presentation of themselves and their skills to their future clients. They systematically visited all administrative bodies in their region, gathered the chiefs, the personnel officers, the supervisors, the union representatives, the joint committees, etc. General gatherings of all personnel in work units also took place. At all these gatherings the team members offered their medical and social services, with the explanation that they were not to take care of sick employees but to help solve work-related problems.

In some of the biggest administrative bodies the social workers were allotted a reception room on the work premises, but in general people had to call for our services at our own office. Each unit with a developed personnel department was visited regularly about four times a year for discussions about absence records and personnel policy questions.

Problems encountered

A certain hesitancy was to be expected on the part of our clients. The service we offered was something new and unusual. There may even have been some suspicion about our true motives. But even allowing for this natural hesitancy, it turned out not to be so easy to get at the real problems. Actually all problems were denied. There was a general cover-up on all levels. We were treated as guests or even as intruders and by what seemed to be a general silent consent it was felt that problems should be kept 'within the family'.

Each team had about 10 000 civil servants to look after in their allotted area (county-wise). That meant about 2000 employees for each social worker. He (or more often she) got to know most of these people within months at least as groups. He learnt which doors to go through and which were better avoided. He felt the emotional climate, modes of communication, prevailing attitudes, etc. He also found people with problems, people who had lost spirit, people who made more trouble than contributions, and all varieties of human reactions to working conditions.

We sooner or later found the problems, or at least many of them, that people at all levels tried to cover up. This descrepancy between 'official' attitudes and internal problems is worth some consideration in this context. Actually it is one of the key problems in preventive mental health work. How does one get past the common denial, how does one get at the taboo topics? We learnt that there is in every organization something we have called 'a twilight zone of reality distortion'. It is within this zone that one finds most of the real stressors, the sources of anxiety of despair, it is mostly here that the emotions are generated which may produce nervous strain or psychosomatic illness.

People tend to blame themselves for shortcomings in the job, rather than to question the organization and its emotional climate. Part of this 'twilight zone' may be unconscious or semiconscious—or perhaps obvious only to a few who prefer to keep their observations to themselves. We shall have reason to return to this phenomenon later in the chapter.

Demonstration of usefulness

The social workers tried to sit in on joint committee meetings and other gatherings, they tried to visit the work premises for various reasons, but most of the information came through people seeking the social workers in their reception rooms, at the jobs, or in our offices.

Sooner or later came the moment when the social worker saw the chance to make an impressive contribution. It could be in the form of a successful transferral of someone to other job assignments or a successful rehabilitation of someone to old activity levels. Once the demonstration had been given, confidence in our organization rose and the seclusive attitudes softened. In the following stage we might even be flooded with requests to take care of 'problem cases'.

To begin with we went about happily making ourselves useful. It was a rewarding feeling to have a number of people waiting for you at the job, to help them sort out their life situations, and to assist in improvements. The more work we got done, the more we were asked to do. It was wonderful—until we understood what was really happening.

Side effects

Actually our own activities turned people into 'problem cases'. It became easy for managers and personnel officers to dump their problems on us—not in order to learn but in order to sneak away from their responsibilities. And even to put the blame upon us for a less successful outcome. 'Take care of him! Don't let him back until he is fit for work!' or sometimes in more subtle terms like: 'I might do him harm if I tell him what I think of him. Why don't you, specialists, tell him that he has got problems?'

We had to make it a rule that no one should be 'ordered' to seek our unit. And we would not agree to be the first to tell an employee that he was in trouble. Such information was the clear responsibility of the closest supervisor of his superiors. Only if a need for our services was felt by the employee himself could we be expected to do anything worthwhile.

Even with these restrictions we increasingly felt that we were working against our better intentions. Through our organization people were branded, often with a diagnosis of some sort. They thereby became scapegoats for trouble which was in fact caused by other people. Attention was distracted from the destructive situation in the organization. All the blame was put upon the victim. And we were the ones who confirmed this vicious misconception. It even became a drawback to seek our services. If someone wanted a transferral, he had better try himself. If we got involved, his chances of being accepted on the new job were reduced. Our clients became suspect!

We were far from practising preventive psychiatry. Somehow we had to find a better method to get at the true sources of the evil. We were just adding to the general cover-up process that contributed to the establishment of a 'twilight zone of reality distortion'. The real stressors and anxiety sources were still chiefly hiding in the taboo field where we could not reach them.

Identification of problems

By chance we got an opportunity to gain some insight into these problems, when we were asked to participate in the organization of a general health control study of state employees. Health check-ups were very popular at that time (1966) and the unions had requested that their members should have this benefit. The government answered by offering a pilot study of 1000 civil servants, before more general measures were contemplated. We saw this study as an opportunity not only to gather information on the health of the employees, but also to get some insight into how they experienced their working conditions. Possibly correlations were to be found.

Three hundred employees were offered, in addition to the health check-up, a chance to participate in an extensive psychological study on a voluntary basis. They were given numbers of test and interview sessions with psychologists. Questionnaires were designed for the occasion and it took the statistician and myself several years to sort out the 300 data pieces we had on all 300 subjects, and to process these data in various cross-tabulations. The results are still digestible only for people with a research interest in this field, and it has been published in Swedish only. Previous family histories, present social activities, working conditions, feelings about same, ambitions for the future, etc., were on record. A few highlights of this study may be mentioned here.

A surprisingly high number of these people, who were leading an active working life, were found to have problems or defects worthy of a medical diagnosis (as judged by a teaching hospital over which we had no influence). Only 9 per cent of the females and 31 per cent of the males escaped a diagnosis. (The apparent sex difference in these and the following figures is virtual and not real, as we were able to determine from our psycho-social data. Females in our administration still have lower positions than most of the males and are therefore drawn from a less fortunate segment of the society. More often than the men they came from broken homes, had a lower education, had experienced more divorces, etc. Females with an academic background and positions equalling those of the men, have health records and absence records similar to those of their male colleagues.) Of the various diagnoses that were given our employee group, neurotic or psychosomatic disorders dominated. Forty-eight per cent of the men and 66 per cent of the women got such a diagnosis.

We checked the absence records and the medical certificate which is mandatory if the absence exceeds seven days. There only 3·6 per cent of the men and 9·9 per cent of the women had a psychiatric diagnosis. The latter figures better fit the prevailing feeling about the magnitude of psychological problems as held in various personnel departments. The former figures are, however, probably closer to the truth. There is evidently an extensive and unrecognized mass of psychic and social problems among these active and seemingly healthy employees.

One of the questions we posed at the outset of this study was: What characterizes the frequently sick employee? In light of the above evidence we had to rephrase the question: Why do they go to work, all these people who could have a medical certificate legalizing a sick leave at any time? They hardly lose economically yet they keep on going to their jobs in spite of their difficulties.

ADAPTATION OF WORKING CONDITIONS

Obviously a health service can never be expected to treat away all problems and resulting diseases. The aim must be rather to alter working conditions in a direction that permits more people with problems and health defects to function in spite of their shortcomings. This conclusion became a cornerstone for further strategic thinking. People do go to work in spite of difficulties to a large extent. It must be our task to increase their possibilities of doing so, rather than to chase diagnoses. The health defect is one thing. What people choose to do with it is another and separate thing. This dichotomy seems to have been neglected. Actually we should help people to dissimulate!

The dimension a person gives his health defect will depend on many things in his total life situation. If he needs a face-saving escape from an unacceptable situation, the defect may come in handy. If, on the other hand, life is attractive and the urge to live it fully is strong, the defect may be considered a nuisance and disturbing bother that must be made the least of.

Motivational factors; positive health

This is where motivational factors come in. Motivation to live, including motivation to work. Preventive medicine must pay greater attention to these qualities of positive health and learn to augment them—learn and teach how to make life richer and more worth living.

Medical education has hitherto centred too much upon the negative aspects of health, the defects and diseases. A diagnosis has been considered essential for further medical action in accordance with science and proven experience. A diagnosis is of course still essential for correct reparative work in an individual case. In preventive health work, at least in preventive mental ealth work, the individual diagnoses are actually of minor importance. More important is a finding that in one working unit people seem to contract various ailments to an extent that they did not do before, or to an extent exceeding other similar working units.

The outcome of a pressing situation may take many forms, depending on the individuals' genetic dispositions, life experiences, and actual habits. Preventive health workers would soon get lost if they tried to investigate all that. Instead the question about the possibly common source must guide the preventive mental health worker.

Can we eliminate something in this work unit that reduces motivation to work and to live? Can we build more elements into the work situation that stimulate its members and make life more appealing? What are the techniques by which changes in this direction may be brought about?

Absenteeism

We learnt from our study that absenteeism is not a conventional medical problem, at least not short-spell absenteeism. One cannot predict from a health check-up if somebody is going to be frequently sick-absent, except in unusual cases. Short-spell absenteeism is instead closely linked to job satisfaction, or rather dissatisfaction.

One interesting group among the frequently sick-absent employees consisted of intellectually gifted women with a Bohemian lack of punctuality; they loathed monotony and rigid schedules. Yet their work position called for disciplined routine. In higher quality job positions their life styles might be creative assets. Is there no way of changing job demands so that assets may be assets in a larger number of jobs? Flexible working hours might save suffering for these people and save lost work days for their organization.

Teaching; change agent techniques

One obvious way to try to bring about changes was to teach. We had access to managers, supervisors, and union leaders. We also got invitations to teach at leadership courses and participate in the training of joint committee members. We tried to teach and inform on a broad scale. Once insight of this sort was made easily available, we thought, knowledge itself must take effect and the process of change will start.

We also glanced at 'change agent' techniques evolved in the growing field of 'organizational development'. This is a branch of the behavioural sciences aiming at improving the efficiency of organizations by facilitating open communication and the personal development of each of its members. We tried roles as change agents with varying success. As one physician put it: 'You don't have to be a psychiatrist in order to tell a supervisor that he should say hello to his co-workers when he comes in the morning'.

It was difficult to structure the task for the social workers when we wanted them to go out in the work places and start up change processes. The role of the physician became also unclear and unfamiliar. The shift from individually oriented activities towards group-oriented did not bring the same intrinsic rewards as previously. Most of us stopped half-way in this shift or even returned to take care of individuals who had been expelled from the organizations in one way or another.

No mandate to change organizations

I can think of several possible reasons for this failure to shift into a more truly preventive type of work. It called for skills that were outside our field of competence. We really had no mandate to change organizations, and no change can be brought about unless some people in the organization strongly want a change.

At this point it seems appropriate to relate our experience of using nurses in this type of work. The employees tended to seek a nurse much more readily than they would seek a social worker—even if the social service were offered at the work premises, and even if the problem were a clear-cut social one. They would seek the nurse for ailments that often turned out to be mental or social problems. For this reason nurses were valuable for the team; they facilitated contacts and discovered problems. The team could use such information that pertained to the environment as an input for preventive activities at group level.

Social workers or nurses

We also experimented with the practice of a nurse paying a home call to each and every one in a unit, on the first or second day of sick absence. As a means of reducing short-term absence rates, the method was surprisingly effective. The experiment was, however, discontinued after a year and a half, because of waning union support.

From our point of view the most important experience from this practice was, however, that the nurses got insight into social problems, including economic, that we had not expected to find within the civil servant group. One problem with the use of nurses in our setting was that they needed doctors to function well. Our physicians had been picked because of interest in psychiatry, social medicine, and preventive work, rather than in regular medical practice. The nurses tended to preserve the individually-oriented curative activities that we were by then trying to avoid. This was the chief reason for not including nurses in the teams that were established after the initial experiences.

The year 1968 was a turning point for political and cultural activities in many Western countries. President de Gaulle was shaken by student riots in France and on university campuses in the United States police were firing at students. Sweden had its share of student occupations of official buildings and other signs of political unrest.

A CAMPAIGN ON MENTAL HEALTH

That same year we happened to launch a campaign on

mental health. It had been planned and prepared for many years by the Swedish insurance company Folksam. The same company had previously organized campaigns on better ergonomy and similar topics. This time they had two renowned psychiatrists write a book each on mental health and how to improve it in the work places. On this scientific basis an extensive educational programme was launched through existing networks of study circles within the biggest employee unions. Well over 30 000 persons were estimated to have taken part in the circle studies.

The campaign was heavily attacked by leftist groups. Counter-pamphlets were published with titles like *How to domesticate people*. The idea behind the reaction was that the campaign only aimed at helping people to adapt to existing conditions—it never questioned these conditions. In the emotional turmoil that was created, the existing and planned expansion of occupational health services also came under attack. 'By quenching the cries of the suffering people and smoothing out the frictions between employees and the work organizations, the health services facilitated a development of society in an inhumane direction.' The term 'manipulation' came to be used whenever employers tried to improve the lot for their employees.

Democratization of working life

Whether or not as a result of this debate, a lot of steps were in fact taken in the following decade towards a more genuinely democratic society, even in workplaces. In Sweden we have had extensive legislation consistently strengthening the position of the employee in relation to his employing organization. Most of this redistribution of power has taken the form of increasing the rights of the employee unions, as being the responsible representatives of the employees. Besides the legislation there have been collective bargaining negotiations that have further increased the power of the unions. Union activities are now permitted in paid working hours, union officials have particular job security, union safety delegates may order the suspension of dangerous job procedures, etc.

Occupational health services are today directed by boards with joint representation from management and employees. In the national administration these health boards are even dominated by employees, who appoint both the chairman and the vice-chairman. We now have a law on co-determination at work, legalizing negotiations on all matters that affect working conditions—including the investment programmes of a company. This right is coupled to corresponding rights to be informed beforehand of any plans to alter working conditions and to participate in the planning of such changes. We shall return to this development later in the text and to similar developments in Norway. For the moment the sketchy description is given only as a background for a better understanding of the more recent strategic considerations within the pilot project and its successor.

The grass-roots approach

It became increasingly clear in the project that it was not only directors and supervisors, or for that matter union representatives, who had to be taught about how to improve working conditions. Our information service and educational activities would never bring about changes if the target was thus limited. Everybody in the working organization had to be taught not how to adjust to working conditions, but how to question these very conditions and how to assume a co-responsibility for necessary changes. To begin with, thoughts like these were looked upon in many quarters as subversive activities. But the political and social development outlined above has provided the platform from which thoughts like these could become a respected reality.

Broadening our competence

We felt within our pilot organization a need to add to our competence skills that were not part of our background training. We needed to know how jobs should be organized better, how to develop a personnel policy, how to teach leaders to function in a better way. We studied personnel administration in order to be able to influence people in responsible positions to better live up to their responsibility and thereby prevent unnecessarily unhealthy conditions. It was no longer our task to solve their personnel problems; we should give them the help they needed to solve the problems themselves. 'Help to self-help'.

Having come that far in our strategic thinking, it was time to report our experience to the government, and thereby in practice set an end to the existence of our pilot organization. For it was no longer a job for doctors and social workers—preventive mental health work seemed to be part of established activities in work organization, personnel administration, leadership, and co-determination.

CREATION OF A GOVERNMENTAL PERSONNEL BOARD

The government concurred with the conclusions of our experiment and created a new board, the personnel board, manned primarily by professional personnel administrators. Through regional branch offices throughout the country it was to provide all local units of the national administration with help to self-help on personnel matters. Only extremely unusual or difficult problems were to be 'taken care of' by this specialist organ. This was all well and good, but somehow it was not enough. People were still having trouble in their job situations and some of them got sick or were in other ways sequestrated (knocked out) from the togetherness in the work units.

From my new position as chief medical adviser to the personnel board I could take up the problem of preventive psychiatry from a new angle. Medical services in industry had expanded during the 1960s and it was bvious in 1971 that demands for similar services could e expected from the civil servants, too, even though ey already had free medical care.

Industrial medicine or an occupational health service as in Sweden defined in an agreement from 1967 etween the employers' organization and the trade nions as consisting of two functions, one medical and ne technical, both with duties primarily in preventive ork with regard to occupational health. Considering nat the national administration mainly employs admini-rative personnel, the need for technical occupational ygiene could be expected to be less than in industry or a the mines. On the other hand we knew from our xperience that there was a considerable mass of mental nd social problems among the civil servants, problems nat to some extent resulted in nervous or psychoso-natic diseases.

ntroduction of psychosocial services

a our planning for the coming occupational health ervices for civil servants, we redefined the concept to nclude not only a medical and a technical function, but lso a social function. Later it became called psycho-ocial.

To make a long story short: there are now ordinances nd collective negotiation agreements on the non-rivate side (that is for employees of the national admini-ration and for local government employees) where ccupational health service is defined as having three inctions: a medical, a technical, and a psychosocial nction. All three aspects work in close co-operation nd under a common steering board with a dominating ersonnel influence.

This health organization is now being built up. There s still some confusion in many quarters about what the sychosocial division should actually do and what quali-ications people recruited to this function should ossess. To me it is clear that they should be change gents with qualifications in behavioural sciences and ot social workers or curators. Otherwise the mistakes of ur pilot organization will just be repeated.

A change agent in the health team has an advan-ageous position from many points of view. He has the upport of a joint board, permitting him to work in a eutral professional situation, and providing for the trust hat he needs for successful work. He has the support rom the other team units, providing him with valuable nput data on group problems. He has the advantage that ur pilot group did not have, of being 'within the family', ince the health service is felt as 'ours' in the work organi-ation and not as an intruder. If he does his job right he lso has an advantage over the doctors and nurses of not aving any personnel contract with anyone in the work rganization. He can fight for truth and insight without ny special considerations for patients or other indivi-lual help-seekers. Everyone in a group can trust his notives and everyone will get the same treatment, in the rocess of establishing consciousness and change pro-esses.

Reality distortion

The causes of fear, anxiety, and other emotions that may mediate nervous and psychosomatic disease are multiple. Basic security, physical and economic, must be estab-lished first of all—but that is not enough. Basic security is usually established for people in an employment situa-tion. Yet, as we have seen, people have problems in their job situations and some of those problems result in loss of well-being and actual disease.

In our opinion a hitherto unrecognized source of stress and disease is to be found in the so-called 'twilight zone of reality distortion' that exists in every organization. Anxiety, frustrations, anger, and disappointments are generated here, yet people prefer not to talk about, to cover it up. To feel lack of trust, to feel humiliated, to have fear of repercussions, are not easy to talk about particularly since emotions like these are often perceived as personal shortcomings that should be hidden from public exposure. Thus taboo zones are generated. People become blind to their own situation, adapt to it by giving up ambitions for a better life, or strive to get away from the present job to a better one. To many organization members this zone may be unconscious or semiconscious. Others who see more clearly prefer to remain silent since they do not think they could achieve any real change. People in power may simply be ignorant about it. Yet as this taboo zone expands, the efficiency of the organization suffers. Contacts are not made, creative contributions are withheld, communication becomes formalized, and people suffer. It seems to be a logical task for a psychosocial expert to minimize this vicious zone of reality distortion. To do this he needs techniques that create insight, promote openness and communica-tion. Such techniques exist and can be found in the literature on 'organizational development' and quality of working life.

QUALITY OF WORKING LIFE; CONFLICTING OBJECTIVES

'Quality of working life' has been defined (Hackman and Suttle 1977) as 'the degree to which members of a work organization are able to satisfy important personal needs through their experience in the organization.' Most obstacles to this satisfaction and reasons for suppression of needs are to be found in the twilight zone discussed here.

Managers usually want to create a healthy climate for their co-workers, but they rarely succeed. It should be clear that the objectives of an organization are not always congruent with the personal needs of its members. The people in power who identify themselves with the objectives of the organization sooner or later may come to resent the efforts to improve working life. Only to the extent that the efficiency of the organization is promoted by individual and collective development will they support the activities wholeheartedly.

Yet from a health perspective it may well be asked why

people should have to sacrifice the satisfaction of important human needs or perhaps even become ill in order to gain money that might—or more often might not—make life worth living in their spare time? There seems to be two steps to consider. One is in the interest of both parties, the organization and its employees, the other is not. With information and insight-promoting methods like those evolved in the organizational development techniques, the efficiency of an organization may be increased at the same time as the quality of working life is improved for the members. But the other step calls for sacrifices from either or both parties. Improvement of working conditions will eventually cost money that may not be repaid by an increase in productivity. Who then is to yield?

So far it has been the employees. Only minimum requirements have been set up by law in most countries. If we really want to fight for the health and well-being of the employees, some sort of power strategy must be resorted to, as a complement to the change agent activities. Requirements for job conditions may be specified directly in a law, as in the recent Norwegian act on work environment. Or the requirements may be formulated by the employees themselves if they are given support in a law, providing for their information and participation in decisions, as is done in the recent Swedish law on co-determination. We shall return to these laws at the end of this paper.

Work and health

Quality of working life is an issue in itself and need not be linked to health aspects in order to be recognized. But on the other hand from a health perspective it is rather essential to see links to quality of working life. Evidence has accumulated over the past decade, in particular, that clearly links poor job experience with diseases, both physical and mental.

A. Kornhauser's (1965) *Mental health of the industrial worker* stands out as one of the pioneer works in this field. More recent reviews may be found (e.g. ICOMH 1976). Myocardial infarction may be mentioned as an example of a disease that has been positively linked to job conditions. It may well be asked if we need more evidence. If there are no definite proofs, there is yet strong reason to believe that a lot of disease has its roots in job conditions. Anxiety, frustrations, anger, and other emotions produced in the job experience will surely take their toll in terms of sleepless nights, ulcers, hypertension, depressions, and suicides.

Work and leisure

We do have proof of a spill-over effect from work experience to leisure activities. People with monotonous, repetitive, short-cycled work tasks, with no margin for personal creativity development and emotional reward, tend to have a similarly empty leisure time. While people who are fortunate enough to have jobs calling for creativity, initiative, and responsibility, also lead a more active life in their spare time. Surveys of white collar workers

point to a correlation between conflicts in the job and neurotic or psychosomatic reactions, high tobacco consumption, and alcohol abuse, with consequent increase in disease risks.

Components of the health concept

We do not have to stretch the health concept in order to make the quality of working life a concern of the health organizations. But in my opinion the WHO definition of health lacks important components. Well-being is too static a concept. Man is a striving, conflict-resolving dynamic creature who cannot be expected to feel permanently well. Ability to cope constructively with reality is one important health component. To be willing and able to strive for life goals: recognition, support for self-esteem, identity, etc.; to feel a motivation to live including a motivation to be active and work, are essential elements of the health concept. Given the right job opportunities, even a handicapped person may use his work as a tool for establishing health as well as a sign of health. In this perspective an extensive literature on work motivation becomes relevant also for health issues. To make work worth doing and life worth living should be objectives of a health organization.

SUGGESTIONS FOR A WHO PROGRAMME

1. There is a need for information about what is meant by health and its links to the quality of working life.
2. There is a need for a broader competence in the field, for professional training and for research.
3. There is a need for legislative action or other means of power demonstration in various countries if real changes are to be brought about.

Need for information

The experience reported in previous sections of this paper indicates that many employees pursue their work in spite of health problems. It is an important aspect of preventive health work to improve the possibilities for doing this. In order to achieve this end, health workers must learn to treat organizations rather than individuals. Preventive mental health workers must learn to become 'change agents', applying skills and techniques from organization development procedures or from group psychotherapy. Their tasks as experts will not be to solve the problems for people, but to help them to solve their problems themselves in a better way—to induce awareness of problems and to encourage efforts to alter working conditions into more humane directions.

'Quality of working life' has, as mentioned, been defined as the degree to which members of a work organization are able to satisfy important personal needs through their experience in the organization. This definition also points to a strategy for mental health work: to make working people aware of their needs and help to augment their chances for job satisfaction. In simple erms, the health worker may have to ask: What can we eliminate in the given work conditions that unnecessarily limits the satisfaction of needs? Can we build in new elements that permit more needs to become satisfied? Permit more people to strive for things that make life worth living as parts of their jobs?

It may be noted in passing that reducing all occupational stress is *not* a goal for this kind of activity. Personal progress and experience of success cannot be won without accumulation of personal resources and strong effort. This kind of constructive stress may well have to be built into many job situations in order to make them healthier.

What are the important personal needs that should be recognized and the satisfaction of which should be promoted? What is man striving for? There is, of course, no universally true answer to that question. It has to be specified at each work unit by the people who are members of it. But they may need indications where to seek. Most people seek security, not only physical and economical; they seek trust, they want to be able to rely on their fellows and to be able to expect support from them when needed. Some seek recognition, support for self-esteem, pride in the product of their efforts. Some seek to become unique individuals, express their personality, develop an identity. Most people want to use a broader part of their capacity, to use not only their muscles, but also their heads and their hearts. They want to understand what they are doing and how their task fits into the bigger production system. Quite a few want to share the responsibility in decisions on questions affecting their working conditions. And still more may well learn to ask for, and grow with, increased responsibility. People who have experienced that seldom want to return to previous conditions.

It is seldom difficult to find elements in working conditions that unnecessarily limit the chances of satisfying these needs. If people feel exchangeable, are given too simple tasks, feel like robots, or look upon pay as the only reward of the job, that is usually easy to verbalize. It may be more difficult to find the more subtle frustrations: lack of trust, derogative treatment by superiors, competition, conformism, fear, and unsupportive activities, etc. To make people aware of such facts may be difficult, partly because of the adaptation process that most employees remaining in an organization have gone through. They often have to deny their needs, give up their ambitions to live a full life, in order to achieve peace within themselves. And they do not want to give up that peace unless they are convinced that a change might be a trustworthy alternative.

The mental health worker must be careful not to impose his own standards, values, and preconceived ideas upon the group. It is the group members' own value systems that have to guide development. Only the people themselves in the organizations can identify the elements that must be changed and only if they decide the alterations themselves will they become a reality. The expert can create forums for discussions. He may, by his presence, legalize discussions of emotions. He may help to trace the emotions to their sources. He may also be able to suggest alternatives when it comes to work technology, work organization, personnel administration, and collaborative leadership styles. But only as conceivable alternatives for the group to choose among.

The expert may also furnish fuel for the discussions by eliciting group statistics on productivity, absence rates (not individually traceable), turnover rates, etc. He may also promote insight by distributing questionnaires with more or less provocative questions. Not that the direct answers are of much value in themselves. But feeding them back to the groups in anonymous form may start up a discussion about how things really are and how they might be instead, thereby initiating the process of change.

Insight-promoting techniques should not be used indiscriminately. Just as in psychotherapy, one has to find out if the patient can stand the truth or if it might disrupt the little normal function that is left. More important: It would be cynical to produce conscious awareness if the insight gained cannot be used for adaptive changes. This is why a power redistribution must precede or accompany the process. The people in power must be willing to share it with the other members of the organization, if any real and lasting change is to take place.

It is the task of the expert to create a climate where information is willingly shared in the interest of realism. A leading principle should be to create prerequisites for informed decisions at all levels, and preferably at as low levels in the organization as possible. The leaders of an organization may be reluctant to accept this principle—especially if it is taken further than serves the interests of organization efficiency and productivity. The health worker, or change agent, may therefore need support from outside sources of power, as has been mentioned earlier in this paper. This is where legislation may be needed. We shall discuss that further below. An important point is, however, that given a power distribution to lower levels in the organization, there are realistic chances with available methods of changing working climates in a healthier direction.

Since the change agent moves in a field of conflicting interests and powers, it is essential that he has a mandate both from the managers and from the employees. This mandate may be established on a contract basis as a temporary consultant. Or it may be provided for more permanently through a joint steering board, such as the boards that now steer the occupational health services in our country. If the WHO is convinced that efforts of this sort are needed in the interest of health and quality of working life, then it seems natural for the WHO to recommend to its member nations to install a function of this sort in the occupational health teams.

Increasing knowledge and competence

There is today no formal training or defined qualifications for the suggested sort of health workers. The job calls for a person trained in the behavioural sciences:

psychologist, sociologist, social worker, or physician with unusual interests in preventive work. In addition to this basic training in behavioural sciences the specialist needs to know about insight-producing techniques such as those used in organizational development or in group psychotherapy. He also needs a personal insight into his own value system and prejudices, so he does not unconsciously impose them on the clients. The training should therefore include a bit of personal analysis. Finally, the specialist is well helped by some knowledge of work organization, personnel administration, and leadership.

It seems to be a task for the WHO to outline the requisite qualifications and influence the member states to start education programmes in this new health profession. The WHO has already given support to research in the field of job-related diseases and other stress reactions.

The suggested applications of new knowledge are, however, not in all respects based upon scientifically proven evidence. There is a great need for scientific testing of the effects of the suggested methods, and the various variations that may be necessary in different work settings. To encourage reseach activities of this sort should be one of the WHO contributions.

Legislation: two examples
As repeatedly stated, the suggested health-promoting changes will perhaps never become a reality unless some supportive legislation is also introduced. This is particularly true in competitive societies, where a threat to the efficiency of an organization, in the interest of the health of its members, may risk the existence of the very same organization. Therefore, an international organ, like the WHO, is in a unique position to suggest similar legislative conditions to its various member nations.

I shall end this paper with a description of two samples, the Norwegian work environment act and the Swedish act on co-determination. Both could serve as models for other countries, even if local traditions may call for changes or alterations. Both have the same ultimate aim but they differ in strategic approaches.

Section 12 of the Norwegian work environment act.

1. General requirements
Technology, work organization, work time (e.g. shift plans) and payment systems are to be designed so that negative physiological or psychological effects for employees are avoided as well as any negative influence on the alertness necessary to the observance of safety considerations. Employees are to be given possibilities for personal development and for the maintenance and development of skills.
2. Design of jobs
In the planning of work and design of jobs, possibilities for employee self-determination and maintenance of skills are to be considered. Monotonous repetitive work and work that is bound by machine or assembly line in such a way than no room for variation in work rhythm is left, should be avoided.

Jobs should be designed in a way that gives possibilities for variation, for contact with others, for understanding of the interdependence between elements that constitute a job, and

for information and feed-back to employees concerning production requirements and results.
3. Systems for planning and control (e.g. automatic data processing systems).
Employees or their elected representatives are to be kept informed about systems used for planning and control, changes in such systems included. They are to be given the training necessary to understand the systems and the right to influence their design.
4. Work under safety risks.
Piece-rate and related payment systems are not to be used where wage systems can influence the safety level.

This is not an authorized translation but it is made by one of the men behind the law, Björn Gustavsen, who presented the philosophy behind it at a mental health conference in New York in May 1977 (Mclean 1977). In the present context the law may well speak for itself.

In Sweden the legislative approach was twofold. There is a new work-environment act coming into force on 1 July 1978. It is a framework law with general statements like: 'Working conditions shall be adapted to man's mental and physical capacities. Jobs shall be designed so that the employees themselves may influence their work situation'. This framework has to be filled in with specifications from two sources. One source is the Board of Occupational Safety and Health. The other source, and for mental health purposes perhaps the most important one, is the outcome of another law, the act on co-determination at work.

The latter act provides for information to employee union representatives on all matters, and on all levels about working conditions. The law gives the right for local unions to negotiate on any matter that may influence their job situation. The parties themselves, the managers, and the employees at the local plants, shall agree on the specifications of job requirements that fit themselves.

It is still too early to judge the relative merits of the Norwegian and the Swedish system. On paper the Swedish system seems more flexible. It gives the local employees a chance to share responsibilities and to grow with it as human beings. It is a little disturbing that the local negotiations have not yet gained momentum, even though the law has been in force since January 1977. The beneficial effects in terms of health might be missed entirely if power is simply shifted from the local directors to central union headquarters. There is, however, a declared intent on the part of the central trade unions to make the planned local self-determination and co-determination a reality.

If co-determination is a necessary prerequisite for successful change processes, it may well be asked if the system of co-determination does not also need the complement of change agent activity in order to function well. So far some unions have not been too eager to let in specialists of the change agent type. In their negotiations they have, however, provided for the right to call in their own specialist consultants. The prospect of two different sets of consultants, one engaged by the employers nd another by the employees, does not seem very attractive.

The WHO should support a development where health and well-being in workplaces are recognized as a joint interest of both parties, and where the necessary expertise must have a positive mandate from both.

SUMMARY

t has been suggested in this paper that the WHO should spread knowledge of how preventive mental health work could be done in an occupational setting. The WHO should point out the links between bad working conditions and impaired health, and its opposite aspects: stimulating working conditions and positive health and life enjoyment.

The WHO should encourage its member nations to provide for specialist services to improve the mental health of employees. The specialist may work either as free consultants contracted jointly by management and employees, or as a part of the occupational health team under the steering of a jointly composed board.

The WHO should also draw up the lines for training and define the competence of the specialists in preventive mental health work. Regular medical training is not adequate for this type of work, which rather should be based upon a competence in behavioural sciences, change agent technology, and group psychotherapy.

The WHO should stimulate research in preventive psychiatry and particularly on its practical applications in occupational settings.

The WHO should encourage the member nations to legislate in a direction that supports the positions of the employees in relation to their employing organization. If possible, the individuals should be given the opportunity to share responsibilities and take part in planning of changes in working conditions.

The job itself must be made a contribution to life content. Work should become a valuable tool for the realization of life goals.

REFERENCES

HACKMAN, J. R. and SUTTLE, J. L. (1977). *Improving life at work. Behavioural science approaches to organizational change.* Goodyear Publishing Co., Santa Monica, California.

ICOMH (1976). International Committee on Occupational Mental Health, Conference in Stockholm, Sweden, August, 1976. (Can be requested from TCO, Box 5252, 102 45 Stockholm, Sweden.)

KORNHAUSER, A. (1965). *Mental health of the industrial worker.* Wiley, New York.

McLEAN, A. (ch. ed.) (1977). Proceedings of a Conference in New York, May 1977, co-sponsored by a number of organizations including the WHO and the ICOMH. (Can be requested from NIOSH (contract number 21-77-0041) or from Dr. McLean, 21 Bloomingdale Road, White Plains, N.Y. 106 05, USA.)

36. COMMUNITY MENTAL HEALTH CENTRE CONSULTATION AND THE WORKING LIFE OF THE COMMUNITY

F. E. SPANER

INTRODUCTION

The Community Mental Health Centre Programme of the United States has been evolving over the eleven-year period since the enactment of the initial enabling legislation in 1963. An integral part of this evolution has been the emergence of the consultation and education services to community mental health centres as an important factor in the treatment and prevention of mental health problems within the community. In recent years consultation and education services of centres have become increasingly concerned with the relationship of the working life of persons residing in the community to their mental health. This paper reviews some of the background and concepts of the community mental health centre programme and some current knowledge about community mental health centre consultation and the working life of the community.

HISTORY OF THE COMMUNITY MENTAL HEALTH CENTRE PROGRAMME

President Dwight David Eisenhower appointed a Joint Commission on Mental Illness and Health in 1955 to study the problem of care and treatment of the mentally ill in the United States. The Commission reported its findings in a report *Action for mental health* in 1961. In 1963 President John Fitzgerald Kennedy sent a message to the Congress of the United States on mental illness and mental retardation in which he urged implementation of the Joint Commission's recommendation that comprehensive mental health services be located in the community, close to where people lived.

The Congress enacted the Community Mental Health Centre Act of 1963 (Title II 1963) which provided Federal support for part of the cost of construction of community-based mental health facilities. The regulations to implement the Act contained the first basic concepts of the programme. These were: (1) that comprehensiveness of service at a minimum included five essential services: consultation and education, emergency, out-patient, partial hospitalization, and in-patient services; (2) community was defined as a geographic portion of a state containing 70 000 to 200 000 persons, called a catchment area, which was determined by the state's mental health planning group in the state's mental health plan; (3) each catchment area could have only one federally supported community mental health centre responsible for providing a comprehensive range

of mental health services to persons residing in the catchment area regardless of age, sex, diagnostic condition, ethnic or cultural background, socio-economic status, or ability to pay; (4) the centre services had to be readily accessible and available to all residents of the catchment area and connected together so as to assure continuity of care; (5) the residents of the community had to be involved in the planning and operation of the centre's programme so as to insure optimal responsiveness of the programme to the specific mental health needs of that particular catchment area. In 1965 the Congress amended the Act to provide Federal support for part of the cost of professional and technical staff for 51 months on a declining basis from 75 per cent Federal support in the first year to 30 per cent in the period immediately prior to termination of Federal participation. Subsequent amendments have extended the range of mental health services encouraged by Federal support to include special programmes for alcoholics, drug abusers, and children. The amendment of 1970 extended the period of staffing grant support from the 51 months to eight years and provided preferential rates of support for community mental health centres serving designated poverty catchment areas.

EVOLVING CONCEPT OF THE COMMUNITY MENTAL HEALTH CENTRE

The initial legislation establishing the community mental health centres programme provided Federal support for part of the cost of construction of a facility to house the centre. It was believed at that time that the facility was the centre. Since July 1965, when the first Federal community mental health centre construction grant was awarded, experience has demonstrated that a community mental health centre is not merely a building, but rather a system of mental health care, a service network. It encompasses both existing community agencies and whatever new ones are needed to assure the provision of a comprehensive range of services to all the persons residing in the catchment area who may be in need of such service.

The full comprehensive range of services is defined in the regulations as consultation and education, emergency, out-patient, partial hospitalization, and in-patient services. Experience has shown that these are not really discrete services; they are a range of time commitments pertaining to the delivery of mental health services. This range is from prevention, attempting to forestall mental health problems in the population (consultation and education service); to immediate responsiveness on a twenty-four-hour-a-day, seven-day-a-week basis whenever an individual, family, or group residing in the catchment area experiences an acute mental health problem (emergency service); to treatment of catchment area residents as needed on an ongoing basis while they continue their day-to-day relationships and obligations (out-patient services); to providing mental health services to persons in need of mental health care either during the day on a five-day-a-week basis, when they are not able to function effectively because of mental health problems related to their daily activities, or provision of mental health care during the evening and night-time hours because they cannot temporarily continue their usual relationships at those times, or provision of mental health care over week-ends for those who have difficulties at those times (partial hospitalization); to twenty-four hour care for persons who cannot function either during the day or evening in their usual settings and must, therefore, have a new setting free from whatever factors have been found by them to be overwhelming (in-patient service).

Each of the above services have permitted community mental health centres to develop special programmes to meet the specific needs of persons residing in their catchment areas. Such programmes have introduced concepts and procedures into community mental health services which have been incorporated into mental health planning. These include such concepts as community involvement, accountabilty, responsiveness, equity, accessibility, availability, and continuity of care, and such procedures for services delivery as satellites, outreach programmes, and utilization of paraprofessionals and indigenous mental health workers.

The Community Mental Health Centres Programme, therefore, is attempting to make a full range of mental health services accessible and available to a total population of a geographically defined service area (catchment area), vest responsibility for this objective in the community, and make the mental health professionals who are charged with implementing these objectives accountable to that community. The attempt to develop such a system on a national basis is relatively new. By 1 July 1974 the Community Mental Health Centre Act made this system of care available to approximately 40 per cent of the people residing in the United States.

CHANGES IN THE DEVELOPMENT OF CONSULTATION AND EDUCATION SERVICES

From 1966 when the first community mental health centre became operational under a Federal staffing grant until 1 July 1974, when approximately 450 community mental health centres were providing comprehensive mental health services as a result of such grants, each has included as part of its comprehensive range of services a consultation and education service. Centres in the early years of the programme focused their consultation and education efforts on informing their community of the kinds of services they had to offer. It seems that each new centre still goes through this stage, and even mature centres have to engage in this informational activity in order to obtain the participation of new community groups in their mental health effort. This first step seems to be part of a natural evolution which permits the CMHC to interact with community agencies who should be aware of its programme and work with it. This is followed by the centre's staff attempting to help community caretakers to identify individuals who have mental health problems whom they can handle themselves, if provided adequate mental health consultation. A next step in the process is helping the staffs of these human service agencies in the community to achieve sufficient understanding of their role in interpersonal relationships so that they can deal with troubled people without the direct support of mental health professionals. Hence, the consultation and education service of the CHMC tries to help community care-givers to identify those whom they can serve directly and those whose problems are beyond their capability. In the latter case the objective is to train agency staffs to make effective referrals to the community mental health centre.

Many consultation and education programmes do not evolve past this stage. A few, however, have been able to achieve a further stage of development by effectively using catchment area demographic and centre utilization data to identify sources of mental health problems. The identification of such problems has, in some instances, led to a dialogue with the relevant community groups to consider possible ways of changing the conditions which may be producing the problems. Consultation and education services have evolved from informing potential referral sources of the centres' services, to helping the community consider, and possibly institute, changes which may reduce the incidence of mental health problems.

AREAS OF COMMUNITY MENTAL CENTRE CONSULATIVE ACTIVITY

The major thrust of the consultation and education services of community mental health centres has been directed toward schools. Over 90 per cent of the federally supported centres report consultation programmes with school systems in their catchment areas. An important factor in this development has been the need for CHMCs to develop sources of non-Federal support as Federal funding participation declines. Many school systems have recognized the value of mental health consultation and have entered into contractual relationships with community mental health centres to help support this service.

The consultation provided to schools has followed the

developmental process described. Initially the centre staff focus their efforts on informing teachers and school counsellors about the centre's services and how they may serve as referral agents. Then they try to help them to handle some of the less acute problems they previously referred. In such instances the mental health consultant is available to provide case consultation should it be needed. As the teachers and counsellors become more effective, they gain confidence and assume a greater role in resolving problems on their own. In addition, as mental health consultants become more familiar with the schools and their mental health problems, the consultants may be able to identify focal points in the system which seem to be producing some of the mental health problems. By helping school authorities to understand how their system may be contributing to mental health problems, they may help them to change conditions to reduce such problems.

Other community agencies with whom community mental health centres have developed consultative relationships are the law enforcement, health, social, and welfare agencies. In addition, community mental health centres have also directed their consultation and education efforts toward attorneys, physicians, clergymen, and governmental officials.

It is only very recently that community mental health centres have attempted to develop consultation and education programmes with industry and employer and employee groups. This has not been an easy development because the Community Mental Health Centres Programme is resident rather than employment-based. The problem involved may be understood when one considers that for optimal effectiveness the catchment area is supposed to include from 70 000 to 200 000 persons. However, in large metropolitan areas the centre's catchment area may contain major portions of the downtown business section or may include large industrial complexes so that the number of persons employed in the catchment area during the forty-hour work week may be as much as ten times the resident population of the catchment area. Community mental health centres have felt that they cannot serve the population which does not reside in the catchment area except for emergencies. In addition, the population which comes into the catchment area for employment may not contribute to the support of the centre and may not have any voice in its operation. The catchment area concept has served to hold community mental health centres accountable to the persons who reside in, pay taxes, and determine the local policies, needs, and priorities of the area. How to effectively provide mental health services to those who enter the area during the work week and how to include them in the centre's decision-making process is yet to be worked out. This issue is intimately related to CHMCs finding effective funding alternatives to declining federal staffing grants. Industrial connections are most likely to develop as they offer opportunities for CHMCs to improve their fiscal viability.

COMMUNITY MENTAL HEALTH CENTRE CONSULATION AND THE WORKING LIFE OF THE COMMUNITY

In order to determine the extent and nature of the mental health consultation that community mental health centres were providing to employers and/or employees in the work setting, the 392 community mental health centres which were operational as of 1 July 1973 were asked to provide the names of their staff responsible for such a programme. Although the question was posed so that no reply was necessary if the centre did not have such a programme, 30 centres replied that they did not have such a programme. These, plus the 207 which did not reply, may be assumed not to have any consultative activity of this kind. An additional 14 centres indicated that although they had no programme at present, they were developing or planning such a programme, and another 14 stated that their relationship to industry was solely to help patients in treatment at the centre to return to an effective working life.

Approximately one-third (127) of the community mental health centres provided the name of one or more staff members who were responsible for the centre's mental health consultation to employers and/or employees in the work setting. Seventy-five (approximately 60 per cent) of these centres were contacted to determine the nature of their programme.

Consultation to industry regarding alcoholism problems

Twenty-eight (37 per cent) of the centres contacted were engaged in industrial alcoholism programmes, or a programme with industry where alcoholism, although not the sole area of concern, was, nevertheless, the major focus. Most of these programmes were stimulated or strongly influenced by the Troubled Employee Programme of the National Institute on Alcohol Abuse and Alcoholism. The community mental health centres in these cases were providing consultation to industry to help supervisors identify and refer for counselling, employees whose productivity had declined. This programme assumes that if an individual is troubled, it will be reflected in a decline in productivity. In many instances, indeed, the troubled individual, whose work performance was suffering, was also found to be using alcohol to excess.

This programme is relatively new, having been initiated approximately eighteen months ago by the Occupational Programmes Branch of the National Institute of Alcohol Abuse and Alcoholism. It has been adopted by some of the community mental health centres surveyed as an effective entrée to industrial mental health consultation. It was also noted by them that this programme has the advantage that referrals from industry may be covered by insurance which can produce much needed third-party reimbursement income for the centre.

Employers are able to accept this programme on the basis that it helps them to keep trained and experienced workers whom they might otherwise lose. Employees find this programme to their advantage since, rather than being fired when their job performance has slipped, they are helped to deal with their problems.

Consultation to industry regarding general mental health problems

The community mental health centre consultative effort in regard to industry has been largely focused on selling the concept to the employer that it is better to try to help troubled employees than to get rid of them. If this thesis is accepted by management, the next step is to obtain their support for a programme to train supervisiors, not to be clinicians or diagnosticians, but to be better supervisors. This programme involves sensitizing supervisors to early signs of declining job performance on the part of a worker, and teaching them how to confront such workers with the evidence of poor performance in a non-punitive, non-threatening manner. The objective of such confrontation is to offer the employee the opportunity to see a counsellor. The employee's dealings with the counsellor are in complete confidence, and it is the counsellor who determines whether a referral to the community mental health centre is appropriate.

Although the community mental health centres contacted have limited their efforts to consultation and education with industry, which facilitates the early detection and referral aspects of mental health problems, some are considering discussions with management regarding aspects of the work setting which have the potential for producing mental health problems. Most of those who have considered initiating such discussions feel that a necessary first step is providing good service on a case basis before attempting to provide consultation on a programme basis.

Consultation to unions

Some community mental health centres contacted, rather than working with employers, are working with unions to develop effective mental health services to the union's members. This is mainly an effort to implement the mental health coverage included in the collective-bargaining contract between the union and the employer. A major union involved in this effort is the United Automobile Workers. Two community mental health centres, one in Michigan and one in New Jersey, have been awarded grants by the National Institute of Mental Health to demonstrate a feasible linkage between them and the work setting where collective bargaining health insurance benefits for 'nervous and mental disorders' are available to workers. Other community mental health centres in those states have become involved as a result of state-wide efforts on the part of the union. In the relationship with the unions, the mental health programmes developed in the plants consider mental health services for the employee to be a right, and it is not necessarily related to the employee's productivity level as in the Troubled Employee Programme. In these cases the employee's receipt of mental health services is not usually initiated by supervisors, but rather is initiated by the employees themselves or their union counsellors. The community mental health centre provides information to union counsellors and employees on the nature of the centre's services and provides training and consultation to counsellors on how to relate to and refer workers who manifest mental health problems.

Consultation to industrial health personnel

Among the community mental health centres contacted, many provide mental health consultation to industrial physicians and nurses of companies located in their catchment area. Such consultation may be either of a direct or indirect nature. It may be for pre-employment screening, assessing the potential mental health impact of contemplated employee transfers, determining whether an individual with mental health problems should remain on the job or be given a leave of absence, or, where a worker has been relieved from duty because of mental health problems, whether he or she is able to return to duty.

Much of this consultation is the traditional type of consultation which an industrial physician might solicit from a psychiatric consultant. The community mental health centre psychiatrist or other members of the staff provide this to industrial health units, either on request or as part of a contractual relationship. This type of consultation is case-oriented. It is conceivable that if the centre staff identifies some significant problem patterns in the plant, it may discuss them with top management to find ways of reducing the problem-provoking factors. However, this is not usually a part of the contractual relationship.

Consultation to community agencies

Although from the inception of the programme, the main consultation efforts of CHMCs have been directed toward providing community agencies with case consultation and programme consultation regarding their clientele, it is only recently that CHMCs are providing consultation to these agencies in regard to the mental health aspects of their work setting. The mental health problems of employees and staffs of human service agencies in the community may affect the mental health of persons who seek their services. Hence it is not only the mental health of the individual employee in the agency which is important—it is also that employee's impact on those whom they serve. For example, consultation and education services to schools have been primarily focused on case or programme consultation regarding the students. New directions indicate consultative activity in regard to school personnel as employees, the school administration as employers, and the school as a work setting. Similar programmes are being initiated with the staffs of law enforcement agencies and social welfare and health agencies.

In each instance, initial consultation by the CHMC is mainly aimed at informing the agency of the centre's services to which their employees are entitled as residents of the catchment area. Since the centre's staff is also engaged in providing consultation to them regarding the mental health problems of their clients, it has been possible to develop other mental health programmes such as seminars and workshops. Some of these have led to an examination of the mental health factors in the agency's work setting.

Consultation regarding vocational rehabilitation

Most CHMCs are involved with industry and the world of work as an integral part of their rehabilitation of persons with mental health problems. This may involve work with and through the established vocational rehabilitation agencies of the community, or it may involve independent efforts on the part of the CHMC to prepare those in treatment for an effective working life. This has included the development of sheltered workshops, group living and work arrangements, specially supervised placements in industry, and follow-up and consultation to supervisors and employers of ex-mental patients.

By consulting with employers and supervisors regarding patients or ex-patients, the centre staff has the opportunity to educate them in regard to mental health principles. On occasion it is found that the same factors which may prevent the exacerbation of mental health problems for the person in treatment may also help prevent potential mental health problems in the work setting for other employees.

When such consultation efforts are successful, and industrial managers and supervisors find the CHMCs mental health consultation to be meaningful, it can in some instances lead to management examining mental health factors within the organization.

SUMMARY

Reports from seventy-five community mental health centres, claiming to have consultation and education programmes with employers or employees in the work setting, indicate major emphases on information giving and soliciting referrals from industry.

Many of them are involved in the Troubled Employee Programme with an emphasis on early detection and treatment of alcoholism which is impairing the performance of workers. The 'troubled employee' orientation is also being applied in some mental health programmes supported by management which address themselves to other than alcoholic problems. Programmes with unions are also developing. Their objectives are similar to the 'troubled employee' programme, but are not focused on diminished productivity as the principal indicator of possible mental health problems. Many centres are also providing mental health consultation to industry by consulting with industrial nurses and physicians. Another reported work setting target for CMHC mental health consultation is human service agencies in the community. Although consultation to them has been and continues to be directed toward helping them with their clients, there is a growing effort to help them deal with mental health problems of their staffs. Community mental health centres are also involved in the vocational rehabilitation of parents and ex-patients, which brings them in contact with employers and supervisors.

It seems that CHMCs are recognizing that, in addition to the family and the school, the work-setting is an important area for mental health services and consultation. If consultation patterns develop in the same way for the work setting as they have for community agencies, it may be expected that case consultation will be replaced by programme consultation.

Community mental health centres need to become knowledgeable of research findings which are applicable to their situation. They also need to develop mechanisms for involving employers and employees in the work setting as part of the community to which they are accountable and from which they receive support.

REFERENCES

Annual CHMC Inventory. Survey and Reports Branch, Division of Biometry, National Institute of Mental Health, U.S.A.

Joint Commission on Mental Illness and Health (1961). *Action for mental health*. Basic Books, New York.

OZARIN, L. D., FELDMAN, S., and SPANER, F. E. (1971). Experience with community mental health centers. *Amer. J. Psychiat.*, **127**, 7.

SPANER, F. E. (1974). New directions in community mental health centre programs. In *Behavior analysis and systems analysis: an integrative approach to mental health programs* (ed. D. Harshbarger and R. F. Maley). Behaviordelia, Inc., Kalamazoo, Michigan.

Statistical Notes, Survey and Reports Branch, Division of Biometry, National Institute of Mental Health, U.S.A.

Title II (1963). Mental Retardation Facilities and Community Mental Health Centers Act of 1963, U.S.A., as amended.

37. FEMALE EMPLOYEES AT WORK: PRESENT PROBLEMS. LABOUR MARKET COUNTERMEASURES

ANNA-GRETA LEIJON

An important part of man's life is work and the condiions thereof. Work is a means of earning a livelihood but it also has the specific quality of paving the way to social communication. Work can satisfy man's basic need to develop and enrich his existence. The conditions of work often determine many other fundamental conditions for the individual. Material circumstances, health, social activities, participation in political and union activities, family and living conditions—all these factors are to diverse degrees connected with the conditions prevailing at work.

The right to work must therefore be a determining base for political reform. All social structures which are not built on full employment mean that conditions of life are curtailed and human resources wasted. The requirements of man at work are also the central area for political action. If man cannot influence the form and content of his work, he experiences work only as a necessity for earning his living on conditions dictated by others. It is therefore a necessary requirement that the workers themselves shall influence the formation of their working conditions, functions, and environment if their work is to serve any purpose for developing and enriching the individual.

SOCIETY'S GROWING RESPONSIBILITY TOWARDS EMPLOYMENT

From the point of view of the function of work for the individual and society, the state has adopted growing responsibility for measures that offer employment to a greater number of persons of working age. The ambition has been to equalize social and economic conditions between individuals, groups, and regions.

During the 1960s, policy measures in the labour market were developed in various directions and received increased resources. Support for both geographical and occupational mobility acquired a more important function together with sheltered employment and more traditional measures against unemployment, such as emergency relief work. A basis for this policy lies in the ambition to increase possibilities of choice for people seeking employment and at the same time facilitate recruitment to firms with stable employment and good wage capacity.

In recent years, the aims of labour market policy have increased. Besides offering employment to those openly seeking work, programmes have been geared to altering the situation for those who are latently unemployed. In

other ways, too, labour market policy has become more positive. A number of measures have been taken to help enterprises adapt their demand so that this will be better suited to the employees' possibilities, instead of just calling for adaptation by those seeking employment. This policy is aimed at opposing the process of elimination on the labour market and, among other things, at strengthening the position of the handicapped. Further, labour market policy has, to a greater degree, been adjusted to break up the remaining traditional labour market classification of occupations and functions between men and women, thereby promoting equality between the sexes.

Towards the end of the 1960s, problems on the labour market were intensified. Changing market conditions, rapid technical development, as well as various efforts of industrial policy in many competing countries, contributed to a more rapid transformation of industry and commerce. A threat to security as regards employment, occupation, and income, was often experienced. Demands for increased efforts by the government were growing. The active economic policy that was then explored, aimed towards contributing to industrial expansion and full employment.

THE TREND ON THE LABOUR MARKET DURING THE 1960s AND 1970s

In spite of declining employment in manufacturing, there has been a considerable increase in total employment in recent years. Through rapid economic growth and various public activities within the community during the 1960s, approximately 300 000 more people were employed. During the period 1965–72, the manpower surveys show that employment increased by 165 000 people. This increase reflects a relatively great net immigration, particularly towards the end of the 1960s, as well as an increasing number of women seeking gainful employment. In the period 1965–72, the participation rate for women rose from 37 to 54 per cent. The state and the municipalities accounted for most of these increases, in the form of hospital personnel, visiting nurses, teachers, and other school personnel. The increased employment contributed both directly and indirectly towards augmenting and distributing the standard of living in a more correct manner.

Behind this expansion on the labour market there was also a conscious effort to tear down employment barriers of various kinds. From the latter half of the 1960s, many industrial countries have noted a tendency towards increased registered unemployment. An earlier trend towards a long-range decline in unemployment appears to have been slowed down or stopped. This description also applies to Sweden. Various factors have been involved.

The efforts of society to develop work for groups that used to seek employment to only a limited extent have helped to boost the supply of manpower. Through a great number of reforms in various areas, total employment has increased continuously. At the same time, registered unemployment has increased, too. This means that some of the latent job-seekers have begun to seek employment actively.

Unemployment has also altered its character as a result of the strength and uneven pace of structural change. Earlier, there was already an imbalance between labour supply and demand and this has become more and more apparent. Even during periods of recession, the demand for personnel, primarily experienced and trained, has been substantial. There may be various reasons why this demand could not, in many cases, be met as rapidly as had been desired. The requirements of vocational training and job experience constitute a short-range obstacle. A special problem is the regional imbalance in supply and demand. In many communities with limited industry and commerce, the demand from firms is often for personnel with other professional specializations and/or vocational training than what those seeking employment have to offer.

At the same time, with the continuously increased demands for job satisfaction, it is apparent that a great number of the unemployed can accept work only under certain fixed conditions with regard to the type of work, work schedule, and the geographical location of the job site, etc. In addition, the traditional outlook regarding the choice of employment for men and women still prevails. The resultant division of the labour market limits the individual's choice of employment and makes for difficult adjustment on the labour market as a whole.

A decisive factor with regard to unemployment is the longer periods of unemployment that prevail. Between 1965 and 1970, the proportion of the unemployed grew for those whose period of unemployment exceeded three months—an increase from 13 to 24 per cent. The shift towards longer periods of unemployment continued into the early 1970s. This lengthening of unemployment periods is an important part of the explanation for the increased number of unemployed. In total numbers, no more persons seem to have been involved in unemployment than before. However, the period required to find new employment is longer now and this means an increase in the number of unemployed registered each time a census is taken.

BRIEF OUTLINE OF WOMEN'S SITUATION ON THE LABOUR MARKET

The situation of women has changed radically over the last twenty years. Between 1950 and 1970 the number of women employed has doubled and the number of married women gainfully employed has quadrupled. Women, today, comprise approximately 40 per cent of the labour force. In 1973, the participation rate (i.e., the portion of the whole population aged 16–74 years that was employed or seeking employment) totalled 55·2 per cent for women and 79·5 per cent for men. For all women aged 20–54 years, single or married, the participation rate is currently above 50 per cent. An interesting phenomenon, which also illustrates the increasing public awareness of the necessary child-care provisions, is that the manpower rate for women with one or two children increased by more than 6 per cent. In 1973, the rate was accordingly 70·8 per cent for women with one child, 59 per cent for women with two children, and 49·2 per cent for those who had three children or more.

Both the participation rate and unemployment for women vary a great deal between different parts of the country. In 1973, the employment rate was, for example, 62 per cent in Stockholm county but under 50 per cent in other areas. In straight figures, the number of employed women has increased by 230 000 from 1965 to 1973. Almost half of the employed women, now totalling more than 1·5 million, are in public administration and other public services. The greatest increase in employment for women is found within hospital care, teaching, and public administration.

The latest recession is of special interest from the women's viewpoint. The number of employed women went on rising even during these years. In earlier recessions, women's participation rate has decreased or stagnated. The recent change is therefore noteworthy. But unemployment among women has also increased a great deal, both totally and relatively. The proportion of women among the registered unemployed has increased gradually in recent years. We can note that an equivalent trend is found in the labour force surveys, where women now constitute more than half of all those seeking employment. This increase of umemployment is, however, accompanied by a decrease of latent job seekers. In other words, women are now leaving the group of latently unemployed and are instead openly registering with the public employment offices. There, in fact, we have an example of a manpower supply that just a few years ago was called 'potential resources'. But the number of latent job seekers is still large and it is not unlikely that they will offer their services actively during the 1970s. The reasons for this change from latent to open unemployment are numerous. I believe that a different attitude is emerging in growing parts of society, a different view towards womens' participation on the labour market. It is no longer self-evident that men should have first choice of available jobs—not even when jobs are hard to get. I think there is another reason for this—the self-confidence of women has increased. Fear of entering the labour market after a longer period of work as a housewife has been reduced once they see that other women have been able to cope with these problems. It is, of course, also quite clear that women are leaving latent unemployment for open unemployment because they really believe that society has possibilities of helping them find work.

A continued increase of women seeking gainful employment will also be noticed during the next decade. But currently, one finds that the labour market is still divided into *one* part mainly for men and *one* dominated by women. Let me illustrate this with a few figures. Over 80 per cent of those employed in the health and sick care sector are women, whereas women constitute only one-fourth of the employed in the manufacturing sector. The changes in this pattern over a period with a substantial increase in the number of women on the labour market have been very limited.

In the occupations dominated by women, wages are much lower on the average than in the jobs when men are in a majority. Women constitute the largest group of low-income earners. However, one can fortunately note that an equalization is going between men and women regarding their average wage level. Among other things, this can be explained by the fact that the last few years' wage negotiations, in both the private and the public sectors, have put the emphasis on low-income earners. The equalization of wages is also proceeding faster in Sweden than in other comparable industrial countries.

THE RIGHT TO WORK—A PREREQUISITE FOR QUALITY

Regarding equality between men and women, the basic question is the problem in the labour market. We must assert women's right to work. We know today that women want to work outside the home, that this is not just a question of financial necessity. In certain families this admittedly is the reason—but this does not suffice to explain the enormous increase in the number of women on the labour market in recent decades. What remains, before we have really succeeded in asserting women's right to work, will not come automatically. It is naturally much easier for both women themselves, and the labour market and employment policies of society to give employment to those women who do not have a family and children. We have now reached the situation where over one-half of all women with pre-school children are employed. But we know that many of them work part-time and we can assume that one of the reasons for this is the lack of community service. To assert women's right to work, it is natural that we are concerned not only with the question of an adequate supply of jobs but also with society's policies concerning residential environment, child care, and communications.

We can also establish that it is easier to place women in jobs in areas where there is a well-differentiated labour market. It is much more difficult in the parts of the country where the economy is one-sided and where there is a substantial domination of jobs which are traditionally regarded as being for men only. I am completely convinced that, in this case, it will not suffice merely to supply adequate job opportunities. We must also, in different ways—more actively than before—seek to match the jobs available with the people applying for them.

AN EXAMPLE OF AN UNBALANCED LABOUR MARKET

This question does not just concern women. To illustrate the problem, I wish to refer to an investigation that was made in the autumn of 1973 in Gothenburg, Sweden's second-largest city. At that time there were over 5000 vacant jobs and 4200 unemployed. But what made it so difficult for the unemployed to take the jobs that were available?

The results showed that approximately 2500 of the unemployed were restricted in various ways. There was a group of approximately 400 persons who were handicapped in some manner, physically, psychologically, or socially. Another group of almost 300 persons did not have the necessary training and 1350 had other obstacles such as high age, etc. Almost 200 people were seeking part-time work and close to 300 had local ties. But, 1700 people had no such obstacles; why, then, could they not take any of the 5000 jobs available? 1000 of them were young, healthy, and well trained, but their training did not coincide with the type of work available just then. They were looking for work in the technical, humanistic, administrative, and office technical fields. In these fields, there were approximately 500 jobs available. But in manufacturing there were 1600 jobs; 1000 people were seeking work in this very sector, but over half of them were women and half of them were over 55 years old and the employers were not too interested in these job-seekers. How, then, should we manage this process of matching jobs and the unemployed?

MEASURES FOR OBTAINING BALANCE AND ASSERTING EVERYONE'S RIGHT TO WORK

We can and should invest in information to employers. Remind them that job-seeking women and older men are certainly not second-rate employees. Also, we can and *should* inform those seeking employment about the labour-market. This is particularly important where women are concerned, since they, to a greater extent than men, lack knowledge of various job duties and working environments because, on average, they have less experience of the labour market than men. We can school those seeking employment for the jobs that are vacant. This we have been doing for a long time and it has been an effective policy. But we can also state that this is not sufficient.

I believe that a pre-condition for accomplishing this adjustment is that we bring labour market policy into the enterprises. At this level, it is necessary seriously to discuss what jobs would be suitable for the job seekers on the local labour market, regardless of when these jobs are vacant. Serious discussions should be held concerning what changes can be made in the job duties if they are not suitable. This can apply to the organization of the work—i.e. who is supposed to do what duties—and it can of course also apply to the work equipment and the technical aids. There are many other items that could be discussed in this connection.

It is probable that today we place too high demands on the people who have the greatest difficulty in fitting into the jobs that are available. In the investigation I referred to, it was established that a number of persons had employment obstacles in one way or another. Not just physical impediments, but also that they were too old. To be too young and without experience is, of course, also a hindrance. A long time in unemployment can in itself become an obstacle in seeking employment. Our discussion thus far has focused mainly on how we, to a greater extent, should adjust demand to the unemployed, or the unemployed to demand. To really solve these problems, we cannot confine ourselves to the small group of unemployed; we must also consider all those who are already employed. We must consider the jobs that are already filled, and this is not so easy when considering the practical issue. This necessitates an internal transfer within the enterprise so that those who are outside can get a job. And it is apparent that from the personnel's point of view, as well as from the management side, there is perhaps the feeling that they have enough problems to cope with for those already employed. Many problems arise in effecting an internal shift within an enterprise in order to create employment for those seeking jobs. This will also put demands on the trade unions. It means that they must be included in the reorganization activity that must take place within the enterprise. We need a combination of mobility on the labour market and within enterprise. This calls for a labour market policy and labour market authorities that operate within the workplaces and not beside them, whether they are public or private. I do not know if one can say that we have found the definite form for this work, but we have at least begun to experiment with adjustment groups within the enterprises.

Adjustment groups are composed of representatives of the Employment Service, trade unions, and employers. These groups promote a positive attitude towards elderly employees and persons with work impediments at various places of work. These adjustment groups are to suggest measures that will make it easier to employ hard-to-place persons at the place of work and make it easier for those already employed to remain with the enterprise. The adjustment groups are the instrument through which we apply the law on employment-promoting measures for elderly and handicapped people that came into force in 1974. The adjustment groups are highly important, above all because they enable us to bring labour market policy into the enterprises—into the individual places of work.

I believe that the adjustment groups will indirectly—but certainly in some cases directly—have great importance for women. Both because here it will be possible to take up discussions concerning female labour with enterprises where men predominate, and indirectly because they promote adjustment between work and employees.

HOW EFFECTIVE ARE THE INSTRUMENTS OF LABOUR MARKET POLICY AS FAR AS WOMEN ARE CONCERNED?

Relief work

A few thoughts regarding other auxiliary means of labour market policy. We can, without exaggeration, state that most of the measures are tailored to a situation where, above all, the unemployment problems of men must be solved. But there has been a marked change in the pattern during the last few years and this must be continued and intensified. We can study relief work where, for a long time, there has been a limited number of women engaged, a few hundred or so, and the work has, above all, been in construction and building. It is gratifying that the labour market authorities during the last few years really have tried to change the type of relief work and expand it into the service sector. So far, this comprises a relatively small part quantitatively, but it is growing. And it is self-evident that such a change cannot be undertaken quickly since it demands, among other things, another kind of planning preparedness than the one people were used to before, particularly in the municipalities. It is also a great deal more difficult to organize relief work in practice in what can be called the operative field. The risks of interfering with normal work, work that belongs to the continuous activities, is greater, and quite naturally it is important for the trade unions that obligations which are the natural responsibility of, for example, the municipality are not replaced by relief work. Nevertheless, I think it can be said that the labour market authorities have begun to find forms of relief work in the service sector—work which is suitable and satisfactory for all—for the responsible bodies, the job seekers and those already employed, and their trade unions. We can establish that, through, for example, the provision of relief work in the nursing sector, a combination has been found that offers, over and above employment, training for those already employed who did not earlier have a chance of gaining competence in the occupation they have had for a number of years.

The labour market authorities thus far have proved to possess the necessary imagination to break old traditions in this way and find new alternatives and new methods to accomplish this part of the fight against unemployment and I am perfectly sure that they will manage to continue this. When it comes to other employment promoting measures carried out within the framework of the labour market policy to moderate a business recession, it is atural that such things as, for example, government orders to industry and other means to advance various kinds of production, may well be directed towards areas where, above all, women can reap the benefits of the increase in employment. As far as I know, the available statistics do not give any clear indication of how these measures have been divided with regard to the effect on men and women. I believe that one can, however, judge that there has not been the same unbalanced distribution as in the case of relief work.

Labour market training

Labour market training is a good method of using a recession effectively, both because in this way people are given employment during the recession and because they become better prepared for periods of full employment—which, naturally, not only for them, but also from the employers' point of view, must be of great value. As far as labour market training is concerned, there is not the slightest doubt that it has been of great importance for women's possibilities of joining the labour market.

We know that the number and share of women in the labour market training programme has increased and now amounts to 47 per cent. The problem which still remains and which we have not yet succeeded in solving satisfactorily, is that even here the distribution of training between objectives is still guided too much by the traditional pattern of sex roles. The labour market authorities have for many years tried to provide information of various kinds to change this attitude and have to a certain extent succeeded in doing so. But it is possible that we must try out new methods to bring about a change in attitude more rapidly. I will refer below to examples of such measures.

Sheltered and semi-sheltered employment

Other measures for solving problems of job-seekers are sheltered and semi-sheltered employment. Here, too, we can note that there is an unbalanced distribution between men and women. Sheltered employment is provided for people with a handicap, at special work sites—above all in sheltered workshops. It is, at present, often the municipality which is responsible for the management of these workshops.

Semi-sheltered employment is found in the regular labour market. By means of government grants which constitute 40 per cent of the wages, handicapped people can be employed under the same conditions as others but do not have to be as productive as their fellow-workers. The grants for semi-sheltered employment have been greatly improved in the last few years and we can also note an increase in the number of places provided for semi-sheltered employment. This is probably a consequence not only of the improved grants but also of the improved information the Employment Service can give about this service. In this case, the places have been concentrated above all in the private market in industrial enterprises and this might well be one of the explanations for the unbalanced distribution between men and women.

It is self-evident that even in other sections of the labour market, for example in municipal administration, there should be space for an expansion of semi-sheltered employment so that people who otherwise have difficulties in obtaining a job in the open market, can be offered jobs there. Concerning sheltered employment, we know that it, too, to a great extent, has been aimed at men rather than women. In this case, it is probable that the concept of men having priority in job seeking has remained stronger here than on the open labour market. A woman who, besides being a woman, has a work impediment is in a difficult position. We can state that exactly the same problem is found regionally as well. As an example, there is quite a difference between the people placed in sheltered employment in the Stockholm area and those placed in an aid area. The people in the Stockholm area who work in sheltered employment have work disabilities, handicaps that are far more serious than those of the workers in the sheltered workshops in the aid area, where probably many of these persons could quite easily seek employment on the open labour market. It is a task for all of us to work for the self-evident right of women with a handicap to receive society's assistance in obtaining a job.

THE COUNCIL TO ADVISE THE PRIME MINISTER ON EQUALITY BETWEEN MEN AND WOMEN

An important instrument for the promotion of women's interests in, among other things, the labour market is the Council to Advise the Prime Minister on Equality between Men and Women that was appointed by Prime Minister Olof Palme at the close of 1972. The Council has, in particular, the task of stimulating and supporting the authorities' work for equality between men and women and stimulating and supporting measures to achieve this purpose in society as a whole, including industry and commerce. In the directives for the work of the Council, women's right to work is emphasized above all.

The Council has at its disposal an advisory committee which include representatives of the organizations on the labour market as well as a reference group of women from various parts of the country. This reference group, which is unique in its kind, has been of great importance for the work of the Council.

The twelve women in the group are not there to serve as spokesmen of a particular organization, nor are they there by virtue of duty or position in society. They are there because it has been presumed that they can give the Council experience and knowledge regarding how employed women and housewives experience their normal day—their problems and joys of work, family, and society. The group has more than fulfilled the expectations the Council had when it was appointed.

OPENING CLOSED INDUSTRIAL DOORS
FOR WOMEN

The Council to Advise the Prime Minister on Equality between Men and Women has taken the initiative in an interesting experiment, the purpose of which is to prepare women for employment within typical 'men-only areas'. The experiment is intended to provide guidelines for continued work to improve the situation for women on the labour market. The experiment has been set up in a number of industrial enterprises representing various categories of industry. Earlier, the unionized work force was composed entirely, or almost entirely, of men. One of the purposes of the experiment was to influence industry towards a new recruitment policy, i.e., to employ women as well. In order to achieve this goal, the enterprises have formed reference groups that have taken up discussions regarding attitudes to female labour as well as questions regarding hours of work, working environment, etc.

In the areas where the industries involved in the experiment are located there has been a lack of so-called traditional opportunities for women. The unemployment registered among women in these areas was high. In addition, the participation rate was low and it could therefore be assumed that there was a substantial latent employment. Employment in industry had never been a realistic alternative for women, partly because in their recruitment policy the industries had always turned to the men, and partly because women themselves had too little knowledge of industrial work and, thus, they would first seek employment in the service sector.

Another purpose of the experiment was therefore to give women a better opportunity to learn about labour market conditions. One-month courses of practical vocational guidance were therefore held in the enterprises concerned. During this time, the women could try the various jobs within the enterprise. The women came into contact with the male fellow-workers, the supervisors, the union representatives, and the Employment Service representatives who often visited the enterprise. During this period, the women were thus given a proper opportunity to decide for themselves if industrial work would suit them.

There are two things which, I believe, are of specific importance in this connection. First, the women came in a group. They did not have to endure the hardships that a lone pioneer often has to face. They could discuss problems and difficulties with one another. Second, the women had the right to try various jobs within the same enterprise. This was considered a natural part of the practical vocational guidance and was not reported as a failure, which would probably have been the case in an ordinary job.

A final appraisal of the experiment cannot yet be made, but we know from the work done so far that it has given many interesting results. Women have shown a greater interest for what was earlier considered typical work for men, and the male workers involved in the participating enterprises think it works well. Employers have gained a positive attitude towards the employment of women and the Employment Service has acquired new knowledge as to how a good service for women can be provided. Thus far, 105 women have taken the practical vocational guidance course and 77 of them are now permanently employed in the industries participating in the experiment. About ten have continued in another kind of labour market training and the rest have not yet decided what their future vocation will be.

The experiment has attracted great attention from the mass media and perhaps this may be one of the reasons why this activity has had substantial effects in the rest of the county. Recently, when a questionnaire was submitted to 122 industries with over 50 employees in the county, it turned out that 70 enterprises had newly employed 363 women during the latter half of 1973. The experiment has been such a success that we are now going to expand it so that experience can be gained from more parts of the country.

The practical course of vocational guidance is carried out in a somewhat different manner alongside this experiment. The training is located at two or three different industries. In 1972, 5600 women started such courses. Many of them received a job directly upon completion of the course. Approximately 1500 went on after three months to some labour market training, 650 of whom attended courses for special occupations; many of these entered courses in office work and nursing, but 220 entered courses in manufacturing jobs, more than 100 of them in engineering work.

SPECIAL MEASURES FOR WOMEN
ARE REQUIRED

The labour market policy we practise has the basic principle that measures shall be the same for men and women. We should not divide policy into one part for men and one for women. Everyone has agreed on this basic principle and I also believe that, in the long run, it is correct. But correct principles can in the short run be unsuitable as a method of work. The Council to Advise the Prime Minister on Equality between Men and Women therefore proposed a few measures especially aimed at women. The Swedish Parliament has decided to sanction these measures proposed by the Government. In brief they are as follows:

First, we will reinforce the Employment Service with one hundred persons whose task will be to concentrate on the problems of women labour. This personnel increase in the Employment Service will, of course, enable the Service to make further efforts in order to find employment for women.

Second, we wish to counteract sex prejudice in personnel recruitment and vocational decisions and for this reason we have decided that during a 3-year trial period, enterprises will be given a special training grant

This means that employers who employ and train men or women in certain capacities dominated by the opposite sex will receive a grant of 5 Swedish kronor per training hour for a period not exceeding six months.

Third, we decided that the conditions for regional support should be altered so that enterprises that receive loans and grants for localization purposes had the obligation of employing both men and women. This change became effective as of 1 July 1974 and meant that at least 40 per cent of the number of job opportunities created in an enterprise receiving government regional support were reserved for either sex.

In the Government's proposal to Parliament on this issue it is said, among other things, that:

The regional support constitutes, in my opinion, an area that is suitable for an experiment of the type the Council has suggested. A basic motive behind the creation of the regional support has been to increase the number of employment opportunities and bring about a more differentiated labour market in those parts of the country, mainly the timber-producing counties, where unemployment and under-employment are most striking. Experience has shown that under-employment in these timber-producing counties is greatest among women. It is therefore of great importance that regional support is organized and utilized in such a manner that it will effectively contribute improving the women's situation on the labour market.

For all forms of support, the main rule already today is that enterprises receiving support shall be able to account for an increased employment. It is, according to my understanding, natural that this demand is made explicit in such a manner that both men and women have the same rights to the new job opportunities that are created through the support of the society. I therefore recommend that an experimental period should now begin according to the principles suggested by the Council.

I am convinced that the difficulties facing us, if we are going to succeed in asserting women's right to work, are quite substantial and place great demands on our means,

demands of another kind than we have been used to. This means we must assert women's right to work even in areas with an one-sided economy. It also means that we must assert women's right to employment even in situations where there is a lack of jobs. To manage this, I feel we must dare to utilize activities other than those we have considered correct before. And, we must expect that this action will naturally be accompanied by many practical difficulties in a period of transition. We must expect to make experiments that may later prove unsuitable and we need not see such efforts as failures—because we know that we also gain experience from them that will be of use in future. We must be prepared to accept that steps taken to bring about equality between men and women on the labour market can have a negative side-effect on other aspects of life, and in certain cases, I believe, we must accept these side-effects and try to overcome them in another way. In other cases it may, of course, happen that these side-effects become too great to be accepted—they may affect equality in other respects in society. But even if we should at first react negatively because the measures do not agree with what we have been used to, we should not be ready to accept this negative reaction, but instead go forward in deepened discussions and also be prepared to take the risks involved.

In closing I wish to say that it is important that we attempt to reach new methods in this way in order to bring about equality between men and women. But the question of equality between men and women can never be isolated from equality within society as a whole. Therefore, it is self-evident that reforms which do not explicitly refer to the relationship men–women are perhaps most important. The work being carried out just now to expand democracy at places of work, increase security of employment, improve the working environment, and strengthen the position not only of the individual, but also of the trade unions within working life, will perhaps be of greater importance for women than the labour market policy measures I have mentioned.

38. QUALITY OF THE WORKING ENVIRONMENT: PROTECTION AND PROMOTION OF OCCUPATIONAL MENTAL HEALTH

LENNART LEVI

HOLISTIC APPROACH TO WORK ENVIRONMENT AND HEALTH

The past few decades have seen a rapidly growing awareness of the impact of the *physical* and *chemical* work environment on man's physical health and well-being. Much less attention has been paid to possible effects of such environmental factors in terms of mental stress and the ensuing mental and psychosomatic ill health. Even less interest has been devoted to corresponding effects of *psychosocial* factors at work, for good or bad (see WHO 1973).

To us, physico–chemical and psychosocial factors must be of equal concern, as they all focus on aspects of health and well-being in total man's interaction with total environment. What should interest us is the general question of whether present conditions and present trends in occupational environmental change do in fact pose a threat to human health or survival, to well-being and to the quality of life, and if so, what is the magnitude of the problem and what could we do about it (see Levi 1977, 1978).

Principal goals of working life
However, before discussing this in any depth, it may be worthwhile to review the principal goals of working life, not primarily in terms of economy or technology but with regard to satisfaction of human needs such as *health*. Health has been defined as not only an 'absence of disease or infirmity' but also 'a state of physical, mental, and social well-being' (ECOSOC 1946). The attainment of health in this broad sense (one could equally well refer to it as 'quality of life') must be one of the principal aims of *all* social activity, both national and local, including the important sector of *working life* and its conditions.

Admittedly, working life also provides income and an output of goods and services. But these things are not ends in themselves; they can only be means of assuring optimum physical, mental, and social well-being for the greatest possible majority and of promoting their health, development, and self-realization. Thus, working life can satisfy human needs directly, through opportunities for creative and stimulating activities and social contacts, as well as indirectly, through the provision of income.

What workers have a right to expect
A good summary of what people have a right to expect from working life is given in a recent resolution from the International Labour Conference (ILO 1975). It states:

that work should respect the worker's life and health; this is the problem of safety and healthiness in the workplace;

that it should leave him free time for rest and leisure; this is the question of hours of work and their adaptation to an improved pattern for life outside work; and

that it should enable him to serve society and achieve self fulfilment by developing his personal capacities; this is the problem of the content and the organization of work.

In essence, this means that work is made the servant and not the master.

However, this is *not* what work amounts to for hundreds of millions of workers all over the world.

Recent changes in working life
Generally, recent changes in working life in economically developed countries can be summarized as a trend towards:

Increasing mechanization, and computerization;
Increasing proportion of shift work;
Increasing proportion of large enterprises;
Increasing anonymity, division of labour, and heterogeneity of life;
Increasingly distant relationships between worker and management, worker and worker, worker and union officials, and producer and consumer.

All this has led to increasing advantages for the young, healthy, highly adaptable, well-educated high-performers, and corresponding disadvantages for those who are physically, mentally, and socially disadvantaged.

In developing countries the picture looks different. Here, a series of dramatic transitions is taking place from agriculture to manufacturing, and from the latter to mass production or even automation. This is more or less the same sequence through which today's developed countries passed in the nineteenth and early-twentieth century. However, the velocity of these transitions differs greatly. Developing countries are undergoing the same process in one-tenth or less of the time taken by the developed countries (see WHO 1971).

Benefits—and costs
Although the economic benefits of present trends in working life are obvious, the satisfaction of some human needs has led to frustration of others. In addition, there is an increased over- or under-utilization of human abilities and a discrepancy between human expectations and perceived outcome, in short a *misfit* between man and his environment.

Discussing various types of person–environment discrepancies some people argue that humans are *adaptable*. They are, indeed, but you can equally say that they are *deformable*. Deformation becomes the price. This price can be expressed in terms of reactions on three levels:

Psychological reactions (e.g. anxiety, malaise, low-spiritedness, apathy, depression, feelings of helplessness, disrupted somatic awareness, defensive reactions of various kinds) (see Levi 1975);
Behavioural reactions (e.g. increased consumption of alcohol, tobacco, drug abuse; prolonged sickness absence, anti-social behaviour, suicide);
Physiological reactions (e.g. an increased activity of adrenal cortex and medulla; psychosomatic diseases) (see Levi 1972; Theorell *et al.* 1972; Cleary 1974; Kagan and Levi 1975; Rahe 1975).

It would seem to have been firmly established that considerable psychological, psychosomatic, and social problems occur among workers in response to person–environment misfit at work. On the other hand, we lack evidence as to who is at particularly high risk in respect to such problems, how grave the problems are, and how they could be prevented.

Nor do we possess any reliable data concerning the *components* of the total situation at work and outside it which are particularly stressful, the extent to which they are amenable to environmental adjustment and/or psychosocial support, and, if they are amenable, at what 'price'.

Common phenomena
But we know that all these reactions are exceedingly common. In a random sample of all Swedes who are gainfully employed, 37 per cent found their work mentally stressful; two out of three said it was characterized by rush and 'wear and tear'; 18 per cent felt it to be monotonous; and 14 per cent reported that they felt mentally exhausted on arriving home from work (Institute for Social Research 1978).

These figures, moreover, are only part of the story. As already emphasized, there are the other indicators of a bad person–environment fit at work and elsewhere, such as alcoholism, suicide, and mental and psychosomatic disorders. These, too, are very common phenomena. Although a causal connection between them and occupational stressors is not clearly proven, it is highly suspected (see Bolinder and Ohlström 1971; Wahlund and Nerell 1976; Levi and Andersson 1975; Levi 1979; Levi and Alaby 1979).

MAN-MADE ENVIRONMENTS CAN BE ADAPTED—BY MAN, FOR MAN

To all this, some people say that technological and economic development cannot be changed. In claiming this, they seem to forget that work environments and processes are man-made. It follows that they can also be adapted—by man, for man. The question is not if, but *how*.

As Trist (1974) indicates, we have two choices: The first is to leave the vast bulk of jobs that must still be done in manufacturing and service industries in the dull and monotonous state in which they exist at present, accepting the need to work as the primary curse, a necessary evil which we must endure; the principal aim then becomes to reduce the amount that has to be done, shortening both working hours and the working week, while maintaining a scale of pay which enables satisfactions to be sought elsewhere.

The alternative would be to redesign jobs and organizational forms so that the majority rather than merely the privileged few can do work which is meaningful and fulfilling, while maintaining a high level of performance (see McLean *et al.* 1977).

Meeting people's psychological requirements
Such a redesignation would imply meeting people's psychological requirements at work other than those specified in a contract of employment (such as wages, hours, safety, security of tenure, etc.). Six such requirements have been listed (Emery 1963) that pertain to the content of a job and which must be met if a new work ethic is to develop:

The need for the job to be reasonably demanding in terms other than sheer endurance, and to provide at least a minimum of variety;
The need to be able to learn on the job, and go on learning;
The need for some area of decision-making that the individual can call his own;
The need for some degree of social support and recognition in the work place;
The need to be able to relate what he does and what he produces to his social life;
The need to feel that the job leads to some sort of desirable future.

Organizational consequences
Translated into organizational terms, measures to satisfy these needs appear to involve two fundmental ideas (Walker 1974).

The first is concerned with a reversal of the trend towards the division of jobs into smaller and smaller elements, each to be performed by a single worker, and its replacement by a trend towards putting together the various functions in a meaningful, integrated whole.

The second concerns modification of the hierarchic organizational structure of the enterprise by arranging for workers to work together in small face-to-face groups, which have a good deal of autonomy, and whose supervisor no longer gives detailed orders, but sees that the group has the resources it needs and handles the group's relations with the rest of the enterprise. Or, as put by Trist (1974), under the principle of self-regulation, only the critical interventions, desired outcomes, and organizational maintenance requirements need be specified by those managing, leaving the remainder to those *doing*.

None of these measures (nor any others) provide a patent solution to all the problems. There are no patent solutions. What is good in *one* respect for *one* individual need not be good in *another* respect for another individual. What we have to do is to find out what is good (and bad) for whom, in what way, when, and under what conditions. A considerable amount of interest, of course, will then focus on measures which are more or less *generally* effective.

Five cardinal principles
To be effective, such measures should be based on five cardinal principles.

First, on a *holistic* (overall) view of man and environment, i.e. equal and integral consideration for physical, mental, social, and economic aspects.
Second, on an *ecological* strategy, i.e. consideration of the interaction between the entire individual and the entire environment (physicochemical and psychosocial) and of the dynamics of the entire system.
Third, on a *cybernetic* strategy, with continuous *evaluation* of the effects (physical, mental, social, and economic) of different working environments and of changes in them; continuous feed-back to decision-makers and the public; and a continuous adaptation and reshaping of the working environment by all concerned in the light of these various types of experience.
Fourth, on a *democratic* strategy, giving the individual the greatest possible *influence* over his own situation and direct, efficient channels of communication to the various decision-makers.
Fifth, on the principle of *mutual support and solidarity* between individuals and groups, with a certain amount of altruism serving as the cement of any community.

These are the strategies. The tactics to improve person–environment fit at work concern the adaptation of environmental demands and opportunities to workers' abilities and needs. Accordingly, our action must focus on several *types* of environmental factors, which can be summarized as follows.

SATISFACTION OF VARIOUS TYPES OF HUMAN NEEDS

Satisfaction of physiological needs and of security and safety is often referred to as 'hygiene'. Attention to such factors is extremely important but not enough. Other environmental factors are connected with satisfaction of other human needs. These include, e.g., salary, number and quality of human contacts, supervision, security at work, and physical factors in the work environment (cf. Baneryd 1976). Unless these aspects are satisfied to some degree, dissatisfaction and unhappiness will occur. As soon as they have been satisfied, additional 'improvements' will not yield any further substantial increment to satisfaction.

Another class of factors is referred to as 'motivational', i.e. related to needs such as ego-experience, self-esteem, and self-appreciation. These include advancement to more stimulating tasks, appreciation of work well done, to be allowed to complete a task, to take responsibility, inherent qualities of the task itself, etc. These factors have a positive influence on the involvement in, and the experience of satisfaction from work.

It follows that, to be successful, an occupational mental health protection and promotion programme must be comprehensive and take into account *all* types of human needs and their satisfaction through environmental adjustments, i.e. by creating a good person-environment fit.

For such a fit to be good, the general organization of the work process is no less important than hygiene factors such as noise and illumination. Organizational factors (see Brännström *et al.* 1975) are those primarily concerned with:

The workers' knowledge of how his part of the work contributes to the finished whole;
The independence and responsibility of the workers; and
Their social contact and collaboration with other employees.

Part of a meaningful whole
The first point means that the work task should be seen to constitute a meaningful whole or at least form an essential part of a production process which is understandable and meaningful to the worker in terms of the relationship between his own contribution on the one hand and the ultimate goals of the production process on the other.

This could be achieved by letting the worker take part in the preplanning, realization, and control of his task. Further, one might wish to consider the amalgamation of several fragmented pieces of the work process into meaningful sequences.

The worker should further be allowed to utilize and develop further his knowledge and skills through the work process and through education and thereby enable him to take over increasingly qualified work tasks. This can be facilitated by choosing the right man for the right job and by rotating workers who so wish between different tasks and positions. Job rotation and job enlargement can also include an increased participation for the worker in the planning and control of his own achievements. It should further include options—but not necessarily demands—for recurrent training and education.

One of the most important ways of learning from

experience is through feedback from the environment. In working life, every worker ought to know the result of his endeavours, i.e. the quality and quantity of his achievements. This is true not only for the individual worker but for the work group as well.

This can be achieved in several complementary ways. One is to allow continuous contact with the preceding and following link in the production chain. Another is to allow the worker to control and check his own results. To this might be added regular reports and evaluations from his supervisors about the quantity and quality of his performance. There should also be some opportunity to discuss with fellow workers and management how work is and should be carried out (see Brännström *et al.* 1975).

Independence and autonomy

Our second point concerns independence and autonomy. This does not mean that every single worker should do whatever he likes, whenever he likes, in any way he likes. This would be to go to one extreme. The other extreme, where man is turned into a passive tool, is equally unfavourable. Work is made much more stimulating, rewarding, and effective if it allows an optimal degree of participation, e.g. in planning the work, influencing the method and work pace, and location of pauses.

This can be accomplished by making the individual worker or work group responsible for carrying out the job, for breaks and for temporary absence from work. Information on the progress of the work will then allow each unit to make the necessary decisions. This might mean that the work pace should be left to the individual or the group to decide. Responsibility and power should be delegated as much as possible to those directly concerned with the production process.

Social contact and collaboration

With regard to our third point it seems clear that one of the great advantages of working life is that it creates the social context for contact and collaboration with other human beings. These are basic human needs. Accordingly, conversation and contact between employees should be made a necessary part of the production process instead of being eliminated. Whenever possible, work should be planned in such a way that its various components could be allocated to relatively small groups of, say, 4–8 people. Speech and eye contact and collaboration between the group members should be encouraged. If this turns out to be impossible for practical reasons, human contact should be facilitated at least during breaks, and opportunities for friendly contact with supervisors and management should be promoted.

becomes humanized and, simultaneously, more smooth and efficient, with mutual solidarity and social support. Extreme, competitive individualism is counteracted and a more communal approach is favoured. This may include tangible support, i.e. concrete assistance such as helping a person complete a task or sharing resources. Another type of support that is favoured is psychological–emotional support, as in lending a sympathetic ear, reassuring, or demonstrating concern and care (Pinneau 1976). For these and other reasons, the mental health of the executive is of particular importance not only in itself but for its effects on other workers. For example, a mildly depressed manager cannot generate enthusiasm in his staff: and an irritable supervisor might be unable to provide any support and instead create stress for those under him. Man's most important environmental factor is—fellow man.

Deprofessionalization: sharing of responsibility

It is often taken for granted that responsibility for the humanization of working life is a matter for a few selected professionals. In our opinion it is more logical, and effective, to see this responsibility as given to each and everyone, although one naturally also has to allocate some specific responsibilities. It is in the interest of all concerned that the work environment is maintained or made optimal in all possible respects to improve person–environment fit and, consequently, health, well-being and productivity.

Much can be accomplished through two universally available tools of measurement and intervention, namely, *listening* and *speaking*. People know best where their own shoe pinches, and they should be allowed and encouraged to tell their own story. Wherever possible, they should further be allowed and encouraged to make their own adjustments with regard to the immediate environment, if this can be done without harm to others.

Implementation now—but with continuous evaluation

Some of these principles and measures are well supported by present knowledge and should be implemented immediately on a general level. Others may be good for some people, under some circumstances and in some respects, but not beneficial or even harmful for others. A third category concerns well-meant but untested, and therefore speculative approaches.

To implement such a programme without delay but at the same time safeguard the public and increase the programme's effectiveness and efficiency, we need continuous *evaluation*. This will allow us to learn from experiences, our successes and mistakes, and thus enable us to correct and improve the programme.

NEEDS SATISFACTION AN INTEGRAL PART OF THE PRODUCTION PROCESS

In these ways, satisfaction of human needs is made an integral part of the production process. Working life

ACQUISITION OF NEW KNOWLEDGE

In many instances, however, our present state of knowledge simply does not allow rational health action even if combined with evaluation. To close such critical gaps, new knowledge must be acquired; i.e. before modifying, and evaluating our modifications, we need to *identify* three classes of phenomena, namely:

High-risk situations (e.g. with regard to occupation, shift work, piece wages, sensory overload);
High-risk groups (e.g. within populations such as working mothers, migrant workers); and
High-risk reactions (e.g. various forms of psychological, physiological, and immunological dysfunction).

Whenever possible, our research strategy should combine

Key hypothesis testing (basic research), with
Evaluation of health actions (applied research), and
Collection of quantified information on the interrelationship and interactions of various parts of the man–environment ecosystem (see Chapter 42).

To provide the necessary data, research projects can often be carried out in three consecutive steps:

Problem identification with survey techniques and morbidity data,
Longitudinal, multidisciplinary intensive studies of the intersection of high-risk situations and high-risk groups as compared with controls,
Controlled intervention, including laboratory experiments as well as therapeutic and/or preventive interventions in real-life settings (e.g. natural experiments; interdisciplinary evaluation of health action).

Some examples of the application of such strategy and tactics to the area of shift work, health, and well-being and of their results are given below.

Examples of research on shift work, health, and well-being

One source of problems in working life is the possible temporal misfit between man and his environment, arising from the altered rest/activity patterns required from subjects with work hours placed outside the conventional daytime range, e.g. shift workers (Akerstedt *et al.* 1977). Such a misfit rests on the assumption of a conflict between endogenous, i.e self-sustained biological rhythms in various psychophysiological functions on the one hand, and environmental demands on these functions on the other.

In our first series of studies we therefore wanted to look into the possibly endogenous properties of the temporal variation of some important physiological and psychological functions, i.e. their persistence in the absence of the normal time cues. To this end, more than 100 normal healthy volunteers of both sexes were exposed to three days and three nights of continuous work. In spite of the strict standardization and equalization of

environmental stimuli, the diurnal rhythms persisted throughout the vigil, with pronounced decreases in adrenaline excretion and in body temperature, shortfalls in performance, and increases in fatigue ratings taking place in the small hours (Levi 1972: Fröberg *et al.* 1975 a, b; Fröberg 1977; Akerstedt and Fröberg 1977). This persistent oscillation under conditions of constant activity, light, food intake, etc. clearly indicates that there is an obvious endogenous component in this oscillation (Akerstedt and Levi 1978).

As a second step, several hundred shift workers presumably exposed to such conflicts between endogenous rhythms and environmental demands were studied with health questionnaire techniques. The results showed higher frequencies of sleep, mood, digestive, and social disturbances among the shift workers than among the day workers. The complaints about well-being reached their peak during the night shift.

In a third step, we studied physiological, psychological, chronobiological, and social reactions in response to the *introduction* of three weeks of night-work in habitual daytime workers. We found that, although the endocrine system does indeed adapt to the environmental demands induced by shift-work by 'stepping on the gas' to keep awake in night-time and 'slowing down' in the day to allow for some sleep, the usual one-week cycle does not suffice for a complete adaptation of turning night into day and vice versa. Not even three weeks of continuous night work are enough to cause an inversion of the circadian functions; the original circadian rhythms flatten out but still persist. In addition, switching from habitual day work to three weeks of night work is accompanied by increases in a number of indices of physiological stress and social problems in the workers and in their families (Theorell and Akerstedt 1976).

In a logical fourth step, night work was not introduced but instead *eliminated*. A group of steel-workers was kept on a continuing 3-shift work whereas a comparable experimental group was switched to 2-shift work, everything else being held constant and equal. In a one-year follow-up we were able to demonstrate that the change to work schedules without night shift brings with it an improvement in physical, mental, and social well-being. The control group who remained on their habitual 3-shift work schedule did not change or even deteriorated with respect to well-being (Akerstedt and Torsvall 1977a, b; 1978).

RESEARCH AND HEALTH ACTION ON THE SHOP FLOOR LEVEL

Accordingly, our programme—not only nationally but also on each shop floor and in each office—must be as follows:

(1) to identify the type and extent of the problems

present, e.g. incidence of mental and psychosomatic disorders, absenteeism, alcohol abuse, labour turn-over, dissatisfaction, and social unrest.

(2) to identify psychosocial and physical/chemical environmental correlates of the various problems.

(3) management, labour unions, occupational safety and health workers, and authorities must consider, together with the workers concerned, which of these environmental influences are likely to be of greatest causal importance and at the same time accessible to change, and which of such changes are feasible and acceptable to all concerned.

(4) to change the work environment in the manner described above on a small and experimental scale to evaluate benefits and side-effects in all possible terms, and on the basis of this to decide what kind of change can be implemented on a wider scale.

(5) such a wider application should be continuously monitored, evaluated, and modified as occasion arises.

To be efficient, the whole procedure (1–5) must be carried out with 'feed back' of results and with *full participation and understanding* of all concerned.

SUMMARY

In summary, occupational mental health protection and promotion should be seen as a means to adapt work environments to man's capacities, needs, and expectations and to help man to find the job and the environment best suited to fit his personal requirements. The work environment should not only avoid exposing man to noxious physical, chemical, biological, and psychosocial influences but also promote health, well-being, development, and self-realization. In addition, and most important, in all these endeavours man must be seen not as a passive object of benevolent expert supervision and action but as an active and respected subject, who often knows better than the experts where his shoe pinches and who is willing and able to make his own considerations and decisions (see WHO 1974).

When we treat machines badly, technocratic protest is immediate and strong because of the obvious economic loss. Human beings have been, and to a considerable extent still are, treated badly in working life and elsewhere, resulting in disease and human suffering. Protest is not very loud and response is far too weak. Now that we have rational guidelines for humanizing work, there should be no further delay in protecting human flesh and blood and—last but not least—the human mind.

REFERENCES

AKERSTEDT, T. and THEORELL, T. (1976). Exposure to night work: relations between serum gastrin reactions, psychosomatic complaints and personality variables. *J. psychosom. Res.*, **20**, 479–84.

—— and FRÖBERG, J. (1977). Psychophysiological circadian rhythms in females during 75 hours of sleep deprivation with continuous activity. *Waking and Sleeping*, **4**, 387–94.

——, ——, LEVI, L., TORSVALL, L., and ZAMORE, K. (1977). *Shift work and well-being.* Rep. No. 63b from the Laboratory for Clinical Stress Research, Stockholm.

—— and TORSVALL, L. (1977a). Experimental changes in shift schedules—their effects on well-being. In *Proceedings of the IVth Symposium on Night and Shift Work, Dortmund, 1977* (ed. J. Rutenfranz, P. Colquhoun, P. Knauth, and S. Folkards). (In press).

—— and —— (1977b). *Medicinska, psykologiska och sociala aspekter pa skiftarbete vid Specialstalverken i Söderfors.* Rapport 2: Sambandsstudier. (Medical, psychological, and social aspects of shift work at the Specialstalverken at Söderfors. Report No. 2: Studies of the relationships). Rep. No. 64 from the Laboratory for Clinical Stress Research, Stockholm.

—— and —— (1978). Experimental changes in shift-schedules—their effects on well-being. *Ergonomics* (In press).

—— and LEVI, L. (1978). Circadian rhythms in the secretion of cortisol, adrenaline and noradrenaline. Editorial in *Eur. J. clin. Invest.*, **8**, 57–8.

BANERYD, K. (1976). Psykosociala effekter av fysisk arbetsmiljö och skyddsförhallanden i arbetet. (Psychosocial effects of physical working environment and occupational safety conditions.) In *Statens offentliga utredningar* SOU 1976:3, p. 10, Stockholm.

BOLINDER, E. and OHLSTRÖM, B. (1971). *Stress pa svenska arbetsplatser: en enkätstudie bland LO-medlemmarna.* (Stress in Swedish working places: A survey study among LO members.) Prisma/LO, Lund.

BRÄNNSTRÖM, J., GÖRANSSON, I., MARTENSSON, L., NILSSON, B., OLSSON, G., and VEIBÄCK, T. (1975). *Generella arbetsmiljökrav för Stalverk 80.* (General criteria for the working environment at Stalverk 80). Arbetsmiljölaboratoriet, Stockholm.

CLEARY, P. J. (1974). *Life events and disease: a review of methodology and findings.* Rep. No. 37 from the Laboratory for Clinical Stress Research, Stockholm.

ECOSOC (1946). The Preparatory Committee of the International Health Conference, E/H/PC/W/2, 21 March, 1946.

EMERY, F. E. (1963). *Some hypotheses about the ways in which tasks may be more effectively put together to make jobs.* Tavistock Institute Doc. No. T813.

FRÖBERG, J. E. (1977). Twenty-four-hour patterns in human performance, subjective and physiological variables and differences between morning and evening active subjects. *Biol. Psychol.*, **5** (2), 119–34.

——, KARLSSON, C.-G., LEVI, L., and LIDBERG, L. (1975a). Circadian rhythms of catecholamine excretion, shooting range performance and self-ratings of fatigue during sleep deprivation. *Biol. Psychol.*, **2**, 175–88.

——, ——, ——, and —— (1975b). Psychobiological circadian rhythms during a 72-hour vigil. *Försvarsmedicin*, **11**, 92–201.

Institute for Social Research (1978). Unpublished data from the 1974 level of living survey, Stockholm.

ILO (International Labour Organization) (1975). *Making work more human. Working conditions and environment.* (Report of the Director-General to the International Labour Conference.) International Labour Organization, Geneva.

KAGAN, A. R. and LEVI, L. (1975). Health and environment—psychosocial stimuli, a review. In *Society, stress and disease* (ed. L. Levi), Vol. II, pp. 241–60. Oxford University Press, London.

LEVI, L. (1972). Stress and distress in response to psychosocial stimuli. Laboratory and real life studies on sympathoadreno-medullary and related reactions. *Acta med. scand. Suppl.* No. 528.

—— (Ed.) (1975). *Emotions—their parameters and measurement.* Raven Press, New York.

—— (1977). Psychosocial stress at work—problems and prevention. In *Reducing occupational stress* (ed. A. McLean, G. Black, and M. Colligan). National Institute for Occupational Safety and Health, Cincinnati, Ohio.

—— (1978). Occupational mental health—its monitoring, protection and promotion. *J. occup. Med.* (In press).

—— (1979). Psychosocial factors in preventive medicine. Paper for the National Academy of Sciences Institute of Medicine, Washington, D.C., for inclusion in a policy statement on disease prevention, requested by the U.S. Assistant Secretary for Health.

—— and ANDERSSON, L. (1975). *Psychosocial stress—population, environment and quality of life.* Spectrum Publications, New York.

—— and ALABY, G. (1979). *Psykisk Hälsovård, Problem och Problemlösningar* (Mental health care: problems and problem solutions). Liber, Stockholm. (In press).

McLEAN, A., BLACK, G., and COLLIGAN, M. (1977). *Reducing occupational stress.* National Institute for Occupational Safety and Health, Cincinnati, Ohio.

PINNEAU, S. R., Jr. (1976). Effects of social support on occupational stresses and strains. (Paper presented at a symposium at the 84th Annual Convention of the American Psychological Association.) Institute of Social Research, University of Michigan, Ann Arbor.

RAHE, R. H. (1975). Life-changes and near-future illness reports. In *Emotions—their parameters and measurement* (ed. L. Levi), pp. 511–29. Raven Press, New York.

THEORELL, T., LIND, E., FRÖBERG, J., KARLSSON, C.-G., and LEVI, L. (1972). A longitudinal study of 21 subjects with coronary heart disease—life changes, catecholamine excretion and related biochemical reaction. *Psychosom. Med.,* **34,** 505–16.

—— and AKERSTEDT, T. (1976). Day and night work: changes in cholesterol, uric acid, glucose, and potassium in serum and in circadian patterns of urinary catecholamine excretion—a longitudinal cross-over study of railroad repairmen. *Acta med. scand.,* **200,** 47–53.

TRIST, E. L. (1974). Work improvement and industrial democracy. In *Commission of the European communities: conference on work organization, technical development and motivation of the individual.* Brussels.

WAHLUND, I. and NERELL, G. (1976). *Work environment of white collar workers—work, health, well-being.* The Central Organization of Salaried Employees in Sweden, Stockholm.

WALKER, K. F. (1974). Improvement of working conditions—the role of industrial democracy. In *Commission of the European communities: conference on work organization, technical development and motivation of the individual.* Brussels.

WHO (World Health Organization) (1973): Occupational mental health—report of a meeting. WHO/OH/73.13.

—— (1974). A/27 Technical Discussions/6, 16 May, 1974.

39. OCCUPATIONAL HEALTH SURVEY IN RESEARCH WORKERS

M. HORVÁTH and E. FRANTIK†

INTRODUCTION

In the area of psychosocial stress the possibilities of prevention in occupational health are more limited than in other aspects of working conditions for the very reason that interference with the social structure meets with greater resistance. Moreover, neither descriptive statistical studies nor experimental research provide an unambiguous basis for intervention, notwithstanding the fact that the additional load on higher nervous functions arising from hurry and other life pressures are commonly suspected to increase the risk of overstepping the adaptational abilities, which in turn leads from states of tension and anxiety to neuroses and psychosomatic disorders. A substantially wider knowledge of underlying physiological and psychological processes will be required to determine the conditions under which the human could work and live for the greater part of his life in a state of well-being, as stipulated in the definition of health by WHO.

The project reported in this chapter forms part of a wider study which also includes socio-economic, organizational, and other aspects of the effectiveness of research. This study is to provide guidance to institutions which co-ordinate research and technical development on how to improve management and the preventive care of research personnel. Our part of this study is designed as a longitudinal survey of working conditions, living regimen, mental and health conditions of managerial and creative workers in research and development.

These occupations do not involve, as a rule, traditional *work hazards*. On the other hand, onesidedness of the work load, lack of physical activity, and primarily the fact that successful creative mental work requires an intensive and sustained high activation of higher nervous functions, appear as certain risk factors. Under adverse circumstances or in predisposed persons the high level of activation may persist and thus disturb the physiological regimen of work and rest. The individual in a state of high activation is more susceptible to other stress factors, especially of a psychosocial nature, under the influence of which activation may change into a state of negative emotional tension. A state of persisting habitual high activation and negative emotional tension interferes with the ability of relaxation and affects unfavourably not only creative performance but also emotional life and interpersonal relations as well as the equilibrium of autonomic regulatory reactions. Habitual high level of activation corresponds phenomenologically with the behaviour pattern type A described by Rosenman *et al.*(1975) in which, according to repeated evidence, there is a higher risk of developing coronary heart disease.

A pilot survey on work and health conditions of scientific workers organized by our laboratory some years ago (Vinař and Frantík 1968) yielded some valuable inspiration for the design of the present study. Data concerning the effect which the amount and type of work has on health, fatigue, and life satisfaction indicated that neither the working hours, nor regular work during holidays and weekends, nor routine and pedagogic activity had substantial effects. On the other hand, an increased proportion of administrative–organizational work was associated with a feeling of worse health, with more circulatory complaints, and more frequent anxiety, tension, depression, and fatigue. Frequent interference with work, especially due to emergency work, and interuptions by phone, visits, and noise, were also correlated with a higher incidence of fatigue and feelings of tension. This correlation was higher in those respondents who had less physical activity than they would have liked. More than 70 per cent of respondents stated that they did not have a sufficient amount of physical activity and simultaneously that they lived more frequently in a state of emotional tension which did not diminish during week-ends and holidays. Forty per cent of respondents mentioned interpersonal conflicts at work which had a negative impact on them. A large proportion of these subjects also lived in a state of emotional tension at home.

Although the correlations cannot be interpreted simply, they have directed attention in the following study to sources of tension in normal working life and to supporting conditions in the way of life.

The new survey was initiated in technical research institutes of the machine industry with a view to an easier expression of productivity.

METHODS

In the first stage 480 research workers have been

† The following workers participated in the development of the project and data-sampling and processing: D. Frantíková, Ed.D., J. Kodýtková, K. Kopřiva, Ph.D., O. Kovalík, M.D., A. Lajčíková, M.D.

External co-operation: A. Appels, Ph.D., Limburg Univ., Maastricht, Holland; K. Švábová, M.D., M. Menčík, M.D., Ph.D., Associate Professor and other posts, Charles University Medical School of Hygiene, Prague, Department of Occupational Medicine; H. Geizerová, M.D., Ph.D., D. Grafnetter, Ing., Ph.D., Institute for Clinical and Experimental Medicine, Prague; M. Vystyd, Ing., Ph.D., Ministry of Technology and Development of the ČSR, Prague.

examined using a combined questionnaire as to their state of health, mental condition, regimen of life, and rest and working conditions; rating scales and structured interviews, laboratory tests of autonomous regulations in conditions of mental and physical stress, clinical examinations of the cardio-vascular and motor systems, and an analysis of diet habits were performed. The professional qualifications and scientific performance of all workers were assessed by a group of raters—senior researchers. Deeper insight was achieved in occupational–psychological interviews which were performed with selected workers, primarily with those who had great discrepancy between the scores of competence and output.

RESULTS

From the medical point of view it is characteristic of the given sample that the *morbidity rate* in research workers has been somewhat lower than among the rest of the employees, although they are older. Analysis of sickness absenteeism and health complaints in this professional group indicated a high incidence of three types of difficulties: (a) psychological ones of various types; (b) complaints about motor and vertebrogenic disorders; and (c) risk factors of coronary heart disease and cardio-vascular symptoms.

In concord with a low morbidity rate for neurosis (1 per cent), we did not meet a high incidence of expressed *psychopathological symptoms* (Fig. 39.1): there was almost no difference between researchers and university students in distress symptom check-list score SCL-90 (Derogatis *et al.* 1973) and both these groups differed substantially from neurotic patients (Bolelouký and Horváth 1974). On the other hand, their score on psychological difficulties in the MHQ scale occupied a middle position between that of psychiatric out-patients and employees of the United Kingdom Energy Authority (UKEA) from the studies of Howell, Crown, and Crisp (Fig. 39.2). Possible correlation with morbidity is illustrated by Howell and Crown's (1971) comparison of average MHQ scores (Crown and Crisp 1970) of several patient groups which showed a higher score for patients who had lost working time as a result of hypertension, allergies, and gastric or duodenal ulcers (Fig. 39.3) and also showed a higher percentage of men with sickness absence for several diseases in MHQ high-scoring categories. In our samples, the average global score increased only slightly with age and in most symptom groups the score did not increase at all or decreased in higher age groups (in obsession).

About two-thirds of respondents mentioned serious work problems which in more than one-half caused frequent or intensive feelings of tension. The respondents who felt tension due to their work believed more frequently that their problems handicapped their work performance, also had problems in their private life, and more often showed psychopathological deviations. Most frequent were increased irritability (80 per cent of the

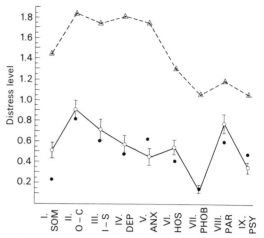

FIG. 39.1. Distress level (SCL-90 group profile) of 88 normal males (M ± SEM), 19 students (black circles), and 23 neurotics (triangles) in the scales: (I) somatization; (II) obsessive – compulsive; (III) interpersonal sensitivity; (IV) depression; (V) anxiety; (VI) anger – hostility; (VII) phobic anxiety; (VIII) paranoid ideation; (IX) psychoticism.

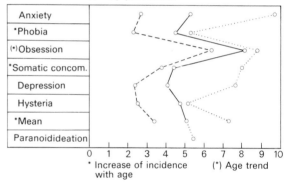

FIG. 34.2. Comparison of MHQ (Middlesex Hospital Questionnaire) scores in 207 research workers (full line), 133 psychotic out-patients (dotted line – Crown and Crisp 1970), and 2352 employees of United Kingdom Atomic Energy Authority (dashed line—Howell and Crown 1971).

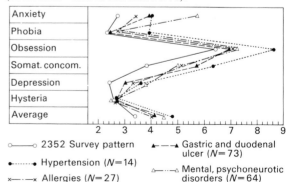

FIG. 39.3. Average MHQ scores of patients who have lost working time as a result of specified diseases compared with means for 2352 survey United Kingdom Atomic Energy Authority employees (from Howell and Crown 1971).

sample), indecision (75 per cent), vague bodily complaints and blunted emotions (60 per cent), and mental fatigue (50 per cent). The lack of an obvious increase in all these complaints except mental fatigue with the years of research activity throws doubts on the causal nexus between them: the higher incidence of psychopathology can hardly be interpreted as a result of the cumulation of work life stresses. It may be hypothesized that these deviations are mostly preformed in subjects who select this type of work and/or indicate defects in the adjustment to the requirements of mental work.

The same hypothesis is valid for the habitual high activation level which was found in about two-thirds of the sample. The assessment was based on both the structured interview (Rosenman et al. 1964) and questionnaire (Jenkins Activity Survey; WHO 1973). The criteria for behaviour pattern Type A/B assessment were adapted under the kind assistance of A. Appels, leading psychologist of the WHO–KRIS Project, and were checked for validity in our population.

The diagnosis of behaviour pattern Type A and high score in JAS questionnaire coincided in one-half of the sample. This subsample differed from the rest in several aspects: it included the greatest part of extraverted and labile subjects (Eysenck Personality Inventory); subjects of this subsample scored higher on the MHQ questionnaire, especially on the anxiety subscale, had more frequent tension, autonomic difficulties and poor relaxation, consumed more coffee and cigarettes, classified their institute less favourably but were generally more satisfied, had a lower scientific competence but a higher scientific output.

The real degree of *hazard of cardio-vascular pathology* associated with the above-mentioned characteristics of this professional group can as yet only be estimated, using literature data from already completed longitudinal studies, e.g. the epidemiological study WCGS conducted by Rosenman et al. (1975), which have shown that the standardized relative risk in persons with behaviour pattern Type A is high in both age groups and on the same level as e.g. cholesterolemia increase by 90 mg per cent or systolic blood pressure by 30 mm Hg (in males 39–49, 50–59 years as intake).

In co-operation with the Clinic of Occupational Medicine (K. Svábová, M. Mencík, and others) most respondents were screened for somatic risk factors with the use of the recommended WHO procedure, adopted for the Czechoslovak National Multifactorial Preventive Study on Myocardial Infarction and Stroke.

Considering only 6 factors (i.e. hypertension ≥ 160/95, hypercholesterolemia ≥ 270, positive glucose tolerance test ≥ 110, smoking of cigarettes ≥ 20, overweight ≥ + 15 kg, and family history of CHD) only 10 per cent of the whole sample had no risk factors and about 60 per cent had two or more. The association of Type A behaviour pattern with the number of other risk factors was not convincing, but there was a positive correlation with hypercholesterolemia and a negative one with hypertension.

Higher occurrence of some cardio-vascular risk factors, especially of behaviour pattern Type A and of low physical activity, in creative research workers provides arguments for specific care of their mental and physical condition.

Our findings approve the presumed ambivalent role of Type A behaviour pattern. Disregarding the component of hostility, which seems to recede in conditions of a society which purposefully moderates the antagonistic forms of competition, the Type A pattern of behaviour cannot be held for an obviously negative phenomenon as shown also by the primarily positive effect of a high level of activity on the productivity of our creative workers. Therefore, one of the aims of our study is to find ways to compensate its adverse psychosomatic effects. This should be also our main contribution to the multifactorial intervention in CHD risk factors, which is the aim of National Multifactorial Preventive Study on Myocardial Infarction and Stroke.

So far we have studied for two years, on a subsample of 50 men, the cardio-protective and relaxing effect of systematic physical exercise and we are introducing a technique of mental relaxation or relaxation–activation training in addition to intervention of other coronary risk factors, active prevention of vertebrogenic difficulties, modification of dietary habits, and psychological counselling service.

SUMMARY

Creative research work is typical of occupations which lack traditional harmful working conditions but require a sustained high level of activation.

The material reported here is the introductory part of a longitudinal study of research and development workers. The aims of the study are:

(a) Epidemiological and laboratory testing of the hypothesis that the persisting high level of activity both due to psychologic stress factors or due to a fixed behaviour pattern (Type A/B of Friedman and Rosenman) might contribute to adverse effects on mental and somatic health;
(b) Identification of and recommendations for the elimination of dispensable sources of 'job pressures' in institutes of technological research and development;
(c) Development of physiological and psychological intervention which should compensate for chronic overactivation and evaluation of the efficiency of this intervention.

In this context the correlation between behaviour pattern and the incidence of ischemic heart disease will be studied in groups where intervention (c) has occurred and in control groups and the results compared with other professions; a laboratory search for physiological components of the state described as a 'high level of activity' will also be conducted.

At present in addition to generating hypotheses:

(1) The validity of the criteria for behaviour pattern assessment were checked in our population by a standardized interview and questionnaire (Jenkins Activity Survey);

(2) The assumption about the primarily positive effect of a high habitual level of activity (behaviour pattern Type A) on the productivity of creative workers was confirmed (e.g. compensation of deficiencies in professional qualifications);

(3) It has been confirmed that there is no simple relation between the characteristic of behaviour type A/B and other personality characteristics (EPI, MHQ, etc.).

REFERENCES

BOLELOUCKÝ, Z. and HORVÁTH, M. (1974). SCL-90 rating scale: First experience with the Czech version in healthy male scientific workers. *Activ. nerv. sup. (Praha)*, **16** (2), 115–16.

CROWN, S. and CRISP, A. H. (1970). *Manual of the Middlesex Hospital Questionnaire (MHQ)*. Psychological Test Publisher, Barnstaple, England.

DEROGATIS, L. R., LIPMAN, R. S., and COVI, L. (1973). SCL-90: An outpatients psychiatric rating scale—preliminary report. *Psychopharmacol. Bull.*, **9** (1), 13–28.

HOWELL, R. W. and CROWN, S. (1971). Sickness absence levels and personality inventory scores. *Brit. J. indust. Med.*, **28,** 126.

ROSENMAN, R. H. *et al.* (1964). A predictive study of coronary heart disease: The Western Collaborative Group Study. *J. Amer. med. Assoc.*, **189,** (1), 103–10. (Appendix: procedures for assessment of behaviour pattern.)

—— *et al.* (1975). Coronary heart disease in the Western Collaborative Group Study: Final follow-up experience of 8 1/2 years. *J. Amer. med. Assoc.* **233** (8), 872–77.

VINAŘ, O. and FRANTÍK, E. (1968). La fatigue et la santé des travailleurs scientifiques. *Travaux du Troisième congrès international de médecine psychosomatique, Toulouse*, pp. 297–300.

WHO (1973) Behavioural and operational components of health intervention programmes. Appendix III—Jenkins Activity Survey, pp. 49–61. *WHO Study Protocol Interregional 0674*. WHO/Kaunas/Rotterdam.

SESSION 5

Objectives and methodology for future research

40. CHANGING TRENDS IN OCCUPATIONAL HEALTH RESEARCH

S. FORSSMAN

INTRODUCTION

Changes in research have been influenced by the now generally accepted wide definition of occupational health. Fifty years ago, occupational health was mainly concerned with occupational diseases and accidents, their prevention and treatment, and with rehabilitation. Occupational health now covers the general health of the working populations in relation to work and the work environment (for definition see ILO/WHO 1953; ILO 1971–2). The recent changes in occupational health research can also be attributed to major factors: changes in the human environment at work with regard to health hazards, stress, and work load, and changes in the working population as far as health, morbidity, age distribution, job adjustment, and job attitudes are concerned.

CHANGES IN THE WORK ENVIRONMENT

It has recently been emphasized that the environment plays a predominant role in man's health, and that rapid technological changes, increased population, and greater concentration of people in urban centres will make it still more important to maintain the environment at a healthful level (Nelson *et al.* 1970).

The technological changes include mechanization and automation not only in industry, but also in forestry, agriculture, and transport. Mechanization will shift more of the load to machines, but will create other forms of stress related to such factors as working postures, noise and vibration, or perception and information overload (Forssman *et al.* 1972a).

However, some operations are difficult to mechanize and may be expected to persist, at least in part; these will probably continue to act as important barriers to the employment of certain groups of persons with limited capacities, such as the middle-aged and elderly. Momentary peak loads seem to be of special importance as limiting factors for the ageing worker.

Monotonous work on assembly lines may be a health problem, but such work may also impose a heavy physiological load even if the job's total energy demands are moderate. The cause may lie peripherally in the muscles as well as in the greater strain imposed on the blood circulation by prolonged standing or other fixed postures. Environmental factors, such as heat, carbon monoxide, noise, and vibrations, may increase the physiological work load.

A new production process may introduce new chemical substances, of which the toxic effects are unknown. In the future it will be important to study not so much the health effects of acute exposure to high concentrations as those of long-term exposure to low levels of chemical toxic substances or physical factors, alone or in combination.

Structural changes occur very often in industrialized countries, so that one type of industry will be expanding and another type may be heavily reduced or even disappear. This will call for the replacement and retraining of workers, who will have to face new professions and new work demands. In Sweden, for instance, the iron foundries, the textile industry, and the stone and quarry industry have been reduced, while the machine industry has been expanding. Small units may merge into large ones, thus creating many psychological problems in adjusting to new working conditions. The very small factories may have a low standard of industrial hygiene, but the employees usually have a low sickness rate and a high level of job satisfaction. These structural changes are seen on a larger scale in developing countries during the process of rapid industrialization and urbanization.

CHANGES IN THE WORKING POPULATION

In many countries during the last decades there have been considerable changes in the working population which have also influenced occupational health research. The age and sex distributions of the working population have changed. The number of middle-aged and elderly personnel in industries has increased to such an extent that in many workplaces in industrialized countries more than 50 per cent are over 45 years of age. This happens especially in industries which are reducing their manpower through mechanization. The reduced need for manpower often results in no employment of new personnel for several years and after some time the average age of employees becomes rather high. Examples of this can be seen in many Swedish industries, for instance, in the iron foundries and stone industries (Forssman *et al.* 1972a).

In many industrialized countries, more women than before are entering the labour market, not only in industries where, traditionally, the major proportion of the employees are women, such as the textile and food industries, but also in other industries such as iron and steel, where women may be employed, for instance, as crane operators.

The change in population morbidity patterns has also been considered by research planners. Infectious diseases are gradually disappearing and psychosomatic diseases and degenerative diseases are assuming increasing importance. Cardiovascular diseases, cancer, and accidents are now the major causes of death in industrialized countries, and this trend is becoming increasingly evident in the developing countries.

Job attitudes and expectations have changed during the last decade in many industrialized countries. Recent studies have shown that anxiety and complaints about the work environment or working conditions are very common among employees (Bolinder *et al.* 1970). The complaints are very often related to repetitive tasks or monotony at work, but also to chemical and physical factors in the work environment. Anxiety is often focused on the possible long-term effects of those chemical and other factors which are believed to influence the incidence of chronic diseases or to result in earlier retirement.

Some years ago, employees' expectations with regard to their work were mainly centred around an adequate income, safety, and health, as well as the elimination of chemical or physical occupational health hazards such as carbon monoxide, lead fumes, silica dust, and dangerous machinery. With the increasing knowledge of the effect of working conditions upon health and with higher living standards and a higher level of education among the working population, expectations have changed. Naturally there is still a strong demand for health and safety at work, but there is now an additional require-ment for comfort and the elimination of unnecessary fatigue. The repetitive and monotonous work that may occur in modern industry has very often resulted in diminished job satisfaction and alienation. The aspira-tions of employees are now focused increasingly on a meaningful job together with a certain amount of in-dependence in carrying out their own tasks and parti-cipation in planning and arranging their own work and working conditions (Forsmann *et al.* 1972a). There is also a strong trend among the 'consumers' of techno-logical development, that is, the working population, to demand more influence on that development. In earlier days, industrial development had mainly considered technological and economic aspects, i.e. highest produc-tion at lowest possible costs. There is now a strong feel-ing that human aspects should also be considered and the humanization of work conditions is now being increas-ingly emphasized in many places.

With mechanization and automation, the need for manpower has often been reduced and, at the same time, the mental demands of jobs have sometimes increased. This has created problems for large groups of the work-ing population, such as the unskilled worker, the ageing worker, and the handicapped, who in many workplaces are gradually being eliminated from the labour market. The unemployed in many industrialized countries are composed mainly of these groups.

The definition of occupational health has been widened, and this is influencing the field of occupational health research. Fifty years ago, occupational health was mainly concerned with health conditions caused only or mainly by work, such as occupational diseases and injuries. A joint ILO/WHO Expert Committee in 1950 decided upon the following broad definition of occupational health:

Occupational health should aim at: the promotion and maintenance of the highest degree of physical, mental and social well-being of workers in all occupations; the prevention among workers of departures from health caused by their working conditions; the protection of workers in their employ-ment from risks resulting from factors adverse to health; the placing and maintenance of the worker in an occupational environment adapted to his physiological and psychological equipment and, to summarize: the adaptation of work to man and of each man to his job.

Research in occupational health is now more and more concerned with the general health of the worker, taking into consideration the influence upon health and work adjustment of his environment at work and also outside work; this will call for more and more interdisciplinary studies.

EXAMPLES FROM DIFFERENT FIELDS OF OCCUPATIONAL HEALTH RESEARCH

There has been increasing interest in research on the work environment, especially its chemical and physical factors.

Industrial toxicology

Previously, studies were mainly devoted to distinctly defined, now 'classical', occupational diseases not occur-ring among the general population. Exposure was very often high and generally the disease could be related to one cause; the work environment factor was dominant and the 'host factor' was of minor importance. Research is now mainly concerned with long-term exposures to low levels of concentrations of one toxic substance, alone or in combination with others. Hence, human factors such as individual susceptibility, genetic factors, and the existence of other diseases may also exert an increasing influence on the disease (Hatch 1973). In experimental toxicology, research is now mainly focused on the mechanism of action, sub-cellular changes, and the effects of long-term exposure, especially with regard to cancerogenicity, teratogenicity, and mutagenicity (Forssman 1977). Such toxicological studies are, however, costly and time-consuming, as can be seen from Table 40.1. Considerable research is now devoted to developing new methods of evaluating toxic effects, for instance, by studying tissue cultures, or by estimating certain enzyme activities.

On the clinical side, research is concentrated on epidemiological studies to establish the influence of

TABLE 40.1

Draft classification on information on toxicity, to be collected for an international information system— occupational health aspects

---

A. *Animal experiments*
1. *Acute*
   (a) Single dose: LD 50
       Mode of application: Oral, intraperitoneal, subcutaneous, inhalation, skin, eye
       Animals: Mice, rats, rabbits, dogs
       Main effects
   (b) Repeated doses: 1–10 days of exposure
       Animals: Mice, rats, rabbits, dogs
       Main effects
2. *Sub-acute*
   30 days of exposure
   Mode of application: Oral, intraperitoneal, subcutaneous, inhalation, skin
   Animals: Mice, rats, rabbits, dogs
   Main effects
3. *Chronic*
   90 days' exposure
   6 months' exposure
   2 years' exposure
   Lifetime exposure
   3 generations exposure
   Animals: Mice, rats, rabbits, dogs
   Main effects, such as chronic intoxication, pathology, biochemistry, cancer, teratogenicity, mutagenicity
4. *Proposed maximal allowable concentration*
B. *Human exposure*
1. *Experiments*
   (a) Acute
   (b) Sub-acute
   (c) Chronic
2. *Occupational exposure*
   (a) Occupation
   (b) Average concentration; range
   (c) Main effects, such as incidence of intoxication, pre-clinical signs, biological tests of exposure (as lead in blood)
3. *Proposed maximal allowable concentration*

Reference (author, title, journal) should be given for each report or study.

work environment as one of several factors contributing to non-occupational diseases. The technique here is to study the morbidity of occupational and non-occupational diseases among workers exposed to occupational health hazards, compared with that of control groups. Such studies have been carried out, for instance, concerning the incidence of lung cancer among mine workers (Jörgenson 1973), among industrial workers and asbestos workers, and also with regard to the incidence of ischaemic heart diseases among workers in the rayon industry exposed to carbon disulphide (Hernberg *et al.* 1973; Nofer *et al.* 1961; Tiller *et al.* 1968; Vigliani and Pernis 1955). Methods for monitoring the work environment in relation to the health of exposed workers were recently studied by WHO Expert Committee World Health Organization 1973).

As exposure to toxic substances has been gradually reduced in many workplaces as a result of technical preventive measures, attention has now been turned to the problems of vulnerable groups such as ageing workers and handicapped workers. As exposure is reduced, it is of increasing importance to select those individuals with high susceptibility and to place then in non-exposed jobs. Research is also being conducted on 'multiple stress' and the combined effect of exposure to several different health factors at work.

Considerable research has been devoted to studies of maximum allowable concentrations (MAC) of toxic substances. Different research methods have been applied in different countries, but more exchange of experience among various research groups will be needed before internationally accepted values can be established WHO Expert Committee, Geneva 1976; see reports World Health Organization 1975, 1977).

Ergonomics

The idea of adjusting work to man was first applied in a systematic way in the early-1950s. Research was at first mainly devoted to the elimination of peak loads, usually heavy physical work combined with heat stress, and 'physical overload'. Industrial psychology was then concerned with developing methods for measuring job demands and individual work capacities and sometimes very sophisticated methods of job placement and vocational guidance. Later, the psychomotor aspects were considered and research focused on the man–machine system and the system of ergonomics (Grandjean 1969; Singleton 1972). Through mechanization the main job demand shifted from heavy physical load to job demand on groups of small muscles requiring precision movements combined with perception and information, usually at high speed. In some work situations, such as at large instrument panels, too much information may sometimes be presented to the human mind and workers may consequently be subjected to a 'psychological overload'. Considerable research on fatigue was also carried out and interesting studies on muscular fatigue, recorded through 'objective' methods such as measuring the concentration of lactic acid, compared the 'objective' fatigue with the subjective feeling of exertion. When ergonomics studies at work evaluated peak loads and related them to certain parts of the work process, the individual worker's own evaluation in ergonomics interviews often established peak loads related to other parts of the work process. Research since then has been centred on establishing tolerance limits, taking into consideration objective measurements as well as individual attitudes, feelings, and subjective evaluation of work. Age seems to be an important factor, not only for the physical and mental work capacity but also for the subjective evaluation of the job demand and of the individual's own work capacity (Forssman 1969).

Mental health

Stress at work, when biological defence mechanisms are triggered by stressors such as psychosocial factors, is studied in many institutes, especially from the aspect of its importance as a cause of or contributing factor to disease or deviation from health or normal behaviour (Levi 1972).

Automation and mechanization usually decrease the occupational hazards from machinery and toxic exposure but increase the health hazards from paced decision-making through perceptional and mental fatigue, sometimes combined with exposure to factors such as carbon monoxide, alcohol, drugs, noise, and vibration (Nelson *et al.* 1970). Some modern work conditions that include mechanized control and inspection work may result in a work 'underload' and 'understimulation'. The health effects of such work conditions are so far very little known and further research is needed.

From the aspect of mental health, the incidence of neurosis in industry, trigger factors at work, and the effects of changing human relations were studied in the early 1950s (Jaques 1951; Ling 1954). During recent years, research has been carried out on attitudes towards work and working conditions, such as chemical and physical factors of work, and monotony. Research has recently also been concerned with the organization of work, the assembly line, piece-rates, etc., recording different signs of maladjustment such as sickness absence, labour turnover, alienation, diminished job satisfaction, and the incidence of psychosomatic diseases (Gardell 1971; Bolinder and Ohlström 1971; Forssman *et al.* 1972a).

The basic needs of man at work were formerly thought to comprise the provision of an adequate income, as well as safety and health at work. During recent years, needs have been changing and people are now not only expecting that these basic needs should be satisfied, but are also seeking jobs that are adequately related to their physical and mental resources, meaningful jobs with a certain freedom in planning, choosing work methods and a suitable pace, and with a certain freedom of performance. People are now also very much interested in having some influence and control over their own work situation and over the planning of new work methods. These changed demands of the working population in many countries have influenced research in this field, which is now dealing with many of these problems. The changing demands seem to be related to the increased standard of living and education, and to the increased knowledge gained from research on man at work (Forssman *et al.* 1972a).

Shift work

Research has also been carried out on some general problems, such as working time and its influence upon health, especially concerning its duration and distribution over a 24-hour period. Night and shift work has been and is being studied; this will be of great importance, as these types of work will be applied more and more for technological as well as financial reasons in mo[...] countries (Proceedings of international symposium o[...] night and shift work 1969, 1971; Studia Laboris et Salut[...] 1969, 1972; Taylor *et al.* 1972; Swedish Work Environ[...] ment Fund 1975).

Accidents

Research on accidents at work has been changing durin[...] the last few decades. The earlier approach was mainl[...] statistical, but later a clinical approach was introduced aiming at a detailed analysis of the accident syndrom[...] (Gemelli 1955; Schulzinger 1956) and the factors at wor[...] or in human behaviour that contributed to the occur[...] rence of an a accident. Recently, research has also bee[...] focused on near-accidents (Lagerlöf *et al.* 1970) and ha[...] also used epidemiological methods, comparing person[...] involved in accidents with control groups (Hagberg 1960 Forssman 1972; Swedish Work Environment Fun[...] 1975).

RESEARCH PROBLEMS OF THE FUTURE

Trends in research during recent years can provide som[...] conclusions for the future. Research will develo[...] towards broader views, studying the workers' genera[...] health and overall adjustment to his work as well as th[...] general influence of work upon man, taking into accoun[...] the physical and mental work load. Concerning occupa[...] tional health hazards, the trend is, and will be still mor[...] in the future, to study both the health hazards at wor[...] and the total body burden resulting, for instance, fron[...] exposure to lead, mercury, noise, fatigue, and stress a[...] work and outside.

Broad interdisciplinary studies of the health problem[...] of various occupations, involving not only medicine, bu[...] also physiology, psychology and sociology, will be[...] needed. Such studies will include, on the human side[...] health, morbidity, sickness absence, job adjustment, jol[...] satisfaction, and attitudes towards work and, on th[...] work environment side, health hazards, physical an[...] mental work load, working time, and job organization[...] Such studies have been carried out in Sweden, fo[...] instance in forestry and agriculture (Kylin *et al.* 196[...] Lindgren 1973). The needs for further research of thi[...] kind in Sweden have been studied by a working grou[...] (Forssman *et al.* 1972b; Forssman 1972).

More national planning in research will be needed. B[...] way of examples, the following may be mentioned:

A 'problem' committee on occupational health[...] organized in the Soviet Union with representatives fron[...] 15 occupational health institutes and under the directio[...] of the U.S.S.R. Institute of Occupational Health i[...] Moscow, discusses major problems of research o[...] occupational health and coordinates the activities of th[...] different institutes.

A special task force on research planning in environ[...] mental health science was organized in the United State[...] and presented a report on health and the environmen[...]

(Nelson *et al.* 1970). The National Institute for Occupational Safety and Health, established in 1970, is planning and organizing research on occupational health hazards, in close collaboration with research laboratories of universities and industries. All available information on an occupational health factor is being compiled and evaluated in 'criteria documents' (Key 1972). A research programme on the humanization of working life has recently been published jointly by the Ministry of Labour and Social Security and the Ministry of Research and Technology of the Federal Republic of Germany (Minister of Labour and Social Security 1974).

In France, a committee is now working to study the future need for research in occupational health and ergonomics, bearing in mind the changes that will take place in industry in the 1980s and is collecting information from other countries before preparing the report, which is the responsibility of Professor A. Wisner, Paris.

In Sweden, the Ministry of Social Affairs and Health requested that a study on present and future needs of research on occupational health be carried out. A report was presented in 1972 by a working group after discussions on these problems with research institutes, medical, science and engineering faculties, industrial and society planners as well as workers' and employers' organizations (Forssman *et al.* 1972b). A study on the future need for research on behavioural sciences and working environment was made in 1973.

It is important, as far as the future is concerned, to discuss the principles of priorities for occupational health research and to study how such priorities are established in different countries. Technical development, especially the design of new production processes and the use of new chemical substances, must be considered in establishing such priorities, as well as expected changes in the structure of industry with regard to type and size, expected changes in society, e.g. in industrialization and urbanization, and expected changes in the working population, e.g. in age and sex distribution and in morbidity.

Concerning research on health factors at work, the seriousness and incidence of diseases related to work conditions, as well as the number of people exposed, must be considered when priorities are being established. In selecting occupations for interdisciplinary. research, such factors should be considered as a high incidence of accidents or occupational diseases, high general morbidity, high sickness absence or labour turnover, high incidence of negative attitudes towards work, recruitment difficulties, and rapid changes in the production process stemming from mechanization and automation, which will usually create difficulties in adjusting to new conditions at work.

The Swedish report mentioned above (Forssman *et al.* 1972b) established the following eleven fields of priorities: industrial toxicology; industrial hygiene engineering eliminating air contamination at work; noise, effects and prevention; climate, especially low temperature and air movement; organization and motivation of work; back diseases; occupational injuries; interdisciplinary health surveys of occupational groups; working time, length and distribution during day and week, especially shift work; sickness absence and labour turnover; the ageing worker.

Of the eleven priority subjects, the following four were selected: industrial toxicology, working time, accidents, and studies of occupational groups. Special committees were established to study and report on research planning in detail. As priority problems, the 'industrial back' and noise at work, regarding which there was a great need for more knowledge and more research, were then added to the fields of priority.

A special fund for research, education, and information on work environment was created in Sweden in 1972. the contributions by the employers to the compulsory insurance of employees against accidents and occupational diseases were raised in 1974 and this increase, which amounts to about U.S. $20 million annually, will be placed at the disposal of this fund.

PRACTICAL APPLICATION OF RESEARCH

It is unfortunately a common experience that when research results are reported there is usually a long delay before they will be applied in practice on the factory floor. Application of research in practice must therefore be specially organized. It must already be considered at the planning stage of research and it should be a responsibility of a specified individual or organization. The reseach worker should participate in the practical application of his results, but the main responsibility must rest with people who have practical experience of production processes or the work environment.

The application of research will usually take place in different stages. The research report must be presented in a language that can be understood by production engineers, foremen, and safety workers, and the main results should then be published and distributed widely to people with practical experience.

It will often be necessary to apply the results of research to practical conditions at the workplace. Pilot studies in factories with the assistance of the research workers will then be of great value.

Manuals and checklists for introducing new methods will have to be produced and training courses for production engineers, designers, foremen, and safety workers should then be carried out. Practical experience of the results of the research and of the pilot studies should then be published, distributed widely, and finally introduced also in the basic training and education at engineers' colleges and in the engineering, science, and medical faculties of universities, so that the results will be introduced in the planning and construction stages of work places of the future.

REFERENCES

BOLINDER, E., MAGNUSSON, E., and NYRÉN, L. (1970). *Risker i jobbet: LO-enkäten, LO-medlemmarnas uppfattning om arbetsplatsens hälsorisker* [Job hazards—A study in job attitudes]. Stockholm. (In Swedish).

—— and OHLSTRÖM, B. (1971). *Stress pa svenska arbetsplatser* [Stress at Swedish work places]. Lund. (In Swedish).

FORSSMAN, S. (1969). *Der ältere Mitarbeiter* [The older worker] In *Bericht über den 11. Kongress für Arbeitsschutz und Arbeitsmedizin 1969* [Report on 11th Congress on industrial, safety and occupational medicine]. Dusseldorf. (In German).

—— (1972). *National planning of occupational health research in Sweden.* Swedish Work Environment Fund, Report No. 3, Stockholm.

BOLINDER, E., GARDELL, B., GERHARDSSON, G., and MEIDNER, R. (1972a). *The human work environment—Swedish experiences, trends, and future problems.*—A contribution to the United Nations Conference on the Human Environment, Royal Ministry for Foreign Affairs, Stockholm.

——, LAGERLÖF, E., and MALMFORS, T. (1972b). *Forskningsverksamheten inom arbetsmiljöomradet* [Research on work environment]. Report Ds S 1972:2, Social Department, Stockholm.

GARDELL, B. (1971). *Production engineering and work satisfaction.* Swedish Council for Personnel Administration, Stockholm.

GEMELLI, A. (1955). Le facteur humain, des accidents dans l'industrie, *Bull. WHO,* **13,** 649.

GRANDJEAN, E. (1969). *Précis d'ergonomie.* Brussels.

—— (1977). Health hazards associated with introducing new chemicals in industry: prevention and control. *Public Hlth Europe* **8,** 115 (WHO Regional Office for Europe, Copenhagen).

HAGBERG, A. (1960). *Olycksfall, individ, arbete, arbetsmiljö* [Accidents, the human being, work, work environment]. Swedish Council for Personnel Administration, Stockholm. (In Swedish).

HATCH, T. F. (1974). Priorities in preventive medicine—where are the highest yields? *Arch. environm. Hlth* **29,** 32.

HERNBERG, S., NARMINEN, M., and TOLONEN, M. (1973). Excess mortality from coronary heart disease in viscose rayon workers exposed to carbon disulfide. *Work environm. Hlth,* **10,** 93.

ILO (1971–72). *Enclyclopedia on occupational health and safety.* Geneva.

JAQUES, E. (1951). *The changing culture of a factory.* Tavistock Publications, London.

Joint ILO/WHO Committee on Occupational Health (1953). Second Report, Geneva (WHO techn. Rep. Ser., No. 66).

JÖRGENSEN, H. S. (1973). A study of mortality from lung cancer among miners in Kiruna 1950–1970, *Work environm. Hlth,* **10,** 126.

KEY, M. (Director of NIOSH) (1972). *Criteria for a recommended standard . . . Occupational exposure to carbon monoxide.* U.S. Department of Health, Education, and Welfare, Washington.

KYLIN, B., et al. (1968). *Hälso- och miljöundersökning bland skogsarbetare* [Study on health and work environment of forestry workers]. National Institute of Occupational Health, AI-report No. 5, Stockholm. (In Swedish with English summary.)

LAGERLÖF, E., GUSTAFSSON, L., and PETTERSSON, B. (1970). Analysis of near accidents in logging. In *Report on Fourth Intern. Congr. on Ergonomics,* Strasbourg.

LEVI, L. (Ed.) (1972). Stress and distress in response to psychosocial stimuli. *Acta med. scand.,* Suppl. 528.

LINDGREN, G. (1973). *Jordbrukets socialmedicin* [Social medicine of agriculture]. Univ. Lund, Report No. 10, University of Lund. (In Swedish).

LING, T. M. (Ed.) (1954). *Mental health and human relations in industry.* H. M. Lewis, London.

Minister of Labour and Social Security (1974). Bundesminister für Arbeit und Sozialordnung) Forschung zur Humanisierung des Arbeitslebens [Research on the humanization of working life]. *Sozialpolitische Informationen* **8,** 1.(In German).

NELSON, N. (chairman) (1970). Man's health and the environment—some research needs. Report of the Task Force on Research Planning in Environmental Health Science. U.S. Department of Health, Education, and Welfare, Washington.

NOFER, J., et al. (1961). Effect of occupational hazard to carbon disulphide on the pathogenesis of arteriosclerosis. *Medycyna Pracy,* **12,** 101. (In Polish with summary in English.)

Proceedings of international symposium on night and shift work (1969). No. 1. (1971). No. 2.

SCHULZINGER, M. S. (1956). *Accident syndrome. The genesis of accident injury. A clinical approach.* Springfield, Illinois.

SINGLETON, W. I. (1972). *Introduction to ergonomics.* WHO Geneva.

Studia Laboris et Salutis (1969). No. 4, Stockholm.

—— (1972). No. 11, Stockholm.

Swedish Work Environment Fund (1975). *Research for a better work environment: A summary of reports on four central research areas.* Liber, Stockholm.

TAYLOR, P., POCOCK, S. J., and SERGEAN, R. (1972) Absenteeism of shift and day workers. *Brit. J. ind. Med.,* **29,** 208.

TILLER, J. R., SCHILLING, R. S. F., and MORRIS, J. N. (1968) Occupational toxic factor in mortality from coronary heart disease, *Brit. med. J.,* **4,** 407.

VIGLIANI, E. and PERNIS, B. (1955). Klinische und experimentelle Untersuchungen über die durch Schwefelkohlenstoffbedingte Atherosklerose. *Arch. Gewerbepath. Gewerbehyg.,* **14,** 190.

World Health Organization (1973). Environmental health monitoring in occupational health. *WHO Tech. Rep. Ser.* No. 535.

—— (1975). *Methods used in the USSR for establishing biologically safe levels of toxic substances,* Geneva.

—— (1977). *Methods used in establishing permissible levels in occupational exposure to harmful agents.* Report of a WHO Expert Committee with the participation of ILO, Geneva.

41. RESEARCH PRIORITIES FOR DEVELOPING COUNTRIES: THE SELECTION AND TRAINING OF SKILLED WORKERS

MAUREEN A. BAILEY

INTRODUCTION

Although the need for skilled workers is great in developing countries, their selection and training has not proceeded at a particularly rapid pace. The percentage of workers who fail to complete training programmes is high and studies have been done which show that this is due to these workers' lack of experience with tools, lack of responsivity to unusual visual and aural stimulation, and generally poor educational preparation for numerical, verbal, and social (i.e., punctuality) components of their jobs. However, some of the skills are learned easily, and other deficits are overcome by a certain percentage of workers regardless of educational background or level of cultural deprivation. Thus there are important differences between worker and task.

Furthermore, it is the consensus of most cross-cultural researchers that the largest differences between industrial and non-industrial peoples are due to familiarity effects that (among children, at least) are easily eliminated with practice (Levine 1970). This line of research goes on to suggest that patterns of child-rearing may be more significant as they affect emotional adaptation rather than the exposure they provide to experiences with stimulating events and objects. Levine has summarized the research demonstrating that severe training in obedience and compliance 'interferes with the capacity for active mastery involved in solving model problems . . .' (Levine 1970, p. 603).

The current findings regarding skilled worker selection and training will be reviewed in order to:

1. Estimate the extent to which the findings could be interpreted to support the possibility that psycho-endocrine factors may also be involved in the failures observed among skilled trainees in developing countries.
2. Outline models for selection and training which would be appropriate if such factors were included.

PREVIOUS WORK

Previous work on stress factors in the training of skilled workers even in industrialized countries is not extensive. Selection factors too are little understood from the point of view of the psychoendocrinology of work as against perceptual-motor skill assessment. Psychomedical assessment currently appears largely confined to ascertaining in a fairly specific way whether the candidate has a disability that would interfere with job performance. Much information has been gleaned regarding stress in learning environments in connection with manned space flights but its generalizable merit for the common variety of problems of selection and training remains to be assessed. Cohen and Margolis (1973) report a review of the literature which is underway to identify psychophysical attributes which can be meaningfully tied to problems of worker safety and health. Interestingly, these researchers are building toward environmental rather than personal standards, and will use the results to recommend allowances in industrial safety to protect worker 'groups' with special characteristics. This is certainly another important way of looking at the problem. If we can expect that 'x' per cent of a group of job applicants will have certain attributes which would cause them to fail in the current training environment, how can that environment be altered to make it possible to utilize a greater portion of available and motivated personnel?

CONCEPTUAL APPROACH

The conceptual issues which formed a background to the present discussion grow out of the need to maintain a distinction between operant and respondent behaviour. Operant behaviour is defined as behaviour that is controlled by its consequences. Respondent behaviour is defined as behaviour that is controlled by its antecedents. A training environment is quintessentially a setting for the development of operant behaviours, but the physical and social attributes of any environment can elicit a large number of respondent behaviours, most of which are irrelevant for the learning of the operant responses required and function more or less as psycho-endocrine 'background noise'. Respondent behaviour can cease to be irrelevant and become intrusive or disequilibrating. It is very tempting to attribute failure to the operant learning history of an individual worker when this occurs because to all intents and purposes he just may not seem to be catching on, or he may be catching on in discrete portions but never consolidate behaviours.

PROPOSED MODEL FOR ASSESSMENT

Having said that the prevocational assessment of perceptual-motor skills is not sufficient to identify the risks of failure due to psychoendocrine factors, what assessment approach can be recommended alternatively? It would be fruitless to recommend physiological screening because individual reactions are not straightforward to interpret. One subject experiencing anxiety may increase his heart rate; another one may decrease it; a third may react primarily with gastrointestinal or muscular reactions. Monitoring of catecholamines excreted in the urine during a trial working experience should provide one satisfactory measure provided mean different values between trial and non-trial work environments were available. Second, some measures of the pattern of child-rearing the individual was exposed to as it would relate to his capacity for active mastery in problem-solving solutions should be designed. Third, a free environment perceptual motor testing might be designed in which the individual could demonstrate his capacity for co-ordinated activities without being made to feel under a microscope, as it were, and the familiarity of the items employed emphasized. (Bicycle wheels being used in some variant of a rotor pursuit task, for example, as against a standard apparatus.) Fourth, some measures of social support or rootedness should be available to describe the applicant's current situation.

Using these four ingredients could result in a physiological, developmental, perceptual motor, and social cross-section of the individual on the basis of which fairly solid predictions could be worked our regarding his capacity to adapt to the demands of the work environment.

TRAINING MODEL

Certain environmentally disequilibrating factors must b carefully controlled in the work environment in an event, but especially, one estimates, for trainees, eve carefully selected ones. Provision for habituation to di crete aspects of the working environment should b made. Noises, lights, shifts in temperature among othe variables, would require special habituation effor *before* an individual was expected to master a task in volving such possibly stress arousing ingredients.

Second one must anticipate failure and build a way c dealing with it into a training environment that does nc create intolerable stress for the worker. As a general ru one might want to make each initial step toward th mastery of a task so small that an errorless path migh eventually be followed. Alternatively, habituation c desensitization to disequilibrating responses to inevi able small failures could be designed into habituation t physical aspects of the environment. A situation coul be engineered to produce failure, the responses to highlighted by the trainer, and effective social/emotion: ways of coping outlined—i.e., take a deep breath, rela: count to ten, etc. Above all the trainee would learn t accept his own physiological response to the demands c the work environment, and this is a very basic ingredien

REFERENCES

Cohen, A. and Margolis, B. (1973). Initial psychological research related to the Occupational Safety and Health Act of 1970. *Am. Psychol.* **28**, 600–6.

Levine, Robert A. (1970). Cross cultural study in child psychology. In *Carmichael's manual of child psychology* (3rd edn) (ed. Paul H. Mussen), Vol II, p. 603. Wiley, New York.

42.   A COMMUNITY RESEARCH STRATEGY APPLICABLE TO PSYCHOSOCIAL FACTORS AND HEALTH

AUBREY R. KAGAN

THE MISSING LINK

Never before in the history of mankind has there been a greater demand for research in the life sciences than in the last 30 years. And never before has there been a greater supply. Great advances have been made at the molecular, cellular, and organ level but very little at the family, industry, parish, or community level. This is not because society has neglected to support epidemiologists, sociologists, behavioural scientists. On the contrary, their numbers, status, and funding have increased at much the same rate as for biochemists, immunologists, and pharmacologists.

A clue to the discrepancy can be found by scanning the literature of the last 30 years or indeed the chapters in this and preceding volumes on *Society, stress, and disease*. Once we move from laboratory studies to the community we hardly ever find hypothesis-testing studies reported. Once we leave clinical trials it is rare to find a report of evaluation of a health or social action. There are innumerable studies showing associations and many speculating on ideas for health or social action or hypotheses of community spread and control of disease. There are rare exceptions where hypotheses have been tested or actions have been evaluated and these are important because they show that it can be done.

The reason given for failure to do so are that—it is unethical; it is technically impossible; it is too expensive; it takes too long. Whilst there is an element of truth in all these objections, the first three can often be overcome and something can be done to mollify the effects of the last. Under such circumstances it becomes unethical and more costly to impose an action of doubtful value, possible dangers, and high cost without evaluation, or to accept an hypothesis without prior test.

THE DIFFICULTIES

Leaving aside the problems which many people would agree can be overcome—ethical, study design, analysis, precision and bias of data, much data from many subjects, follow-up—and which have been considered elsewhere. I would like to concentrate here on a group of difficulties which are due to the large number of interacting or confusing variables, the long period of observation necessary, and the absence of proven mechanisms. The last three conditions lead to two difficulties and these suggest three remedies which are the basis of the research strategy that we will propose.

The difficulty of controls

Any evaluation or hypothesis test requires study controls. When the *end effect follows quickly* upon the action, the *mechanism is known,* and the effect of the *treatment is dramatic,* it is sufficient to study a few cases and to use the subjects as their own controls e.g. reduction of mortality by 50 per cent in 6 patients with tuberculous meningitis was conclusive evidence that streptomycin was of value in preventing death in this condition. Previously the mortality was 100 per cent. The mechanism of disease progress through the tubercule bacillus was known and seen to diminish with successful treatment. When the end effect does not follow swiftly upon the action, the mechanism is not known and there may be many interacting variables which could affect the result e.g. the use of cervical smear to prevent cancer of the neck of the womb, it is useless to use the subject as her own control. Unfortunately this is the situation with most of the problems we wish to tackle. *Testing a hypothesis or evaluating an action by comparing the observed effect of the action with what was expected is unsatisfactory unless the chances are extremely low that any factor other than the one under test will affect the results.* Unfortunately the conditions we are concerned with have many powerfully effective interacting variables.

Limited number of factors studied

In most cases the only reasonable controls are those provided by random assignment. But the random control design which makes it possible to evaluate a rather small number of factors by neutralizing the effect of many others gives us limited knowledge, i.e. limited to those factors we have tested. This is fine in some respects but, if, as is likely, it takes 1–5 years to come to a conclusion, the danger is that at the end of that time we will have a solution for the problem as it existed 1–5 years ago but social conditions may have changed so that the variables we have examined and know how to manipulate are no longer of interest and other and as yet untested variables need to be considered. Another 1–5 years to test the new variables may see us end up as before. The greater the rate of social change the more likely is this to be the case.

THE PROBLEM

The problem is how to make suitably controlled trials to evaluate health actions or test hypotheses in situations where the studies will take a long time and where the interacting variables are numerous, powerful, and insidious in action. It has been suggested that since there are many interacting factors one can consider the man–environment–disease complex as a system and apply the rules of systems analysis. The idea is to translate the relationships between the elements of the system into mathematical terms and by bringing these terms together to simulate the real situation. Then simulated manipulation on any one or more elements of the system will, on computer analysis, indicate what would be the effect on health, or show the end result may be modified in the direction required when changes of a specified kind in any of the interacting variables take place. This approach certainly has been shown to work in some ballistic and industrial problems. Unfortunately this has never been shown to work in any biological problem more complex than optimizing appointment systems or ambulance services. Indeed a prerequisite for its applicability seems to be a good understanding of the total system and a detailed understanding of the relationships between the parts of the system. This is just what is lacking in the problems with which we are concerned.

THE SOLUTION

Systems analysis would be the answer if it could be made to work. How can we approach this objective with the maximum, but still very doubtful, chance that it will work and at the same time ensure that our effort will be productive in some way. I think we must find a way of obtaining a better understanding of the whole system and at the same time obtain a detailed quantitative inter-relationship of many parts of the system. If we can combine this somewhat speculative approach with an activity that will be of undoubted value and if the combined approach costs little more than the last part we will have achieved a research strategy that is in itself efficacious and efficient.

(1) An activity that will be of undoubted value to a community is evaluation—for safety, efficacy, and cost—of a new health or social action. Such actions are foisted on the unsuspecting public by administrators, with the best intentions in the world, often without knowing, or having any means to know, whether they do good or harm, or learning from their successes or mistakes. All that is usually known for certain is that something must be done and it will be expensive. So the first and non-speculative approach in our research strategy is, in selected situations, to offer to *evaluate* such *health/social actions* in terms of who is benefited and to what degree (efficacy); who is harmed and to what degree (safety); and the cost. This will usually be in the form of a randomized controlled trial.

(2) Understanding is advanced by testing hypotheses. But some hypotheses are likely to advance understanding more than others. Into this category come hypotheses of mechanism, e.g. the demonstration of a viral and bacteriological mechanism for the spread of a large number of diseases unlocked the door to their control.

So the *second approach in our research strategy is to attempt to identify key hypotheses and, if there are any, to test them within the framework of the evaluative study mentioned above.*

(3) During the evaluative and hypothesis testing studies resulting from a combination of approaches (1 and (2) above it should be possible to obtain information that shows *quantitative relations between factors or elements of the health system thought to be relevant to the outcome.* These factors may have been excluded deliberately by the study design from interfering with the purpose of the first two approaches but they can be identified and assessed for little additional cost within the framework of the first two approaches.

In summary our research strategy consists of combining three aproaches:

(1) Evaluate one or more health/social actions;
(2) Test one or more key hypotheses;
(3) Identify, assess, and show quantified relationships between factors (or elements) thought to be of importance in the system as a whole.

The first approach is highly likely to be of immediate practical value. The value will be limited to the action studied and to some extent to the community studied. We could describe it as a low risk, moderate yield, moderate cost approach. The second approach is more speculative. It is, however, likely to advance understanding of the problem in general and could provide a means of simplifying further research. We would describe it as a medium risk, high yield, low cost (because covered by the first) approach.

The third approach is most speculative of all. It is probable that the findings will not be of immediate practical value. More likely similar data will need to be obtained from a number of studies and combined before conclusions on interrelationships can be hypothesized in the form of mathematical equations. A simulation model would then be constructed and tested against the retrospective data. It is unlikely that reasonable fit would be obtained without modification. If modification led to good retrospective fit and the modifications were based on a rational process, the modified simulation model could be tested in prospective studies and whether or not it could be used, and if so, the limits of it use, would be demonstrated. If there was no fit to retrospective data, or if fit could not be obtained by rational modification, or if the modified model did not fit in prospect, the attempt to simulate would have failed.

In spite of all these 'ifs' and the highly speculative nature of this approach we believe it to be the approach to 'systems analysis' of complex biological processes most likely, or perhaps one should say least unlikely, to succeed. The cost will be almost completely offset by the advantages of the associated evaluative studies. We could describe it as a high risk, enormous yield, low cost approach, when taken in conjunction with the other two.

APPLICATION TO PSYCHOSOCIAL FACTORS AND HEALTH

Let us see if we can translate this research strategy into something more specific in relation to the psychosocial stress occupational health system.

Our concept (see Figure 42.1) is that many different kinds of social situation (box 1) may give rise to a small number of different kinds of psychological stimulus (box 2) which in some subjects (box 3) will give rise to a pathogenic mechanism which under some conditions of duration, intensity, or frequency (box 4) will give rise to a wide variety of precursors of disease (box 5) or eventually predispose to a wide range of disease (box 6). Interacting variables will accelerate or reverse this tendency (box 7).

1. *Health/social actions to be evaluated* (box 1; Fig. 42.1) would be selected from those proposed to reduce a perceived or objective 'worker–environment' misfit (cf. Chapters 7 and 16). For example:

Diminution in perceived physical hazards which carry a psychological as well as physical element (noise, odour, climate);
Diminution in mismatch between circadian stress hormone levels and work time (cf. Chapter 13);
Diminution of monotony of work;

Increase in worker participation in decision-making; (cf. Chapter 12);
Increase in flexibility of working hours.

2. *Key hypotheses to be tested* would be those concerned with the mechanism (box 4) Fig. 42.1, or nature of pathogenic stimuli (box 2) Fig. 42.1., e.g.:

'Selye stress' is a common pathway by which stimuli from social situations cause disease;
Disease occurs only if 'Selye stress' is prolonged or frequent;
Disease occurs only if the normal response (the equivalent of 'flight or fight') does not follow 'Selye stress';
'Selye stress' is not a disease mechanism at all but merely an index of response to stimulus;
Disease occurs only if there is a difference between expectation and the situation as perceived;
Disease occurs only if there is a difference between expectation and the situation as perceived and there is an increase in frequency, intensity, or duration of 'Selye stress'.

3. *Factors or elements of the system whose interrelationships are to be quantified* (box 7) Fig. 42.1 would be selected from those thought to be of importance but which are not the object of study in the evaluative or hypothesis testing approach e.g.:

Confidence or support from spouse, family, friends, community services;
Availability, attitudes to, nature, and use of health services;

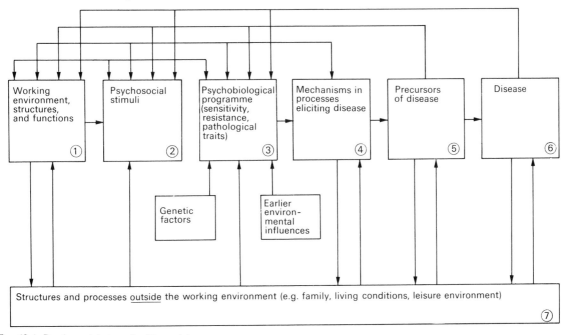

Fig. 42.1. Psychosocial stress–health model.

Participation in the local social network;
Life change;
Psychological and physical malfunctions.

4. *The basic study design* would consist in identifying subjects in several work places in which the study is to take place and to assess certain aspects of their psychobiological programme (box 3, Fig. 42.1) before the study commences e.g. current satisfactions, life change, psychological and physical malfunctions, stress hormone response to a load test.

Subjects (or workplaces) can then be assigned to treatment or control at random or stratified with reference to one or other of the psychobiological programme factors.

Change in social situation, satisfactions, stimuli, stress hormones, interacting factors, precursors of disease (box 5), and disease (box 6) will be monitored in the 'treated' and in the 'control' groups by 'bias-free' or 'bias-known' methods. These will represent 'precursors' and 'disease' at individual, family, worker group, and work institution levels.

At the end of the first stage of the study (3 months to 1 year) some of the controls will be transferred to the 'treated' group and the study continued to the next stage (3 months to 1 year).

PROGRAMME OF RESEARCH IN PSYCHOSOCIAL FACTORS AND DISEASE

The research strategy outlined and briefly related to occupational studies forms the basis of the Programme of the Laboratory for Clinical Stress Research into Psychosocial Factors and Disease in the Community. The programme aims to evaluate a wide variety of health actions and to test key hypotheses in a wide range of subjects. Thus a study is now being completed of day care in 3-year-old children. Studies of the type outlined above for 'working life' are in the planning stage. Projects on retirement in old age are now being proposed. Studies on health education in late adolescence and crisis care in family life will be considered.

It is hoped that the strategy proposed, applied on a wide front with the co-operation of our colleagues from many institutions and laboratories, will enable science to transfer the 'psychosocial stress health' system from an exciting, but not very practical, laboratory exercise to public health measures that will reduce morbidity and increase well-being in much the same way as understanding of bacterial and viral spread of disease has reduced mortality in the past.

43. HUMANIZATION OF WORKING LIFE— SYNOPSIS OF DISCUSSION

AUBREY R. KAGAN

BACKGROUND

From the 'law of self-interest and survival of the fittest' to 'industrial democracy and support of the under-privileged'
Lambo referred to the WHOs commitment to 'engage in a broad combined strategy of social and health action and economic advances which will improve the conditions of people who exist at the bottom of the social and economic pyramid in many of our contemporary societies'. He considered that work not only had a role in providing the economic basis for this but that it might also prove capable, on a broad scale, of strengthening man's sense of competence and well-being directly.

McLean spoke of the trend in many industrial nations to move from the protestant ethic of 'work for work's sake' towards the Buddist philosophy of 'minimizing suffering of the individual'—in modern jargon 'increasing well-being'. Leijon thought that the latter should be the objective of work. Surveys had shown in Sweden that salaried employers had to a large extent 'built up their knowledge and value through their work' whilst 'manual workers had been worn out and broken'.

New laws were in action or preparation to enable employers to increase job satisfaction through participation in decision-making. This industrial democracy would be a source of satisfaction in itself but it should also lead to improved conditions of work and a better quality of social communication for all and particularly those who at the moment are underprivileged.

Batawi demonstrated that although physical conditions of work left much to be desired and needed improvement one could often find a friendly 'family atmosphere' in small factories in developing countries. He argued that developing and industrial countries had much to learn from each other. Levinson, pointed out 'the dearth of knowledge to make recommendations for legislation'. It was a challenge to us all to obtain the kind of knowledge which can be applied in the way the Swedish Government proposed and thus to encourage less *avant garde* governments to act in an appropriate way but *on the basis of knowledge.*

PSYCHOSOCIAL STRESSORS

Thus it was not surprising that although much needs to be done in some countries and some things need to be done in all countries to improve physical conditions, the emphasis was on psychosocial factors.

Small is beautiful

Edström and Forssman referred to earlier studies in Sweden in which small workshops (less than 10 workers) with known poor physical conditions were investigated, and the workers found to be unusually healthy and happy.

Batawi referred to WHO studies on health in small industries in 12 developing countries. In spite of bad physical conditions there was evidence that the 'psychological climate was good'. Rates of absenteeism were lower and feelings of identification with the work and being part of the establishment were greater than in larger industrial settings. There was a better 'face to face' relationship between management and workers.

Levinson reported studies in small groups in the United States which showed that such people were more likely to see the whole of the problem with which they were concerned and also that there was 'a good deal of supportive interaction. If people are sick or have other difficulties others will mobilize around them'. French regarded the findings of higher level of absenteeism, more strikes, and greater labour turnover in large organizations, in Britain, compared with small organizations, as supportive of the notion that small industries had a better psychological climate but he pointed out that it might not be the size of the organization *per se* that was the important explanatory variable. Henry and Groen mentioned the tendency of animals and humans, respectively, to form small groups, Corson advised against drawing the conclusion from this that there was something magic about the size.

Lazarus agreed that whilst there were pros and cons for the small and big groups the limiting conditions were not understood. Levinson's studies had shown that 'there can be just as much anguish in small as in larger organizations, particularly with regard to leadership, rivalry, and focus'. Corson thought that the important factor was not the size of the group but that people could get to know each other and what was going on. Henry pointed out that 'recognition' was a key factor for animal groups and size would affect this.

Belov reported studies in the Soviet Union which showed that workers there feel they have more influence in large organizations than in small factories. This might be because the union pressure is greater in large factories. Further they have more influence over the remote top manager than their immediate supervisor. French pointed out that this would teach us to be cautious in generalizing without considering 'conditioning variables in the larger social context'.

Various participants indicated that size also affected attitudes of, and relations to, leadership and worker participation in discussions on how the work would be done (see below) and through this whether work is seen as a stressor or a source of satisfaction.

Worker participation and 'person–environment fit'
Gardell has shown (Chapter 33) that in 9 Swedish industries the majority of workers felt they had insufficient say on how they should do their own work but a smaller percentage were dissatisfied with their influence on the organization's policies. French quoted results from cross-cultural studies in Austria, England, Israel, Yugoslavia, Norway, Sweden, and the United States on this subject. On the whole these studies supported the notion that a worker's participation in deciding how he did his own work or the small team deciding how it did its own work resulted in greater satisfaction, less absenteeism, and need not decrease productivity. However it was not a simple matter of more participation—more satisfaction, etc. Subjective person–environment fit was important. Thus in Yugoslavia direct worker participation was encouraged by government policy. The expectation amongst the workers was much higher than in other countries. What they thought they were getting, however, was much less. The result was discontent and poor effects on absenteeism and productivity.

Individual–group conflict in priorities
French's notion of subjective person–environment fit as a source of satisfaction and misfit as a source of dissatisfaction was similar to Levi/Kagan's notion of 'difference between what the person thought he should have and what he thought he had got'. It was necessary in using this concept to remember that what is wanted is not always biologically useful (French, Kagan), i.e. does not correspond to objective fit (French), and that what is wanted and needed by one individual or group may conflict with others (Kagan, French).

French pointed out that there were sources of stress in applying the value principle in industrial democratization.

Each individual had a right to have some influence on altering his work environment in such a way as to improve its ability to meet his needs and improve his (person–environment) fit and his health. On the other hand, there are serious problems in conflict resolution which we felt we would have to deal with in the future when we come to one of the final topics we will deal with, and that is, the application of any knowledge to improve health. At that point, whose values are going to get applied, and when they conflict, how are we going to resolve that? We've talked as if the value conflict between the individual and the group was essentially between the individual and the firm, but there also may be conflicts between the individual and his union. Perhaps the union has goals for the individual or priorities with respect to goals that are different from his own. For example, in work life he may want most self-actualization, an interesting and exciting and challenging job, and his union is fighting to get for him more pay, shorter hours, and safer working conditions.

Kagan thought the prevention of a stressor situation would require knowledge equally available to all, priority rules acceptable to all, and compromise solutions based on this.

Relations to, and attitudes of, leadership
The question of relations to leadership was closely bound up with knowing and respecting the leader for his ability and for his intentions.

In the small organization everyone knew the boss; everyone could and did speak to him. The boss's needs and intentions were often closely related to the workers. As Levinson pointed out, in

large organizations the leadership is often focused on the external world. For example, the head of an insurance company is rarely much interested in insurance, he sees himself as a financier and his reference group are financiers. He is often preoccupied with his position in that kind of atmosphere. The head of a petroleum company, until fairly recently, was rarely concerned about selling gasoline, and gasoline stations, but was more pre-occupied with raw petroleum, and his social position. That external focus in turn, means that the second layer of command becomes heavily dependent on the nuances of acceptance or rejection by the top management. They look upward. If you ask executives or managers how they know how they are doing, their point of reference will be their superiors, not their subordinates. As a result there is a big gap between upper middle management or the officer level and lower middle management which, in turn, has to support first level supervision of the foremen. Employees depend on the foreman in the same way that in a small amount organization the unit depends on the boss, and looks to the boss for leadership. The foreman, in turn, depends on his first level supervision, but with that gap, and the inattention from top level, they get little information, little that is correct, little that is supportive, and the foreman representing the organization can not adequately support his people. As a consequence, the foreman representing the organization inadequately represents it for reasons beyond his control. It is this phenomenon, rather than bureaucracy *per se*, that gets in the way, that contributes to the alienation. And the underlying assumption about who these people are who work in this organization is often one of condescending contempt, or the organization would not be organized that way, and the motivational system would not be set up that way. So the combination of these things contributes to the whole issue of alienation, and lack of concern, low morale.

Corson felt that by decentralization and better information systems large organizations could retain the productivity of the large group and regain the psychological advantages of the small group.

Change as a stressor
Levinson drew attention to the increasing likelihood of white collar workers becoming obsolete due to the changing requirements of their jobs—change in responsibility and also 'what people have to know to fulfil the new requirements'. And this could return several times in a workers lifetime. Retraining, in his view, was not likely to be an adequate answer. In some respects this was like the total cultural change that a person from a

developing country meets when he enters industry. The totally alien disciplines based on straight lines and need to work to times set by a clock are difficult to adapt to. It was a curious reflection that in developed countries the movement was towards flexible hours and in developing countries away from them.

Forssman referred to the reverse process—adapting the work situation to the changing needs of ageing workers (see Chapter 15). He indicated that individual variation in change of capability increased in range with ageing and that made it more difficult to predict for the group as a whole. The worker was unlikely to report the gap between his ability to perform and his perception of what he could manage.

Lind referred to the need to change work conditions without loss of pay or status and at the same time to maintain interest and productivity and allow for promotion and the influx of new ideas. Change in social and cultural conditions often acted adversely for the migrant worker (Groen, Bailey) and change in attitude (Kagan) or lack of change in attitudes as well as social backing (Leijon) often acted adversely on women at work.

Boredom, repetitive work, machine pacing

French referred to the importance of defining variables such as 'boredom' which in subgroup discussion had been referred to in terms of 'understimulation', 'lack of responsibility', 'repetitive work'. In the Michigan studies it had been found necessary to differentiate all these factors and even to divide 'responsibility' into two subgroups—for people and for things. Subjective excess of the former was related to elevated serum cholesterol whilst excess of the latter was not.

Henry, reporting his subgroup discussion, said that the subject of boredom had arisen through discussion of alienation. Whether a repetitive job was seen as boring or monotonous depended on interaction of many factors in the work setting, the individual's characteristics, and the social environment in which 'the task and the worker were enmeshed.' Examples of the first were: small or large works, type of supervision, whether the work was rapid, frequent, or machine-paced, opportunities for social interaction whilst doing the work. Examples of personal variables were age, experience, expectations, identification of the worker with his employers, workmates, other. With regard to the social environment, Henry reported for his subgroup, a large number of factors:

whether the society itself favoured the extended family, or whether it was a nuclear or even a broken family type of situation; whether the worker is in his own traditional homeland and within sight of the structures and the areas in which he was born and perhaps even his parents were born, or whether he is a migrant, just arrived, and in an alien culture. These, too, might have an influence on his attitude towards his task; whether the system around him was a stable social and political system, or whether it was unstable, with much crime and violence; it is not worthwhile putting a lot into a thing if it gets stolen from you; the philosophy, itself, of the community,

whether it was a co-operative humanitarian philosophy or an intensely competitive, dog-eat-dog philosophy, such as is found in deteriorated social groups; and finally, the question of whether the society had traditionally established sets of norms and customs which were unhesitatingly supported, or whether it was what you might call an anomic or normless community such as is often found in the megalopolitan situation. Now, these aspects of anomie are not just abstractions. We thought that these can be assessed and given at least some sort of a rating scale.

French felt that the latter recitation was interesting but in no case could he guess the direction of Henry's hypothesis: for instance 'Does repetitive work produce more boredom in an extended family than a nuclear one' or vice versa? Henry replied that these social factors were speculative with regard to boredom but he had shown that in several communities social characteristics likely to contribute to anomie were associated with disease.

Gardell felt very doubtful that boredom produced disease and had not been able to establish that personal factors were related to preference for or ability to stand monotonous tasks. On the other hand he felt that there was sufficient evidence that frequently repeated tasks of short duration paced by machine were so unpleasant to so many people that they ought to be abolished. Selye wondered if boredom was akin to sensory deprivation. Henry felt that in the bored state this was probably the case and that the worker was both denied sensory stimulation and shut himself off from such stimulation. Whether there was risk for disease or not was speculation but in some jobs boredom of the worker could lead to a dangerously inadequately performed task. Levinson said that boredom was not limited to the factory floor. It was often seen in management, professional people, and professors; in his view the danger occurred when they had mastered the 'technical tasks and not yet encountered novel challenges'. Groen said

We have some experience with doctors. The College of Family Practice in Holland made some studies of this. They isolated mainly two causes, and it is interesting how these are related to the boredom in industrial workers. In the first place they were apparently inadequately prepared for the task. They started their practices anticipating to see and do in their practice what they have been taught to do in hospital. Well, actually, they thought that if a person comes to you with, say, a problem of sleeplessness, that if you give them a sleeping tablet you will be successful, but you are not; the person comes back and wants another tablet. You expect that if a person with constipation comes, you only have to give him a laxative, but it doesn't help; in a short while he is back. And so, it is the same repetition and it makes them, then, feel helpless and inadequate.

The second reason was related to that. They are taught in the hospital that if you examine an abdomen, you'll find a nice big tumour, because they think it is a nice finding; they feel rewarded by the finding. Here you have a beautiful carcinoma; you can send the patient to the surgeon; you have done something. But tummy after tummy, abdomen after abdomen, and the liver is normal, the spleen is normal, nothing to be discovered. It is even worse when you listen to a heart. In the hospital they listen to hearts and then, you hear murmurs:

345

sshhh boom, sshhh boom, or mitral stenosis rrrrrrum boom boom, rrrrrum boom boom, but in practice it is always boom boom, boom boom, and this won't alternate like the industrial work.

Do psychosocial factors predispose to chemical intoxication?

The interplay of psychological and physical factors in such stressors as noise, smell, dirt, etc, was pointed out by several participants. Horváth drew attention to experiments on rats in his laboratory which indicated that when exposed to carbon disulphide the rats showed symptoms of intoxication at an earlier stage if also subjected to a psychological stressor which induced fear. This could be of particular importance in conditions in which psychoneurotic complaints were the early signs of intoxication. It could be that they were the symptoms of a general stress response which, in Selye's terms, 'conditioned the body' to overreact to the chemical toxin.

PSYCHOSOCIAL FACTORS AND HEALTH CARE: ACTION NOW

The discussion was concerned with action which could be recommended on the basis of present knowledge to reduce mental physical and social disability. The participants realize that some of the proposals were untried and many of the situations were complex. They therefore proposed measures which could be taken to learn from the inevitable mistakes that would be made in instituting new approaches (see Feasability and Evaluation below).

General

'Declaration of psychosocial health rights of the worker'. Under this heading Groen reported the following proposals of his subgroup:

1. The protection of health and well-being of the worker is of equal interest to management, to the worker, to the state, and the society at large. An increase in productivity at the cost of the health and well-being of the worker is an inhuman aim and any attempt or research to improve productivity should, therefore, be accompanied by a study of its effect on the worker. This applies both when private enterprise or a government is the employer. This principle, of equal interest to the health of the worker and to management, is a basis on which worker and employers and government representatives could start common efforts. Adequate pay and working hours need not *per se* be the subjects of political or economic strife when it is realized that they are a fundamental human right and a necessary condition for the health of the worker. In the past this principle has not been sufficiently taken into account and as a result the industrialization of the so-called developed countries in Europe, America, and Asia has often been achieved at the cost of the well-being, health, and even the lives of the workers. It is hoped that developing countries will better protect their workers from this fate during their transition to industrialization.

2. In particular, no worker should be dismissed, without adequate compensation, because of illness. Adequate social insurance laws should protect his health and see to it that disease is not automatically associated with poverty. Similarly, legislation and agreements between trade unions and employees should protect the worker from poverty and impairment of health as a result of unemployment which may follow economic catastrophes like economic depressions or energy crises.

3. Handicapped workers should not be excluded from work by too strict medical entry examinations, unless this would be in their own interest so as not to perform work which is damaging to them from the point of view of their handicap. A physician, therefore, should not exclude workers from participation in work only because of the often unfounded fear that they are so-called bad risks for the company or for their state agency. On the contrary, such handicapped workers can be usefully employed in certain jobs which are within their capacities. This also applies for special groups like middle-aged or elderly workers.

4. Occupational medicine, until recently practised primarily in the service of the companies or the state, should regard itself as a part of health services with its main aim directed towards the health protection, both curative and preventive, of the workers. An industrial physician, therefore, regardless of whether his salary is paid by the government or the company, should regard himself like every other doctor to be in the first place in the service of his patients and of those whose health he tries to protect by preventive activities. Industrial and occupational medicine are becoming more and more a form of community medicine.

5. Occupational physicians should not, therefore, limit their task to detection and prevention of the typical occupational diseases, but should more and more be aware of their function in the detection of early signs of physical, mental, and social manifestations of stress which, more than commonly realized, can be the result of the conditions under which many people are forced to perform their work, both manual and intellectual. The early detection and prevention of these work stresses occupy a central place in both research and regular activity of the occupational physician.

6. Occupational physicians should be members of multi-disciplinary teams including personnel administrators, human engineers, ergonomists, work psychologists who co-operate with the management and especially with the workers themselves, or their representatives. The aims of such teams are to carry into practice the general concept that a satisfactory fit of the worker to the job and of the job to the worker should be achieved by taking into account needs of productivity, the conditions in which the work is performed, and the health of the worker. Especially the common aim of

346

educing absenteeism from work should be pursued by both decreasing disease and precursors of disease and by increasing the gratification of the worker and his motivation for his task.

Etzioni added the right of a worker to be informed of the hazards of the occupation at the time of employment.

Biological basis for a psychosocial contract. Henry, reporting for his subgroup, said that they had defined the components of the work setting and social environment and then listed and contrasted favourable and unfavourable factors for each component. The same could be done for interactions designed to improve the situation. These factors are mentioned under specific problems below. The generalization behind it was, in Henry's view, close to that of the 'Stockholm's Stressor' (Kagan–Levi model). As you move from favourable to unfavourable factors you get a situation where the individuals involved are not having their expectations met, and disturbances of the basic attachment instinct of the organism are induced.

Both animal work as well as human studies show that this is a situation of high stress. When expectations are disappointed and loss of status is felt in the system, there is a stimulation of the stress mechanisms, the corticosteroids are increased, and there is a decrease in the gonadotrophins. Under favourable conditions, corticoid levels are at a lower level and gonadotrophins at a higher level and self-esteem is satisfied. In the unstable, competitive environment there is great difficulty in establishing and feeling a sense of security in the hierarchy which, again, all animals and man, as much as, and more, perhaps than any, seek: It could be called part of the territorial instinct but it is not territory in man so much as hierarchy and, of course, in primates, too, the social status which is so important in determining roles. And if these are constantly shifting, then you get the arousal of these instinctual mechanisms which are what Paul McLean has described as species-preservative instinctual drive mechanisms. These are disturbed. Then, in turn, you get the eliciting of those responses, not only of the classical Selye response with the corticosteroids and the defence alarm fight – flight response, in the attempt to avoid the loss of status and position. The sympathetic adrenal medullary system is activated as the individual attempts to avoid this subordination and loss of self-esteem.

Lazarus thought this model useful but that the factors should be expressed in a continuum rather than as favourable and unfavourable and Batawi thought there was some possibility of producing a score. Henry said that he had this in mind, and that for example unfavourable factors in one setting (e.g. work) might be compensated for by favourable factors in another (e.g. social). Levinson thought that this approach gave

a biological base to the concept of psychological contract which has to do with expectations, particularly, the way they are met, especially unconscious expectations, that is, people's needs for settings which support their psychological make-ups, but which they cannot, themselves, specify in words. And they therefore come to organizations with these implicit contracts

which, if then violated, that is, when the organization in effect changes its personality or its ways of meeting expectations, causes them to kick up a fuss which Dr. Henry has now specified in biological terms. So the interaction and interrelationship between person and organization becomes a much more significant kind of relationship than the historic employer–employee relationship on an economic exchange basis.

Developing countries. Kagan and McLean felt that in principle the problems of developing and developed countries were similar though there were some important practical differences. Batawi and Corson pointed out that one of the most important practical differences was that the developing countries still had an opportunity to learn from the mistakes of the developed. Groen pointed out that the problems in several developing countries in which he had worked were different in each. The common belief that starvation and infectious disease were the only major problems was completely false.

Such problems as transition to industrial states or social problems are indeed very great, and physicians who train to go to so-called developing countries should get at least as much training in these psychosocial factors we are discussing today as in nutrition and infectious disease.

Batawi and Groen referred to the enormous cultural economic and political difficulties in putting such knowledge into effect in developing countries and Corson referred to the difficulties and failure experienced in developed countries in putting into effect well known methods, e.g. for preventing pollution by industry.

Specific

Many participants contributed to and supported the following proposals:

(a) *Social isolation.* 'Where the conditions on the job cause social isolation—for example, the noise is so excessive that a worker cannot communicate with his fellow workers—then we should recommend the use of job rotation.'

(b) *Flexible working hours.* 'The working hours should be made more flexible. In particular, the time of starting and stopping work should not be a specific hour of the day, but a worker should be provided with the option of coming to work anywhere between, say, 8 o'clock in the morning and 10 o'clock in the morning so that there is flexibility.'

(c) *Shift work.* 'Where ill effects of shift work have been demonstrated, we should recommend changes in the patterns of shift work.'

(d) *Machine paced repetitive work.* Gardell was of the opinion that this gave rise to so much dissatisfaction that it should be abolished, at least for frequently repeated operations of short duration (up to 2 min or so).

(e) *Worker participation.* 'Because participation may have bad effects or good effects depending on various conditions, e.g. in the personality of the individual, any programme of participation to improve health, well-being, etc. should be individualized. No standard programme affecting all individuals the same way will be effective. Because the conditioning variables also include various situational factors from the widest culture down to the immediate question of what kind of level of participation this individual is used to, any programme of participation must be adapted to these conditions.

Further, any programme of increasing participation has to be concerned with timing. If changes are introduced too fast they could be expected to have less positive effects or even negative effects.

Also we must develop indicators of excessive misfit. 'Excessive misfit' implies we have a suspicion that just a little bit of misfit is a good thing. Levels of aspiration and motivation set at a little bit higher than the present condition may be a healthy situation for the human being. So, we must have indicators of excessive misfit with regard to participation and democratic relations. We must have ways to correct excessive misfits.'

(f) *Education and training.* McLean reporting subgroup discussion said:

We feel there needs to be a great deal more flexibility, a great deal more imagination, in the educational system at large, in the community, as well as within the employing groups. The point was made, and I think there was general agreement, that key education today should be a broad, general education with the work organization subsequently assuming responsibility for the specialized education for specific tasks. And this over a lifetime, for we clearly recognize that careers these days will be in the nature of five to seven years, rather than for a lifetime and the educational process must take place between careers for the most part.

Second, the point was made, and I think agreed to, that much greater efforts should be made to expose children, in the educational years, of seven or eight on, to various work experiences so that they can, indeed, begin to make more intelligent choices than at this point in time for at least their first career.

Third, there was the recommendation that there be a lifetime career guidance system established with career centres to aid individuals in initial career choice, in subsequent career choice, and in terms of what they will be doing with their retirement years.

Fourth, and finally, under the broad rubric of education, there should be an educational system to stimulate greater awareness—and this is the point, I think, that Dr. French's group was discussing but we broadened it somewhat—greater awareness of psychosocial work factors by individuals such as industrial engineers, such as occupational health professionals, such as physicians in the community who rarely have been inside a factory or a work place. And, contrariwise, there should be much broader exposure to occupational health professionals, to concerned behavioural scientists — exposure to concepts of management technique and practice.

B. Hamburg said that her subgroup had also been in agreement with these proposals, but had given perhaps an even greatest emphasis to education:

One reason is that the workers who are the unhappiest and who are the lowest paid and whose mortality, just to take an indicator which is, of course, extremely meaningful, are the ones with the least education. And we took a view of education that was perhaps the broadest of any of the groups because keeping in mind the developing nations we would like to make a recommendation that there be universal compulsory education in all countries. We were interested in the process of education as well as the content. We believe there is sufficient evidence that the way in which a student is taught has an outcome in the way he will perform on his job and the expectations that he will have.

Either by accident or perhaps otherwise, it has been the case that there has been a rote kind of education with a rigid teacher, often almost tyrannical, and, as I say, either accidently or not this has turned out to be a useful model of the work situation in which you have a rote kind of job and you have a boss who is acting in the role of a supreme authority. And we believe that there should, then, be a de-emphasis on rote learning and encouragement of initiation and participation in the learning process.

We believe there can be training for careers that begin in the kindergarten stage and grade one. And I think that there are reasons that are important in the developed nations as well as the undeveloped nations, and the reasons are different. In the industrial and post-industrial nations many of the important jobs are not visible to children.

The jobs that are visible to children are garbage men, doctors who are giving them jabs, shop-keepers, etc., but there are many many more important jobs which will be their ultimate careers which are not visible to them. I think that as early as kindergarten and the early grades that children can be taken to visit and begin to learn about this; as they proceed in the school, at age appropriate levels, then it is important that they have actual work experience.

In the developmental kind of model that Dr. Levinson proposed, there is an early stage in a work career in which you have a sampling, a testing out. And in the schools in our area we have what is called exploratory experience which is an elective in the school in which they get a grade and get credit. Beginning at 12 years of age a certain portion of the school day is spent over a sufficient period of time, a number of months, a whole term, as a member of a work group. The students are allowed to spontaneously choose what experience they want and it is usually the case that the experiences are widely divergent.

They will work in an office, in a laboratory, in a carpenter shop, in a veterinarian hospital as a veterinarian assistant, in a teaching role with children, etc. And over the period of time and at the end of their school career they have learned what are realistic job expectations, who are the kinds of people that are one's colleagues in these situations, the amount of isolation, the amount of interaction with others. I think this is important in our industrialized world.

In the less industrialized countries I think it is very important to institute this as a part of the schooling. Because it will be in keeping with the apprentice kind of model which perhaps will be in that culture. Further in the instance of the industrialized occupations which are new to the culture, you would want your students to have this opportunity for a practical introduction, observation, and example of the new career which has not previously existed in their culture.

All have put a lot of emphasis on the importance of the interpersonal relations at every level from the manager to his employee, employee to employee, and the worker in his relation to the outside world, to the community context. We ave at the present time had an emphasis in our teaching on the cognitive content of education. And there is a substantial body of work, in America at least, which indicates that we can also teach the interpersonal, the communication, the affective aspects of education and that it is personally enhancing at the time to the student and obviously would have significance in his role as a worker later.

Selye has been actually teaching his stress model in the schools in Canada. I think it is important that this could be included as an item in the curriculum at a secondary school level. We need to teach them about alcoholism, about drugs related occupationally to the use of drugs as an occupational hazard under stress and the impairments in terms of career aspirations if one becomes involved with the heavy use of these, and all the other aspects of the use of these.

And again, I think the school may be a model in which we can train them in participation in a social network, actually using the school as model, how to initiate some changes in a school curriculum which the students would like to have, how to get changes in the school rules. I think there is evidence in terms of our experiences with the schools in the San Francisco, California, area that there is a generalization, a carry-over of these kinds of learnings which we would not ordinarily associate with a school curriculum but I think is an important potential of the school situation.

We have viewed, as was mentioned, I believe, by Dr McLean, learning as a lifelong process, and so we include here the later vocational guidance and the special education of worker representatives. And I believe that you, Mr. Daniels-son, can probably speak as to the impact of that. Knowledge is power, and presumably these workers with their special education are then empowered to act, on behalf of their fellow workers. We believed, in terms of the mobility of the worker, or just his ability to change his job if it did not suit the person in terms of the kind of a match that we have been hearing about, that there ought to be opportunities for on the job training that would enable him to have a move.

Addressed particularly to the underdeveloped or developing nations, we believe that where there now exist adults who are illiterate, that there ought to be some time allotted in the work place and during the hours of work in which they could have some education in reading and writing and the computational skills which will enable them to function better.

Several participants felt there should be education for supervisors, management, and leaders in psychosocial factors, work psychology, etc. McLean said:

We spent a good deal of time during the week focusing on leadership, particularly focusing on first level and middle management, and one point that emerged today which I think has particular applicability to areas such as ILO, is the need to recognize in any given culture the role of the father in the family and the characteristics which constitute a successful father in that particular culture, and to apply some of these same characteristics when one begins to look for a first line supervisor or a foreman; one who is a particularly good father who at least or clearly recognizes the characteristic, understands the role of father, by and large tends to make a better foreman.

Levi thought that a 'mother' figure might be equally appropriate. Levinson thought this was not likely to be the case at the present time and Danielson thought it was a matter for the 'near future'.

(g) *Data bank*. Levi underlined the need to 'collect, store, and disseminate information in the area of psychosocial factors and health in working life'. McLean, agreeing on the necessity, pointed out that much was going on in this field and as a first move it would be desirable to know 'who is doing what now'. McLean and Horváth thought that a central agency would be rather slow because of delay in receiving the journals from some nations and further delay in their translation. They thought that regional centres would overcome these difficulties and then 'the computers at each centre would talk to each other'. Selye pointed out that he had 'collected all the stress literature irrespective of language ever since 1936 in all fields to which the concept has been applied'.

Science and administrators

Need. McLean voiced the opinion of many when he spoke of

the need to build in to responsible agencies ways of taking advantage of existing scientific knowledge—to have expert information available to the leadership of work organizations of countries or communities. Not that we feel that we should impose that knowledge, of course, but that it should be made somehow more readily available.

Hamburg spoke of a two-way relation—'the interface between the work place and the scientific community'.

The shift work research here in Sweden is a nice example of it, brought up by an earlier group. On the one hand, how do you stimulate scientific interest in investigating this problem? And on the other hand, when it becomes investigated, say here in Stockholm, and important results are found, how are those results fed back, not only to Sweden but to the work place in other countries? It might be shift work this year and something else five years from now and something else twenty years from now. This is a very long-term problem, a continuing long-term need to have an adequate interface between the scientific community and the work place. Now spontaneous interaction may be sufficient to take care of it, but if the problems are very important in terms of human suffering you may need a more systematic mechanism to facilitate communication and mutual benefit. And let me give two or three examples. In one country it might be that the ministry of health, let's say together with the ministry of labour, might set up something called a 'work stress council' which would include both biological and social scientists, would include engineers, union management, etc., a sufficiently diverse composition so that the group could scan the area broadly to detect major problems and major opportunities—not to overlook them. Similar considerations might apply on an international level to WHO: In some countries it might not be a governmental body that would do this job, but one of the science research councils that might do the job, but it does seem to me it is worth considering some systematic mechanism for covering the interface between the scientific community and the work place.

Difficulties. In addition to political and economic barriers between scientist and administrators there were genuine difficulties due to the complexity of the

349

problems, conflict in values and priorities, and often inadequacy of scientific knowledge. The large number of interacting but only partly dependent factors mitigate against the obvious solution being the correct one. For instance it is known that social support by a person's immediate supervisor is good for his health. French referred to two studies in which attempts to provide this were made through supervisor training programmes.

Both studies showed that during the course of the training, the supervisors, at least in their verbal behaviour, were greatly changed, but after they got back on the job they not only regressed to where they started out, but indeed were worse.

This was because 'their boss did not approve and wouldn't permit it'. Further

We can't consider only fit and misfit with respect to participation, because there are trade-offs between any valued outcome variables for an individual. The individual may like more participation but he would like even more to have certainty and no ambiguity in his job, and maybe the two are contradictory, so that we have to consider in any practical programme the outcomes at the physical, physiological, health levels, the outcome at the social level, and within each of those a variety of dimensions, and what is the total trade-off of all of those before we can end up saying: this programme will, on the whole, have good effects rather than bad effects.

In addition to the conflict in priorities of various benefits for the individual there are likely to be conflicts between individual and between interests of different groups, e.g. the work group, the families, the trade unions, the employers, the community. There was a real risk that, as French put it, 'the value conflicts and the trade-offs involved become highly institutionalized in organizational structures'.

Further, as Gardell pointed out, 'people with the least influence in their own jobs are least interested in changing that situation'. And this is only an example of the generalization that 'resistance to change is strongest in those who are in greatest need'. Hamburg said that

'hereditary ascription of status and hereditary access to opportunities is less stressful for the individuals than achievement, motivation, and struggle to enter the meritocracy. It is also probably true that it is less stressful for individuals to have their expectations met even if their expectations are low than to have their expectations unmet, to experience surprises, uncertainty, and so on. However, value conflict comes into this very soon, and there are trade-offs of a very consequential kind.

If the expectations are low and are met and there is a certain apathetic satisfaction connected with that, it is entirely possible that most of us here, I suspect, would nevertheless not envision that as a particularly desirable condition. We might wish to find more opportunities for people who have such low expectations even though there may be difficulty in the transitional period. It is just to remind you, stress is also challenge; opportunities even of a very creative kind are often difficult, hard to implement, and stressful for a while. The time scale is important. If the time scale is not unduly long—and what will be unduly long varies from one case to another—but if it is not unduly long, there is

no reason to believe that the consequences of the stress mobilization will be pathogenic and there is no reason to believe that the price will be too high for the creative response to the challenge even though it is difficult in the short run. But even beyond the short run, there are some very difficult value questions of people who do not fit the low stress model, who, for one reason or another, suffer a great deal, but nevertheless accomplish a great deal. Would the world have been better off if Eugene O'Neill, suffering as much as he did, had not written the plays that he did? And so on. So it is a reminder of a theme that has recurred in this series that we are not aiming to relieve stress to the point that some kind of vegetative existence is the outcome. In terms of, I should think, the prevailing values in these volumes, we are quite willing to accept a certain amount of stress, and even probably a certain amount of stress-induced pathology in order to implement other values that may have higher significance.

Solution. In view of these difficulties and the inadequacy of present scientific knowledge to resolve them, Kagan proposed a community research strategy (see Chapter 42) which would evaluate health or social actions from the point of view of advantages and disadvantages to the various interests at the same time as testing more fundamental hypotheses. The results of such small-scale studies would enable administrators to learn from mistakes. As French said, 'It would provide the basis for trial- and error-learning'—the kind of cybernetics system described by Corson and Corson (see Chapter 29). Svane thought that this was a clear offer to government agencies. Kagan felt that the strategy would be successful if it was carried out in co-operation with all concerned and if all concerned were informed of the results. Only in this way could an informed compromise decision be reached on how to use the new knowledge. Further he felt that this strategy should be applied to all the recommendations made in the 'Specific' section above.

Recommendations for legislators

(a) *General.* Danielsson said that he realized that the problems under consideration were complex but would nevertheless suggest that recommendations to lawmakers should be concrete. He agreed with French that in principle one should avoid unnecessary constraints 'and leave as many options open to the person as possible'.

McLean speaking for a subgroup said the

goal was to remove the status of employees as chattels in work organizations, to enhance participation in the job itself, and to enhance the meaningfulness of work. As we considered this we identified one trend which I think is significant, and a trend which I suspect may make some of our recommendations a little more likely to come into existence. That trend was the concept of the corporate employer as increasingly a public trust with greater public and greater employee representation at meaningful policy-making levels.

We recommend that first

legislation quite specificaly include the requirement of social indicators as part of the ongoing monitoring process in these agencies. It seems quite reasonable that such indicators can be recommended in a context of identifying within that piece of legislation concern for the psychosocial factors on the job.

Second that legislation charge a capable agency, perhaps one to be created by the legislation, a competent agency, with the development of indicators of job satisfaction as well as with the techniques to measure the effectiveness of that job satisfaction on a monitoring basis. Mechanisms, we recognized, will take time to develop. They cannot be created by legislation. But the model in operation in several companies, including your own agency with concern for physical environment, can, we suspect, be modified to evaluate psychological factors as well.

Finally, we feel legislation is required to effect changes in many countries as regards the use of various economic means to foster increased choice and opportunity for employees.

(b) 'Portable pensions'. McLean said that in the United States

today, the benefit programmes in each work organization tend to be quite different and quite unique. In many organizations it takes five to twenty years of employment before you have any entitlement, for instance, to retirement programmes. There is a tendency to reward individuals with increasing benefits on the basis of the length of stay, on the basis of senility. They are *tied in*, they feel locked in, they don't feel free to move to another job, they don't feel free to move on to train for another job. There aren't provisions for that.

If you move the benefit programme outside of the individual organization, to say, a federal or state or other agency, and if vesting is on a year by year basis regardless of where one works, and if the benefits are essentially uniform across the board, it would tend to obviate this sort of restriction. It would tend to promote a much wider range of choice of occupation for individuals.

With portable pension or benefit plan of 'relatively uniform character and with a vesting in such programmes outside the specific work organization, we feel that much greater freedom would be created to foster a flexibility in moving to more fulfilling work should the individual employee be so inclined'.

Danielsson pointed out that such a scheme had been introduced in Sweden 15 years ago to cover all workers, all employees, and all self-employed. Prior to its introduction there had been 'a hot political debate' between two sides—those in favour of the 'compulsory scheme covering everybody', and those in favour of a more voluntary scheme. The basis reason for the compulsory scheme which was accepted was so that people should not be slaves where they work. They could carry their rights with them.

B. Hamburg took this idea further.

I think there is an equally great problem of the portable network of support—well, the fact that it is not portable. In situations in which the workers are mobile or migrant it is important that their sources of interpersonal support and gratification should be extended beyond the nuclear group. This is also important for cases in certain developing nations and in our own country where people are removed out of the nuclear group. It is not uncommon in a number of the developing

nations that a man will leave everyone and go into an urban area and become an isolated individual on a job. A responsibility must be taken to meet his needs and to supply him with a network of social underpinnings and support.

FUTURE RESEARCH

The meeting of applied and basic research
Engström introducing the discussion said that 'The social sciences are more and more in the focus of national as well as international interest'. He considered

The crucial problem is that we need both the free creative type of science and also to a larger and ever increasing extent research which is coupled to needs. And at the moment there seems to be a little bit of no man's land between these two groups so one of the very essential points here is to bring them into contact with each other.

Substantive and methodological needs
French speaking for a subgroup said:

We have reviewed a variety of substantive problems where further research is needed. These arise from the importance of social problems of working life in this and other countries, and they also come out of previous research. . . . This whole field of psychosocial factors is at a beginning stage and we cannot expect any project nowadays to answer all the problems. . . . We also still need a good deal of methodological research, that is, our methods of research need to be improved. There are a whole series of causal links and mechanisms that need to be studied and they need to be put together in single studies, not only studied separately, one link at a time. This has rarely been attempted and we will need to develop new methods and research strategies to deal with such problems.

Our group distinguishes three levels of approach. (1) What are *the content* problems requiring further research? (2) What are *the theoretical* problems requiring further research? (3) What are *the methodological* problems?

Under *content* we distinguish evaluation of programmes and techniques, for example, systems like job rotation to avoid social isolation, or flexible hours of work, or various schemes of representative democracy, or various schemes of direct democracy which we have discussed. All these need further evaluative research. Secondly, still on content problems, we have identified a large number of pathologies and disabilities requiring further research. These would include things like psychosomatic diseases, dissatisfactions in work, low self-esteem stemming from work, or specific occupations that are problematic like air traffic controllers or miners.

Now, moving to the *theoretical* problems, I would like to discuss these at three levels. We have, first, a set of problems of conceptualization where we are asking what is the nature of the variables we are talking about. We have second a whole series of specific simple hypotheses simply saying one independent variable, one stressor, for example, has a given effect on one strain, for example, on blood pressure. And third we have more complex theoretical models that involve more than two variables.

Amongst the first class, those problems of conceptualization of occupational stresses, one is how should we conceptualize a whole set of variables such as participation, control, the control structure, power, autonomy, etc. A second one, how should we

351

properly conceptualize a set of variables that include role ambiguity, future ambiguity, knowledge of results, feedback of information, uncertainty, etc. These include concepts used in animal experiments, human experiments, groups, and so forth. A third one, how should we conceptualize coping techniques and defence mechanisms? Can we go beyond Anna Freud? Now, moving to the area of hypotheses, I will give only a couple of examples of a great many here—'Stress at work can be compensated for by favourable factors at home or in recreation. Stress at work spills over into family life with negative effects on the family life, for example, causing divorce.' Now, hypotheses of this sort are very important but mostly untested.

With respect to theoretical models, I would like to talk about three levels. First, there are a whole host of simple statements to the effect that occupational stress causes strain in the individual depending on the level of moderator variables, and the whole question of whether these really are moderator effects, or main effects of those variables needs to be investigated. Second, a lot of us have studied simple models, three variables in a causal sequence. For example, the goodness of objective fit between the person and his environment influences the goodness of subjective fit which in turn influences strains within the individual. That is a three variables sequence. Finally, we have overall theoretical models such as the model used here in the group in Stockholm, or such as the model of person – environment fit presented in my paper. I would add that nobody has ever tested that model or ever attempted to. We have only dealt with a couple of the variables at a time.

With regard to the *methodological* problems, I think our group would go along with many of the other suggestions here about the needs for interdisciplinary methods, the needs for evaluation-type models. I would also go along with the need for more field tryouts and experiments. Incidentally our group has just finished a field experiment—a controlled test of the effects of group discussion methods. This is exactly what Dr. Groen recommended (see below) a study of the effects of group discussion methods in reducing job stresses and measuring their effects on heart rate, blood pressure, biochemical determinations, and other risk factors in coronary heart disease.

Levinson, summarizing subgroup recommendations said:

(1) *The hierarchical* system with reward or punishment as the motive was *not the only model* although this was assumed to be the case in Industrial Engineering

This may well fit cultures which are heavily governed by internal social structures which highly differentiate social status and distribution of authority. They may not fit other kinds of cultures which do not operate in the same way. But we have taken these for granted and I want to put a big question mark on them. I think it may well be possible to think of production processes built around the naturally cohesive groups of different cultures. We need more research on compensation and authority systems to support, and to fit more closely, given subcultures.

(2) I think we need to do more work on *differentiating value systems* of people and fit such value systems to the tasks and organizations and processes for which they are more effective. That is, there is not much point in talking about self-actualization to groups of people who may primarily be interested in solely earning money. Next it seems to me that we have to learn something about how to go about changing such value systems. That is, there are people who have reactive value systems, i.e. move when they are stimulated in some fashion but who do not assume responsibility for their own behavioural outcomes, but

who, in the kinds of societies towards which we are moving, may indeed need to assume more responsibility or be destroyed in the process by events beyond their control. So we need to know something about how does one awaken that kind of responsibility and acquire experiences in coping with those forces.

(3) We need more study of *adult stages of adaptation.* We have a great deal of information about stages of development in children, ranging from the stages in conceptual development that Piaget has pioneered in, to stages in psychosexual development, and stages in moral development. We don't have much information about adults. Yet adults do not merely exist as extensions of their respective childhoods. They go through vicissitudes of their own and those vicissitudes need both exploration and explanation. We have just begun to scratch the surface of those transitional issues. There are points at which people need help and support as well as understanding, and as was pointed out yesterday, we need to know more about these for women as well as for men. We need to know something about the developmental sources of organizational vulnerability. By that I mean, for what reasons in childhood development do people seek omnipotence as executives of organizations, or conversely do people seek roles in organizations which demand of them that they be martyrs and all of the differentiations in between. And how can such information be used both for the continuous career guidance to which we referred yesterday as well as to ameliorate those distortions in development which in turn may make for continued unhappiness and mental ill health?

(4) We need studies of *career choice alternatives.* That is, how do people most easily shift, and to what kinds of activities? While this may seem irrelevant to the developing countries now, as they become industrialized the same issues will arise.

(5) We need experiments and studies on *adult technical re-education,* as people are required to change from one occupation to another with increasing technical obsolescence.

(6) We need to know what the *steps* are *in cultural change,* particularly for developing countries so that the necessary supports can be mobilized and that technical advances can be made without too much injurious effect on indigenous populations. We need to know what are the conditions for the mobility of children. That is, in an increasingly mobile society, both within nations and across nations when families have to move for occupational reasons, what do we know, what can we know about times that are optimum for movement of children of given ages and times when perhaps they should not be moved? Or when families move, how can they be moved with the kind of support which will insure their preservation rather than their destruction?

(7) We need to know how to create, if not evolve, *social structures in migrant* groups, in *temporary societies,* so that people need not be cast adrift simply because they have to go away from their home bases for work. And we have to know something, it seems to me, increasingly about social architecture in the sense of how do we architecturally create work places which are conducive to maintaining not only individual values, but the cultural values of the groups that I mentioned earlier that would support their social cohesion.

Henry said:

I have a specific proposal on the question of the social environment from the point of view of trying to get *an index of the degree of disturbance.* There are certain parameters which are indicative of social strain which have been mentioned such as violence, competition, broken family, rootlessness due to migration, what one might call future shock due to culture shift, and so on. These can be scored and communities can be evaluated and given a score by a team involving sociologists, say, and anthropologists, and perhaps an economist, and given a score.

And then, at the same time, but quite independently and without knowledge by either group of the other, you can make a blood pressure survey of the community. In a healthy organism that is not under social strain, the blood pressure will not change with age.

The hypothesis is that if the blood pressure line that you would plot as you go from 20 to 80 years shows a gradient, then the steepness of this is an expression of the extent to which the social stimulation is being excessive. And it should be possible to get a regression line showing a correlation between the score of the community and the rate of rise of the blood pressure.

At the moment in Western communities we have just experienced a shift in opinion about what is a tolerable rate of rise. It used to be thought that the rise could be one millimetre per annum. So that roughly speaking, just very roughly, a young fellow would start at about a systolic pressure of about 100 and by the time he was 60 nobody got very excited if it was 160. Recently work has shown that this rate of rise is unacceptable. And if you have a blood pressure of 160 systolic at age 60 there is an unacceptable level of myocardial infarction, kidney failure, and strokes. And so the Western world, as you know, is making extensive blood pressure surveys in attempting to keep this down. The proposal is that this blood pressure rise will be found to be related to the extent of social stimulation of the society or of the social group within the society that is being observed.

Groen giving a personal summary of subgroup discussions said the following programmes were recommended:

1. Further *methodological improvements*. For instance the impressive work done here in Stockholm by Dr. Frankenhaeuser and Dr. Levi in the laboratories on catecholamine excretion and other parameters in the blood as an objective sign of stress certainly should be combined with a study of pulse rate to see if the latter correlates sufficiently enough with these parameters to see whether it can be used to provide continuous monitoring with simpler apparatus. Similarly the pioneer work of Dr. Petersén on trying to record certain electroencephalographic parameters needs development and that, then, could also be a very important objective measure of how work affects the worker.

The interesting animal experiments of Dr. Henry could perhaps be adapted more to the actual working conditions by having running belts in the cage and the animal might be required to, say, press a handle to avoid a shock. And then one can present these signals on the belts just as in the actual work situation in an unpredictable, monotonous way that only very few signals come in so as to imitate understimulation and to have many erratic signals. And it will be interesting to see whether some of the stress phenomena and stress diseases of the human could in such a way be reproduced in animals and thereby, the latter would be used for intervention studies.

2. Work has been presented here on the results of questionnaires given to workers; on listening to workers' symptoms like fatigue, irritability, impotence, insomnia, and so on; studying objective medical signs like serum cholesterol, free fatty acids, inteferon levels in the blood, immunoglobulins; and measuring the non-specific indicators like pulse rate, blood pressure, catecholamine excretion, and so on. And all these could be *combined with a study of absenteeism and productivity.*

We underline the need for *interdisciplinary research* in which occupational physicians work together with work psychologists, ergonomists, and so on, as already stressed in Chapter 19.

3. We felt there was a great need for *controlled intervention studies, aimed at producing a better fit between the worker and the job*, and the job and the worker. In this respect, we are very curious to know what would be the effect of *regular discussion groups*. As you know a great source of problems is the alienation of one worker from another, in general the alienation of man from his fellow man in this society. At previous conferences I have tried to advocate discussion groups for future parents. Actually we all need discussion groups and the healthy effect of discussion groups on our own feelings was very well expressed in the group over which I had the honour to preside. So if one has discussion groups for workers, one might judge the results of such a programme by these objective measures both of a biological nature and of questionnaires or absenteeism.

A special case for such discussion groups which I would feel can be made is the prevention of coronary heart disease. Now this is not, strictly speaking, a problem of industrial research only. But industrial research may form an excellent field in which to study this. One can, for instance, choose certain factories and divide them into two groups, one to be subjected to the intervention, and the other not to be subjected to the intervention, serving as a control. And introduce in one factory discussion groups for the workers and especially for the wives of the workers and discuss there such problems as diet, smoking, and conditions in the work. And then the industrial physicians could co-operate in the following up, not only cholesterol levels, but also the incidence of coronary heart disease in one company compared to the other one. Such a programme is at present in preparation in the Netherlands.

4. Next, we also endorse Dr. Forssman's proposal to devote special psychosomatic studies to certain *diseases* which are *responsible* for the *absenteeism* in factories. And here we agree with him that especially the headache, and the so-called industrial back, the low backache in workers, are diseases which up to now have had insufficient attention from the medical profession as far as their aetiology and the problem of prevention is concerned. We have in Holland at present such a group which calls itself 'the low back group'.

5. We feel that only a small minority of doctors are fit to be research workers. There are a lot of people who do so-called research but just try to confirm what another fellow did before them. Now, in industry, it seems to us that there is a mine of potential research workers among the workers who work in the industry. That is to say, in every industry there are foremen or other people who could not study, did not have the privilege of an academic career because of the social situation of their parents, but who in the actual work situation distinguish themselves by ingenuity, originality, perseverance, reliability, in other words, just those psychological characteristics which are so important for a good research worker. So that, as a recommendation to support research, I would recommend the *use of non-academicians recruited from workers who distinguish themselves in industrial research*.

Kroes summarized the discussion of a subgroup.

I would like to summarize four points which came out of our subgroup discussion.

(1) *Use of present knowledge for demonstration and evaluation.* One of them is the question of what do we need for research. And I think our group, maybe more than some of the others, made the point we already have a lot of information. We have techniques available. We have measurement instruments. We have a great deal of information. This needs to be passed on. But we now need action-oriented programmes which I think can have a substantive impact on the job environment. Present technique could be used for demonstration programmes of application and evaluation of alternative approaches in evaluation.

If we find a group that is very stressed and we find that we cannot redesign the job, how do we lower the stress? What techniques do we use? Do we use job enrichment of one sort? Do we use behaviour modification, which is a very bad word I see this morning? Or do we use sensitivity training? Which is the most effective and what components of any one are effective?

(2) We emphasize the need for the *multidisciplinary approach,* not only between disciplines, but *also within disciplines.* The work of Johansson and Gardell is an excellent example, I think, of intra-discipline co-operation between laboratory and field psychologists.

(3) We need to develop *educational programme packages.* There are a tremendous number of occupational psychiatrists and physicians around but they really don't have a good grasp of the stress area. What they need is a programme specially developed for the purpose. These are research questions because you just don't sit down and write a programme. You have to see what is the best, what information you need. And I don't mean to just emphasize the physician. You need research programme packages for the physician, the workers, the managers, the wives, and what have you. And you need it through-out the life cycle.

(4) Research is part of a wider milieu. There is always that next step after research. There is *research and dissemination.* I think oftentimes we forget this. How do we translate the research or the main points from any one research so it can be applicable elsewhere? Several people have cried for information in this conference about developing countries. What can we use, how can we help them? So what do we learn in an industrial programme in one country and how can it be applicable elsewhere, and such? We have to learn and pay attention to dissemination.

Petersén pointed out that the *study of a large number of physiological responses under usual working conditions by telemetering* was available to many laboratories—not just for space research—and should be combined with studies of psychological and social parameters. Frankenhaeuser was concerned about the use of advanced instrumentation now being used at the boundaries between biological and behavioural science. This was of particular importance in relation to 'brain, behaviour, and stress diseases' and in general in assessing harmful influences encountered in working life.

According to the OECD, research in brain and behaviour is, as they put it, on the threshold of making dramatic progress, thanks mainly to advances in instrumentation. So there is now a vast body of new knowledge emerging and at the same time the field of application will, of course, widen. The knowledge gained in this field is of such a nature that it can bring great benefits to societies, but also at the same time there are great risks involved since it is so difficult to assess the long-term consequences. I am wondering whether, perhaps we need an *international body* that would sort of systematically scan the advances in *brain and behaviour research considering in particular the long-term social consequences.*

Engström summarized recommendations from Lazarus and Levinson as the need to be sure to *include indigenous workers* in the planning and carrying out of research. Levi and Kagan thought that requests for applied research should come from representatives of all those concerned and be investigated with the aid of all concerned and reported back to all concerned.

Groen had recommended the *inclusion of 'wives'* as part of the study of men at work. Levinson thought this might be an unacceptable invasion of privacy and gave examples of American experience. Groen said his recommendation was

based in the first place on two pieces of work, one which was done in industry in Holland and has been well documented and published. Questionnaires were distributed to the workers about how they liked their work, what they felt was wrong with the work, and so on. And then the wives of the workers were invited to visit the factory in groups. They were shown the factory from the basement to the rooms where the executive worked and they could stay for a while with their husbands in their work. And they could also attend a demonstration and a small lecture about the purpose of the factory, and so on. And then these same questionnaires were again administered to the workers and questionnaires were administered to the wives about how they liked this procedure.

It was highly significant that the workers said that the wife was, since the visit, more interested, asked questions when they came home in the evening: how has it been? What happened there? Did you meet Mr. So and So? How is Mr. So and So's wife who was ill? And it was a great encouragement for the worker to have his wife interested in the evening when he came home in what he had done during the day. And I suppose all of us who have the privilege that our wives are interested in our lives, in our work, can realize what this means. Those of us who are doctors know the tremendous help the wife of a country doctor can provide. And the reverse: those of us who know how much it means for a working wife that her husband is interested in her work can realize how important this is.

I repeated this experiment when I was director of a small hospital in Holland shortly after the war. And the workers in the first place were shown around the hospital because in a hospital there are people working in the laundry department, working in the kitchen; they have never seen the operating theatres; they have never seen the X-ray machines. And both these workers and the wives of doctors, of nurses, of so-called technical workers were shown around the hospital. And the wives became very proud of the function of the husband in the hospital. The so-called lower personnel, porters for instance, realized what happiness it was to work in an institution which served humanity. This research was not documented by questionnaires but it was so evident that I still can recommend it to everybody.

There have been discussion groups going on already in Gothenburg, for instance, in which it was realized that if you want to change the nutrition habits of the worker, you must do this with the help and co-operation of the wife who cooks for him. It is no use that he changes his nutrition. The whole family must change nutrition. Similarly, smoking habits: smoking is very often a substitutive mechanism for lack of gratification in other fields. And we have been using this very much so in our attempts to get rid of smoking. So partly documented by experience of scientific nature, partly by everyday experience, I feel that such an attempt should be encouraged.

Finally, we speak about alienation; alienation of the worker from his product, alienation of the worker from his fellow workers. There is a tremendous amount of alienation going on in the families.

French referred to the need 'once we have some knowledge of how psychosocial factors affect health and well-being' to apply this knowledge.

I would like to make the following specific recommendation to the WHO. The WHO should set up a *centre for research on the application and utilization of knowledge about psychosocial stressors and their effects on health and well-being in industry*. I would like to recommend, secondly, that such a centre, of course, have in it members from many disciplines, the basic sciences that are represented here, and also what I will have to call social engineers such, as we do not have them in the social sciences and it will be necessary for them to be involved in the problems of studying the process of utilization.

RESEARCH STRATEGY

Batawi endorsed the view expressed by several participants that the *industrial setting presented many advantages for real-life and action-oriented research*. He reminded the meeting of the need and possibilities for studies in developing countries.

Svane said that his institute gave certain *priorites in deciding what kind* of research to support:

First of all we think that people who are young are better to study than people who are older, from the point of view that you have a longer time span for studying alterations assumed to be better if you want to make controlled studies.

We turn to as large groups or large problems as possible. We want to define the problem seen, for instance, from an economic point of view, and try to make priorities according to the extent of the problems.

We want to find research objects where the independent variables are tangible, practically or politically.

We find and define the consumer groups quite clearly and we find channels—it may be governmental agencies—to the consumer groups before starting the project.

It is essential to have controls for independent variables. And we tend to try to establish study designs so that we are only working in one dimension and controlling for covariation in other dimensions, preferably, if it is possible, in a mathematically-oriented statistical model.

Engström, referring to the community research strategy proposed by Kagan (see Chapter 42 and the section of this synopsis on 'Science and Administrators'), said that

many of the applied research problems that we were discussing appeared uninteresting and unglamourous to sophisticated scientists. Nevertheless such research was of the greatest importance – amongst other things as a 'stepping stone to convincing policy-makers'.

He therefore endorsed the notion of *combining applied and basic research* as this would attract scientists of high quality and obtain the necessary high scientific standard for the applied studies. The need for identifying key mechanisms and the practical value of this was clear.

In social problems the chain of fundamental research, applied research, and development, does not exist in the classical linear manner. The feedback loops are, and should be more, intense.

Closer communication between the consumer, whether it is a worker or an administrator, and research workers should prove stimulating for both. But for this to work, *communication has to be in jargon-free, simple, and understandable terms.*

INDEX

369

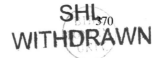